Alopecia

Alopecia

MARIYA MITEVA, MD

Assistant Professor
Department of Dermatology and Cutaneous Surgery
University of Miami Miller School of Medicine
Miami, FL, United States

ELSEVIER

ELSEVIER

3251 Riverport Lane
St. Louis, Missouri 63043

ALOPECIA   ISBN: 978-0-323-54825-0

Content Strategist: Kayla Wolfe
Content Development Manager: Kathy Padilla
Content Development Specialist: Jennifer Horigan
Publishing Services Manager: Deepthi Unni
Project Manager: Nadhiya Sekar
Designer: Gopalakrishnan Venkatraman

Printed in United States of America

Last digit is the print number: 9 8 7 6 5 4 3 2 1

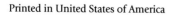

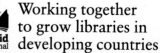

Working together to grow libraries in developing countries

www.elsevier.com • www.bookaid.org

List of Contributors

Ralf Paus, MD, FRSB
Professor of Dermatology
Director
Dermatology Medicine & Science Training Program
Department of Dermatology & Cutaneous Surgery
University of Miami Miller School of Medicine
Miami, FL, United States
Professor of Cutaneous Medicine
Director of Research
Centre for Dermatology Research
University of Manchester
Manchester, United Kingdom

Penelope A. Hirt, MD
Research Fellow
Department of Dermatology & Cutaneous Surgery
University of Miami Miller School of Medicine
Miami, FL, United States

Antonella Tosti, MD
Fredric Brandt Endowed Professor of Dermatology
Miller School of Medicine
University of Miami
Miami, FL, United States

Matilde Iorizzo, MD, PhD
Dermatology Private Practice
Bellinzona, Switzerland

Luis Garza, MD, PhD
Associate Professor
Department of Dermatology
Johns Hopkins School of Medicine
Baltimore, MD, United States

Rachel Sennett, MD, PhD
Resident, Mount Sinai St. Luke's and West
Icahn School of Medicine at Mount Sinai
New York, NY, United States

Rodney Sinclair, MBBS, MD, FACD
Chairman
Department of Dermatology
Epworth Hospital
Melbourne, VIC, Australia

Aisleen Diaz, BS
Ponce Health Sciences University School of Medicine
Ponce, PR, United States

William C. Cranwell, MBBS(Hons), BMedSc(Hons), MPH&TM
Clinical Research Fellow
Department of Dermatology
Sinclair Dermatology
Melbourne, VIC, Australia

Rodrigo Pirmez, MD
Dermatologist
Hair Diseases Unit
Instituto de Dermatologia Professor Rubem David Azulay
Santa Casa da Misericórdia do Rio de Janeiro
Rio de Janeiro, Brazil

Ralph M. Trüeb, MD
Professor
Center for Dermatology and Hair Diseases
Wallisellen, Switzerland

Ncoza C. Dlova, MBChB(UKZN), FCDerm(SA), PhD(UKZN)
Professor
Head of Dermatology
Dean School of Clinical Medicine
Nelson R Mandela School of Medicine
University of KwaZulu Natal
Durban, South Africa

Nonhlanhla P. Khumalo, MBChB, FCDerm, PhD
Professor
Head of Dermatology
Groote Schuur
University of Cape Town
Cape Town, South Africa

Renée A. Beach, MD, FRCPC
Assistant Clinical Professor
Dermatology
Women's College Hospital
University of Toronto
Toronto, Canada

Paradi Mirmirani, MD
Regional Director
Hair Disorders
Dermatology
The Permanente Medical Group
Vallejo, CA, United States

Yanna Kelly, MD
Dermatologist
Ada Trindade Dermatology Clinic
São Paulo, SP, Brazil

Lynne J. Goldberg, MD
Jag Bhawan Professor of Dermatology and Pathology &
    Laboratory Medicine
Boston University School of Medicine
Boston, MA, United States

Sergio Vañó-Galván, MD, PhD
Professor
Head of Trichology Unit
Dermatology Department
Ramon y Cajal Hospital
Madrid, Spain

Sebastian Verne, MD
Research Fellow
Department of Dermatology and Cutaneous Surgery
University of Miami Miller School of Medicine
Miami, FL, United States

Lawrence A. Schachner, MD
Department of Dermatology and Cutaneous Surgery
Miller School of Medicine
University of Miami
Miami, FL, United States

**Kiasha Govender, MbChB(UKZN), FCDerm(SA),
    Mmed(Dermatology)**
Consultant Dermatologist
King Edward Hospital
Durban, South Africa
Honorary Lecturer
Nelson R Mandela School of Medicine
Durban, South Africa

Kate E. Oberlin, MD
Chief Resident
Department of Dermatology and Cutaneous Surgery
Miller School of Medicine
University of Miami
Miami, FL, United States

Nayoung Lee, MD
Chief Resident
Dermatology and Cutaneous Surgery
University of Miami
Miami, FL, United States

Laila El-Shabrawi-Caelen, MD
Professor
Department of Dermatology
Medical University
Graz, Austria

Debora C. de Farias, MD
Dermatologist
Universidade Federal de Santa Catarina
Florianópolis, Brazil

Rita Rodrigues-Barata, MD
Dermatologist
Dermatology Department
Ramon y Cajal Hospital
Madrid, Spain

David Saceda-Corralo, MD, PhD
Dermatologist
Dermatology Department
Ramon y Cajal Hospital
Madrid, Spain

Bianca M. Piraccini, PhD
Professor
Dermatology
Department of Experimental, Diagnostic and Specialty
    Medicine
University of Bologna
Bologna, Italy

Michela Starace, MD
Dermatology
Department of Experimental, Diagnostic and Specialty
    Medicine
University of Bologna
Bologna, Italy

Aurora Alessandrini, MD
Dermatology
Department of Experimental, Diagnostic and Specialty
    Medicine
University of Bologna
Bologna, Italy

Aron G. Nusbaum, MD
Dermatologist
Miami Hair & Skin Institute
Miami, FL, United States

Anna J. Nichols, MD, PhD
Department of Dermatology & Cutaneous Surgery
University of Miami Miller School of Medicine
Miami, FL, United States

Jose A. Jaller, MD
Research Fellow
Department of Dermatology and Cutaneous Surgery
Miller School of Medicine
University of Miami
Miami, FL, United States

Giselle Martins, MD
Dermatologist
Dermatology Department
Santa Casa Hospital
Porto Alegre, Brazil

Gil Yosipovitch, MD
Professor of Dermatology
Director Miami Itch Center
Department of Dermatology & Cutaneous
    Surgery
University of Miami
Miami, FL, United States

Natasha A. Mesinkovska, MD, PhD
Assistant Professor of Dermatology and
    Dermatopathology
University of California Irvine
Irvine, CA, United States

Nisha S. Desai, MD
Assistant Professor of Dermatology
Oregon Health & Science University
Portland, OR, United States

Robin Unger, MD
Assistant Professor
Dermatology
Mt. Sinai Hospital
New York City, NY, United States

Dorota Korta, MD, PhD
Dermatology
University of California Irvine
Irvine, CA, United States

Ruel Adajar, MD
Assistant
Hair Transplant
Walter Unger MD PC
New York, NY, United States

Jade Fettig, MD
Department of Dermatology
Boston University School of Medicine
Boston, MA, United States

Daniel Callaghan III, MD
Department of Dermatology
Boston University School of Medicine
Boston, MA, United States

Laura Miguel-Gomez, MD, PhD
Dermatologist
Dermatology Department
Ramon y Cajal Hospital
Madrid, Spain

Jannett Nguyen, MD
Dermatology
University of California Irvine
Irvine, CA, United States

Suchismita Paul, MD
Chief Resident
Department of Dermatology and Cutaneous Surgery
University of Miami
Miami, FL, United States

Maria Fernanda Reis Gavazzoni Dias, MD, PhD
Professor of Dermatology
Department of Dermatology at Fluminense Federal
    University
Chair of the Alopecia Outpatient Clinic at Antonio
    Pedro Federal Hospital
Niterói, Rio de Janeiro, Brazil

Flor MacQuhae, MD
Research Fellow
Department of Dermatology and Cutaneous Surgery
University of Miami Miller School of Medicine
Miami, FL, United States

Preface

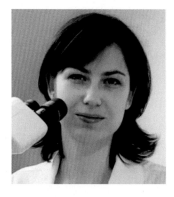

Alopecia is a collective effort of some the finest hair experts in the world to create a book that provides the most updated information about hair disorders and their management. It is designed as a manual containing easy to find clinical, trichoscopic, and pathologic information on most common hair disorders.

The book is organized in 29 chapters. It takes the reader on a journey from basic science of the hair follicle, hair biology, and hair cycling to the most advanced aspects of management and new treatment modalities.

Special highlights of this edition include the following:

- **Basic knowledge** on healthy hair, hair pathology, and hair and scalp dermatoscopy (trichoscopy) enriched with high-quality visual information
- **Updated information** on most common nonscarring and scarring alopecia along with experts' recommendations
- **Hot topics** such as scalp itch, novel off-label treatment modalities for hair loss, medications for hair loss in clinical trials, hair cosmeceuticals, and hair supplements
- **Practical information** on hair weathering and hair changes due to drugs
- **Research data** in different aspects of alopecia

I would like to thank all my friends who worked with me on this book. We spend hours every day in diagnosing, treating, and helping patients with hair disorders for which there is no cure today. If we can rephrase the great Louis Pasteur who had said *"Chance favors the prepared mind,"* our mind is already prepared; it is time to find the cure for Alopecia!

Mariya Miteva, MD
Assistant Professor of Dermatology
Department of Dermatology and Cutaneous Surgery
University of Miami Miller School of Medicine
Miami, FL, United States

Contents

1 **Healthy Hair (Anatomy, Biology, Morphogenesis, Cycling, and Function),** *1*
Penelope A. Hirt, MD and Ralf Paus, MD, FRSB

2 **Hair Pathology: The Basics,** *23*
Mariya Miteva, MD

3 **Hair and Scalp Dermatoscopy (Trichoscopy),** *43*
Rodrigo Pirmez, MD and Antonella Tosti, MD

4 **Alopecia Areata and Alopecia Areata Incognita,** *59*
Matilde Iorizzo, MD, PhD and Antonella Tosti, MD

5 **Androgenetic Alopecia,** *67*
Rachel Sennett, MD, PhD and Luis Garza, MD, PhD

6 **Telogen Effluvium,** *83*
William C. Cranwell, MBBS(Hons), BMedSc(Hons), MPH&TM, and Rodney Sinclair, MBBS, MD, FACD

7 **Trichotillomania,** *95*
Aisleen A. Diaz, BS and Mariya Miteva, MD

8 **Frontal Fibrosing Alopecia,** *103*
Rodrigo Pirmez, MD and Yanna Kelly, MD

9 **Fibrosing Alopecia in a Pattern Distribution,** *115*
Ralph M. Trüeb, MD and Maria Fernanda Reis Gavazzoni Dias, MD, PhD

10 **Central Centrifugal Cicatricial Alopecia,** *127*
Kiasha Govender, MBChB(UKZN), FCDerm(SA) and Ncoza C. Dlova, MBChB(UKZN), FCDerm(SA), PhD(UKZN)

11 **Traction Alopecia,** *135*
Renée A. Beach, MD, FRCPC and Nonhlanhla P. Khumalo, MBChB, FCDerm, PhD

12 **Lichen Planopilaris,** *143*
Nisha S. Desai, MD and Paradi Mirmirani, MD

13 **Discoid Lupus Erythematosus,** *151*
Jade Fettig, MD, Daniel Callaghan III, MD, and Lynne J. Goldberg, MD

14 **Folliculitis Decalvans,** *161*
Laura Miguel-Gómez, MD, PhD, David Saceda-Corralo, MD, PhD, Rita Rodrigues-Barata, MD, and Sergio Vañó-Galván, MD, PhD

15 **Dissecting Cellulitis of the Scalp,** *167*
David Saceda-Corralo, MD, PhD, Laura Miguel-Gómez, MD, PhD, Rita Rodrigues-Barata, MD, and Sergio Vañó-Galván, MD, PhD

16 **Acne Keloidalis Nuchae,** *173*
Rita Rodrigues-Barata, MD, Laura Miguel-Gómez, MD, PhD, David Saceda-Corralo, MD, PhD, and Sergio Vañó-Galván, MD, PhD

17 **Erosive Pustular Dermatosis of the Scalp,** *179*
Rita Rodrigues-Barata, MD, David Saceda-Corralo, MD, PhD, Laura Miguel-Gómez, MD, PhD, and Sergio Vañó-Galván, MD, PhD

18 **Hair and Scalp Disorders Associated With Systemic Disease (Secondary Alopecia),** *183*
Sebastian Verne, MD and Mariya Miteva, MD

19 **Hair Loss in Children,** *193*
Kate E. Oberlin, MD and Lawrence
A. Schachner, MD

20 **Hair and Scalp Infections,** *207*
Giselle Martins, MD and Mariya Miteva, MD

21 **The Itchy Scalp,** *219*
Nayoung Lee, MD and Gil Yosipovitch, MD

22 **Scalp Psoriasis,** *229*
Laila El-Shabrawi-Caelen, MD

23 **Hair Weathering,** *235*
Débora C. de Farias, MD

24 **Hair Changes due to Drugs,** *245*
Bianca M. Piraccini, PhD, Michela Starace,
MD, and Aurora Alessandrini, MD

25 **Novel Treatment Modalities for Hair
Loss,** *259*
Aron G. Nusbaum, MD and Suchismita Paul, MD

26 **Clinical Trials and Hair Loss,** *267*
Jose A. Jaller, MD, Flor MacQuhae, MD, and
Anna J. Nichols, MD, PhD

27 **Hair Cosmeceuticals,** *285*
Giselle Martins, MD and Maria Fernanda Reis
Gavazzoni Dias, MD, PhD

28 **Hair Supplements,** *295*
Jannett Nguyen, MD, Dorota Z. Korta, MD,
PhD, and Natasha A. Mesinkovska, MD, PhD

29 **What Should the Hair Clinician Know
About Hair Transplants?,** *305*
Robin Unger, MD and Ruel Adajar, MD

INDEX, *317*

Healthy Hair (Anatomy, Biology, Morphogenesis, Cycling, and Function)

PENELOPE A. HIRT, MD • RALF PAUS, MD, FRSB

INTRODUCTION

The human hair follicle (HF) represents a complex (mini-)organ with a somewhat complicated morphology, which involves several cell types of diverse embryologic origin. How the human HF functions in health and disease remains quite incompletely understood, and most of our knowledge arises from studying microdissected and denervated human scalp HF under organ culture conditions[1] and from concepts synthesized as the result of hair research in mouse models. This insufficient understanding of human HF biology, explains, in part, why many hair disorders are still poorly controlled from a therapeutic perspective. Moreover, the genetic basis of the regulation and dysregulation of human HF cycling is poorly understood.

Hair research started around the 19th century with the discovery of fungi as the cause of tinea, and later the role of *Malassezia* was described in seborrheic dermatitis of the scalp.[2] Although the striking hair phenotypes seen in many mouse mutants have long inspired and helped to advance basic hair biology research,[3] the discovery of epithelial HF stem cells (HFSCs) in mice[4] and the dissection of epithelial-mesenchymal interactions during HF development and cycling[2] have promoted hair research in general. The development of minoxidil in the 1980s and finasteride in the 1990s as treatments for androgenetic alopecia greatly encouraged human hair research.[2] Most recently, the introduction of Janus kinase inhibitors into the treatment of alopecia areata[5,6] has served as another example for how therapeutic interventions have propelled human hair research. It is expected that this will continue to be the case in the future.

This chapter synthesizes some basic facts and principles of hair biology, with an emphasis on the human scalp HFs.

EMBRYOLOGY

In utero, the future distribution and phenotype (long scalp hair and short eyebrow hair) of HFs over the surface of the body is already genetically determined.[7]

Interestingly, many of the homologs of the molecular signals governing these events in mammals were first discovered in drosophila (fruit flies).[7-10] The precise spacing and distribution of HF is also established by genes expressed very early in utero, creating gradients of inhibitory and stimulatory molecules, which determine where, and where not, the HFs will develop in the epidermis and which type of HF will grow.[7-12]

Around 5 million HFs are thought to be present in the surface of the body at birth.[7] Follicle formation occurs once in a lifetime of an individual, so a mammal is born with a fixed number of HFs.[7] However, in exceptional circumstances, for example, after sufficiently large skin wounds, postnatal HF neogenesis is possible in some mammals.[13,14] Nevertheless, the size of the follicles and the hair shafts they produce can change with time, mostly under the influence of hormones such as androgens.[7-10,15]

Human HF formation begins around the third month of gestation and is initiated in the eyebrow and scalp regions, progressing caudally.[16] HF development is the result of neuroectodermal–mesodermal interactions and requires input from the HF's distinc stem cell populations epithelial, neural crest, and mesenchymal.[11,16-18]

Early in fetal skin development, specific foci of the primitive epidermis become capable to generate HFs.[14] The basic requirements for HF development are the interactions between the epidermis and the underlying mesenchyme[16,19,20]. These requirements are intrinsic to the epidermal-mesenchymal exchanges; hence, HF production does not need intact hormonal or neural circuits.[20] This explains why HFs can develop de novo from organ culture fragments of fetal skin.[14,21]

HFs develop in a periodically patterned manner, with several models having been proposed to explain the spontaneous emergence of such patterns[11,12]:

Stages of Hair Follicle Formation

HF formation has been divided into eight distinct developmental stages (0–8)[20] (Fig. 1.1). Induction comes from the dermis (stages 0–1); however, while

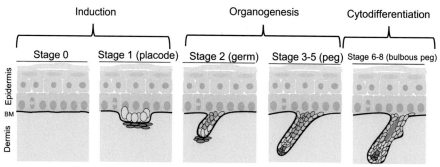

FIG. 1.1 Embryonic hair follicle (HF) development. HF development can be divided into three phases: induction, organogenesis, and cytodifferentiation and eight morphologic stages. Induction (left column): at stage 0, prior to HF placode formation, interactions between the epidermis and the underlying dermis involve local activators overriding inhibitors, creating an inductive field. In subsequent stages, the hair placode becomes visible and downward growth is initiated, while at the same time forming the dermal condensate and the future dermal papilla. Organogenesis (middle column) and cytodifferentiation (right column): in the stages 3–8, the orientation of the follicle is defined (peg stage), and the different hair lineages develop (bulbous peg). (Image modified from Schneider MR, Schmidt-Ullrich R, Paus R. The hair follicle as a dynamic miniorgan. *Curr Biol.* 2009;19(3):R132–R142.)

the underlying molecular controls are reasonably well-defined in mice, they remain quite unclear in human fetal skin.[20] The induction process results in the placode formation, followed by organogenesis (stages 2–5) and cytodifferentiation or maturation (stages 6–8), each phase requiring specific molecular interactions.[20]

Mesenchymal cell aggregation below the epidermis is one of the first steps in HF formation.[20] Specialized fibroblasts interact with the epidermis and become enlarged and elongated, inducing the focal growth of hair placodes in defined, regularly spaced areas of the overlying epidermis (stages 0–1) (Fig. 1.1).[7,16,20] The hair placode starts to become morphologically apparent once epidermal keratinocytes start to focally proliferate and assume an upright position to form a small epithelial ingrowth into the dermis.[20] Hair placode formation is followed by condensation of specialized fibroblasts with inductive properties in the underlying mesenchyme.[16] The interactions between the epithelial hair placode and this mesenchymal condensate induce proliferation in both structures. Hair placode and mesenchymal proliferation stimulate the process of shaping of the follicular dermal papilla (DP) in the mesoderm and the downgrowth of the ectodermal placode.[16]

Stage 2 is characterized by the formation of the hair germ, which occurs due to keratinocyte proliferation, because of cyclin D1 upregulation.[16] Stages 3–4 result in the peg stage, where the most proximally located keratinocytes begin to enfold the DP, followed by the bulbous peg stage (stage 5–8), when distinct strata of epithelial differentiation within the HF becomes morphologically evident (Fig. 1.1).[16]

As a critical event, during stage 5, HF keratinocytes begin to form a central tube that will differentiate into the inner root sheath (IRS) (Fig. 1.1).[16] These keratinocytes are the first epithelial cells in the HF that have the ability to terminally differentiate.[16] In the center of the tube, the hair shaft will originate from terminally differentiated HF keratinocytes, i.e., trichocytes.[16] The IRS is surrounded by cylindrical layers of outer root sheath (ORS) cells.[16] The IRS formation is a decisive step in HF morphogenesis, because it is a critical prerequisite for orderly hair shaft formation.[7,15,16]

There are other important events during stage 5, such as the migration of immune cells to the distal follicle epithelium and the perifollicular mesenchyme.[16] Langerhans cells and T cells migrate to the distal follicular epithelium (predominantly γδ T cells in mice and αβ cells in humans).[16] Mast cells and macrophages home to the perifollicular mesenchyme, which is the connective tissue sheath (syn.: dermal sheath) of the HF.[16] Current understanding is that the secretion of chemoattractants, such as interleukin (IL) 8 cytokines, and distinct adhesion molecule expression patterns by HF keratinocytes may play a major role in determining this homing of immunocytes onto the HF.[16] However, more research needs to be done to better understand how these important events are controlled. Also, during stage 5, melanin production is initiated in the HF pigmentary unit, and keratinocytes in the distal HF epithelium differentiate into sebocytes or precursors of the apocrine gland.[16]

Molecular and Genetic Basis of Hair Follicle Embryogenesis

There are many molecules controlling HF development through the communication of the epidermis and dermis. These include members of the Wnt family, whose activity is tightly controlled by Wnt antagonists such as Dkk-1, sonic hedgehog, as well as members of the transforming growth factor (TGF) β/bone morphogenetic protein (BMP), fibroblast growth factor (FGF), and TNF families.[11,12,16,19,20]

Not every epidermal keratinocyte will become a follicular keratinocyte, which results in hairless spaces between the regular arrays of HF.[11,12,20] This is now known to be controlled by changes in the local gradient of HF activators and inhibitors.[11,12,16,20,22] Wnt, Eda-A1, and Noggin are hair placode–inducing signals, whereas BMPs are HF-inhibiting signals.[12,20]

The molecular controls of HF induction and morphogenesis have mostly been studied in mice[16]; therefore, caution is advised as to assuming that the very same controls also operate during human HF development. However, it is widely assumed that key regulatory principles are conserved between mammalian species, including human skin, with fundamental pointer to gene relevant in HF development being derived from rare human genetic disorders.[23]

Activation of Wnt signaling is indispensable for the initiation of hair placode formation.[24] In guard hairs, EdaA1/EdaR and transcription factor NF-κB activity induces local epidermal cell proliferation.[19,25,26] Wnt/β-catenin and Noggin/Lef-1 are responsible for inhibiting the expression of the adhesion molecule E-cadherin;[16,27] thus, decreasing the local cell adhesion that is necessary for normal placode downgrowth.[16,28] BMP and Wnt are also important for HF cycle regulation, where these signals tend to have opposite effects.[12]

At the end of its morphogenesis phase, the HF has a cyclically remodeled inferior (proximal) region, including the bulge, and a "permanent" superficial (distal) region. Nevertheless, it has long been clear that this is an illusion based on simplistic histochemical analyses, because even the so-called "permanent" part of the HF, including the bulge, undergoes significant hair cycle–dependent remodeling events, such as focal apoptosis.[29]

Once fully formed, the follicle enters its first genuine cycle. HF cycle begins with a short phase of regression (catagen), followed by a state of relative rest (telogen), and then resumes its production of a hair shaft (anagen).[20,30] In human HFs, cycling occurs already in utero and the first "test hair shaft" (lanugo hair) is shed into the uterine fluid. On the other hand, in mice, HFs enter into hair cycling only much later, after the first 2 weeks of postnatal life.[29]

It is known that during the early postnatal period regulatory T (Treg) cells accumulate in the skin and that germ-free neonates have fewer skin Treg cells.[31] Scharschmidt et al. recently showed that HF development induces the accumulation of Treg cells in neonatal mouse skin, which becomes predominantly localized to HFs.[31] These authors also observed that commensal microbes augment Treg cell accumulation.[31] Ccl20 was identified as an HF-derived, microbiota-dependent chemokine, and its receptor, Ccr6, was found to be expressed by Treg cells in neonatal skin.[31] Presumably, this Ccl20-Ccr6 pathway mediates Treg cell migration in vitro and in vivo.[31] Together with the recent discovery that Treg cells are actually important regulators of murine HF cycling,[32] introducing Treg cells and their interaction with the skin microbiome as novel regulators of HF cycling in mice, thus joining perifollicular mast cells, macrophages, and γδ T cells, which had previously been shown to regulate murine HF cycling.[33-35] In spite of, it is yet unclear under which conditions and to which extent these immune cells also contribute to the regulation of human HF cycling.

ANATOMY AND CYTOLOGY OF THE PILOSEBACEOUS UNIT

Anatomically, the HF is traditionally divided into three portions—inferior follicle (bulb and suprabulbar regions), isthmus (including the bulge), and infundibulum—(Fig. 1.2).[20] However, this represents a rather crude and simplistic division of the HF, which surely displays more than just three functionally distinct epithelial levels.[36-38]

In the hair matrix (the main proliferation compartment of the anagen hair bulb), it has been noted long ago that a horizontal line can be drawn across the widest portion of the papilla, known as the Auber's critical level (Fig. 1.2). This functional line delimitates the most proliferative activity within the HF, which is localized to the bulb.[36]

The architecture of HFs is chiefly characterized by its cylindrical nature, with two major epithelial tissue cylinders (ORS, IRS) folding around the central hair shaft, which forms the core of this stringently compartmentalized epithelial tissue column (Fig. 1.2). Two interlocking cuticles (of the hair shaft and that of the IRS) form a slippage plane via which the upward-moving hair shaft is guided to skin surface.

This complex architecture represents an ingenious solution that evolution has found for the challenge to, first, have a relative soft epithelial tissue column grow down into the dermis (during HF morphogenesis and during the development of each new anagen phase) and,

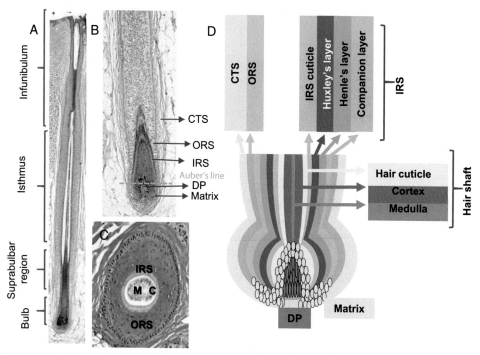

FIG. 1.2 Morphology of the hair follicle (HF). **(A)** Sagittal section through a human scalp HF in anagen stage showing the three portions of the HF—inferior follicle (bulb and suprabulbar regions), isthmus, and infundibulum. **(B)** Sagittal section through the inferior portion of the HF in anagen stage showing the *bulb* where the dermal papilla (DP) is located, which is an onion-shaped indentation made up mainly of inductive fibroblasts. The *suprabulbar* portion is also observed, with the concentric layers of the outer root sheath (ORS), inner root sheath (IRS), and the connective tissue layer sheath (CTS). Note that below the level of the widest diameter of the DP (Auber's line), hair matrix keratinocytes undergo maximal proliferation **(C)** Axial section through the isthmus showing the hair shaft with its medulla (M) and cortex (C) surrounded by the IRS and the ORS. **(D)** Schematic drawing showing concentric layers of the ORS, IRS, and shaft in the bulb. The IRS is composed of four layers: companion layer (CL), Henle's layer, Huxley's layer, and the IRS cuticle. The CL cells are tightly bound to the Henle's layer, but not to the ORS.

to then, radically change the growth direction of two central terminally differentiating tissue columns (the IRS and the hair shaft) into an upward movement. The most central of these columns is further processed into a hardened, avital and surprisingly resilient proteinaceous fiber: the hair shaft, which must be safely guided out of the skin, so as not to cause a foreign body granuloma.[14,39] The latter task is mainly mastered by the IRS, a rigid tissue cylinder that affects hair shaft packaging and curvature,[40] but likely has many additional, yet ill-understood functions. As such, the interlocking cylinders of HF epithelium accomplish a minor miracle of bioarchitecture.

The *hair bulb* is predominantly composed of hair matrix keratinocytes, which proliferate and terminally differentiate, moving toward the epidermis. At the base of the bulb, there is an onion-shaped indentation known as the follicular dermal papilla (DP) (Fig. 1.2).

The DP of human HFs is made up mainly of inductive fibroblasts that enfolded a central capillary loop and are embedded into an extracellular matrix. This extracellular matrix has more in common with a typical basement membrane-type matrix than with the matrix found in the interfollicular dermis—likely to facilitate bidirectional communication between DP fibroblasts and hair matrix keratinocytes.[12,31] Cell division in the DP is a rare event and probably occurs only once during the earlier stages of anagen development.[31]

The *suprabulbar* portion of the inferior follicle is characterized by concentric layers surrounding the hair shaft, which are the IRS, ORS, the vitreous layer, and the connective tissue sheath (dermal sheath).[7] Hair matrix cells get funneled into their final shape by the rigid ISR[7] (Fig. 1.2).

Hair matrix cells are characterized by round nuclei with prominent nucleoli and a high mitotic rate.[36,41] Their complex regulation in the human HF remains unknown. CIP/KIP family member proteins (p21CIP1, p27KIP1, and p57KIP2) have a supportive role in the regulation of their cell cycle endoreplication, differentiation, progression/arrest, and apoptosis stimulating hair bulb growth and hair shaft formation during anagen VI.[36]

Melanocytes are interspersed among the innermost layer of hair matrix keratinocytes[7] and differ in many respects from epidermal melanocytes and the HF pigmentary unit.[42,43] These melanocytes produce melanin, the hair pigment, which is deposited in the cortex of the hair shaft.

The cells of the ORS above the hair bulb are rich stores of glycogen, which results in a clear-cell phenotype, and possess a basal layer with palisading pattern.[41] Whether these long-known glycogen stores in the ORS service the metabolic needs of the HF is a subject of ongoing investigation. Interestingly, ORS keratinocytes not only generate the key growth factors that regulate human HF cycling, namely the anagen-promoting and -prolonging Insulin-like growth factor (IGF) type 1 (IGF1) and the catagen-inducing TGFβ1 and TGFβ2,[20] but also are rich in mitochondria with high metabolic activity.[44,45] These cells physiologically express a distinct array of keratins (namely keratin 6 and 16), adhesion molecules, cytokines, growth factors and growth factor receptors,[7,8,46] as well as an astounding variety of neurohormones, neuropeptides, neurotransmitters, and neurotrophins.[47] Taken together, this suggests that ORS keratinocytes may well operate as the "powerhouse" of HFs and the second main regulatory center of HF activity besides the DP.

Although ORS cells emigrate from the follicle under conditions of wounding and are capable to regenerate the epidermis after injury or loss,[7] their physiologic direction of migration and differentiation appears to be centripetal, i.e., horizontally direct toward the IRS. Strikingly, ORS do not terminally differentiate and their exact fate from their proliferation in the basal layer toward the innermost layer of the ORS remains poorly understood and ill-studied. The ORS also contains melanoblasts, Langerhans cells and Merkel cells (specialized neurosecretory and mechanosensory cells).[7]

Further, distally lies a special region in the ORS known as "the *bulge*," a specialized niche for epithelial and melanocyte stem cells (Fig. 1.2). It consists of a cluster of distinct cells that have the properties of epithelial stem cells—slowest-cycling and the longest-lived epithelial cells within the HF. These cells are located near the insertion of the arrector pili muscle (APM).[4,7] Contrary to the often reverberated belief that the bulge of human HFs is morphologically nondistinct (in contrast to the prominent bulge of murine HFs), it can often be identified by trochanter-like protrusions of the ORS.[48] Immunohistologically, these HF epithelial stem cells in the bulge are positive for cytokeratin 15 and the "no-danger" signal CD200 and negative for the gap junction protein connexin 43.[38] Epithelial stem cells in the bulge may also serve as a reservoir for epidermal and sebaceous gland cells.[4,49] However, the human HF harbors several additional epithelial progenitor cell populations.[37,38] Moreover, the bulge is also the seat of melanocyte stem cells,[50] whereas amelanotic melanoblasts are also found interspersed along the ORS.[43]

The bulge continues into and forms the lower portion of the *isthmus* (Fig. 1.2). The isthmus is inferiorly delimited by the insertion of the arrector pili muscle (APM) and superiorly by the sebaceous gland duct. At this level, the IRS (keratinized) detaches and is shed, whereas the ORS progressively thins as it merges with the infundibular epithelium. The *infundibulum* is the area above the entrance of the sebaceous duct and it is in continuity with the follicular ostium[20,51] (Fig. 1.2). Infundibular cells keratinize with an intervening granular layer, so-called infundibular or epidermoid keratinization.[41] This region is likely to play a central, but as yet ill-understood, role in the pathogenesis of several dermatoses that affect the HF.[51]

Immunologic Components of the Hair Follicle

The HF displays a complex immune system, with immunologically "privileged" matrix and bulge cells that lack major histocompatibility complex (MHC) class I expression and create an immunoinhibitory tissue milieu.[7,15,52–54] This property enables the HF to limit the risk of activating autoreactive T cells through autoantigen presentation[7,15,52,54] and dampens the activities of natural killer cells and other innate immune cells patrolling the skin for the detection of "danger signals."[54] The HF mesenchyme also harbors important immune cells, such as perifollicular macrophages, mast cells, Treg cells, γδ T cells, and others that not only act as the effector arm of the immune system but, also profoundly affect HF function, which has been observed in mice.[7,15,32–35,52]

In fact, malfunctioning of HF immune privilege is an essential prerequisite for HF autoimmune diseases to develop. For instance, collapse of the hair bulb immune privilege is a predisposition and a requirement for the development of alopecia areata,[55] and bulge immune privilege collapse is a key element in the pathobiology of cicatricial alopecias, such as lichen planopilaris.[56] Moreover, the immunocyte composition, number, location, and activity in murine skin changes strikingly during HF cycling, having an immune-permissive phenotype during telogen and an immune-suppressive phenotype in anagen.[53,57] For example, type IV immune responses can only be elicited in mouse skin when the HFs are in telogen but not in anagen stage.[53,57] Furthermore, the expression of a member of the β-defensin family is higher in telogen than in anagen skin,[58] and messenger RNA levels for IL-1α and IL-1β (hair-growth inhibitory cytokines) peak during telogen in murine skin.[59] Interestingly, the differential hair cycle–dependent release of chemokines from defined regions of the HF epithelium controls Langerhans cell migration within mouse skin.[30,60] Even though it has not been formally documented, that similar phenomena occur in human skin, there is little reason to believe that HF cycling does not have an impact on the immune status of human skin as well.

Other Constituents of the Pilosebaceous Unit

Other structures associated with the HF are the APM, the sebaceous gland, and the apocrine sweat gland, all of which are summarily described as the pilosebaceous unit (Fig. 1.3). However, this name may be a misnomer: at least in human scalp skin, the coil of the eccrine gland is closely associated with the HF, located slightly below the level of the bulge, and both the HF and the eccrine gland coil are intimately embedded into a cone of intradermal adipocytes, all of which may be an integral component of the follicular unit.[61] This may explain, in part, why the follicular unit extraction has provedn to be a superior technique in modern hair transplant surgery.[62]

The APM is responsible for perpendicular pull forces acting on the HF and thus for piloerection. Contrary to conventional depictions of this muscle, it typically slings around the HF at the level of the bulge, attaching to the follicular stem cells, often encircling two or three HFs within a distinct follicular unit[63,64] (Fig. 1.3). This proximal attachment was observed to be lost or miniaturized in androgenic alopecia and has been proposed to get lost when hair loss becomes irreversible.[64] The distal end of the human APM has a "C"-shaped structure that connects to the dermal-epidermal junction and anchors to the basement membrane of the ORS,[64] which often shows stem cell–rich epithelial protrusions in this zone ("follicular trochanter").[48]

The duct of the sebaceous gland inserts into the upper (distal) ORS at the level where the IRS ends. In this critical juncture of two epithelial cell lineages (HF vs. sebaceous epithelial cell differentiation), the gland's contents, i.e., sebum, are emptied into the hair canal. Sebum is the result of the holocrine secretion of terminally differentiated sebocytes. Abnormalities in this "neuralgic" HF region just above the isthmus and the insertion of the sebaceous gland duct (a.k.a. "infundibulum", as mentioned earlier) play a key role in the development of both acne vulgaris and acne inversa/hidradenitis suppurativa.[51,65]

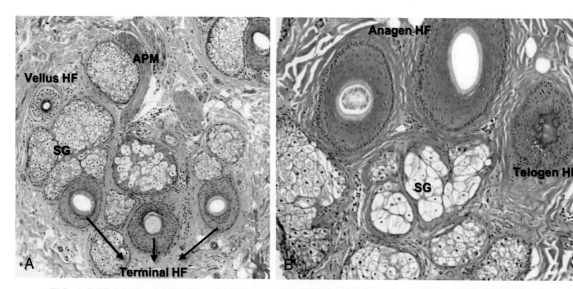

FIG. 1.3 Histologic picture of the pilosebaceous unit. **(A)** The pilosebaceous unit is formed by the arrector pili muscle (APM), the sebaceous gland (SG), and the apocrine sweat gland. However, contrary to conventiional wisdom, the coil of the eccrine gland may also form part of the follicular unit (61). Vellus hair follicle (HF) and terminal HFs are also observed. **(B)** The differences in the morphology of a HF during the anagen stage versus the telogen stage are appreciated. (Images courtesy of Mariya Miteva)

It is often forgotten that the pilosebaceous unit, as a sensory organ, is closely integrated into central nervous system (CNS) functions and, receives trophic and neuroinflammatory signals from the CNS in health and disease.[66-71] For example, the ORS in human HFs, including its stem cell zone (bulge), is densely innervated and is also richly equipped with mechanosensory Merkel cells.[66-71] Moreover, neurotrophins produced by the HF epithelium control HF innervation and affect the development and growth of both mouse and human HFs.[66-71] Also, in mice, the innervation of HFs is being rhythmically remodeled in dependence of HF cycling.[66-71] Finally, substance P, nerve growth factor–dependent neurogenic inflammation, and the action of mast cells can inhibit hair growth.[66-71]

Most recently, Jonsson et al. studied the relation between HF density (HFD) and affective touch perception in humans.[72] Individuals were stroked on the forearm and rated the pleasantness and intensity.[72] Discriminative touch measurements were also assessed. HFD was determined using the cyanoacrylate skin stripping method.[72] It was shown that women rated affective touch stimuli as more pleasant and had higher tactile acuity; women also showed a higher HFD than men, which was explained by body size and weight.[72]

A particularly exciting recent development in this field is that human HFs can also sense their environment not only via sensory nerve fibers and Merkel cells but also by the expression of proteins that are sensitive to visible light. Buscone et al. detected the expression of the photoreceptors OPN2 (rhodopsin) and OPN3 (panopsin, encephalopsin) in distinct compartments of skin and in anagen HF.[73] Treatment with $3.2\,J/cm^2$ of blue light with 453 nm central wavelength prolonged anagen phase in ex vivo HF.[73] In contrast, HF treatment with $3.2\,J/cm^2$ of 689 nm light (red light) did not significantly affect hair growth ex vivo.[73] Also, silencing of OPN3 in the ORS cells resulted in altered expression and gene expression patterns and abolished the stimulatory effects of blue light ($3.2\,J/cm^2$; 453 nm) on proliferation in the ORS cells.[73] This experiment proved that OPN2 and OPN3 are expressed in human HF and that 453 nm laser has a positive effect on hair growth ex vivo, likely via interaction with OPN3.[73] Thus, human scalp HFs can engage in direct physical "sensing" of visible light, independently of established neurosensory circuits.

TYPES OF HAIR FOLLICLES

The human body, apart from areas of glabrous skin, is covered with HFs. There are many types of hair shafts produced in the body—lanugo, vellus, and terminal—(Fig. 1.3).

Lanugo hairs are the first body hairs formed in the fetus.[14] Lanugo is a very thin, soft, and usually unpigmented hair. It is normally shed before birth, but it can be present during the first weeks of age.[14] Lanugo are vellus hair by definition but are often longer than the vellus shafts of the adult.[14]

The vellus hair shaft is short, thin, fine, and very slightly pigmented, usually with no medulla and absence of APM (Fig. 1.3).[14,74,75] Tiny vellus follicles can have large sebaceous glands (face).[14,74] It develops over most of the integument during childhood, except the lips, retroauricular area, palmoplantar skin, some external genital areas, the umbilicus, and scar tissue. A vellus follicle is defined as a small HF that extends no deeper than the upper dermis and produces a shaft no wider than its IRS.[14] Vellus hair is most easily observed on children and adult women.[14]

Terminal hairs are thick, long, and dark, as compared with vellus hair (Fig. 1.3). Androgens are crucial to human HF/shaft patterning.[14] Sexual maturity is characterized by the growth of body hair in adolescence, usually seen on a greater extent in men than in women. With maturity and exposure to androgens, regional human HFs switch in morphology from vellus follicle to terminal follicles that produce terminal hair shafts.[14] Terminal hair differs depending on the region where they are located and its sensitivity to androgen: androgen dependent (axilla), androgen insensitive (eyebrow), and androgen independent but androgen sensitive (scalp vertex in susceptible individuals).[14]

Intermediate hairs are produced by HFs that are in the process of terminal-to-vellus or vellus-to-terminal transformation.[76]

HAIR FOLLICLE CYCLING

Each HF goes continuously through three stages: anagen (growth), catagen (involution), and telogen (rest) (Fig. 1.4). Numerous growth factors and its receptors are crucial for normal HF cycling.[7,46,77] HF cycle is controlled locally and organ-autonomously by an intrafollicular oscillatory system that is not completely understood,[44,78,79] in which intrafollicular changes in the activity of the peripheral clock are likely to play an important role.[80] The HF is continuously engaged in the registration, transduction, interpretation, and processing of signals from the inside and outside environment, leading to the modulation of hair cycling, hair shaft growth, and hair pigmentation.[14,20,44,78,79] These signals are delivered cutaneously, systemically, and environmentally.[47] The circadian clock system also participates in the control of HF cycling, so the central clock triggers neuroendocrine controls over

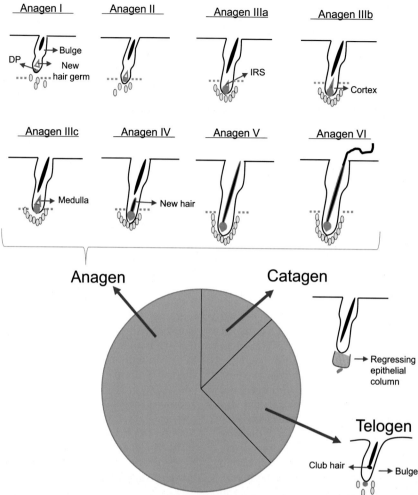

FIG. 1.4 Stages of the HF cycle. The hair cycle is divided into three phases: anagen (growth phase), catagen (regression phase), and telogen (resting phase). **Anagen** is subdivided into six subphases. At anagen I
a small DP, a secondary hair germ shaped as a triangle, and an initiation of proliferation at the base of the
germ are seen. At anagen II the DP has a wide stalk (compared to telogen and anagen I), and there is an
enlarged secondary hair germ. At anagen III an enlarged, oval-shaped DP (compared to anagen II), a newly
formed small matrix (4–5 cell layers thick), small IRS, and a hair shaft that lacks pigmentation are seen.
Also, a newly formed hair bulb enters into the adipose layer. Anagen III is subdivided into three subphases.
Anagen IV is characterized by a prominent matrix, stratified ORS, and a mature hair shaft that reaches the
level of the sebaceous gland. In anagen V there is a large, onion-shaped DP and significantly increased
pigmentation (compared to anagen IV) and a mature hair shaft that reaches the hair canal. In anagen VI HFs
achieve their maximum size, and the hair shaft tip extends far above the skin surface. **Catagen** represents
the regression phase, during which the lower, cycling portion of the HF is degraded, bringing the DP into
close proximity to the bulge. **Telogen** is characterized by a very small DP and a short secondary hair germ
that lacks apoptotic cells. The entire length of the telogen HF rests in the dermis.
DP, dermal papilla; HF, hair follicle; IRS, inner root sheath. (Image modified from Schneider MR, Schmidt-
Ullrich R, Paus R. The hair follicle as a dynamic miniorgan. Curr Biol. 2009;19(3):R132–R142; Oh JW,
Kloepper J, Langan EA, et al. A guide to studying human hair follicle cycling in vivo. J Invest Dermatol.
2016;136(1):34–44.)

the different stages of the HF.[47] For instance, molting occurs in response to seasonal climate changes.[47]

HF cycling has been largely described in mice;[81] however, this chapter focuses on HF cycling in human scalp skin.[39]

Anagen Stage

Anagen is the phase of HF growth that starts after the termination of the quiescent phase (telogen),[7] The cells secondary germ cells located immediately below in the bulge start regenerating the lower HF These cells must receive a signal to proliferate, differentiate into the epithelial lineages, and produce the hair shaft.[7,14,17,49]

Phases of anagen stage

The anagen stage has been divided into six subphases[14,39,82] (Fig. 1.4). With the exception of anagen VI (the duration of which dictates the shaft length), the length of the anagen subphases I–V does not differ between the HF from different body areas.[14,83]

In *anagen I*, HFs look very similar to the ones seen in telogen but the secondary hair germ becomes triangular or crescent-shaped and begins to extend and wrap around the DP (which is still condensed and ball-like and may contain melanin clumps)[39] (Fig. 1.4). The transcriptional activation starts in anagen I, specifically in the cells of the papilla and the secondary hair germ (a cluster of epithelial cells at the base of the telogen follicle).[14]

In *anagen II*, the secondary hair germ undergoes proliferation-driven thickening and elongation; the proximal portion forms a new hair matrix, which is still unpigmented, crescent-shaped, and only partially encloses a small ball-shaped DP.[39] HFs resides above the dermal/adipose boundary.[39] The bulge region's epithelium still contains melanin deposits.[39] (Fig. 1.4).

In *anagen III*, the hair matrix is 4–5 cell layers thick.[39] It encloses at least 60% of the DP.[39] DP becomes enlarged and oval-shaped.[39] In this stage, HFs develop a hair shaft and IRS and the hair bulb reaches and extends into the adipose layer[39] (Fig. 1.4). Three anagen III substages can be differentiated based on hair shaft appearance: anagen IIIa, IIIb, and IIIc.[39] Importantly, during this stage the hair shafts still lack visible pigmentation, even though HF melanogenesis in the HF pigmentary unit starts in anagen IIIc.[84] In anagen IIIa, the shafts lack a visible cortex. In anagen IIIb and IIIc shafts have a visible cortex. In anagen IIIc hair shafts are long, reaching approximately twice the length of the hair matrix[39] (Fig. 1.4). Lastly, the bulge

epithelium of HFs retains a pleated appearance, and the DP still contains occasional melanin clumps.[39]

In *anagen IV*, the hair shafts are fully mature, with a visible medulla, cortex, and cuticle, and the hair tip reaches the level of the sebaceous gland duct[39] (Fig. 1.4). Also, melanin production is fully reactivated, and hair shafts become pigmented.[39] The hair bulb reaches down to the upper dermal adipose layer. The hair germ proliferates as an epidermal finger into the dermis, reaching their destined depth[14] (Fig. 1.4). Once the secondary hair germ cells reach their maximum depth, a reverse of growth direction occurs and the cells located in the central cylinder progress distally (outward), forming the IRS and the hair shaft.[14]

During *anagen V*, the connective sheath trail disappears and the hair bulb extends further into the adipose layer, the tip of the hair shaft finally enters the hair canal, and the DP becomes onion-shaped[39] (Fig. 1.4). Finally, pigmentation is present down to Auber's line.[39]

Lastly, in *anagen VI*, the hair bulb is located deep in the dermal adipose layer and the hair shaft is visible above the skin level.[39] Also, hair matrix contains the maximum amount of melanin. Compared to anagen V, the DP is maximally enriched in extracellular matrix[39] (Fig. 1.4).

Regulatory pathways/molecules

Although the molecular pathways that regulate murine HF cycling are getting increasingly well-defined,[12,20,30,85] much less is known about the corresponding pathways in the human system, even though it is widely assumed that many of these are conserved between mice and humans. During early anagen, stem cell progeny in the hair matrix (transient amplifying cells) maintains active Wnt signaling and β-catenin throughout anagen.[20] Cells in the precortical hair matrix stop proliferating and initiate terminal differentiation.[20] Many regulators of hair cycling have been discovered, such as GATA3, Cutl1, and BMPs for IRS formation; Sox9 and SHH for ORS; and Wnt/β-catenin, VDR, Notch, BMPs, and Foxn1 for the hair shaft development.[20,86] The termination of the anagen stage is thought to be mainly controlled by the upregulation of fibroblast growth factor 5, TGFβ1, and TGFβ2 and the downregulation of IGF-1.[7,87]

Hair follicle stem cells are key protagonists during anagen development

The HF is a regenerating system and, as such, must contain stem cells. Because the HF bulb shows significant cell division, it was previously thought that stem cells were located there.[14,88] However, the bulge region (situated in the isthmus level) is now identified as the main seat of adult epithelial HF stem cells (HFSCs) in both mice and humans, even though additional epithelial progenitor cell populations are found elsewhere in the human HF.[17,20,37,38,89–91]

In vivo marking studies in mice have greatly enhanced our understanding of the function of stem cells of the function of stem cells.[17,92] HFSCs show two directions of flow: upward and downward. The upward flow directs out of the bulge into the epidermis and occurs in response to epidermal injury. The downward flow is induced by a periodic signal from the DP, at the beginning of each hair cycle.[17]

The "bulge activation hypothesis" states that at the onset of anagen, a subset of HFSCs gets activated. The cells generated become transiently activated matrix cells after migrating to the base of the follicle. In vivo studies confirmed the ability of these stem cells to give rise to all cell lineages of the mature HF, sebaceous glands, and epidermal cells.[20,93,94] Therefore, major damage can result in permanent injury to the stem cells and in their inability to produce new lineages, clinically resulting in alopecia.[20,95,96] After giving rise to the new hair-producing cells, stem cells return to a dormant state. It is important to mention that an extended quiescent phase and the long life span of the stem cells makes them prone to multiple genetic mutations, and to retain carcinogens, developing tumors.[20,89,92] Lastly, after an injury to the bulge, slightly more differentiated cells reproduce and relocate to the base of the follicle, called the secondary germ.[97] Probably, this is an effort to maintain the integrity of the stem cells by inducing direct descendants of these cells to revert to a stem cell phenotype.[92]

Catagen Stage

During catagen, the HF goes through an involution process that is driven by programmed cell death (apoptosis) in the majority of HF keratinocytes but spares the stem cells.[7,29] Follicular melanogenesis also terminates during catagen, and some of the differentiated melanocytes of the HF pigmentary unit undergo apoptosis.[7,98] Bulge HFSCs are able to escape apoptosis.[20] Ultimately, the lower HF becomes reduced and condensed to an epithelial strand, and the DP moves upward, coming to rest underneath the HF bulge and the secondary hair germ[14,20,81,85,99] (Fig. 1.4).

Phases of catagen stage

Catagen has been divided into eight subphases in murine, beginning with late anagen and ending in early telogen.[14,81] In humans, catagen is best subdivided into three stages: early catagen (I–IV in murine), mid-catagen (V–VI in mice), and late catagen (VII–VIII in mice).[39,81]

Catagen starts with the withdrawal of the papilla fibroblast projections from the basement membrane.[14] In *early catagen*, there is matrix and DP volume reduction and a complete cessation of HF pigmentation.[39] DP becomes more condensed and almond-shaped. Termination of melanogenesis[39,43,84] results in the proximal end of the hair shaft being depigmented, and there may be some melanin incontinence into the DP.[14] Bulbar epithelial cell division ceases, and massive epithelial cell apoptosis starts in well-defined regions of the regressing HF.[14]

In *mid-catagen*, the lower follicle shrinks progressively and withdraws as an epithelial strand; the residual matrix is only one to two cell layers thick and partially wraps around the condensed DP.[39] The club hair becomes prominent as a "brush" and resides above the dermal/adipose boundary.[39] This process is followed by thickening of the vitreous membrane and lower connective tissue sheath, followed by the condensed papilla moving distally.[14,39,43,100] Lastly, the IRS regresses and disappears.[39]

In *late catagen*, the matrix disappears, the DP becomes condensed and ball-shaped, and the epithelial strand is shortened (about half the length of that of mid-catagen HFs).[39] Also, the thickened connective sheath increases in size ("dermal streamer").[39] In late catagen, apoptotic cells can also be found in the shrinking sebaceous gland.[39] The ultimate goal of catagen is to eliminate the old hair shaft factory and to ensure that the new follicle can form from the stem cells of the bulge and the inductive powers of the papilla.[14]

During the anagen-catagen transformation, there is infiltrate of activated mast cells in the perifollicular space.[101] Also, in early catagen in the rat (but not the mouse[52]), there is a light mononuclear cell infiltrate.[102] The role of these proinflammatory cells is not completely clear. It is thought that they may phagocytose excess basement membrane of the shrinking bulb and/or apoptotic cells of the regressing lower follicle.[14] Nonetheless, there is increasing insight into various immunocyte populations being much more intimately involved in the control of HF cycling than long thought (as discussed earlier).

Regulatory pathways/molecules

Catagen is a highly controlled process. The signals governing the human HF to enter catagen stage are not completely understood, but must ultimately affect the apoptotic machinery of HF keratinocytes and genes that control catagen-associated tissue remodeling processes.[14,28,29,103,104] Accordingly, molecules of the apoptotic cascade are expressed and active in the HF. For example, in mice, IL-1β converting enzyme is expressed within the cells of the proximal follicle.[29] Bcl-2 is expressed in the epithelium of the earliest stages in the surrounding mesenchyme, in the matrix epithelium adjacent to the papilla, and in the bulge region in mouse and human follicles.[28,29,103,104] Immediately before catagen and throughout the anagen-catagen transformation period, TGF-β1 transcripts are found within the follicular epithelium.[14] Transcripts for TNF-β are also expressed during catagen.[105] In addition, c-*myc*, c-*myb*, and c-*jun* (transcription factors associated with the induction of apoptosis in other systems)[14] change immediately before or during catagen.[105] The expression of heat shock proteins (HSP27, HSP60, and HSP72) in late anagen and catagen suggests a role for these proteins in the regression process.[14]

In organ-cultured human HFs, IGF-1, insulin, TGFβ-1 and -2, 17-β estradiol, dihydrotestosterone (DHT), thyroid hormones, thyrotropin-releasing hormone (TRH), corticotropin-releasing hormone (CRH), adrenocorticotrophin (ACTH), P-cadherin-mediated signals, glutamine, hair cycle–dependent changes in intrafollicular clock activity, NF-κB activity, and many other signaling pathways have all been shown to be involved in regulating the anagen-catagen transformation in ex vivo models.[47,80,106–108] Also, environmental factors, such as stress-associated neuropeptides, chemicals, trauma, and dexamethasone, can induce the HF to enter the catagen stage.

Telogen Stage

During late catagen and early telogen the hair shaft matures into a club hair and eventually sheds from the follicle, usually during washing or combing the hair; this process also occurs in an active regulated process called exogen (discussed in the later section).[7] The percentage of HF in telogen stage varies substantially depending on the region of the body: 40%–50% of follicles on the trunk are in telogen at any time, whereas only 5%–20% of scalp follicles are traditionally assumed to be residing in this stage.[7]

Telogen was previously thought to be a quiescent stage. Today, it is appreciated that the HF is highly active during telogen in several respects and shows complex biological activities for the "active" maintenance of the hair fiber and the response to its loss.[30] Moreover, telogen coincides with major changes in gene expression activity. The HF shows a "refractory" and a "permissive/competent" subphases that differ in

their responsiveness to anagen-inducing stimuli from the surrounding dermal adipocytes.[20] In telogen, the DP comes to rest directly under the two main epithelial stem cell populations of the HF: the secondary hair germ, and the bulge, allowing direct interactions between these stem cells and the inductive fibroblasts of HFs.[20,79]

As catagen ends, the IRS gets shorter until it forms a band around the telogen shaft base.[14] Trichilemmal keratinization starts in the area where the ORS and hair cuticle touch, which adds a supportive base to the periphery of the lower shaft. The lower end of the catagen shaft is embedded in keratinized cells that bind it to the trichilemmal sac.[14,109] Consequently, the telogen shaft base folds into the trichilemmal sac just below the duct of the sebaceous gland, where the pilary canal–exposed ORS undergoes trichilemmal keratinization. Then, the coating cells enlarge vertically, enucleate, and form dense K17-containing keratin without forming a granular layer, embedding and anchoring the shaft[110] (Fig. 1.4).

Telogen is often cited to last several months in terminal scalp HFs[111] and that 5%–20% of all terminal scalp HFs are in telogen under physiologic circumstances. Recent analyses, however, question this, because clinical examination methods, such as trichogram and phototrichogram, cannot reliably distinguish late catagen from telogen HFs. Thus, the percentage of catagen HFs may even be higher than that of telogen HFs.[39]

Regulating pathways/molecules

The refractory phase is characterized by the upregulation and activation of BMP 2/4.[20,112] In the competent phase, the bulge stem cells become highly sensitive to anagen-inducing factors,[20,112] BMP signaling is turned off, and Wnt/β-catenin signaling is turned on before anagen starts.[20]

The termination of telogen phase is likely controlled by an inhibition–disinhibition system that has been reviewed elsewhere; once the concentration of stem cell activators has reached a threshold, anagen is initiated.[30,78,79,81,112–121]

Bulge stem cells and secondary hair germ cells from early and mid-telogen follicles are kept quiescent during the "refractory" period of telogen. This is achieved because of an active signaling process through BMP4 release from the DP, BMP6 and FGF18 from K6-positive niche cells, and BMP6 from subcutaneous fat cells.[30,118] However, as for all hair cycle controls, it is unclear whether these murine HF biology concepts are applicable to human HFs.

Exogen

Exogen is defined as the process in which the club hair shaft of the telogen follicle is shed spontaneously (likely actively) from its mooring in the HF.[122] Although mechanical forces can release old hair shafts passively, it has been established in mice that hair shaft shedding may mainly be an active process termed exogen.[14,122] Because exogen can occur independently of the three traditionally recognized hair cycle phases, as the timing of club fiber release is variable,[123] it is debatable whether exogen should be viewed as a distinct hair cycle phase or simply as an active process of hair shaft shedding.

Animals have a protective mechanism to minimize the possibility of shedding the protective fur before new fur is available; this is why new hairs grow before old ones shed.[14] Because the shedding phase occurs independently of telogen and anagen stages, it is probably regulated by different mechanisms. A correlation between a sexual cycle and the molt in animals has been established.[14] For instance, in sheep the parameters inducing the molt have been defined to be: light (primarily), temperature, nutrition, hormonal, and genetic factors.[14] Although hair shedding is influenced by systemic factors (e.g., endocrine signals) and environment dynamics (light, temperature, and nutrition), it is generally believed that there is significant local control of hair shedding, because each fiber grows to a specific, location-dependent, predetermined length, for an exact period of time, before being shed.[14]

Higgins et al. found a positive correlation between the amount of tissue remaining on the club fiber after plucking and the time remaining for natural release.[123] In early anagen, a total of 66% of murine exogen club fibers had substantial quantities of cellular material, although none was devoid of attached material.[123] On the other hand, in late anagen, 81% of exogen club fibers plucked from follicles had very little or no cellular material attached.[123] These findings invited to subdivide exogen into "early exogen" and "late exogen", with shedding of the club fiber signaling the end of the latter phase.[123]

Surrounding the attachment site of the hair club are located cells rich in desmosomes (desmoglein) and K14.[14] Although the loss of DG3 may not describe the mechanism of exogen,[124] it does indicate that tight junctions are important for telogen hair shaft anchorage.[14] Later work proposed that a plasminogen activator/inhibitor concentrates to the cells in the area of the club hair attachment site[125] and that a chymotryptic enzyme is expressed in the sebaceous gland and pilary canal.[126] It was also evidenced that lysosomal proteases

such as cathepsin L are involved in the regulation of exogen,[127] at least in mice. In any case, it is now assumed that proteolytic pathways are implicated in the process of club hair formation and shedding.[14,127]

Another finding that supports the role of enzymes in the exogen phase is the observation of patients with acquired immune deficiency treated with protease inhibitors who suffer from hair loss, which might be related to the modulation of the protease-antiprotease systems on exogen.[14] Lipid bonding may also play a role, because lipids have been found to be necessary to the adhesion of cuticle cells.[14]

The exogen phase appears to be affected in several dermatoses. For example, in trichostasis spinulosa, the infundibulum of an HF becomes dilated with retained hair shafts from previous cycles, presumably as a result of an abnormally delayed exogen process.[14]

Kenogen

Kenogen (from the Greek κενός meaning empty) describes an empty follicle in telogen after the club fiber has been extruded.[111,128,129] When a hair is shed during exogen, any HF that is already in its anagen IV phase is anticipated to replace it swiftly.[111] However, sometimes, under physiologic conditions, this does not happen, so the HF enters into the so-called "kenogen", whose exact duration appears to be quite variable and dependent on the presence of male or female pattern baldness.[111,129,130]

Differences of Hair Follicle Cycling in Various Anatomic Locations

Hair cycle length for each phase may vary among different body areas. Unlike other mammals, human hair growth and shedding occurs in a mosaic pattern and it is not synchronized. At any given time, a certain location-dependent percentage of hairs will be in one of the three main hair cycle stages, with the duration of anagen in the scalp having been calculated to last 4–7 years, catagen 2–3 weeks, and telogen approximately a few months.[83] Although, recent research suggests that these traditional assumptions have to be questioned and reexamined.[39]

In any case, anagen duration determines the length of the hair shaft.[7] Therefore, HFs in different areas of the body produce hair shafts of different length,[7] with terminal scalp HFs having a much longer growth cycle than HFs in other body regions. The hair on the scalp grows about 0.3–0.4 mm/day or about 6 in/year. As opposed to the putative anagen duration of 4–7 years on the scalp,[83] HFs from other regions of the body, such as eyebrow, hands, ears, chest, arms, and legs, have shorter anagen ranging from 4–7 months.[83]

Seago et al. investigated the activity of HFs in arms and legs and concluded that they are androgen-dependent.[131] They described that the hair growth rate of thigh HFs was significantly higher in males than in females, whereas on the arms the difference was not statistically significant. The percentage of hairs in telogen was significantly higher in females than in males on the thigh, but not on the arm.[131] The duration of the anagen period was longer in males than in females for the thigh, but not for the arm and also demonstrated that on the thigh the fully grown hair is three times longer in males than in females.[131] The growth rate was 12 times greater in males, and most of the difference is produced by a longer anagen phase, which is 25 times greater.[131] On the upper arm, the hair was 14 times longer and the duration of anagen phase was 13 times greater in males than in females.[131]

Loussoran et al. performed a longitudinal study aiming to measure and compare the hair growth profiles of young adults without alopecia living in the five continents. It was observed that hair growth rate slightly decreased (by 0.4 cm/year, $P<.001$) in subjects older than 26 years.[132] Hair growth appeared significantly lower at the nape in men compared to women, by a few 0.1 mm/month ($P<.001$), and both genders showed hairs that grow slightly faster on the vertex, by a few μm/year compared to on the nape and temple ($P<.001$).[132]

Hair Follicle Metabolism During Cycling and Role of Oxidative Damage

Although human scalp HFs in anagen primarily are thought to engage in aerobic glycolysis and glutaminolysis,[133] it also engages in substantial mitochondrial energy metabolism.[44] Most recently, Lemasters et al. studied the energetics of growing HFs through mitochondrial and oxidative metabolism. Mitochondrial membrane potential ($\Delta\Psi$), cell viability, reactive oxygen species (ROS), and secretory granules were assessed.[45] It was shown that in growing follicles, the lower bulb epithelial cells had high viability, and the mitochondrias were polarized.[45] ROS and $\Delta\Psi$ were strongest in the sites for formation of the outer cortex/cuticle of the hair shaft.[45] By contrast, in DP fibroblasts, polarized mitochondria produced minimal ROS.[45]

Moreover, the human HF uses complex systems for regulating oxidative damage, such as the expression of ROS scavenging enzymes, such as catalase, synthesizes melatonin,[47] and expresses nuclear factor (erythroid-derived 2)-like 2 (Nrf2), a "master regulator" of genes controlling cellular redox homeostasis. Current understanding is that Nrf2 may have a therapeutic role in diseases with impaired redox balance.[134]

HAIR SHAPE AND HAIR SHAFT COMPOSITION

Hair curliness is predetermined in the bulb and is linked to asymmetry in the hair matrix, the curvature of the IRS, and changes in the specific composition of hair shaft keratins.[40,135,136] Also, some structural proteins are expressed differently depending on the shape of the HF including K38,[136,137] K82,[136] and insulin-like growth factor–binding protein 5.[135,138] Interestingly, hair shape can be pharmacologically modified in vivo, by EGFR and IFNα-2b[139] pathway inhibitors.[135,140] Curly hairs have an elliptical shape in cross-section, enabling them with bidirectional bending stiffness.[40]

Alibardi reported the localization of hair keratins, two high-sulfur keratin-associated proteins, and sulfhydryl oxidase in the human hair.[141] He showed that sulfur-rich KAP1 is mainly cortical and a diffuse labeling is present in differentiating cuticle cells.[141] Sulfhydryl oxidase is diffusely present in differentiating cortical cells and is weak in cuticle cells and absent in medulla and IRS.[141] Lastly, sulfur-rich K26 was only detected in the exocuticle and endocuticle.[141]

MELANOGENESIS IN THE HAIR FOLLICLE

Melanogenesis is the complex process by which the pigment melanin is produced in melanosomes by melanocytes. There are two distinct types of melanin: black to brown eumelanin and yellow to reddish-brown pheomelanin.[142] The ratio of eumelanin to pheomelanin determines the color of the hair, skin, and eyes.[142] Both pigments derive from the same common precursor produced from L-tyrosine by the action of tyrosinase.[143] Melanogenesis in the HF, in contrast to the continuous melanogenesis observed in epidermal melanocytes, only takes place during anagen III–VI[20] and shares some controls with their epidermal counterparts.[144–146] Melanogenesis in human HF also underlies distinct controls not found in the epidermis, such as stimulation by TRH.[144]

NORMAL HUMAN SCALP CHARACTERISTICS IN DIFFERENT RACES

General features of the HF and hair shaft vary depending on the ethnic backgorund. Loussouran et al. measured and compared the hair growth profiles of young adults without alopecia in the five continents.[132] Twenty-four various human ethnic groups were included and hair growth patterns in three different scalp areas (vertex, occipital and temporal) of 2249 young female and male adults (18–35 years) were observed.[132] Natural hair color was assessed from the nape, which is less prone to ultraviolet (UV)-induced discoloration and it was matched to a scale ranging from 1/black to 10/pale blond.[132] Matching was also done for the eight types of reference scale (from 1/straight to 8/highly curly).[83]

It was found that the total hair density (THD) varies from 233 ± 74 hairs/cm^2 (French) to 153 ± 30 hairs/cm^2 (South-African) ($P<.001$).[132] Interestingly, THD was lower in men, but only in the vertex area, by some 19 hairs/cm^2 less than women ($P<.001$). Comparing the three scalp areas, hair density followed the following area gradient: temple < nape < vertex ($P<.001$). T% (ratio of telogen hair density vs. THD) ranged from $8 \pm 6\%$ (Danish) to $14 \pm 7\%$ (Thai) ($P<.001$).[132] Average hair growth rate was another parameter considered in the previous study. It ranged from $272 \pm 37\,\mu m/24\,h$ (South-African) to $426 \pm 39\,\mu m/24\,h$ (Korean) ($P<.001$).[132]

Hair diameter was also assessed yielding median diameters from $69 \pm 8\,\mu m$ (French) to $89 \pm 7\,\mu m$ (Chinese) ($P<.001$); this echoes the tendency toward increased diameter amongst Asians.[132] No significant difference in hair diameter was observed between the three scalp areas.[132]

The last two parameters were hair color and curliness. Seventy-four percent of the subjects in the study showed head hair of darker tones (1–4), whereas lighter tones (8–10) represented 4%.[132] T% showed a tendency to decrease when hair tones increased above 6 (from $11 \pm 5\%$ to $7 \pm 4\%$, $P<.001$). Likewise, the diameters of hairs with tones >6 showed significantly lower values than hairs with tones <6, i.e., $72 \pm 9\,\mu m$ vs. $81 \pm 10\,\mu m$, respectively, $P<.001$.[132]

Commo et al. intended to determine melanin content and composition in human eumelanic hair from different ethnicities and at different ages.[147] They found that eumelanin contents (total melanin values) were significantly higher in African-American hairs, followed by East Asian and Caucasian hairs.[147]

HUMAN SCALP IN DIFFERENT AGES

With age, there is a progressive decrease in the optimal functioning and reserve capacity of all the organs in the body, including the skin and hair.[148] Hair provides partial natural UV protection to the underlying skin in the scalp; therefore, bald scalp shows features of both intrinsic and extrinsic aging.[149]

Matsumara et al. studied the role of HFSCs in the aging process.[150] It was observed that the loss of HFSC is related to HFs miniaturization and hair loss in wild-type mice and in humans.[150] In vivo fate analysis of HFSCs revealed that the DNA damage

response in HFSCs causes proteolysis of type XVII collagen (COL17A1/BP180), a critical molecule for HFSC maintenance.[150] These authors also demonstrated that COL17A1 in HFSCs have a major role in the regulation of the aging process of HFSC.[150]

Senescence features have been studied through scalp-biopsy analysis,[151] macrophotography,[152] and phototrichograms.[153] Some of them are: hair loss, gray hair, color vanishing, decreased scalp water content, decreased transepidermal water loss, decreased hair density and diameter, thinning of the hair, decreased sebum secretion, decreased incidence of dandruff and increased redness[154]

Hair density decreases with age. Sinclair et al. studied scalp biopsies from 928 women between 13 and 84 years old.[152] It was found that for every 1-year unit increase in age, there is a decrease in the total number of HFs of 0.093 ($P<.001$).[152]

Another feature of senescence HFs is the decrease of hair diameter after certain age. Hair diameter increases with age from infancy through the teenage years, reaches a plateau and does not change from age 20 to 49 years, and decreases after the age of 50 years.[151] This phenomenon has been described in many studies in populations of different ethnicity.[151] In Korean women, the average hair diameter was highest in their 20s, maintained steadily until 50 years, and then decreased significantly.[151] Japanese women showed a tendency to increase hair diameter until their 40s and then declined with age.[151]

In contrast, sebaceous gland number and size have not been noted to change with age, although sebum production decreases by approximately 60% over the adult life span.[152,155] In women older than 40 years, the number of people having severe dandruff decreased.[151]

Hair graying is the most noticeable sign of aging in humans. Hair graying mechanisms are not completely understood. The current understanding is that the irreversible stage of graying results from defective self-maintenance of melanocyte stem cells.[156] Melanocyte stem cells share the same niche with HFSCs. Zhang et al. showed that β-catenin is expressed in melanocytes, being significantly increased during anagen and telogen skin of aged mice, when compared to the anagen and telogen skin of young mice, respectively.[157] Zhang et al. proposed that increased Wnt signaling promotes excessive differentiation of melanocytes, leading to fatigue of melanocyte stem cells and, eventually, graying of the hair in aged mice.[157]

With aging, there is also a 15% reduction in eccrine gland number, 10%–20% decrease per decade of active melanocytes, 20%–50% reduction in Langerhans cells, 20% loss of dermal thickness in the elderly, 50% reduction in mast cells, and 66% reduction in Pacinian and Meissner's nerve end organ corpuscles.[158]

Aging is also associated with increased incidence of male and female pattern hair loss (MPHL and FPHL). The follicular changes in MPHL and FPHL are very similar and they all end with follicular miniaturization. Common findings include progressive reduction in the duration of anagen and prolongation of the latent period of the hair cycle (only in men).[159] It is a matter of ongoing debate on how MPHL and FPHL can be reliably distinguished from intrinsic HF senescence and how both contribute to the so-called "senescent alopecia".[160,161] Interestingly, cultured human DP fibroblasts derived from HFs of males undergoing MPHL exhibit markers of advanced cellular senescence compared to DP cells from nonbalding male HFs.[162]

DIFFERENCES BETWEEN HUMANS AND MOUSE HAIR FOLLICLES MORPHOLOGY AND CYCLING

As we have already mentioned, major differences exist between mouse and human HF morphology, especially for those located on the scalp. The most obvious difference is regarding the length and size of HFs. Human scalp follicles are significantly larger, reaching lengths of 5 mm, compared with mouse pelage follicles, which are only 1 mm long.[92] Moreover, human HFs lose up to 80% of their lower tissue volume during catagen and posses only one hair per follicle.[89] Human HFs grow for years rather than weeks.[89]

Rodents also posses specialized HFs, for which no human equivalent exists, such as vibrissa (whisker) HF. Vibrissa are larger than pelage follicles; unique in their cycling behavior; are innervated by large sensory nerves, whose neurons communicate with the sensory cortex; and are surrounded by cavernous blood-filled sinus.[89,92,163]

In mice, HF cycling is initiated about 17 days postpartum.[20] At this time, the HF spontaneously undergoes catagen.[20] The first catagen lasts 2–3 days and is followed by the first telogen, which lasts several days and usually more than 3 weeks in the second telogen, increasing in length with each additional HF cycle.[20] HF morphogenesis continues throughout early postnatal life in mice, which is why it is routinely misinterpreted as "first anagen", but the first real anagen does not occur until 4 weeks after birth.[20] In mice, the initial waves of pelage HF cycling are highly synchronized, but with time, distinct groups of coordinated HF cycling ("domains") show distinct patterns of HF cycling, which become more dispersed and fragmented as the mouse ages.[20,112]

In contrast, human HF cycle long before birth, i.e., in utero, and shed their first "test hair shafts" (lanugo hair) into the amniotic fluid. In human fetal skin, HF cycling is synchronized and becomes asynchronous soon after birth, following its own ("mosaic") cycling pattern in individual HFs.[20] A partial and temporary resynchronization of adult human HFs can be seen, e.g., in connection with major hormonal abnormalities, systemic illness, chemotherapy, and after the transplantation of autologous occipital scalp HFs to frontotemporal skin.

Another key contrast between murine and human HFs is that mouse usually retain their hair shaft during HF cycling, whereas humans do not. Therefore, even major hair cycle abnormalities in mice do not necessarily lead to alopecia. Interestingly, the presence of alopecia in murine skin invariably indicates that HFs in the alopecic areas have suffered some degree of damage that hinders the usual mooring of hair shafts in the hair canal.[164]

NEUROENDOCRINOLOGY OF THE HAIR FOLLICLE

HFs are not only prominent target tissues for an astounding variety of neuromediators, but also are able to synthesize them.[47] These endogenous and intrafollicular synthesized neurohormones, neuropeptides, and neurotransmitters are likely to participate in the control of HF cycling and link the latter to environmental inputs. Possibly, the rich neuromediator expression in the HF epithelium reflects the shared neuroectodermal embryologic origin with the CNS.[47] The neuromediators may be produced as prohormones such as proopiomelanocortin (POMC) and processed within the HF to their respective neuropeptides (e.g., α-melanocyte stimulating hormone [αMSH], ACTH, and β-endorphin) or directly translated from intrafollicular transcribed genes (e.g., TRH,[38] CRH, and prolactin).[44,47] Neuromediators may also be synthesized enzymatically (e.g., melatonin).[47]

Previous studies had pointed out the presence of a hypothalamic–pituitary–adrenal (HPA) axis in mammalian skin.[100,165–167] The functional significance of this peripheral HPA axis equivalent system is not completely understood. Evidence in murine HF in vivo showed that HF expresses CRH and its receptors, which have a high sensitivity to glucocorticoid targets.[47,168–170] Also, in human HF organ culture the presence of a fully functional peripheral HPA axis equivalent was observed.[47,171] Like in the hypothalamus, HF epithelium transcribes CRH and its receptors, and defined regions of human HF epithelium express CRH protein.[47,169–172] Exposure of the HF to CRH upregulates POMC transcription and protein processing into melanocortins (same as ACTH and αMSH in the pituitary). In addition,

ACTH stimulates intrafollicular cortisol synthesis.[47] Interestingly, as in the HPA axis, a negative feedback mechanism occurs in the HF after stimulation by cortisol, which downregulates intrafollicular CRH protein expression.[47,171]

The peripheral HPA axis may serve as a fast response to stressors.[47,167,171,173] UV-induced stress downregulates ACTH expression in human HF.[47,174] Furthermore, POMC-derived products (ACTH and αMSH), β-endorphin, and possibly even POMC itself are pigment-stimulatory neuropeptide hormones that have an effect on melanocytes in the epidermis and the HF.[42,47,175] Melanin production reflects a stress response mechanism, because melanin absorbs UV irradiation, and is an effective free radical scavenger.[47,176]

ACTH also has other effects on the HF besides inducing pigmentation. ACTH production is hair cycle–dependent and induces anagen and premature anagen termination in mice. The effect on the anagen stage of HF cycle may be mediated by the properties of ACTH as a mast cell secretagogue.[35,47,101] Moreover, CRH, which is also a human hair growth inhibitor[47,171,173] and a strong mast cell secretagogue, can activate perifollicular mast cells in the connective tissue sheath of human HF and promote the maturation of their progenitor cells in the HF mesenchyme.[47,101] Lastly, it has been established that the bulb and bulge region during anagen represent zones of relative immune privilege, which helps to protect HF-associated autoantigens from immune recognition and autoimmunity, especially the stem cell zone of the HF and the pigment-producing hair shaft factory in the anagen hair bulb. Interestingly, the neuropeptide αMSH has potent immunosuppressive effects and likely plays a key role in HF immune privilege maintenance by suppressing MHC class I expression by HF keratinocytes.[47,177,178]

Besides the adrenal hormones, thyroid hormones (T3 and T4) also directly regulate human HF biology.[38] This is achieved through anagen prolongation, HF pigmentation, hair matrix keratinocyte proliferation, and modulation of intrafollicular keratin expression.[47,179] Also, T3 and T4 stimulate K15 expression and modulate other functions of human HF epithelial stem cells in situ.[47,180] Human scalp HFs transcribe TSH receptor (TSH-R), which is primarily expressed by the HF mesenchyme at the protein level.[38] TSH-R stimulation increases the transcription of selected keratins and of TSH target genes, such as those encoding thyroglobulin and thyroid transcription factor 1.[47,181] This suggests that human HF exhibits some TSH responses that are typically present in the thyroid gland. Moreover, T3, T4, TSH, and TRH all stimulate the mitochondrial activity of human scalp HFs ex vivo.[44]

In addition, testosterone and DHT act through androgen receptors, e.g., in the DP, increasing the size of HF in androgen-dependent areas such as the beard during adolescence and in older men can cause miniaturization of follicles in the scalp (resulting in androgenetic alopecia).[7,182] Miranda et al. showed that women's intermediate facial follicles respond to men's higher androgen levels with the production of more hair, demonstrating that androgen receptors are present in vivo within these follicles.[182]

CONCLUSIONS

In this chapter, we reviewed key aspects of human HF physiology, with additional pointers taken from the biology of mouse HFs, from human HF development during fetal life, to its mature morphology, cycling, regulatory molecules, and differences between races and aging. Yet, despite more than a century of systematic research, human HF functions in health and disease remain quite incompletely understood, which explains in part why many hair disorders are still poorly controlled from a therapeutic point of view. However, since hair research has attracted the interdisciplinary attention of many life scientists in recent decades, our understanding of this complex (mini)-organ steadily increases, and new targets for therapeutic intervention continue to be uncovered.

REFERENCES

1. Langan EA, Philpott MP, Kloepper JE, Paus R. Human hair follicle organ culture: theory, application and perspectives. *Exp Dermatol.* 2015;24(12):903–911.
2. Messenger AG, Botchkareva NV. Unraveling the secret life of the hair follicle: from fungi to innovative hair loss therapies. *Exp Dermatol.* 2017;26(6):471.
3. Nakamura M, Schneider MR, Schmidt-Ullrich R, Paus R. Mutant laboratory mice with abnormalities in hair follicle morphogenesis, cycling, and/or structure: an update. *J Dermatol Sci.* 2013;69(1):6–29.
4. Cotsarelis G, Sun TT, Lavker RM. Label-retaining cells reside in the bulge area of pilosebaceous unit: implications for follicular stem cells, hair cycle, and skin carcinogenesis. *Cell.* 1990;61(7):1329–1337.
5. Liu LY, Craiglow BG, Dai F, King BA. Tofacitinib for the treatment of severe alopecia areata and variants: a study of 90 patients. *J Am Acad Dermatol.* 2017;76(1):22–28.
6. Xing L, Dai Z, Jabbari A, et al. Alopecia areata is driven by cytotoxic T lymphocytes and is reversed by JAK inhibition. *Nat Med.* 2014;20(9):1043–1049.
7. Paus R, Cotsarelis G. The biology of hair follicles. *N Engl J Med.* 1999;341(7):491–497.

8. Chuong CM, Jung HS, Noden D, Widelitz RB. Lineage and pluripotentiality of epithelial precursor cells in developing chicken skin. *Biochem Cell Biol.* 1998;76(6):1069–1077.

9. Kratochwil K, Dull M, Farinas I, Galceran J, Grosschedl R. Lef1 expression is activated by BMP-4 and regulates inductive tissue interactions in tooth and hair development. *Genes Dev.* 1996;10(11):1382–1394.

10. Zhou P, Byrne C, Jacobs J, Fuchs E. Lymphoid enhancer factor 1 directs hair follicle patterning and epithelial cell fate. *Genes Dev.* 1995;9(6):700–713.

11. Glover JD, Wells KL, Matthaus F, et al. Hierarchical patterning modes orchestrate hair follicle morphogenesis. *PLoS Biol.* 2017;15(7):e2002117.

12. Wang Q, Oh JW, Lee HL, et al. A multi-scale model for hair follicles reveals heterogeneous domains driving rapid spatiotemporal hair growth patterning. *Elife.* 2017;6.

13. Hansen LS, Coggle JE, Wells J, Charles MW. The influence of the hair cycle on the thickness of mouse skin. *Anat Rec.* 1984;210(4):569–573.

14. Stenn KS, Paus R. Controls of hair follicle cycling. *Physiol Rev.* 2001;81(1):449–494.

15. Paus R, Foitzik K, Welker P, Bulfone-Paus S, Eichmuller S. Transforming growth factor-beta receptor type I and type II expression during murine hair follicle development and cycling. *J Invest Dermatol.* 1997;109(4):518–526.

16. Schmidt-Ullrich R, Paus R. Molecular principles of hair follicle induction and morphogenesis. *Bioessays.* 2005;27(3):247–261.

17. Christiano AM. Epithelial stem cells: stepping out of their niche. *Cell.* 2004;118(5):530–532.

18. Sieber-Blum M, Grim M, Hu YF, Szeder V. Pluripotent neural crest stem cells in the adult hair follicle. *Dev Dyn.* 2004;231(2):258–269.

19. Mikkola ML. Genetic basis of skin appendage development. *Semin Cell Dev Biol.* 2007;18(2):225–236.

20. Schneider MR, Schmidt-Ullrich R, Paus R. The hair follicle as a dynamic miniorgan. *Curr Biol.* 2009;19(3):R132–R142.

21. Hardy MH. The development of mouse hair in vitro with some observations on pigmentation. *J Anat.* 1949;83(4):364–384, 363 p.

22. Maini PK, Baker RE, Chuong CM. Developmental biology. The Turing model comes of molecular age. *Science.* 2006;314(5804):1397–1398.

23. Duverger O, Morasso MI. To grow or not to grow: hair morphogenesis and human genetic hair disorders. *Semin Cell Dev Biol.* 2014;25–26:22–33.

24. Andl T, Reddy ST, Gaddapara T, Millar SE. WNT signals are required for the initiation of hair follicle development. *Dev Cell.* 2002;2(5):643–653.

25. Headon DJ, Overbeek PA. Involvement of a novel Tnf receptor homologue in hair follicle induction. *Nat Genet.* 1999;22(4):370–374.

26. Schmidt-Ullrich R, Aebischer T, Hulsken J, Birchmeier W, Klemm U, Scheidereit C. Requirement of NF-kappaB/Rel for the development of hair follicles and other epidermal appendices. *Development.* 2001;128(19):3843–3853.

27. Jamora C, DasGupta R, Kocieniewski P, Fuchs E. Links between signal transduction, transcription and adhesion in epithelial bud development. *Nature.* 2003;422(6929):317–322.

28. Magerl M, Tobin DJ, Muller-Rover S, et al. Patterns of proliferation and apoptosis during murine hair follicle morphogenesis. *J Invest Dermatol.* 2001;116(6):947–955.

29. Lindner G, Botchkarev VA, Botchkareva NV, Ling G, van der Veen C, Paus R. Analysis of apoptosis during hair follicle regression (catagen). *Am J Pathol.* 1997;151(6):1601–1617.

30. Geyfman M, Plikus MV, Treffeisen E, Andersen B, Paus R. Resting no more: re-defining telogen, the maintenance stage of the hair growth cycle. *Biol Rev Camb Philos Soc.* 2015;90(4):1179–1196.

31. Scharschmidt TC, Vasquez KS, Pauli ML, et al. Commensal microbes and hair follicle morphogenesis coordinately drive Treg migration into neonatal skin. *Cell Host Microbe.* 2017;21(4):467–477.e465.

32. Ali N, Zirak B, Rodriguez RS, et al. Regulatory T cells in skin facilitate epithelial stem cell differentiation. *Cell.* 2017;169(6):1119–1129.e1111.

33. Castellana D, Paus R, Perez-Moreno M. Macrophages contribute to the cyclic activation of adult hair follicle stem cells. *PLoS Biol.* 2014;12(12):e1002002.

34. Kloepper JE, Kawai K, Bertolini M, Kanekura T, Paus R. Loss of gammadelta T cells results in hair cycling defects. *J Invest Dermatol.* 2013;133(6):1666–1669.

35. Paus R, Maurer M, Slominski A, Czarnetzki BM. Mast cell involvement in murine hair growth. *Dev Biol.* 1994;163(1):230–240.

36. Purba TS, Brunken L, Peake M, et al. Characterisation of cell cycle arrest and terminal differentiation in a maximally proliferative human epithelial tissue: lessons from the human hair follicle matrix. *Eur J Cell Biol.* 2017;96(6):632–641.

37. Purba TS, Peake M, Farjo B, et al. Divergent proliferation patterns of distinct human hair follicle epithelial progenitor niches in situ and their differential responsiveness to prostaglandin D2. *Sci Rep.* 2017;7(1):15197.

38. Purba TS, Haslam IS, Poblet E, et al. Human epithelial hair follicle stem cells and their progeny: current state of knowledge, the widening gap in translational research and future challenges. *Bioessays.* 2014;36(5):513–525.

39. Oh JW, Kloepper J, Langan EA, et al. A guide to studying human hair follicle cycling in vivo. *J Invest Dermatol.* 2016;136(1):34–44.

40. Westgate GE, Ginger RS, Green MR. The biology and genetics of curly hair. *Exp Dermatol.* 2017;26(6):483–490.

41. Ho J, Bhawan J. Folliculosebaceous neoplasms: a review of clinical and histological features. *J Dermatol.* 2017;44(3):259–278.

42. Paus R. A neuroendocrinological perspective on human hair follicle pigmentation. *Pigment Cell Melanoma Res.* 2011;24(1):89–106.

43. Tobin DJ. The cell biology of human hair follicle pigmentation. *Pigment Cell Melanoma Res.* 2011;24(1):75–88.

44. Vidali S, Knuever J, Lerchner J, et al. Hypothalamic-pituitary-thyroid axis hormones stimulate mitochondrial function and biogenesis in human hair follicles. *J Invest Dermatol.* 2014;134(1):33–42.
45. Lemasters JJ, Ramshesh VK, Lovelace GL, et al. Compartmentation of mitochondrial and oxidative metabolism in growing hair follicles: a ring of fire. *J Invest Dermatol.* 2017;137(7):1434–1444.
46. Danilenko DM, Ring BD, Pierce GF. Growth factors and cytokines in hair follicle development and cycling: recent insights from animal models and the potentials for clinical therapy. *Mol Med Today.* 1996;2(11):460–467.
47. Paus R, Langan EA, Vidali S, Ramot Y, Andersen B. Neuroendocrinology of the hair follicle: principles and clinical perspectives. *Trends Mol Med.* 2014;20(10):559–570.
48. Tiede S, Kloepper JE, Whiting DA, Paus R. The 'follicular trochanter': an epithelial compartment of the human hair follicle bulge region in need of further characterization. *Br J Dermatol.* 2007;157(5):1013–1016.
49. Rochat A, Kobayashi K, Barrandon Y. Location of stem cells of human hair follicles by clonal analysis. *Cell.* 1994;76(6):1063–1073.
50. Tanimura S, Tadokoro Y, Inomata K, et al. Hair follicle stem cells provide a functional niche for melanocyte stem cells. *Cell Stem Cell.* 2011;8(2):177–187.
51. Schneider MR, Paus R. Deciphering the functions of the hair follicle infundibulum in skin physiology and disease. *Cell Tissue Res.* 2014;358(3):697–704.
52. Paus R, van der Veen C, Eichmuller S, et al. Generation and cyclic remodeling of the hair follicle immune system in mice. *J Invest Dermatol.* 1998;111(1):7–18.
53. Paus R, Nickoloff BJ, Ito T. A 'hairy' privilege. *Trends Immunol.* 2005;26(1):32–40.
54. Paus R, Bulfone-Paus S, Bertolini M. Hair follicle immune privilege revisited: the key to alopecia areata management. *J Invest Dermatol Symp Proc.* 2018;19(1):S12–S17.
55. Gilhar A, Etzioni A, Paus R. Alopecia areata. *N Engl J Med.* 2012;366(16):1515–1525.
56. Harries MJ, Meyer K, Chaudhry I, et al. Lichen planopilaris is characterized by immune privilege collapse of the hair follicle's epithelial stem cell niche. *J Pathol.* 2013;231(2):236–247.
57. Hofmann U, Tokura Y, Ruckert R, Paus R. The anagen hair cycle induces systemic immunosuppression of contact hypersensitivity in mice. *Cell Immunol.* 1998;184(1):65–73.
58. Geyfman M, Gordon W, Paus R, Andersen B. Identification of telogen markers underscores that telogen is far from a quiescent hair cycle phase. *J Invest Dermatol.* 2012;132(3 Pt 1):721–724.
59. Hoffmann R, Happle R, Paus R. Elements of the interleukin-1 signaling system show hair cycle-dependent gene expression in murine skin. *Eur J Dermatol.* 1998;8(7):475–477.
60. Nagao K, Kobayashi T, Moro K, et al. Stress-induced production of chemokines by hair follicles regulates the trafficking of dendritic cells in skin. *Nat Immunol.* 2012;13(8):744–752.
61. Poblet E, Jimenez-Acosta F, Hardman JA, Escario E, Paus R. Is the eccrine gland an integral, functionally important component of the human scalp pilosebaceous unit? *Exp Dermatol.* 2016;25(2):149–150.
62. Avram MR, Finney R, Rogers N. Hair transplantation controversies. *Dermatol Surg.* 2017;43(suppl 2):S158–S162.
63. Poblet E, Ortega F, Jimenez F. The arrector pili muscle and the follicular unit of the scalp: a microscopic anatomy study. *Dermatol Surg.* 2002;28(9):800–803.
64. Torkamani N, Rufaut N, Jones L, Sinclair R. The arrector pili muscle, the bridge between the follicular stem cell niche and the interfollicular epidermis. *Anat Sci Int.* 2017;92(1):151–158.
65. Hinde E, Haslam IS, Schneider MR, et al. A practical guide for the study of human and murine sebaceous glands in situ. *Exp Dermatol.* 2013;22(10):631–637.
66. Botchkarev VA, Botchkareva NV, Peters EM, Paus R. Epithelial growth control by neurotrophins: leads and lessons from the hair follicle. *Prog Brain Res.* 2004;146:493–513.
67. Paus R, Arck P. Neuroendocrine perspectives in alopecia areata: does stress play a role? *J Invest Dermatol.* 2009;129(6):1324–1326.
68. Paus R, Peters EM, Eichmuller S, Botchkarev VA. Neural mechanisms of hair growth control. *J Investig Dermatol Symp Proc.* 1997;2(1):61–68.
69. Peters EM, Arck PC, Paus R. Hair growth inhibition by psychoemotional stress: a mouse model for neural mechanisms in hair growth control. *Exp Dermatol.* 2006;15(1):1–13.
70. Peters EM, Hansen MG, Overall RW, et al. Control of human hair growth by neurotrophins: brain-derived neurotrophic factor inhibits hair shaft elongation, induces catagen, and stimulates follicular transforming growth factor beta2 expression. *J Invest Dermatol.* 2005;124(4):675–685.
71. Peters EM, Liotiri S, Bodo E, et al. Probing the effects of stress mediators on the human hair follicle: substance P holds central position. *Am J Pathol.* 2007;171(6):1872–1886.
72. Jonsson EH, Bendas J, Weidner K, et al. The relation between human hair follicle density and touch perception. *Sci Rep.* 2017;7(1):2499.
73. Buscone S, Mardaryev AN, Raafs B, et al. A new path in defining light parameters for hair growth: discovery and modulation of photoreceptors in human hair follicle. *Lasers Surg Med.* 2017;49(7):705–718.
74. Blume U, Ferracin J, Verschoore M, Czernielewski JM, Schaefer H. Physiology of the vellus hair follicle: hair growth and sebum excretion. *Br J Dermatol.* 1991;124(1):21–28.
75. Headington JT. Transverse microscopic anatomy of the human scalp. A basis for a morphometric approach to disorders of the hair follicle. *Arch Dermatol.* 1984;120(4):449–456.
76. Miranda BH, Tobin DJ, Sharpe DT, Randall VA. Intermediate hair follicles: a new more clinically relevant model for hair growth investigations. *Br J Dermatol.* 2010;163(2):287–295.

77. Tobin DJ, Gunin A, Magerl M, Paus R. Plasticity and cytokinetic dynamics of the hair follicle mesenchyme during the hair growth cycle: implications for growth control and hair follicle transformations. *J Investig Dermatol Symp Proc.* 2003;8(1):80–86.

78. Al-Nuaimi Y, Goodfellow M, Paus R, Baier G. A prototypic mathematical model of the human hair cycle. *J Theor Biol.* 2012;310:143–159.

79. Paus R, Foitzik K. In search of the "hair cycle clock": a guided tour. *Differentiation.* 2004;72(9–10):489–511.

80. Al-Nuaimi Y, Hardman JA, Biro T, et al. A meeting of two chronobiological systems: circadian proteins Period1 and BMAL1 modulate the human hair cycle clock. *J Invest Dermatol.* 2014;134(3):610–619.

81. Muller-Rover S, Handjiski B, van der Veen C, et al. A comprehensive guide for the accurate classification of murine hair follicles in distinct hair cycle stages. *J Invest Dermatol.* 2001;117(1):3–15.

82. Muller-Rover S, Peters EJ, Botchkarev VA, Panteleyev A, Paus R. Distinct patterns of NCAM expression are associated with defined stages of murine hair follicle morphogenesis and regression. *J Histochem Cytochem.* 1998;46(12):1401–1410.

83. Saitoh M, Uzuka M, Sakamoto M. Human hair cycle. *J Invest Dermatol.* 1970;54(1):65–81.

84. Slominski A, Wortsman J, Plonka PM, Schallreuter KU, Paus R, Tobin DJ. Hair follicle pigmentation. *J Invest Dermatol.* 2005;124(1):13–21.

85. Krieger K, Millar SE, Mikuda N, et al. NF-kappab participates in mouse hair cycle control and plays distinct roles in the various pelage hair follicle types. *J Invest Dermatol.* 2017.

86. Nguyen H, Rendl M, Fuchs E. Tcf3 governs stem cell features and represses cell fate determination in skin. *Cell.* 2006;127(1):171–183.

87. Rosenquist TA, Martin GR. Fibroblast growth factor signalling in the hair growth cycle: expression of the fibroblast growth factor receptor and ligand genes in the murine hair follicle. *Dev Dyn.* 1996;205(4):379–386.

88. Alexeev V, Igoucheva O, Domashenko A, Cotsarelis G, Yoon K. Localized in vivo genotypic and phenotypic correction of the albino mutation in skin by RNA-DNA oligonucleotide. *Nat Biotechnol.* 2000;18(1):43–47.

89. Cotsarelis G. Epithelial stem cells: a folliculocentric view. *J Invest Dermatol.* 2006;126(7):1459–1468.

90. Fuchs E, Tumbar T, Guasch G. Socializing with the neighbors: stem cells and their niche. *Cell.* 2004;116(6):769–778.

91. Purba TS, Haslam IS, Shahmalak A, Bhogal RK, Paus R. Mapping the expression of epithelial hair follicle stem cell-related transcription factors LHX2 and SOX9 in the human hair follicle. *Exp Dermatol.* 2015;24(6):462–467.

92. Cotsarelis G. Gene expression profiling gets to the root of human hair follicle stem cells. *J Clin Invest.* 2006;116(1):19–22.

93. Oshima H, Rochat A, Kedzia C, Kobayashi K, Barrandon Y. Morphogenesis and renewal of hair follicles from adult multipotent stem cells. *Cell.* 2001;104(2):233–245.

94. Morris RJ, Liu Y, Marles L, et al. Capturing and profiling adult hair follicle stem cells. *Nat Biotechnol.* 2004;22(4):411–417.

95. Harries MJ, Meyer KC, Paus R. Hair loss as a result of cutaneous autoimmunity: frontiers in the immunopathogenesis of primary cicatricial alopecia. *Autoimmun Rev.* 2009;8(6):478–483.

96. Mobini N, Tam S, Kamino H. Possible role of the bulge region in the pathogenesis of inflammatory scarring alopecia: lichen planopilaris as the prototype. *J Cutan Pathol.* 2005;32(10):675–679.

97. Ito M, Kizawa K, Toyoda M, Morohashi M. Label-retaining cells in the bulge region are directed to cell death after plucking, followed by healing from the surviving hair germ. *J Invest Dermatol.* 2002;119(6):1310–1316.

98. Slominski A, Paus R, Plonka P, et al. Melanogenesis during the anagen-catagen-telogen transformation of the murine hair cycle. *J Invest Dermatol.* 1994;102(6):862–869.

99. Ito M, Kizawa K, Hamada K, Cotsarelis G. Hair follicle stem cells in the lower bulge form the secondary germ, a biochemically distinct but functionally equivalent progenitor cell population, at the termination of catagen. *Differentiation.* 2004;72(9–10):548–557.

100. Slominski A, Wortsman J, Tobin DJ. The cutaneous serotoninergic/melatoninergic system: securing a place under the sun. *FASEB J.* 2005;19(2):176–194.

101. Maurer M, Fischer E, Handjiski B, et al. Activated skin mast cells are involved in murine hair follicle regression (catagen). *Lab Invest.* 1997;77(4):319–332.

102. Westgate GE, Craggs RI, Gibson WT. Immune privilege in hair growth. *J Invest Dermatol.* 1991;97(3):417–420.

103. LeBrun DP, Warnke RA, Cleary ML. Expression of bcl-2 in fetal tissues suggests a role in morphogenesis. *Am J Pathol.* 1993;142(3):743–753.

104. Stenn KS, Lawrence L, Veis D, Korsmeyer S, Seiberg M. Expression of the bcl-2 protooncogene in the cycling adult mouse hair follicle. *J Invest Dermatol.* 1994;103(1):107–111.

105. Seiberg M, Marthinuss J, Stenn KS. Changes in expression of apoptosis-associated genes in skin mark early catagen. *J Invest Dermatol.* 1995;104(1):78–82.

106. Kloepper JE, Baris OR, Reuter K, et al. Mitochondrial function in murine skin epithelium is crucial for hair follicle morphogenesis and epithelial-mesenchymal interactions. *J Invest Dermatol.* 2015;135(3):679–689.

107. Ohnemus U, Uenalan M, Inzunza J, Gustafsson JA, Paus R. The hair follicle as an estrogen target and source. *Endocr Rev.* 2006;27(6):677–706.

108. Samuelov L, Sprecher E, Tsuruta D, Biro T, Kloepper JE, Paus R. P-cadherin regulates human hair growth and cycling via canonical Wnt signaling and transforming growth factor-beta2. *J Invest Dermatol.* 2012;132(10):2332–2341.

109. Vandevelde C, Allaerts W. Trichilemmal keratinisation: a causal factor in loosening the murine telogen club hair from the trichilemmal sac. *J Anat.* 1984;138(Pt 4):745–756.

110. Pinkus H, Iwasaki T, Mishima Y. Outer root sheath keratinization in anagen and catagen of the mammalian hair follicle. A seventh distinct type of keratinization in the hair follicle: trichilemmal keratinization. *J Anat.* 1981;133(Pt 1):19–35.

111. Rebora A. Pathogenesis of androgenetic alopecia. *J Am Acad Dermatol.* 2004;50(5):777–779.

112. Plikus MV, Mayer JA, de la Cruz D, et al. Cyclic dermal BMP signalling regulates stem cell activation during hair regeneration. *Nature.* 2008;451(7176):340–344.

113. Chase HB. Growth of the hair. *Physiol Rev.* 1954;34(1):113–126.

114. Paus R, Stenn KS, Link RE. Telogen skin contains an inhibitor of hair growth. *Br J Dermatol.* 1990;122(6):777–784.

115. Petho-Schramm A, Muller HJ, Paus R. FGF5 and the murine hair cycle. *Arch Dermatol Res.* 1996;288(5–6):264–266.

116. Suzuki S, Ota Y, Ozawa K, Imamura T. Dual-mode regulation of hair growth cycle by two Fgf-5 gene products. *J Invest Dermatol.* 2000;114(3):456–463.

117. Weger N, Schlake T. Igfbp3 modulates cell proliferation in the hair follicle. *J Invest Dermatol.* 2005;125(4):847–849.

118. Woo WM, Oro AE. SnapShot: hair follicle stem cells. *Cell.* 2011;146(2):334–334.e332.

119. Lindner G, Menrad A, Gherardi E, et al. Involvement of hepatocyte growth factor/scatter factor and met receptor signaling in hair follicle morphogenesis and cycling. *FASEB J.* 2000;14(2):319–332.

120. Bullough WS, Laurence EB. Epidermal chalone and mitotic control in the Vx2 epidermal tumour. *Nature.* 1968;220(5163):134–135.

121. Marks F, Richter KH. A request for a more serious approach to the chalone concept. *Br J Dermatol.* 1984;111(suppl 27):58–63.

122. Stenn K. Exogen is an active, separately controlled phase of the hair growth cycle. *J Am Acad Dermatol.* 2005;52(2):374–375.

123. Higgins CA, Westgate GE, Jahoda CA. From telogen to exogen: mechanisms underlying formation and subsequent loss of the hair club fiber. *J Invest Dermatol.* 2009;129(9):2100–2108.

124. Koch PJ, Mahoney MG, Cotsarelis G, Rothenberger K, Lavker RM, Stanley JR. Desmoglein 3 anchors telogen hair in the follicle. *J Cell Sci.* 1998;111(Pt 17):2529–2537.

125. Lavker RM, Risse B, Brown H, et al. Localization of plasminogen activator inhibitor type 2 (PAI-2) in hair and nail: implications for terminal differentiation. *J Invest Dermatol.* 1998;110(6):917–922.

126. Ekholm E, Sondell B, Stranden P, Brattsand M, Egelrud T. Expression of stratum corneum chymotryptic enzyme in human sebaceous follicles. *Acta Derm Venereol.* 1998;78(5):343–347.

127. Tobin DJ, Foitzik K, Reinheckel T, et al. The lysosomal protease cathepsin L is an important regulator of keratinocyte and melanocyte differentiation during hair follicle morphogenesis and cycling. *Am J Pathol.* 2002;160(5):1807–1821.

128. Pierard-Franchimont C, Pierard GE. Teloptosis, a turning point in hair shedding biorhythms. *Dermatology.* 2001;203(2):115–117.

129. Rebora A, Guarrera M. Kenogen. A new phase of the hair cycle? *Dermatology.* 2002;205(2):108–110.

130. Guarrera M, Rebora A. Kenogen in female androgenetic alopecia. A longitudinal study. *Dermatology.* 2005;210(1):18–20.

131. Seago SV, Ebling FJ. The hair cycle on the human thigh and upper arm. *Br J Dermatol.* 1985;113(1):9–16.

132. Loussouarn G, Lozano I, Panhard S, Collaudin C, El Rawadi C, Genain G. Diversity in human hair growth, diameter, colour and shape. An in vivo study on young adults from 24 different ethnic groups observed in the five continents. *Eur J Dermatol.* 2016;26(2):144–154.

133. Kealey T, Williams R, Philpott MP. The human hair follicle engages in glutaminolysis and aerobic glycolysis: implications for skin, splanchnic and neoplastic metabolism. *Skin Pharmacol.* 1994;7(1–2):41–46.

134. Haslam IS, Jadkauskaite L, Szabo IL, et al. Oxidative damage control in a human (mini-) organ: Nrf2 activation protects against oxidative stress-induced hair growth inhibition. *J Invest Dermatol.* 2017;137(2):295–304.

135. Bernard BA. The hair follicle enigma. *Exp Dermatol.* 2017;26(6):472–477.

136. Thibaut S, Gaillard O, Bouhanna P, Cannell DW, Bernard BA. Human hair shape is programmed from the bulb. *Br J Dermatol.* 2005;152(4):632–638.

137. Thibaut S, Barbarat P, Leroy F, Bernard BA. Human hair keratin network and curvature. *Int J Dermatol.* 2007;46(suppl 1):7–10.

138. Sriwiriyanont P, Hachiya A, Pickens WL, et al. Effects of IGF-binding protein 5 in dysregulating the shape of human hair. *J Invest Dermatol.* 2011;131(2):320–328.

139. Bessis D, Luong MS, Blanc P, et al. Straight hair associated with interferon-alfa plus ribavirin in hepatitis C infection. *Br J Dermatol.* 2002;147(2):392–393.

140. Agero AL, Dusza SW, Benvenuto-Andrade C, Busam KJ, Myskowski P, Halpern AC. Dermatologic side effects associated with the epidermal growth factor receptor inhibitors. *J Am Acad Dermatol.* 2006;55(4):657–670.

141. Alibardi L. Ultrastructural localization of hair keratins, high sulfur keratin-associated proteins and sulfhydryl oxidase in the human hair. *Anat Sci Int.* 2017;92(2):248–261.

142. Ito S, Wakamatsu K. Quantitative analysis of eumelanin and pheomelanin in humans, mice, and other animals: a comparative review. *Pigment Cell Res.* 2003;16(5):523–531.

143. Simon JD, Peles D, Wakamatsu K, Ito S. Current challenges in understanding melanogenesis: bridging chemistry, biological control, morphology, and function. *Pigment Cell Melanoma Res.* 2009;22(5):563–579.

144. Gaspar E, Nguyen-Thi KT, Hardenbicker C, et al. Thyrotropin-releasing hormone selectively stimulates human hair follicle pigmentation. *J Invest Dermatol.* 2011;131(12):2368–2377.

145. Hardman JA, Tobin DJ, Haslam IS, et al. The peripheral clock regulates human pigmentation. *J Invest Dermatol.* 2015;135(4):1053–1064.

146. Samuelov L, Sprecher E, Sugawara K, et al. Topobiology of human pigmentation: P-cadherin selectively stimulates hair follicle melanogenesis. *J Invest Dermatol.* 2013;133(6):1591–1600.

147. Commo S, Wakamatsu K, Lozano I, et al. Age-dependent changes in eumelanin composition in hairs of various ethnic origins. *Int J Cosmet Sci.* 2012;34(1):102–107.

148. Kim SN, Lee SY, Choi MH, et al. Characteristic features of ageing in Korean women's hair and scalp. *Br J Dermatol.* 2013;168(6):1215–1223.

149. Sinclair RD. Management of male pattern hair loss. *Cutis.* 2001;68(1):35–40.

150. Matsumura H, Mohri Y, Binh NT, et al. Hair follicle aging is driven by transepidermal elimination of stem cells via COL17A1 proteolysis. *Science.* 2016;351(6273):aad4395.

151. Sinclair R, Chapman A, Magee J. The lack of significant changes in scalp hair follicle density with advancing age. *Br J Dermatol.* 2005;152(4):646–649.

152. Birch MP, Messenger JF, Messenger AG. Hair density, hair diameter and the prevalence of female pattern hair loss. *Br J Dermatol.* 2001;144(2):297–304.

153. Robbins C, Mirmirani P, Messenger AG, et al. What women want - quantifying the perception of hair amount: an analysis of hair diameter and density changes with age in caucasian women. *Br J Dermatol.* 2012;167(2):324–332.

154. Kim JE, Lee JH, Choi KH, et al. Phototrichogram analysis of normal scalp hair characteristics with aging. *Eur J Dermatol.* 2013;23(6):849–856.

155. Jacobsen E, Billings JK, Frantz RA, Kinney CK, Stewart ME, Downing DT. Age-related changes in sebaceous wax ester secretion rates in men and women. *J Invest Dermatol.* 1985;85(5):483–485.

156. Nishimura EK, Granter SR, Fisher DE. Mechanisms of hair graying: incomplete melanocyte stem cell maintenance in the niche. *Science.* 2005;307(5710):720–724.

157. Zhang Z, Lei M, Xin H, et al. Wnt/beta-catenin signaling promotes aging-associated hair graying in mice. *Oncotarget.* 2017;8(41):69316–69327.

158. Yaar M, Gilchrest BA. Ageing of skin. In: Freidberg EM, Eisen AZ, Wolff K, et al., eds. *Fitzpatrick's Dermatology in General Practice.* New York: McGraw-Hill; 1999:1697–1706.

159. Olsen EA, Messenger AG, Shapiro J, et al. Evaluation and treatment of male and female pattern hair loss. *J Am Acad Dermatol.* 2005;52(2):301–311.

160. Torres F. Androgenetic, diffuse and senescent alopecia in men: practical evaluation and management. *Curr Probl Dermatol.* 2015;47:33–44.

161. Whiting DA. How real is senescent alopecia? A histopathologic approach. *Clin Dermatol.* 2011;29(1):49–53.

162. Upton JH, Hannen RF, Bahta AW, Farjo N, Farjo B, Philpott MP. Oxidative stress-associated senescence in dermal papilla cells of men with androgenetic alopecia. *J Invest Dermatol.* 2015;135(5):1244–1252.

163. Bertolini M, Meyer KC, Slominski R, Kobayashi K, Ludwig RJ, Paus R. The immune system of mouse vibrissae follicles: cellular composition and indications of immune privilege. *Exp Dermatol.* 2013;22(9):593–598.

164. Sundberg JP, Peters EM, Paus R. Analysis of hair follicles in mutant laboratory mice. *J Investig Dermatol Symp Proc.* 2005;10(3):264–270.

165. Slominski A, Paus R, Mazurkiewicz J. Proopiomelanocortin expression in the skin during induced hair growth in mice. *Experientia.* 1992;48(1):50–54.

166. Slominski A, Wortsman J, Kohn L, et al. Expression of hypothalamic-pituitary-thyroid axis related genes in the human skin. *J Invest Dermatol.* 2002;119(6):1449–1455.

167. Slominski A, Wortsman J, Luger T, Paus R, Solomon S. Corticotropin releasing hormone and proopiomelanocortin involvement in the cutaneous response to stress. *Physiol Rev.* 2000;80(3):979–1020.

168. Paus R, Heinzelmann T, Schultz KD, Furkert J, Fechner K, Czarnetzki BM. Hair growth induction by substance P. *Lab Invest.* 1994;71(1):134–140.

169. Ito N, Ito T, Betterman A, Paus R. The human hair bulb is a source and target of CRH. *J Invest Dermatol.* 2004;122(1):235–237.

170. Slominski A, Pisarchik A, Tobin DJ, Mazurkiewicz JE, Wortsman J. Differential expression of a cutaneous corticotropin-releasing hormone system. *Endocrinology.* 2004;145(2):941–950.

171. Ito N, Ito T, Kromminga A, et al. Human hair follicles display a functional equivalent of the hypothalamic-pituitary-adrenal axis and synthesize cortisol. *FASEB J.* 2005;19(10):1332–1334.

172. Kauser S, Slominski A, Wei ET, Tobin DJ. Modulation of the human hair follicle pigmentary unit by corticotropin-releasing hormone and urocortin peptides. *FASEB J.* 2006;20(7):882–895.

173. Slominski AT, Zmijewski MA, Zbytek B, Tobin DJ, Theoharides TC, Rivier J. Key role of CRF in the skin stress response system. *Endocr Rev.* 2013;34(6):827–884.

174. Lu Z, Fischer TW, Hasse S, et al. Profiling the response of human hair follicles to ultraviolet radiation. *J Invest Dermatol.* 2009;129(7):1790–1804.

175. Rousseau K, Kauser S, Pritchard LE, et al. Proopiomelanocortin (POMC), the ACTH/melanocortin precursor, is secreted by human epidermal keratinocytes and melanocytes and stimulates melanogenesis. *FASEB J.* 2007;21(8):1844–1856.

176. Paus R. Migrating melanocyte stem cells: masters of disaster? *Nat Med.* 2013;19(7):818–819.

177. Brzoska T, Luger TA, Maaser C, Abels C, Bohm M. Alpha-melanocyte-stimulating hormone and related tripeptides: biochemistry, antiinflammatory and protective effects in vitro and in vivo, and future perspectives for the treatment of immune-mediated inflammatory diseases. *Endocr Rev.* 2008;29(5):581–602.

178. Ito T, Ito N, Bettermann A, Tokura Y, Takigawa M, Paus R. Collapse and restoration of MHC class-I-dependent immune privilege: exploiting the human hair follicle as a model. *Am J Pathol.* 2004;164(2):623–634.

179. van Beek N, Bodo E, Kromminga A, et al. Thyroid hormones directly alter human hair follicle functions: anagen prolongation and stimulation of both hair matrix keratinocyte proliferation and hair pigmentation. *J Clin Endocrinol Metab.* 2008;93(11):4381–4388.

180. Tiede S, Bohm K, Meier N, Funk W, Paus R. Endocrine controls of primary adult human stem cell biology: thyroid hormones stimulate keratin 15 expression, apoptosis, and differentiation in human hair follicle epithelial stem cells in situ and in vitro. *Eur J Cell Biol.* 2010;89(10):769–777.

181. Bodo E, Kromminga A, Biro T, et al. Human female hair follicles are a direct, nonclassical target for thyroid-stimulating hormone. *J Invest Dermatol.* 2009; 129(5):1126–1139.

182. Miranda BH, Charlesworth MR, Tobin DJ, Sharpe DT, Randall VA. Androgens trigger different growth responses in genetically identical human hair follicles in organ culture that reflect their epigenetic diversity in life. *FASEB J.* 2017.

CHAPTER 2

Hair Pathology: The Basics

MARIYA MITEVA, MD

SCALP BIOPSY

Scalp biopsies are performed often in the hair practice to establish the diagnosis and to assess for disease activity in scarring alopecias. Usually one or two scalp biopsies are obtained, although data exist that accurate diagnosis is achieved in 98% who had triple horizontal biopsies versus 79% with a single horizontal biopsy.[1] The biopsy in patchy nonscarring alopecia is taken from the patch, and the biopsy in diffuse nonscarring alopecia is obtained usually from the parietal scalp or the midscalp because this is considered the optimal site to assess for follicular miniaturization especially in early female pattern hair loss.[2] If the patient parts the hair in the middle, the biopsy is obtained usually 1–2 cm laterally to avoid visible scarring. The 4-mm punch is used to obtain biopsies in nonscarring alopecia because the follicular counts have been established in 4-mm punch biopsies. In scarring alopecia, the optimal specimen is obtained by using a dermatoscope to guide the site for the biopsy (dermoscopy-guided scalp biopsy).[3] When using this technique, a 3-mm punch is usually sufficient for the diagnosis, especially in biopsies from the hair margin in frontal fibrosing alopecia.

HORIZONTAL (TRANSVERSE) SECTIONS

The histopathologic analysis of scalp biopsies is complicated by the anatomic complexity of the follicular structures and the different stages of the hair cycle.[4] Although vertical sections are the conventional method for processing of skin biopsies, horizontal sections are superior in the evaluation of the diameter of the hair follicles and the hair cycle.[5] Both horizontal and vertical sections have advantages and disadvantages and therefore should be interpreted together. However, if only one biopsy is obtained, horizontal sections should be performed. They allow for the assessment of the follicular architecture and the performance of hair counts in nonscarring alopecia as well as for detecting focal disease in scarring alopecia.[6] There are several methods of processing horizontal sections, and a number of instructive publications exist on the topic.[1,4,7–13]

Most of the literature is based on using the horizontal sections technique as described by Headington in 1984.[4] The punch biopsy is bisected into two halves that are embedded in the same cassette and cut together (Fig. 2.1). Although the optimal area of bisection is still discussed among experts,[4,8,14] the isthmus level is generally used to evaluate the follicular architecture and the presence or absence of sebaceous glands and to perform hair counts and ratios. The follicular architecture is preserved when it contains between 10 and 14 follicular units (hexagonal structures outlined by a loose collagen network and comprised of 3–4 terminal and 1 vellus follicle with the attached sebaceous glands and arrector pili muscles). If the specimen is correctly bisected, up to 20 sections are usually sufficient to assess the follicle along its entire length.[13]

HAIR FOLLICLES AND HAIR COUNTS: *THE BASICS*

The morphologic characteristics of the follicles in horizontal sections can be assimilated to easy-to-memorize images of objects, plants, and animals to facilitate understanding.[15]

The hair follicle is an epithelial structure that produces the hair shaft (keratinized nonviable material) through phases of growth and regression. Based on the hair diameter, the follicles are divided into three groups: terminal hairs that are thicker than 0.06 mm; intermediate hairs that measure between 0.03 and 0.06 mm, and vellus hairs that have a thin diameter of less than 0.03 mm. The growing phase of the hair follicle is called anagen, and *anagen follicles* constitute about 85% of all follicles. They are characterized by concentric arrangement of the follicular epithelial layers, which include an inner root sheath (pink and compact layer that keratinizes at the isthmus level), an outer root sheath (pale cells containing glycogen), and a connective tissue sheath (a thin layer of loose collagen primarily of type I, vessels, and fibroblasts) (Fig. 2.2A).

Catagen follicles are in transitional phase to regression, which lasts about 2–3 weeks. They count for

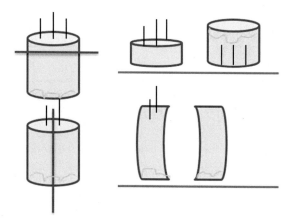

FIG. 2.1 A schematic presentation of the Headington technique for horizontal sections (upper row) versus vertical sections. The horizontal sections enable assessment of all follicles in a 4-mm punch biopsy at several levels.

less than 1% of all follicles in the normal scalp. In catagen, the hair shaft retreats upward, the outer root sheath shrinks, and it contains apoptotic cells (Fig. 2.2B).

Telogen follicles are in regression phase that lasts about 3 months; the telogen club hairs are situated at the bulge level and account for up to 15% of all follicles in the normal scalp The involuting hair shaft presents as bright and degenerated serrated keratin mass in the middle of the shrunken outer root sheath (Fig. 2.2C). The telogen germinal unit (TGU) is formed below the telogen club, consists of trichilemma that is somewhat convoluted and surrounded by palisading basaloid cells (Fig. 2.2D). All catagen and telogen follicles are counted together (telogen count). Terminal follicles are rooted in the subcutaneous tissue or deep dermis, whereas vellus follicles are rooted in the upper dermis. *Vellus follicles* have very thin hair shafts, no medulla, and no pigment (Fig. 2.3A).

Follicular (fibrous) streamers are residual fibrovascular whorled structures representing the impermanent lower third of the hair follicle below the bulge region[16] that may show many small blood vessels and remnants of trichilemmal gray vitreous membrane (Fig. 2.3B). They are not included in the follicular counts. In advanced androgenetic alopecia (AGA), the streamers may contain Arao-Perkins bodies, which represent small aggregates of degenerated elastic material[17]; in alopecia areata and trichotillomania they may contain pigmented casts[18] and in scarring alopecia, fragmented hair shafts.[19]

LEVELS ALONG THE FOLLICULAR LENGTH
- *Hair bulbs*: hair matrix cells and melanocytes surround the dermal papilla (fibroblasts and blood vessels) (Fig. 2.4A); in African Americans the hair bulbs have golf-club shape (Fig. 2.4B).
- *Isthmus*: attachment site of the sebaceous duct and the arrector pili muscle (Fig. 2.4C)
- *Infundibulum*: the follicles open at the surface in common ostia that contain 2–3 hair shafts; the infundibulum is lined by epidermis with a granular layer and basket-weave keratin that is continuous with the interfollicular epidermis (Fig. 2.4D)

FOLLICULAR COUNTS
Follicular counts are performed at all levels and the final sum of all follicles detected from the bulbar level to the infundibulum is reported; the ratio of terminal:vellus follicles is given in numbers and the telogen count in percentage. Care should be taken not to count twice or more times the same follicles at different levels. In a 4-mm punch biopsy, from the midscalp of normal controls, there is a preserved follicular density of about 10–14 follicular units, 40 hairs (3 follicles/mm²) comprising 35 terminal hairs (93.5% anagen and 6.5% telogen), 5 vellus hairs,[2] and about 2 fibrous streamers.[16] These counts differ among races, with biopsies from normal scalp in African Americans showing significantly lower follicular density than Caucasians of about 21.5 ± 5.0 total follicles[20] and biopsies from Asians showing even lower density than African Americans (16.1 ± 3.6 total follicles).[21]

Table 2.1 summarizes the findings that are usually included in reports of horizontal sections.

NONSCARRING ALOPECIA
Nonscarring alopecia is characterized by preserved follicular architecture, composed of terminal and vellus follicles and sebaceous glands, organized in follicular units.

Alopecia Areata
The histopathologic features of alopecia areata depend on the stage of the current episode as described by Whiting in 2003.[22] In the *acute stage*, the growing terminal anagen follicles are characterized by peribulbar lymphocytic infiltrate (known as "the swarm of bees"), which is noted around terminal follicles in early episodes and around vellus follicles in repeated episodes.[22] (Fig. 2.5A). The infiltrate is composed of both CD4 and CD8+ T-cell lymphocytes, with CD8+ NKG2D+ T-cell lymphocytes being predominant. Increased number

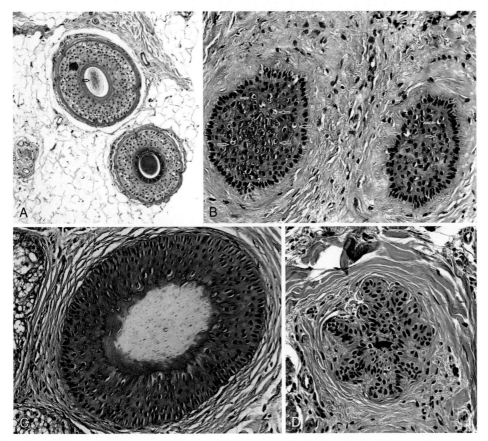

FIG. 2.2 **(A)** Anagen follicles, suprabulbar level in the subdermis: the hair shaft with its medulla, cortex, and cuticle is in the middle (*black arrow*); the outer root sheath is between the inner root sheath (*red arrow*) and the connective tissue sheath (*blue arrow*). **(B)** Catagen follicles. Note the absence of hair shaft and the presence of numerous apoptotic cells (*yellow arrows*). **(C)** Telogen follicle. Note the central bright keratinized mass of the regressing hair shaft resembling a red flame. **(D)** Telogen germinal unit. This palisading remnants of thin follicular epithelial strands resemble a leaf from the dwarf umbrella tree.

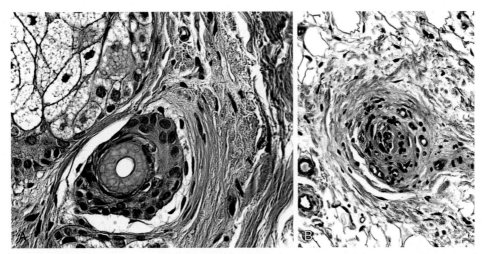

FIG. 2.3 **(A)** Vellus follicle: the hair shaft is very thin (in this particular section it is not present because of the processing of the tissue); compared to the terminal anagen hair in Fig. 2.2A. **(B)** A fibrous streamer in the subdermis; a biopsy from alopecia areata demonstrates the presence of small vessels and pigmented casts.

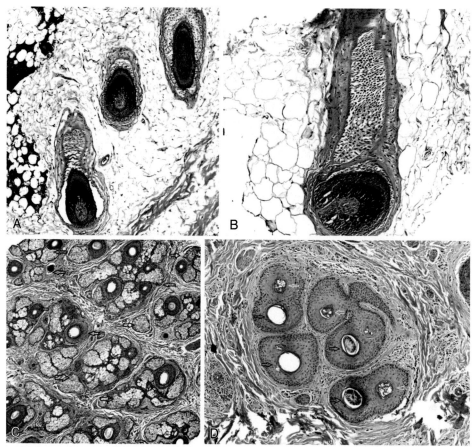

FIG. 2.4 **(A)** The terminal anagen follicles have their bulbs rooted in the subdermis. **(B)** In African Americans the follicular bulbs are asymmetric and twisted to one side resembling a golf club. **(C)** Level of the isthmus: note the follicular units (*black arrows*) separated by thin collagenous stroma. Each unit contains terminal, vellus follicle(s) and sebaceous lobules. **(D)** At the infundibular level the ostia of two or three follicles usually merge and open together at the surface (resembling a skeleton or a monkey face). In this case, the infundibular ostia contain hairs shafts (*black arrows*), sebaceous duct (*yellow arrow*), and acrosyringeal ostium (*blue arrow*).

TABLE 2.1
A Biopsy Report on Horizontal Sections Based on Average Counts in Normal Scalp

Follicular Units	12
Follicular density	38
Terminal anagen follicles	31
Terminal catagen and telogen follicles	2
Vellus (anagen + telogen) follicles	5
Fibrous streamers	2
Terminal:vellus ratio	≥4:1
Telogen count (%)	Up to 15%

of telogen follicles is noted because the affected anagen follicles cycle through catagen into telogen, which results in decreased anagen:telogen ratio (see Fig. 2.5A). The dystrophic hairs observed on trichoscopy, including the exclamation mark hairs, are in fact telogen follicles. There are also pigmented casts as coarse amorphous clumps of melanin in the fibrous streamers and within the dilated infundibula[18] (Fig. 2.5B). In fact, pigmented casts in the hair canals of miniaturized/vellus hairs has been described as a clue to alopecia areata versus trichotillomania[18] (Fig. 2.5C). Nanogen follicles can be numerous in alopecia areata: these are detected in the mid- and upper dermis as minute follicles with mixed features of anagen, catagen, and telogen that cycle faster and may show remnants of pink inner root sheath but no hair shaft[23] (Fig. 2.5D).

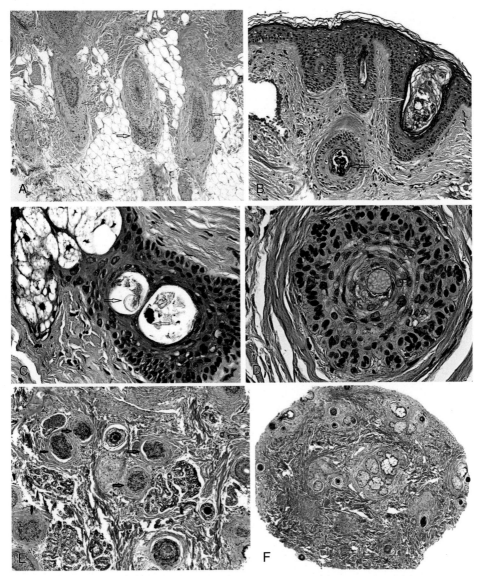

FIG. 2.5 **(A)** In the acute stage of alopecia areata, there is peribulbar lymphocytic infiltrate ("swarm of bees", *black arrows*) and increased number of telogen follicles (*red arrows*). **(B)** Pigmented casts can be observed in the follicle at any level from the fibrous streamer to the infundibulum: note the brown clumps of melanin in the ostium (*black arrow*). The adjacent dilated infundibulum (*red arrow*) contains keratin and sebum and corresponds to the *yellow dot* on trichoscopy. **(C)** Pigmented casts (*red arrow*) in a vellus follicle (*black arrow*) is a clue to alopecia areata because in trichotillomania the pigmented casts result from trauma to terminal follicles only. **(D)** Nanogen follicles are small follicles which show features of anagen/catagen and telogen: in this follicle the hair canal is filled by remnants of the inner root sheath. **(E)** Subacute stage alopecia areata is characterized by increased telogen count (telogen follicles and telogen germinal units are marked with a *black arrow*). A nanogen follicle is marked with the *yellow arrow*. **(F)** Chronic stage alopecia is characterized by significantly decreased follicular density and decreased terminal:vellus ratio. In this specimen there are only 13 vellus follicles.

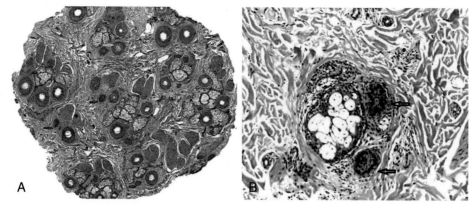

FIG. 2.6 **(A)** This is a biopsy from alopecia areata incognito that demonstrates increased number of telogen follicles (*yellow arrow*), small telogen follicles at the isthmus level and above (*black arrows*), and borderline follicular miniaturization (the terminal anagen is marked with a *red arrow* and the vellus follicle with a *blue arrow*). **(B)** An example of two small telogen follicles at the isthmus.

In the *subacute stage*, there is decreased follicular density with reduced number of anagen and increased number of catagen follicles. Thus, the telogen count may be significantly increased and includes catagen, telogen follicles, and TGUs (Fig. 2.5E). Inflammatory cells such as lymphocytes and eosinophils may persist in the fibrous streamers.

In the *chronic stage*, there is decreased number of terminal follicles and increased number of miniaturized follicles leading to significantly decreased terminal:vellus ratio of average 1.3:1 and the biopsies may resemble those of AGA (Fig. 2.5F). There is usually no inflammation or mild inflammatory infiltrate can be noted around the bulbs of the miniaturized follicles in the upper dermis. The same is noticed also when alopecia areata relapses early in the recovery stage.[24] A biopsy for horizontal sections in the chronic stage alopecia areata can help with the prognosis because mean count of less than one follicle per 1 mm^2 is considered as little likelihood for regrowth.[24]

Alopecia Areata Incognito

The diagnosis is complex and is based on (1) the clinical presentation of abrupt onset of diffuse hair loss in women with no clinical and laboratory findings to suggest acute telogen effluvium; (2) strongly positive pull test result for early telogen hairs, and (3) the pathologic findings for preserved number of follicular units but decreased follicular density with increased telogen count (mean count of 37%) and borderline terminal:vellus ratio for follicular miniaturization (3.3:1)[25] (Fig. 2.6A, Table 2.2). The pathologic

TABLE 2.2
Hair Counts and Ratios in Horizontal Sections From Scalp Biopsies in Women With Diffuse Nonscarring Alopecia[25]

Hair Counts	CTE (n = 21)	AGA (n = 25)	AAI (n = 46)
Follicular units	11	10	10
Terminal follicles	28	17	19
Vellus/miniaturized follicles	3	8	8
Fibrous streamers	4	6	6
Anagen:telogen ratio (%)	85.3:14.7	84:16	63:37
Terminal:vellus ratio (%)	10.8:1	2.4:1	3.3:1

AAI, alopecia areata incognito; *AGA,* androgenetic alopecia; *CTE,* chronic telogen effluvium.

diagnosis requires horizontal sections. A common finding is the presence of dilated infundibular openings as well as increased number of TGUs, and/or small basaloid aggregates of cells with round, irregular, or polygonal shape; lack of hair shaft; and no apoptosis in the outer root sheath, referred to as "small telogen follicles" (Fig. 2.6B). These are telogen follicles bisected just above the level of the vestigial hair bulb and below the level of the cornified club. According to Rebora, alopecia areata incognito occurs when alopecia areata affects patients with high percentages of telogen hairs on the scalp. In such cases, early anagen VI hairs are

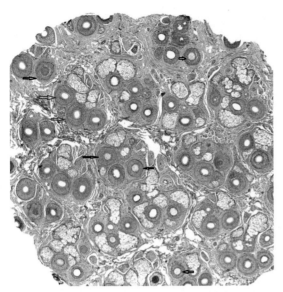

FIG. 2.7 Chronic telogen effluvium: at the level of the isthmus there is preserved follicular density ("busy slide": examples of the telogen follicles are marked with the *black arrows*, the anagen follicles are marked with the *red arrows*, and the vellus follicles with the *yellow arrows*) with no features for follicular miniaturization. The telogen count is usually up to 15%; in acute telogen effluvium, the telogen count may be increased.

scarce and therefore only isolated anagen hairs can be damaged producing diffuse shedding rather than patchy hair loss.[26]

Chronic Telogen Effluvium

The histologic findings in horizontal sections are indistinguishable from those in the normal scalp. There is no or slightly decreased follicular density with normal, and even increased, terminal:vellus ratio of 9:1 as well as normal telogen count (up to 15%) (Fig. 2.7; Table 2.2).[27] Biopsies from acute telogen effluvium are rare and show normal terminal:vellus ratio but increased telogen count.

Androgenetic Alopecia

These are the most common hair biopsies in the dermatopathology practice. The main pathologic finding is the presence of follicular miniaturization (Fig. 2.8A, Table 2.2). There is decreased terminal:vellus ratio of less than 4:1 in biopsies obtained in men.[8] The average terminal:vellus ratio in 219 horizontally sectioned biopsies from women with AGA showed an average ratio of terminal to vellus hairs of 2.2:1.[2] The telogen count may be slightly increased to about 19%–20%.

It is also common to see perifollicular lymphocytic infiltrate and mild fibroplasia at the infundibular level in biopsies from AGA, which can be mistaken for features of scarring alopecia and overcalled as lichen planopilaris (LPP) (Fig. 2.8B). This feature has been shown to correspond to the peripilar sign on trichoscopy.[28] Advanced cases of AGA show features of focal atrichia (increased number of noncycling fibrous streamers), which can also be overdiagnosed as features for scarring alopecia (Fig. 2.8C).

A recent study demonstrated maintenance of contact between miniaturized follicles in alopecia areata versus loss of contact between the arrector pili muscle and the bulge in AGA. This may explain the potential for complete regrowth in AA. In AGA the loss of contact may reflect changes in stem cell biology that also underlie irreversible miniaturization.[29]

Trichotillomania

The horizontal section of a biopsy from trichotillomania shows increased telogen count of up to 70%, the majority of which are catagen follicles (Fig. 2.9A). They are usually grouped together, which may reflect the clinical mechanism that in trichotillomania terminal hairs are rarely plucked individually but rather in bunches of hairs. The differential diagnosis includes alopecia areata, particularly the subacute stage, and pressure-induced alopecia. Several clues point to the diagnosis: (1) trichomalacia (fragmented or distorted hair shafts in the follicular canal) is present in about 40% of the biopsies[30]; the inner root sheath also appears detached or in cases of missing hair shafts, it appears collapsed and fills the hair canal (Fig. 2.9B); (2) pigmented casts are black clumps of melanin usually with peculiar shape of twisted, linear ("ziplike"), and "buttonlike" pigment aggregations that are encountered in 100% of the biopsies at different follicular levels from the papilla and traumatized bulb to the follicular ostium[18] (Fig. 2.9C). The "sprinkled" hair powder reported on trichoscopy[31] most likely corresponds to pigmented casts in the infundibulum; (3) the hamburger sign refers to vertically oriented split, which contains proteinaceous material and erythrocytes and in horizontal sections it is reminiscent of a hamburger within a bun.[32] These features can be seen also in biopsies from lichen simplex chronicus (see Lichen Simplex Chronicus section).

SCARRING ALOPECIA

The pathology of primary cicatricial alopecia is characterized by altered follicular architecture with decreased

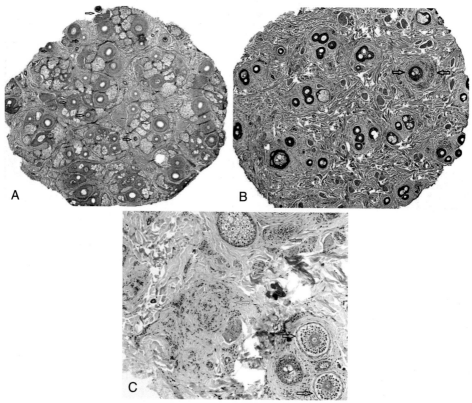

FIG. 2.8 **(A)** Androgenetic alopecia: at the level of the isthmus there is follicular miniaturization. There is increased number of vellus follicles (*black arrows*) and decreased terminal:vellus ratio of 1:1 in this particular specimen. The terminal anagen follicles are marked with the *red arrow* and the terminal telogen follicles with the *yellow arrow*. **(B)** A classic case of androgenetic alopecia at the level of the infundibulum: mild fibroplasia and lymphocytic infiltrate can be seen at this level and should not be overdiagnosed as lichen planopilaris. **(C)** Advanced androgenetic alopecia shows areas devoid of follicular units (focal atrichia, *blue arrows*), which can be difficult to distinguish from true follicular scars in scarring alopecia. At the level of the isthmus, in this section, there are two vellus follicles (*black arrows*) and a fibrous streamer (*red arrow*).

follicular density and loss of follicular units (follicular drop-out), including loss of the sebaceous glands. Dermoscopy-guided biopsies are helpful to identify the optimal site for the biopsy, and horizontal sections are superior to vertical sections to detect focal involvement. In the early active disease, there is follicular inflammation that, depending on the type of the predominant cells, can be primarily lymphocytic (primary lymphocytic cicatricial alopecia) or of mixed cell type (primary neutrophilic cicatricial alopecia). On horizontal sections two clues for the diagnosis are the "eyes and goggles" signs, which refer to compound follicular structures assessed at the level of the isthmus or below that are reminiscent to big owl's eyes (when the fusion is between the connective tissue sheath of the affected adjacent follicles) or to goggles (when the fusion is between the outer root sheaths of the affected adjacent follicles).[33]

Discoid Lupus Erythematosus

Vertical sections of scalp biopsies are similar to the biopsies from skin lesions. On horizontal sections there are several findings at different levels. At the level of the bulb, in the subcutaneous fat there is perivascular and periadnexal (perieccrine and perifollicular) infiltrate of lymphocytes and plasmacytoid dendritic cells. They often aggregate in germinal centerlike collections and may contain dilated blood vessels usually rich in erythrocytes as well as erythrocyte extravasations (Figs. 2.10A and B). This feature has been correlated to the follicular red dots on trichoscopy.[34] The infiltrate also affects the upper follicular levels in an interface dermatitis pattern (Fig. 2.10C). The sebaceous glands are absent but there is usually no prominent perifollicular fibrosis as seen in LPP, although a recent study reported a LPP variant in

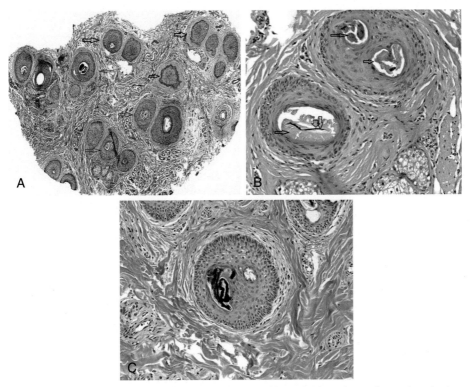

FIG. 2.9 **(A)** In trichotillomania the horizontal sections reveal increased number and grouping of catagen/telogen follicles (*black arrow*). There are pigmented casts of various shapes (*red arrows*). **(B)** Trichomalacia in trichotillomania: only fragments of hair shafts and their inner root sheath are visible in the hair canal (*black arrows*). There is a "zip" like black pigmented cast (*red arrows*). **(C)** The pigmented casts in trichotillomania have peculiar shape.

18% of their horizontal sections from scalp biopsies of discoid lupus erythematosus.[35] There is interface dermatitis along the dermoepidermal junction, with pigment incontinence and thickened basement membrane, which is noted in almost all cases (see Fig. 2.10C).[35] The follicular infundibula are plugged by keratin (Fig. 2.10D). The dermis and subdermis may appear pale and loose because of diffuse deposition of mucin, which can be highlighted with special stains. In LPP, the deposition of mucin is associated with the perifollicular fibrosis and does not involve the interfollicular dermis.[36] The anagen: telogen count varies from normal to diminished.[35,37]

Lichen Planopilaris and Frontal Fibrosing Alopecia

LPP and FFA are lymphocytic cicatricial alopecias that have similar pathologic features but differ by the clinical presentation.[38] There is altered follicular architecture, with areas of follicular drop-out and absent sebaceous glands. The main pathologic finding is the presence of perifollicular lichenoid lymphocytic infiltrate, which can be encountered also at the lower follicular levels but is most pronounced at the level of the isthmus[6] (Fig. 2.11A). The infiltrate can invade the outer root sheath in a more interface pattern. There is perifollicular concentric fibrosis with some increased level of mucin referred to as mucinous fibrosis.[5] Horizontal sections and dermoscopy-guided scalp biopsies are helpful to make the diagnosis in subtle cases[39] (Fig. 2.11B). There are a few pathologic findings that can help distinguish LPP from FFA: (1) in FFA there are usually more apoptotic cells in the outer root sheath[40] (Fig. 2.12A); (2) a recent publication showed that compared to LPP, FFA more often showed inflammation and fibrosis extending below the isthmus into the dermis and even subdermis (93% vs. 62%, respectively)[41] (Fig. 2.12B); (3) the inflammatory infiltrate in FFA is usually milder[40] and affects anagen, telogen, and vellus follicles ("the follicular triad", see Fig. 2.12B)[42]; (4) the affected follicles in FFA more often show a cleft between the outer root sheath and the connective tissue

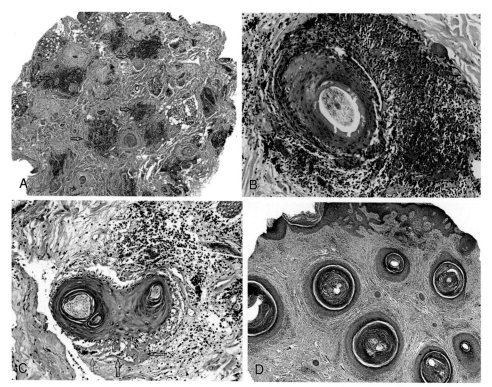

FIG. 2.10 **(A)** Discoid lupus erythematosus: at the suprabulbar level there are nodular (germinal-center–like) aggregates of lymphocytes and plasmacytoid cells (*black arrows*) in perivascular and periadnexal distribution. Most follicles are in telogen stage. **(B)** "Follicular red dots" in discoid lupus erythematosus: note the presence of dilated blood vessels and red blood cells extravasation in the inflammatory aggregate. **(C)** Discoid lupus erythematosus: interface dermatitis involving the follicular epithelium: there is significant vacuolar damage (*yellow arrows*), pigment incontinence (*blue arrow*), and thickened basement membrane (*black arrows*). Note the loose pale mucinous stroma with dilated vessels and mild inflammatory infiltrate. **(D)** The follicular infundibula in discoid lupus erythematosus are often plugged by keratin plugs.

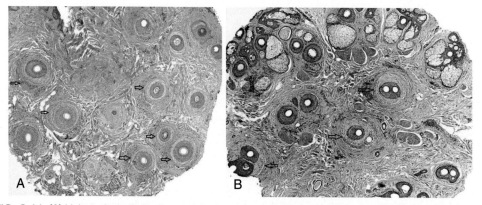

FIG. 2.11 **(A)** Lichen planopilaris: there is follicular drop out (*yellow arrow*) and almost all follicles show perifollicular lichenoid lymphocytic infiltrate and perifollicular fibrosis. The sebaceous glands are absent. **(B)** This case of lichen planopilaris demonstrates the superiority of horizontal sections in detecting focal features for the diagnosis: the affected follicular structures (goggles) are marked with the *black arrows*. Note the preserved follicular architecture at the periphery, including intact sebaceous glands.

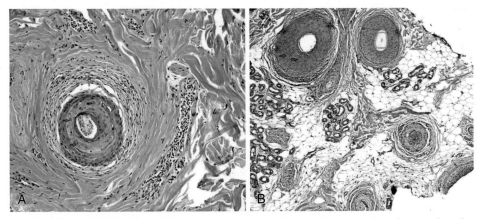

FIG. 2.12 **(A)** Frontal fibrosing alopecia demonstrates more often increased number of apoptotic cells (*black arrow*) in the outer root sheaths. Note the cleft (*red arrow*) between the follicular epithelium and the concentric fibrosis and within the layers of the fibrosis (*yellow arrow*). **(B)** In this case of frontal fibrosing alopecia, the inflammation extends to the subdermis and affects an anagen follicle (the *black arrow* points to the apoptotic cells) and a telogen follicle (*red arrow*). There are fragmented hair shafts within fibrous streamers (*blue arrow*).

sheath or the connective tissue sheath and the inflammatory infiltrate (unpublished data) (see Fig. 2.12A).

Central Centrifugal Cicatricial Alopecia

This is a diagnosis exclusively made in African American women. Scalp biopsies from African Americans demonstrate golf-club–shaped bulbs, elliptical shape of the hair shafts, asymmetric outer root sheaths, and paired grouping of hair follicles.[19] In central centrifugal cicatricial alopecia, on horizontal sections there is altered follicular architecture with areas of follicular drop-out. The follicular density is decreased and in most cases there is diminished terminal:vellus ratio of about 2:1.[43] The affected follicles show perifollicular concentric fibrosis and rarely mild perifollicular lichenoid lymphocytic infiltrate (Fig. 2.13A). Often they form "goggles" that correspond to pairs of follicles fused by their outer root sheaths and surrounded by concentric fibrosis (Fig. 2.13B). The sebaceous glands are focally preserved and often surround vellus follicles[43] (Fig. 2.13C). Naked hair shafts (small hair fragments) are found in the dermis as single structures or within epithelioid granulomas (Fig. 2.13D). Premature desquamation of the inner root sheath of unaffected follicles is observed in most cases[44] as well as in lamellar hyperkeratosis/parakeratosis in the hair canal.

Traction Alopecia

Early cases may show overall preserved follicular architecture with only focal areas of follicular

drop-out and increased catagen/telogen count. In developed cases of traction alopecia, there are areas of follicular drop-out on a background of preserved sebaceous glands (Fig. 2.14A). The difference with primary lymphocytic scarring alopecia is in the preservation of the sebaceous glands and the absence of perifollicular inflammation and fibrosis. One study looked at the ratio of Langerhans cells to T-lymphocytes in scalp biopsies from LPP and traction alopecia and found 1.28 ratio for the LPP group versus 0.59 for the traction alopecia group, which supports the concept that there is an immune component in the pathogenesis of LPP, whereas most traction alopecias are not primarily immune related.[45] In traction alopecia the terminal:vellus ratio is significantly decreased, with vellus follicles outnumbering the terminal follicles.[19] In some cases, only sebaceous glands mark the site of the follicular units (Fig. 2.14B).

Folliculitis Decalvans

There is dense perifollicular but also interfollicular infiltrate of mixed cell origin (lymphocytes, histiocytes, neutrophils, and plasma cells). The main finding is the presence of compound follicular structures (corresponding to the tufts) arising from the fusion of the outer root sheaths of variable number of follicles but usually more than four (Fig. 2.15A). This feature is best appreciated at the infundibular level where the infundibula of the affected follicles merge. Some ostia may be plugged by scale crusts and

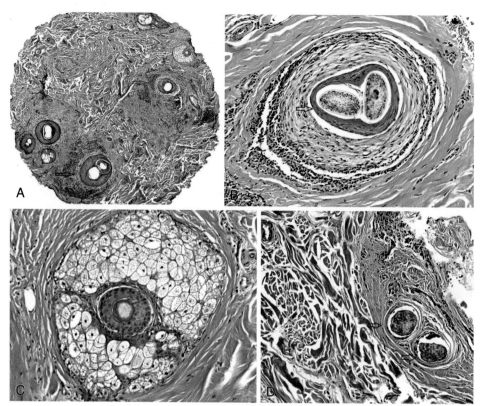

FIG. 2.13 **(A)** Central centrifugal cicatricial alopecia: at the isthmus level the follicular architecture is altered with areas of follicular drop out. Compound follicular structures (goggles, *black arrow*) or individual follicles (*red arrow*) show perifollicular lichenoid infiltrate and fibrosis. Focally preserved sebaceous lobule "hugs" a vellus follicle (*yellow arrow*). **(B)** Goggles in central centrifugal cicatricial alopecia: the inner root sheath is missing and only very thin outer root sheath is present (*black arrow*). There are concentric layers of fibrosis between the outer root sheath and the lichenoid infiltrate (*red arrow*). **(C)** In horizontal sections of central centrifugal cicatricial alopecia, there is usually a solitary follicular unit with preserved sebaceous lobules surrounding a vellus follicle in a "hug." **(D)** Naked (fragmented) hair shafts in the dermis and subdermis can often be found in biopsies from central centrifugal cicatricial alopecia.

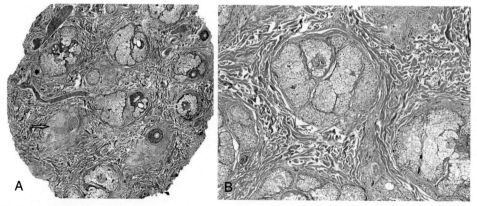

FIG. 2.14 **(A)** Traction alopecia. At the level of the isthmus there is focal follicular drop-out (*black arrow*) and preserved sebaceous glands. The vellus follicles (*yellow arrows*) outnumber the terminal follicles. Note the absence of perifollicular inflammation and fibrosis. **(B)** In this specimen from traction alopecia, only sebaceous glands mark the sites of the follicular units. No follicles are present.

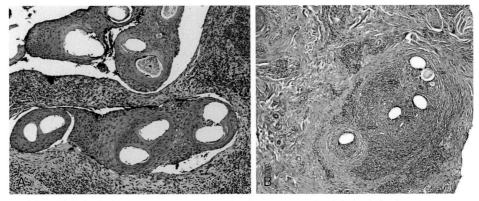

FIG. 2.15 **(A)** Folliculitis decalvans. In this specimen, at the level of the infundibulum there are two compound follicular structures consisting of six and five follicles, respectively, fused by their outer root sheaths and surrounded by dense mixed cell inflammation. **(B)** In folliculitis decalvans, naked hair shafts (*red arrows*) can be found surrounded by mixed cell inflammatory infiltrate or within granulomas (*black arrows*).

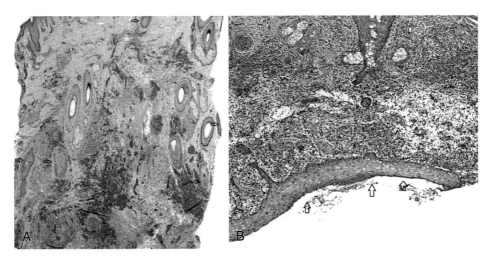

FIG. 2.16 **(A)** Dissecting cellulitis of the scalp: in this vertical section, there is dramatic dense mixed cell infiltrate with edema and red blood cell extravasation, occupying the lower portion of the dermis (below the isthmus) and the subdermis. The telogen follicles are increased (*black arrow*). **(B)** Dissecting cellulitis of the scalp: sinus tract in the dermis (*black arrow*); there is granulomatous infiltrate (*yellow arrow*) and edema with granulation tissue (*blue arrow*).

aggregates of neutrophils (neutrophilic pustules).[46] There is perifollicular fibrosis and sebaceous glands are absent in the affected follicular units. The lower follicular segments are usually spared by the inflammation.[46] Foreign-body giant cells containing small hair fragments (naked hair shafts) can be seen in advanced stages (Fig. 2.15B), and there is prominent follicular drop-out.

Dissecting Cellulitis of the Scalp

Biopsies from early disease show dense and diffuse mixed cell infiltrate, occupying the lower portion of the dermis and the subdermis. The infiltrate also contains giant cells, edema, dilated vessels, and red blood cell extravasation. The majority of the follicles are in telogen, and the sebaceous glands may still be preserved at that stage (Fig. 2.16A). If treatment is initiated at this early stage, there is a chance of regrowth.[47] Developed cases demonstrate follicular drop-out, absence of sebaceous glands, sinus tract formation (epithelial structures surrounding the abscesses in the dermis) (Fig. 2.16B), and epithelioid granulomas with naked hair shafts in the dermis. The differential diagnosis includes inflammatory tinea capitis (kerion); the mixed cells infiltrate is mostly in the lower portion of the specimen in dissecting cellulitis of the scalp, whereas it extends from the surface to the subdermis in kerion.[48]

Acne Keloidalis Nuchae

Most specimens from acne keloidalis nuchae usually come from excisions of symptomatic lesions and therefore they are assessed on vertical sections. There are large areas of keloidal collagenous stroma in the dermis with entrapped hair shaft fragments. Focal aggregates of lymphocytes, neutrophils, histiocytes, and many plasma cells can be observed (Fig. 2.17).

Erosive Pustular Dermatosis of the Scalp

The pathology of erosive pustular dermatosis of the scalp (EPDS) is nonspecific and is usually considered a diagnosis of exclusion. There is diffuse dense mixed cell infiltrate in the dermis, and subcorneal pustules are found in the interfollicular epidermis. A recent study of 20 cases from EPDS revealed three different pathologic patterns, depending on the disease duration.[49] In patches of less than 1 year duration, the follicular density was normal with increased catagen count. The epidermis showed psoriasiform changes, and there was mixed cells infiltrate with slight fibrosis in the dermis. The late stage, lasting more than 2 years duration, showed laminated, compact orthokeratosis and thin epidermis; follicular drop-out and absence of sebaceous glands; slight mixed inflammatory infiltrate; and diffuse and severe fibrosis in the dermis. The intermediate stage, lasting between 1 and 2 years, showed "intermediate" changes of progression to scarring alopecia.

MISCELLANEOUS

Seborrheic Dermatitis

Classic seborrheic dermatitis is rarely biopsied. It may be encountered as a concomitant finding in the scalp biopsies from patients with other primary hair disorders, mostly AGA. The main findings are acanthosis (sometimes psoriasiform) with spongiosis and infundibular and periinfundibular ("shoulder") parakeratosis (Fig. 2.18). There is mild perivascular lymphocytic infiltrate in the upper dermis. Yeast forms of *Pityrosporum* can be found in the stratum corneum. The sebaceous ducts are dilated, and the sebaceous glands are hypertrophic.

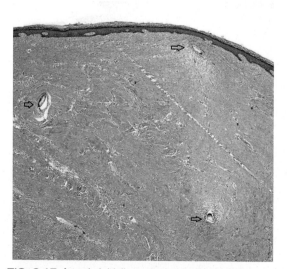

FIG. 2.17 Acne keloidalis nuchae: naked hair shafts (*black arrows*) surrounded by mild inflammatory infiltrate are entrapped in the keloidal stroma.

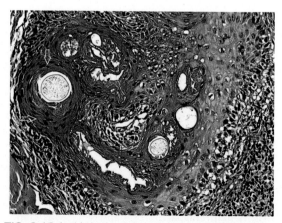

FIG. 2.18 In this horizontal section of seborrheic dermatitis at the level of the infundibulum, the ostia of several follicles merge and open together at the surface. The follicular epithelium shows spongiosis (*red arrow*) and infundibular parakeratosis (*yellow arrows*). The ostia of the sebaceous ducts are dilated (*blue arrows*). There is inflammatory infiltrate in the upper dermis.

Scalp Psoriasis

Classic plaques of scalp psoriasis are also rarely biopsied. There is psoriasiform acanthosis (uniform hyperplasia) with confluent parakeratosis, neutrophils in the stratum corneum (Munro microabscesses), and dilated vessels with perivascular infiltrate in the upper dermis. Necrotic keratinocytes can be found in the epidermis. The sebaceous glands show atrophy[50] and present as thin epithelial stands (mantle structures) or as small sprouts of hypoplastic sebaceous lobules (Fig. 2.19A). There is increased telogen count in horizontal sections (Fig. 2.19B). Prominent eosinophils and plasma cells have been found in scalp biopsies of patients who developed psoriatic alopecia (alopecia areata–like) reactions after treatment with tumor necrosis alpha inhibitors.[51]

Lichen Simplex Chronicus

In horizontal sections, there is usually preserved follicular architecture with preserved terminal: vellus ratio. The sebaceous glands are usually diminished in size and number (unpublished data). At the level of the infundibulum, the outer root sheaths form jagged acanthotic projections, which together with the hair canal in the middle resemble a gear wheel[52] (Fig. 2.20A).

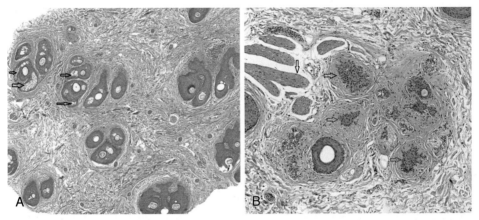

FIG. 2.19 **(A)** In this horizontal section of scalp psoriasis at the level of the isthmus there are only focally present hypoplastic sebaceous glands (*black arrows*). The follicular epithelium shows acanthosis. **(B)** In this horizontal section from scalp psoriasis at the level of the isthmus (the arrector pili muscle is marked with the *black arrow*), this follicular unit is composed of telogen follicles (*red arrows*) and atrophic sebaceous glands (*yellow arrows*).

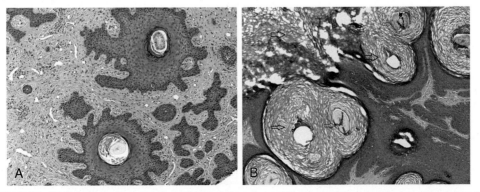

FIG. 2.20 **(A)** Lichen simplex chronicus: horizontal sections at the level of the infundibulum show jagged acanthosis of the follicular epithelium, which together with the hair canal in the middle resembles a gear wheel. **(B)** Lichen simplex chronicus at the infundibulum: there is follicular and interfollicular ortho- and hyperkeratosis (*black arrows*). Note the hamburger sign (*red arrows*).

The infundibular ostium shows hyperkeratosis. There is often fragmentation of the hair shafts because of repeated trauma by rubbing and scratching. The "hamburger sign" can be detected (Fig. 2.20B). If sections through the infundibulum are available, the interfollicular epidermis shows thick layers of orthokeratosis and hyperkeratosis as in acral skin.

Tinea Capitis

In tinea capitis caused by ectothrix infection (*Microsporum canis*), the hyphae and spores cover the outside surface of the hair shaft, which results in destruction of the cuticle. In tinea capitis caused by endothrix infection (*Trichophyton tonsurans*), the inside of the hair shaft is invaded only by rounded and boxlike arthrospores and not by hyphae (Fig. 2.21A).

In inflammatory tinea capitis (kerion) caused by *M. canis*, *Trichophyton mentagrophytes*, *T. tonsurans*, *Trichophyton rubrum*, and *Microsporum gypseum*, there is an abscess extending from the surface into the dermis and subdermis composed of dense mixed cell inflammatory infiltrate of neutrophils, plasma cells, eosinophils, lymphocytes, and histiocytes, as well as giant cells. The infiltrate involves the follicles and the surrounding dermis and subdermis (suppurative granulomatous folliculitis) (Figs. 2.21B and C). The special stains may be falsely negative in up to 50% of the cases.

Syphilitic Alopecia

In scalp biopsy from the moth-eaten patches of nonscarring alopecia in secondary syphilis, there is reduced

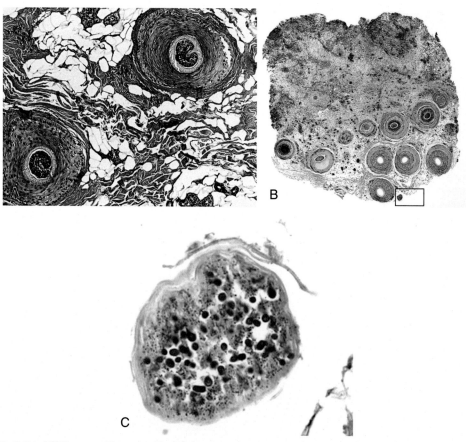

FIG. 2.21 **(A)** Tinea capitis caused by *Trichophyton* spp.: note the spores within the hair shafts. **(B)** Inflammatory tinea capitis (kerion): there is dense mixed cell inflammation in the lower dermis and subdermis mimicking the pattern in dissecting cellulitis of the scalp. In this case, after numerous serial sections only a single hair shaft was found positive for spores by the periodic acid–Schiff stain (rectangle). **(C)** The PAS positive spores within the affected hair shaft in kerion.

number of anagen follicles and an increased number of catagen and telogen follicles. The pathology can be indistinguishable from acute stage alopecia areata because presence of peribulbar lymphocytic infiltrate, widened infundibular ostia, and pigment casts has been observed in both[53] (Fig. 2.22). In syphilitic alopecia,

the inflammatory infiltrate is both perifollicular and perivascular. Scattered plasma cells may point to the diagnosis. In one study on scalp biopsies from moth-eaten alopecia of syphilis, these were present in 75%.[53] Immunohistochemistry can highlight the *Treponema pallidum* in the hair follicles.

Permanent Alopecia After Chemotherapy

Most cases of permanent alopecia have been reported with busulfan and docetaxel. A recent study identified incidence of 16% among children treated with busulfan prior to bone marrow transplant.[54] The incidence for docetaxel is unknown. In the last years, more and more cases have been reported and encountered in the hair practice. The pathologic findings are not specific and require clinical correlation and assessment of horizontal sections. There is an overall nonscarring pattern with a preserved number of follicular units and lack of fibrosis (Fig. 2.23A). The hair counts reveal decreased number of terminal follicles, with increased telogen count, and increased number of miniaturized velluslike follicles, with a terminal to vellus ratio of 1:1.[55] Branching strands of follicular epithelium: TGU-like structures are noted in groups in some cases (Fig. 2.23B). There is increased number of fibrous streamers in both reticular dermis and subcutis. The pathologic findings of permanent alopecia after chemotherapy could be misdiagnosed as AGA without the proper clinical information.

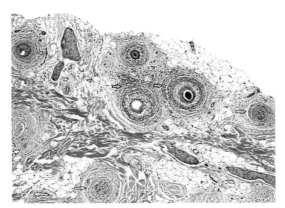

FIG. 2.22 This horizontal section from moth-eaten alopecia in syphilis is indistinguishable from alopecia areata, acute stage. There is swarm of bees like infiltrate in bulbar distribution (*black arrows*) and increased telogen count (*red arrows*). After the diagnosis was confirmed serologically and the biopsy was revisited individual plasma cells were detected in some fibrous streamers which can be a clue to the diagnosis.

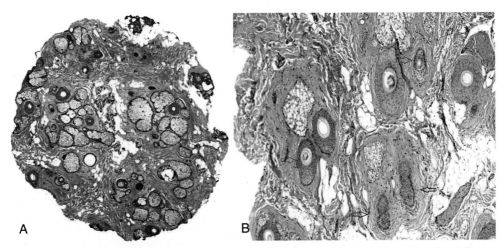

FIG. 2.23 **(A)** Permanent alopecia after chemotherapy with docetaxel: in this horizontal section at the level of the isthmus there is decreased follicular density but overall preserved follicular architecture with significantly increased number of vellus and telogen follicles. This biopsy can be diagnosed as androgenetic alopecia. **(B)** Grouping of telogen follicles (*black arrows*) are increased in many specimens from permanent alopecia after chemotherapy; vellus follicles are marked with *red arrows*.

REFERENCES

1. Sinclair R, Jolley D, Mallari R, Magee J. The reliability of horizontally sectioned scalp biopsies in the diagnosis of chronic diffuse telogen hair loss in women. *J Am Acad Dermatol.* 2004;51(2):189–199.
2. Whiting DA. Scalp biopsy as a diagnostic and prognostic tool in androgenetic alopecia. *Dermatol Ther.* 1998;8:24–33.
3. Miteva M, Tosti A. Dermoscopy guided scalp biopsy in cicatricial alopecia. *J Eur Acad Dermatology Venereol JEADV.* 2013;27(10):1299–1303.
4. Headington JT. Transverse microscopic anatomy of the human scalp. A basis for a morphometric approach to disorders of the hair follicle. *Arch Dermatol.* 1984;120(4):449–456.
5. Stefanato CM. Histopathology of alopecia: a clinicopathological approach to diagnosis. *Histopathology.* 2010;56(1):24–38.
6. Sperling LC. Scarring alopecia and the dermatopathologist. *J Cutan Pathol.* 2001;28(7):333–342.
7. Whiting D, ed. *The Structure of the Human Hair Follicle. Light Microscopy of Vertical and Horizontal Sections of Scalp Biopsies.* New Jersey: Canfield Publishing; 2004.
8. Whiting DA. Diagnostic and predictive value of horizontal sections of scalp biopsy specimens in male pattern androgenetic alopecia. *J Am Acad Dermatol.* 1993;28(5 Pt 1):755–763.
9. Whiting DA. Histopathology of alopecia areata in horizontal sections of scalp biopsies. *J Invest Dermatol.* 1995;104(5 suppl):S26–S27.
10. Sinclair R, Jolley D, Mallari R, et al. Morphological approach to hair disorders. *J Investig Dermatol Symp Proc.* 2003;8(1):56–64.
11. Sperling LC, ed. *An Atlas of Hair Pathology with Clinical Correlations.* Vol. 1. New York: The Parthenon Publishing Group; 2003.
12. Templeton SF, Solomon AR. Scarring alopecia: a classification based on microscopic criteria. *J Cutan Pathol.* 1994;21(2):97–109.
13. Frishberg DP, Sperling LC, Guthrie VM. Transverse scalp sections: a proposed method for laboratory processing. *J Am Acad Dermatol.* 1996;35(2 Pt 1):220–222.
14. Solomon AR. The transversely sectioned scalp biopsy specimen: the technique and an algorithm for its use in the diagnosis of alopecia. *Adv Dermatol.* 1994;9:127–157. discussion 158.
15. Miteva M. A comprehensive approach to hair pathology of horizontal sections. *Am J Dermatopathol.* 2013;35(5):529–540.
16. Horenstein MG, Jacob JS. Follicular streamers (stelae) in scarring and non-scarring alopecia. *J Cutan Pathol.* 2008;35(12):1115–1120.
17. Alopecia Pinkus H. Clinicopathologic correlations. *Int J Dermatol.* 1980;19(5):245–253.
18. Miteva M, Romanelli P, Tosti A. Pigmented casts. *Am J Dermatopathol.* 2014;36(1):58–63.
19. Miteva M, Tosti A. 'A detective look' at hair biopsies from African-American patients. *Br J Dermatol.* 2012;166(6):1289–1294.
20. Sperling LC. Hair density in African Americans. *Arch Dermatol.* 1999;135(6):656–658.
21. Lee HJ, Ha SJ, Lee JH, Kim JW, Kim HO, Whiting DA. Hair counts from scalp biopsy specimens in Asians. *J Am Acad Dermatol.* 2002;46(2):218–221.
22. Whiting DA. Histopathologic features of alopecia areata: a new look. *Arch Dermatol.* 2003;139(12):1555–1559.
23. Sperling LC. *An Atlas of Hair Pathology with Clinical Correlations.* New York: Parthenon Publishing; 2003.
24. Dy LC, Whiting DA. Histopathology of alopecia areata, acute and chronic: why is it important to the clinician? *Dermatol Ther.* 2011;24(3):369–374.
25. Miteva M, Misciali C, Fanti PA, Tosti A. Histopathologic features of alopecia areata incognito: a review of 46 cases. *J Cutan Pathol.* 2012;39(6):596–602.
26. Rebora A. Alopecia areata incognita: a hypothesis. *Dermatologica.* 1987;174(5):214–218.
27. Whiting DA. Chronic telogen effluvium: increased scalp hair shedding in middle-aged women. *J Am Acad Dermatol.* 1996;35(6):899–906.
28. Deloche C, de Lacharriere O, Misciali C, et al. Histological features of peripilar signs associated with androgenetic alopecia. *Arch Dermatol Res.* 2004;295(10):422–428.
29. Yazdabadi A, Whiting D, Rufaut N, Sinclair R. Miniaturized hairs maintain contact with the arrector pili muscle in alopecia areata but not in androgenetic alopecia: a model for reversible miniaturization and potential for hair regrowth. *Int J Trichol.* 2012;4(3):154–157.
30. Lachapelle JM, Pierard GE. Traumatic alopecia in trichotillomania: a pathogenic interpretation of histologic lesions in the pilosebaceous unit. *J Cutan Pathol.* 1977;4(2):51–67.
31. Rakowska A, Slowinska M, Olszewska M, Rudnicka L. New trichoscopy findings in trichotillomania: flame hairs, V-sign, hook hairs, hair powder, tulip hairs. *Acta Dermatovenereologica.* 2014;94(3):303–306.
32. Royer MC, Sperling LC. Splitting hairs: the 'hamburger sign' in trichotillomania. *J Cutan Pathol.* 2006;33(suppl 2):63–64.
33. Miteva M, Torres F, Tosti A. The 'eyes' or 'goggles' as a clue to the histopathological diagnosis of primary lymphocytic cicatricial alopecia. *Br J Dermatol.* 2012;166(2):454–455.
34. Tosti A, Torres F, Misciali C, et al. Follicular red dots: a novel dermoscopic pattern observed in scalp discoid lupus erythematosus. *Arch Dermatol.* 2009;145(12):1406–1409.
35. Chung HJ, Goldberg LJ. Histologic features of chronic cutaneous lupus erythematosus of the scalp using horizontal sectioning: emphasis on follicular findings. *J Am Acad Dermatol.* 2017;77(2):349–355.
36. LaSenna C, Miteva M. Special stains and immunohistochemical stains in hair pathology. *Am J Dermatopathol.* 2016;38(5):327–337.

37. Whiting DA. Cicatricial alopecia: clinico-pathological findings and treatment. *Clin Dermatol.* 2001;19(2):211–225.

38. Kossard S, Lee MS, Wilkinson B. Postmenopausal frontal fibrosing alopecia: a frontal variant of lichen planopilaris. *J Am Acad Dermatol.* 1997;36(1):59–66.

39. Baquerizo Nole KL, Nusbaum B, Pinto GM, Miteva M. Lichen planopilaris in the androgenetic alopecia area: a pitfall for hair transplantation. *Skin Appendage Dis.* 2015;1(1):49–53.

40. Poblet E, Jimenez F, Pascual A, Pique E. Frontal fibrosing alopecia versus lichen planopilaris: a clinicopathological study. *Int J Dermatol.* 2006;45(4):375–380.

41. Wong D, Goldberg LJ. The depth of inflammation in frontal fibrosing alopecia and lichen planopilaris: a potential distinguishing feature. *J Am Acad Dermatol.* 2017;76(6):1183–1184.

42. Miteva M, Tosti A. The follicular triad: a pathological clue to the diagnosis of early frontal fibrosing alopecia. *Br J Dermatol.* 2012;166(2):440–442.

43. Miteva M, Tosti A. Pathologic diagnosis of central centrifugal cicatricial alopecia on horizontal sections. *Am J Dermatopathol.* 2014;36(11):859–864; quiz 865–857.

44. Sperling LC, Sau P. The follicular degeneration syndrome in black patients. 'Hot comb alopecia' revisited and revised. *Arch Dermatol.* 1992;128(1):68–74.

45. Hutchens KA, Balfour EM, Smoller BR. Comparison between Langerhans cell concentration in lichen planopilaris and traction alopecia with possible immunologic implications. *Am J Dermatopathol.* 2011;33(3):277–280.

46. Annessi G. Tufted folliculitis of the scalp: a distinctive clinicohistological variant of folliculitis decalvans. *Br J Dermatol.* 1998;138(5):799–805.

47. Tosti A, Torres F, Miteva M. Dermoscopy of early dissecting cellulitis of the scalp simulates alopecia areata. *Actas Dermo-sifiliográficas.* 2013;104(1):92–93.

48. Isa-Isa R, Arenas R, Isa M. Inflammatory tinea capitis: kerion, dermatophytic granuloma, and mycetoma. *Clin Dermatol.* 2010;28(2):133–136.

49. Starace M, Loi C, Bruni F, et al. Erosive pustular dermatosis of the scalp: clinical, trichoscopic, and histopathologic features of 20 cases. *J Am Acad Dermatol.* 2017;76(6).1109–1114. e1102.

50. Werner B, Brenner FM, Boer A. Histopathologic study of scalp psoriasis: peculiar features including sebaceous gland atrophy. *Am J Dermatopathol.* 2008;30(2):93–100.

51. Doyle LA, Sperling LC, Baksh S, et al. Psoriatic alopecia/alopecia areata-like reactions secondary to anti-tumor necrosis factor-alpha therapy: a novel cause of noncicatricial alopecia. *Am J Dermatopathol.* 2011;33(2):161–166.

52. Quaresma MV, Marino Alvarez AM, Miteva M. Dermatoscopic-pathologic correlation of lichen simplex chronicus on the scalp: 'broom fibres, gear wheels and hamburgers'. *J Eur Acad Dermatol Venereol JEADV.* 2016;30(2):343–345.

53. Jordaan HF, Louw M. The moth-eaten alopecia of secondary syphilis. A histopathological study of 12 patients. *Am J Dermatopathol.* 1995;17(2):158–162.

54. Bresters D, Wanders DCM, Louwerens M, Ball LM, Fiocco M, van Doorn R. Permanent diffuse alopecia after haematopoietic stem cell transplantation in childhood. *Bone Marrow Transplant.* 2017;52(7):984–988.

55. Miteva M, Misciali C, Fanti PA, Vincenzi C, Romanelli P, Tosti A. Permanent alopecia after systemic chemotherapy: a clinicopathological study of 10 cases. *Am J Dermatopathol.* 2011;33(4):345–350.

Hair and Scalp Dermatoscopy (Trichoscopy)

RODRIGO PIRMEZ, MD • ANTONELLA TOSTI, MD

INTRODUCTION

Dermatoscopy, or epiluminescence microscopy, has been widely used in dermatology for the evaluation of pigmented skin lesions. More recently, dermatoscopy has been used in the evaluation of hair and scalp disorders, allowing visualization of morphologic structures not readily visible to the naked eye, including changes to hair shaft thickness and shape, as well as perifollicular and interfollicular features.[1] In 2006, the name *trichoscopy* was first proposed for the use of dermatoscopy in the diagnosis of hair and scalp disorders.[2]

HOW TRICHOSCOPY HELPS THE CLINICIAN

Trichoscopy is a readily accessible method, easily performed in the clinical setting and with affordable options of handheld devices available in the market. It is noninvasive, easy, fast, and helpful also in combination with other diagnostic tools. Several papers have attested the benefits of performing trichoscopy-guided scalp biopsies; it can be used to select the best biopsy site, by rapidly identifying typical signs of the disease and allowing accurate pathologic assessment.[3,4]

Trichoscopy is also useful in the follow-up, allowing the clinician to monitor signs of disease activity and to adjust drug regimen accordingly (Fig. 3.1).[5] Some authors have suggested that trichoscopy may be even superior in the follow-up of patients with alopecia when compared with other traditional methods. Seo J et al. have demonstrated that patients with alopecia areata (AA) treated with steroid injections received less injections and had less risk of developing cutaneous atrophy when disease activity was monitored by trichoscopy than patients who had the same treatment and were monitored by the hair pull test.[6] In the same scope, some trichoscopic features may also have prognostic value. As an example, patients with discoid lupus presenting follicular red dots (FRDs) should be treated aggressively, as this feature represents the possibility of

hair regrowth.[7] On the other hand, white or milky-red areas lacking follicular openings (Fig. 3.2) denote scarring, and patients have little or no chance of recovering their hair even if treated.

Currently, application of trichoscopy has broadened beyond primary hair and scalp disorders, and trichoscopic features of dermatologic and systemic diseases with secondary scalp involvement have already been described.[8–11] Additional uses of the method include evaluation of conditions affecting body hair,[12,13] as well as benign and malignant scalp lesions.[14]

TRICHOSCOPY DEVICES AND THEIR PARTICULARITIES

To perform trichoscopy, the clinician may opt from a variety of instruments available, each one with its advantages and drawbacks. Handheld dermatoscopes usually allow a 10-fold magnification, which is usually satisfactory for the daily practice. In addition, lower magnifications have the benefit of providing a better overview of a large scalp area.[15] Such dermatoscopes are generally considered quite cost-effective. On the other hand, digital dermatoscopes with magnifications from 20- to 100-fold and higher provide better visualization of fine details, specially hair shaft defects and changes in scalp vessels. Such devices are usually equipped with photo storage software applications, allowing comparison of "before and after" pictures among other resources, but their cost is considerably higher. Practical options are mobile-connected dermatoscopes, which allow photography usually at a magnification of 10–20×. Cheaper videodermatoscopes (VM) that can be connected to any computer via USB are also available. A study by Verzì et al.[16] compared low-cost VM available on the internet for nonmedical uses with standard medically marketed VM. They found that both were able to adequately evaluate hair shafts, but because of problems with color, brightness, and resolution, low-cost VM were inferior when used to analyze

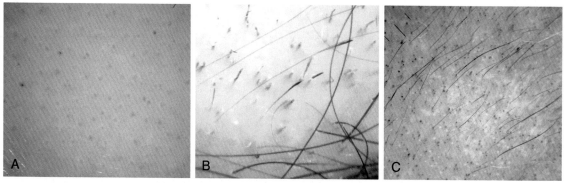

FIG. 3.1 Trichoscopic images of different stages of alopecia areata (AA). **(A)** *Yellow dots* in a Caucasian patient with stable disease. **(B)** *Black dots*, broken hairs and exclamation mark hairs, typical trichoscopic features of active AA. **(C)** Short regrowing hairs in a black patient responsive to therapy. Note the impregnation of hair follicle openings by anthralin.

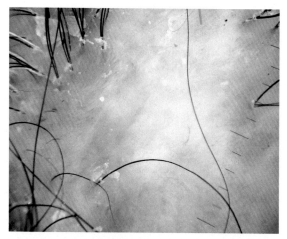

FIG. 3.2 Milky-red areas lacking follicular openings in a patient with scarring alopecia.

scaling and yellow and white dots. The authors concluded that low-cost VM should not be routinely used for reliable scalp trichoscopy.

Some variants that are inherent to the device being used and that should be considered when performing trichoscopy include (1) type of light being used (polarized vs. nonpolarized); (2) use of immersion fluid; and (3) contact versus noncontact lenses. Both polarized and nonpolarized lights can be used in trichoscopy, but nonpolarized devices will require the use of an immersion fluid to cancel out reflections from the stratum corneum. The use of immersion fluids, on the other hand, will hamper evaluation of scaling conditions and visualization of vellus and white hairs (as they "disappear" when a fluid is used). The reader should keep in mind

that "elimination" of scaling with immersion fluid is sometimes desirable, as excessive scaling may interfere with visualization of other trichoscopic features. Personally, we always start with dry dermatoscopy and then use an immersion fluid if we judge necessary. The choice of the immersion fluid (water, gel, alcohol, etc.) is a matter of personal choice. Contact will always be necessary if an immersion fluid is being used. For trichoscopy, we routinely use contact dermatoscopy because without contact, hair shafts will show up in different heights, and focusing the image becomes a challenge. An exception is when detailing the vascular pattern is important because pressure provoked by contact dermatoscopy may mask visualization of vessels.

HOW TO EVALUATE THE PATIENT

Examination of the scalp will depend on the type of hair loss.[17]

In diffuse alopecia, it is always important to part the hair at the midline and photograph at least three sites: frontal and middle scalp and vertex. We usually take two pictures from each site, one with low (20×) and another one with higher magnification (40–50×). Hair diameter variability, a sign of androgenetic alopecia (AGA), may be better appreciated at higher magnifications. Because the occipital scalp is normally spared in AGA, control pictures can be taken from this site for comparison. In diffuse hair loss, trichoscopy from the temporal region usually does not add new information.

In patchy alopecia, it is important to examine the center of the patch to establish whether hair follicle openings are present (nonscarring) or not (scarring) (Fig. 3.3). Signs of disease activity may be present either at the center or at the periphery of lesions, depending on

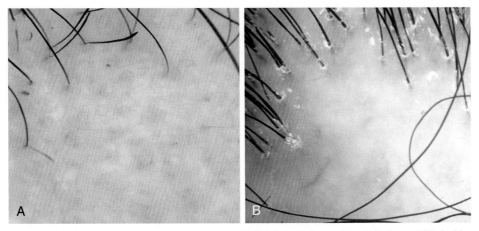

FIG. 3.3 **(A)** Patient with alopecia areata showing hair follicle openings without shafts and filled with sebum, forming yellow dots. **(B)** Lack of follicular openings in a patient with lichen planopilaris, a lymphocytic scarring alopecia.

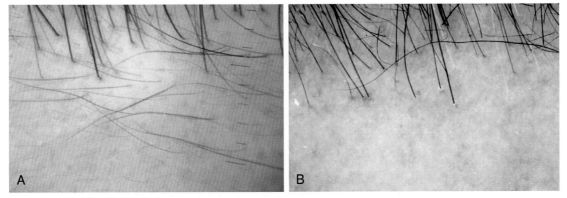

FIG. 3.4 Trichoscopy from the frontal hairline shows **(A)** presence of vellus hairs in a patient with androgenetic alopecia. **(B)** Loss of vellus hairs in the hairline, which is a marker of frontal fibrosing alopecia.

the etiology. Therefore, both areas should be checked. In addition, it is important to evaluate the apparently normal scalp surrounding alopecic patches, for early signs of disease activity may already be present in trichoscopy, even before hair loss becomes clinically evident.

In marginal alopecia, it is essential to check for the presence of vellus hair. Loss of vellus hair in the hairline is a typical sign of frontal fibrosing alopecia (FFA) and quite helpful in the differential diagnosis with AGA and traction alopecia, especially in early cases (Fig. 3.4).

When patients complain of hair breakage or that their hair would not grow, hair shafts should be examined, and trichoscopy has satisfactorily replaced optical microscopy in most of these cases. For hair shafts, it is interesting to use polarized light and higher magnifications (at least 70×), and shafts can be examined directly

in the patient or hair fragments can be obtained and later examined with the dermatoscope. In such cases, the clinician should look for causes of hair breakage such as trichorrhexis nodosa, commonly seen in hair weathering, or hair shaft defects that may signal a congenital condition, such as the typical constrictions of monilethrix.[18]

Trichoscopic examination of the eyebrows is also important. Many hair disorders also affect the eyebrows, and trichoscopy of this area can be quite useful, especially in very early cases of FFA when the scalp is still preserved or in cases of hair loss restricted to this region, as we can see in some patients with AA, for example. Hair shaft disorders such as trichorrhexis invaginata might be only detectable in the eyebrows.

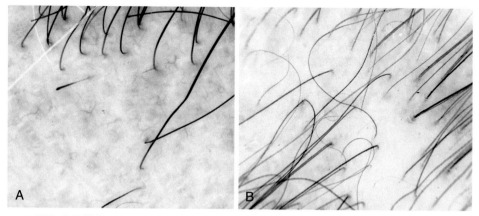

FIG. 3.5 *Yellow dots* in patients with **(A)** alopecia areata and **(B)** androgenetic alopecia.

TRICHOSCOPIC SIGNS AND PATTERNS

Classification of trichoscopic structures according to their location on the scalp helps dermatologists to become familiarized with signs and patterns that characterize each disease. In this regard, trichoscopic features can be grouped as follows[19]:

1. Follicular
2. Peri- and interfollicular
3. Vascular
4. Hair shaft

It is important to stress that an isolated trichoscopic sign will hardly be diagnostic of a given condition; one should analyze the context in which such sign is present. In addition, having in mind the pathologic correlation of each feature will be helpful in the diagnostic process.

Follicular Signs

In trichoscopy, the skin which is a three-dimensional structure will be observed as a two-dimensional image. For such, many of the follicular structures will be perceived as dots.

Yellow dots

Yellow dots represent empty hair follicles filled with sebum and keratin debris. Attached to each hair follicle is a sebaceous gland. Sebum is normally conducted outside of the hair canal onto the cutaneous surface. In conditions such as AA, in which hair follicles become empty, without hair shafts, the follicular infundibula become filled with sebum and keratin debris. In patients with long-standing AA, yellow dots can have a regular distribution on the scalp, representing the distribution of follicular units (Fig. 3.5A). Patients with AGA may also have yellow dots. In these patients,

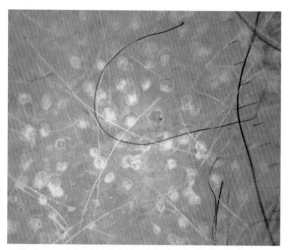

FIG. 3.6 Keratotic plugs in a patient with discoid lupus erythematosus.

thinning hair will also allow sebum to be collected in the follicular infundibula. However, because hair thinning is a slowly progressive and heterogeneous process in the scalp, distribution of yellow dots will not be as regular and normally as numerous as in AA (Fig. 3.5B). Of note, yellow dots are more easily seen in patients of lighter skin types but not in patient with darker types owing to the contrast of color.[20]

Keratotic plugs

Keratotic plugs result from follicular hyperkeratosis and correspond to widened infundibula filled with yellowish/whitish keratotic masses. They are a typical feature of discoid lupus erythematosus (DLE) (Fig. 3.6).[21] Isolated keratotic plugs may also be found in dissecting cellulitis.

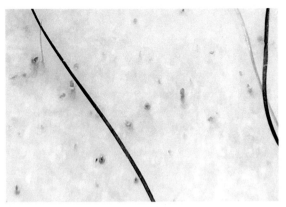

FIG. 3.7 *Black dots* in a patient with active alopecia areata.

Black dots

Black dots, also known as cadaverized hairs, are shafts broken before scalp emergence.[22] They are found in about 50% of patients with AA and are a sign of disease activity.[5] In AA, the inflammatory infiltrate causes weakening of shafts leading to their breakage and formation of black dots (Fig. 3.7). Other types of injury such as ischemia and cytostatic drugs may also result in weakening of hair shafts, and for such, black dots are not a specific trichoscopic sign. Other conditions in which they may be found include chemotherapy-induced alopecia,[23] pressure-induced alopecia,[24] trichotillomania, dissecting cellulitis,[25] and tinea capitis, among others. A few black dots can be seen in scarring alopecias, particularly FFA.

Red dots

FRDs are erythematous, polycyclic, concentric structures regularly distributed in and around the follicular ostia. They were described by Tosti et al.[7] as a trichoscopic feature of discoid lupus (Fig. 3.8) of the scalp and positively correlated with better chance of hair regrowth. Histologically, they correspond to widened infundibulum plugged by keratin and surrounded by dilated vessels and extravasated erythrocytes. Surrounding each hair follicle there is a vascular network that because of skin atrophy and vasodilation may become visible in these patients and be perceived as an FRD through trichoscopy. As latter suggested,[26] their presence may be an indicative that the follicular structure is still viable, explaining why patients with FRDs have a better change of regrowing hair.

White dots

White dots were originally related to follicular fibrosis in patients with scarring alopecia.[27] However, later,

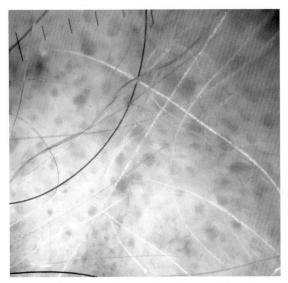

FIG. 3.8 Follicular *red dots* in discoid lupus erythematosus.

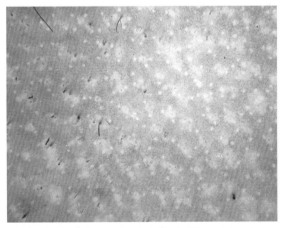

FIG. 3.9 Alopecia areata in a patient of African descent. Note pinpoint *white dots* regularly distributed on the scalp in between follicular units.

they were also described in AA patients with dark skin types, representing follicles lacking hair shafts.[20] Such patients also presented with smaller, isolated white dots in between follicular units corresponding to eccrine gland openings, which were named pinpoint white dots.[28] Pinpoint white dots are found isolated and regularly distributed on the scalp, whereas white dots may be found in groups of two or three, representing the follicular units (Fig. 3.9). Such differentiation, however, is not always evident in patients with alopecia.

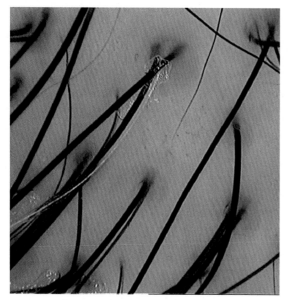

FIG. 3.10 The peripilar sign in a patient with early andro-genetic alopecia.

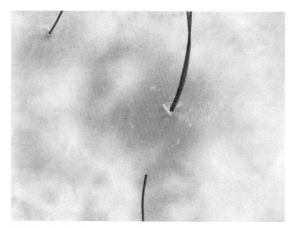

FIG. 3.11 Perifollicular erythema and scaling in a patient with scarring alopecia.

Loss of follicular openings

Loss of follicular openings is the hallmark and the *sine qua non* feature of scarring alopecias (Fig. 3.3A). They represent end-stage disease in areas in which they are present and hair regrowth will no longer be possible. One possible pitfall are patients with long-standing AA. In these patients, follicular openings may be difficult to visualize, misleading the clinician.

Peri- and Interfollicular Patterns

Peripilar sign

The peripilar sign is a perifollicular brown halo (Fig. 3.10). It has been described in patients with AGA, especially in early stages, and linked to superficial mild perifollicular lymphocytic infiltrate.[29] However, its exact mechanism of formation is not clear.

Perifollicular erythema

Perifollicular erythema is usually a sign of disease activity. It is commonly found in scarring alopecia and is important for diagnosis and disease monitoring, especially in alopecias in which the inflammatory process is predominantly folliculocentric (Fig. 3.11).

Scaling (perifollicular/interfollicular)

Scaling can only be appreciated with dry dermatoscopy because immersion fluids hydrate the scales and they become no longer visible by trichoscopy. Scaling is a common finding in many inflammatory scalp disorders. Their color, location, and arrangement may vary according to the underlying condition. Interfollicular scales can be seen in psoriasis, seborrheic dermatitis, tinea capitis, and discoid lupus, for example. In psoriasis, scales are whitish and often referred as argentic, whereas in seborrheic dermatitis, they may have a yellowish hue (Fig. 3.12A and B).[19] White perifollicular scaling is characteristic of lichen planopilaris (LPP) and its variants, including FFA, signalizing disease activity. In LPP, scales may embrace the proximal hair shafts, forming tubular structures (Fig. 3.13). Once they detach from the scalp, they form hair casts that move freely along the hair shafts.[19] Compared with that of LPP, scaling in FFA tends to be subtler. Perifollicular scales may also be seen in DLE, usually associated with interfollicular scaling. Yellowish scaling surrounding hair tufts may be part of the picture in folliculitis decalvans.

Hyperpigmenation

Different patterns of hyperpigmentation may be found on the scalp. The honeycomb pattern is a constitutional feature in patients with dark skin types and is the two-dimensional representation of the wavy epidermal-dermal junction architecture (Fig. 3.14).[20] The hyperchromic lines correspond to the rete ridges, whereas the thinner suprapapillary dermis is perceived as the hypochrromic areas. This pattern may also be seen in patients with lighter skin types, signaling sun exposure. Pigment incontinence has two main patterns of presentation on the scalp: (1) speckled blue-gray dots and (2) blue-gray dots in a target pattern. The latter is a consequence of an interface dermatitis process restricted mainly to the perifollicular area, as seen in LLP (Fig. 3.15), whereas the former indicates a

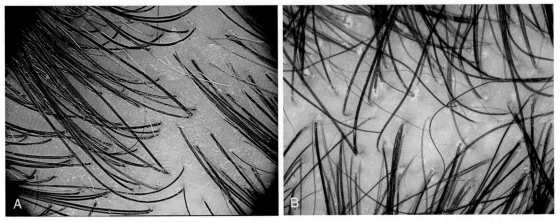

FIG. 3.12 **(A)** Seborrheic dermatitis with scales that may have a yellowish hue. **(B)** Psoriasis scales that are white and often referred as argentic.

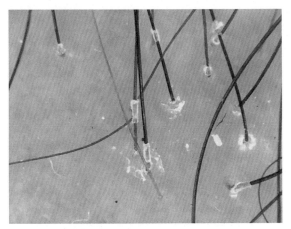

FIG. 3.13 Tubular perifollicular scaling in a patient with lichen planopilaris.

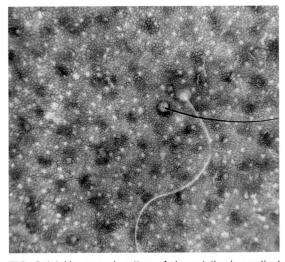

FIG. 3.14 Honeycomb pattern of pigmentation in a patient of African descent with lichen planopilaris.

widespread process affecting the interfollicular region, like in DLE (Fig. 3.16). Both patterns are only seen in patients with dark skin types.[30]

White-gray halo

Peripilar white-gray halos surrounding the emergence of hairs shafts were described as highly specific and sensitive for central centrifugal cicatricial alopecia (CCCA) and were observed in all clinical stages (Fig. 3.17).[31] In pathology, they corresponded to lamellar fibrosis surrounding the outer root sheath. In our experience, they may also be seen in FFA, affecting dark-skinned patients.

Vascular Patterns

There is a variety of vascular patterns on the scalp. Although some may be characteristic, none of them seem to be specific of any condition. Vessels are better appreciated at higher magnifications (>40×) and using an immersion fluid. Simple red loops and thin arborizing vessels can be found in the normal scalp, especially in the occipital and temporal regions, and represent the papillary loops and the underlying vascular plexus, respectively (Fig. 3.18). Thick arborizing vessels are characteristic of DLE (Fig. 3.19) but may also be found in other conditions such as steroid-induced atrophy.[32] Twisted red loops, also known as coiled or glomerular-like vessels, are very characteristic of psoriasis, particularly if present in groups (Fig. 3.20).[19] Numerous giant enlarged capillaries should raise the suspicion of a connective tissue disorder (Fig. 3.21).[33]

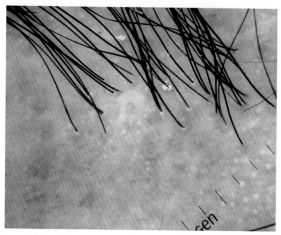

FIG. 3.15 *Blue-gray dots* in target pattern in a dark-skinned patient with lichen planopilaris.

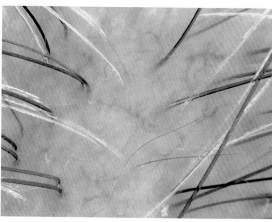

FIG. 3.18 Trichoscopy from the temporal region of a normal scalp showing thin arborizing vessels.

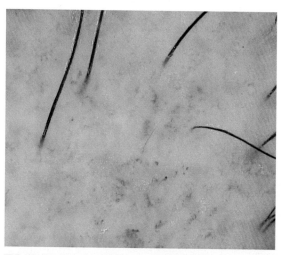

FIG. 3.16 *Blue-gray dots* in a speckled pattern in a patient with discoid lupus.

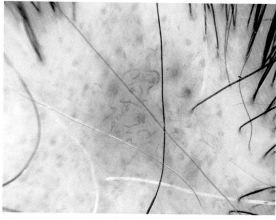

FIG. 3.19 Discoid lupus erythematosus presenting with thick arborizing vessels. Note also the presence of follicular *red dots* at the periphery of the lesion.

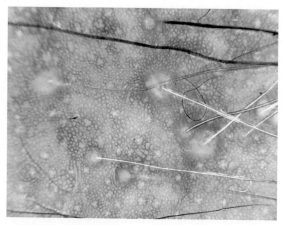

FIG. 3.17 *White-gray halo* in a patient with central centrifugal cicatricial alopecia.

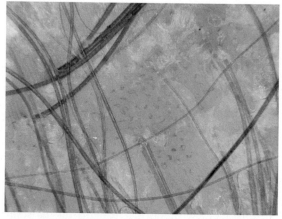

FIG. 3.20 White scales and twisted loops in a patient with psoriasis.

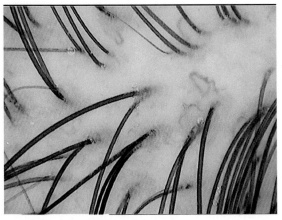

FIG. 3.21 Markedly enlarged capillaries in a patient with connective tissue disorder.

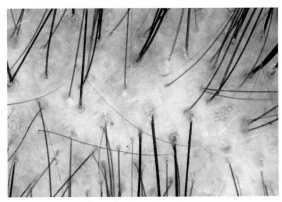

FIG. 3.23 Patient with androgenetic alopecia showing hair shaft diameter variability. Note also areas with honeycomb pattern of pigmentation suggesting sun exposure.

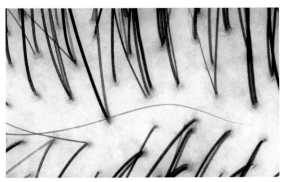

FIG. 3.22 Thickness of hair shafts is quite homogenous in the normal scalp.

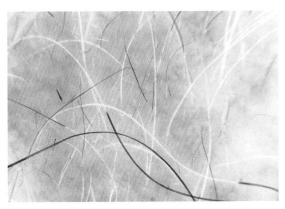

FIG. 3.24 Very thin hair shafts in a patient with active alopecia areata.

Hair Shafts

In the healthy scalp, hair follicles are arranged in groups of two or three, forming follicular units. Hair shaft thickness may vary, but it tends to be quite homogenous throughout the different scalp areas (Fig. 3.22). Different conditions may cause changes in hair thickness, length, and shape, as we will discuss in the following section.

Hair shaft diameter variability

A healthy scalp may have up to 20% thin hairs. Presence of more than 20% thin hairs on trichoscopy is a marker of AGA and represents the process of hair follicle miniaturization (Fig. 3.23).[34] Increase in hair shaft diameter variability is also known as anisotrichosis. In daily practice, there is no need to establish exact measures of hair shaft diameter and a rough estimative (thin vs. thick hairs) is normally enough to reach

a diagnosis. Disturbance of the hair follicle cycle and function in AA may also lead to the formation of thinner hair shafts (Fig. 3.24).

Short regrowing hairs

There are at least four types of short regrowing hairs (SRHs) that may be appreciated through trichoscopy. Isolated SRHs of normal thickness may be eventually seen in healthy individuals and are due to physiologic hair shedding. In patients with telogen effluvium, there will be an increased number of such hairs and they will be present in the whole scalp (Fig. 3.25). They may also be observed in clusters in regrowing patches of AA. SRHs have a thick base with a thin distal end.

On the other hand, thin SRHs in a number of six or more may be present in the frontal scalp of patients with AGA (Fig. 3.26).[35]

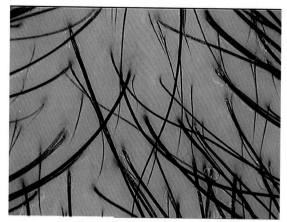

FIG. 3.25 Several short regrowing hairs of normal thickness in a patient with telogen effluvium.

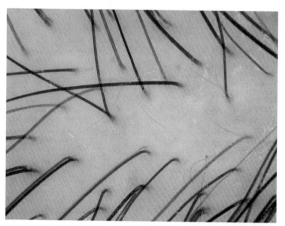

FIG. 3.26 Thin short regrowing hairs in a patient with female pattern hair loss.

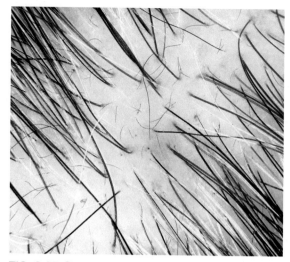

FIG. 3.27 Short regrowing hairs in a patient with alopecia areata incognita.

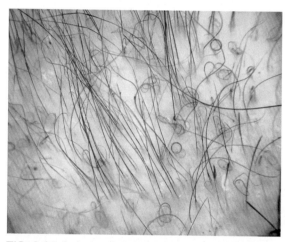

FIG. 3.28 A cluster of circle hairs in a patient with alopecia areata.

Thin SRHs were also described in patients with AA incognita.[36] Rudnicka et al. have proposed the name "dark lines" in this case by observing that such hairs were thin throughout their length and were generally dark, sometimes darker than the patient's natural hair color (Fig. 3.27).[37]

Regrowing circle hairs (or pigtail hairs) are short, evenly coiled hairs. Isolated circle hairs may be found in AGA, but clusters of circle hairs are very characteristic of AA (Fig. 3.28). It has been suggested that they result from the rapid regrowth from a hair follicle that is still not completely recovered. We have also observed them in still viable areas of scarring alopecia.

Broken hairs

Broken hairs may result from a variety of disorders and are normally a sign that the clinician is dealing with an ongoing condition. Diseases affecting hair shaft production such as AA may weaken hair shafts causing breakage (Fig. 3.29). External damage as seen in hair weathering may increase hair shaft fragility, leading to breakage as well. A classical trichoscopic feature of patients with weathering is trichorrhexis nodosa: whitish nodes along the hair shafts that break causing a brushlike fracture[38] (Fig. 3.30). Intentional plucking of hairs in patients

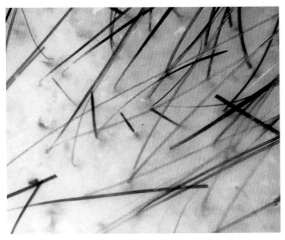

FIG. 3.29 Broken hairs in a patient with alopecia areata.

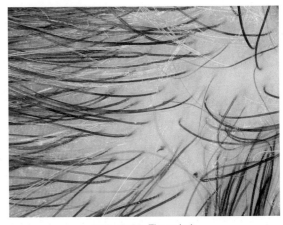

FIG. 3.31 Flame hair.

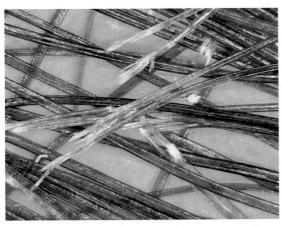

FIG. 3.30 Trichorrhexis nodosa in a patient with severe hair weathering.

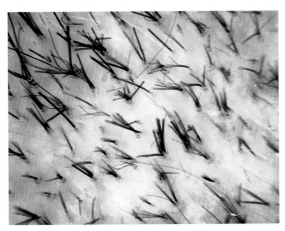

FIG. 3.32 Several broom hairs in a patient with trichoteiromania.

with trichotillomania will, of course, cause hair breakage. Several names have been created depending on the aspect of the fractured hair. Nonetheless, recognizing that they are broken hairs rather than memorizing the different names is more important. Flame hairs were originally described as a specific feature of trichotillomania,[39] but recently they have also been found in chemotherapy-induced alopecia, radiotherapy-induced alopecia, CCCA, and traction alopecia (Fig. 3.31).[40] Broom hairs are short broken hairs with split ends. They are not specific, but in patients with trichoteiromania (alopecia caused by compulsive scratching of the scalp) they can be the predominant feature (Fig. 3.32).[41]

Exclamation mark hairs and coudability hairs

Even though exclamation mark hairs are not pathognomonic of AA, they are very typical of this condition. They are telogen hairs that got broken at their distal end. The rapid transition from anagen to catagen and telogen causes proximal narrowing of the hair shaft, producing their characteristic shape (Fig. 3.33).[42] Their presence is a marker of disease activity. They have also been described in chemotherapy-induced alopecia.[23] Coudability hairs look very similar to exclamation mark hairs; there is narrowing of the proximal hair shaft, but they are not broken at their distal end (Fig. 3.34). Like exclamation mark hairs, they are an indicator of active AA but may be found in chemotherapy-induced alopecia as well.[43]

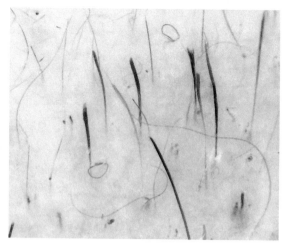

FIG. 3.33 Exclamation marks are telogen hairs with broken distal ends and proximal narrowing of the hair shaft. Note also *black dots* and broken hairs.

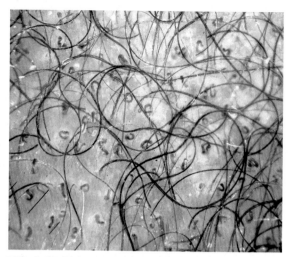

FIG. 3.35 Male child of African descent with tinea capitis presenting with multiple comma hairs.

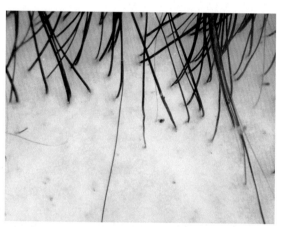

FIG. 3.34 Note in the center of the image a hair shaft presenting narrowing of its proximal portion, known as coudability hair. *Black dots* are also present. This image was taken from an expanding patch in a patient with active alopecia areata.

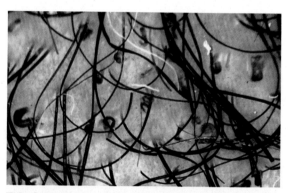

FIG. 3.36 Trichoscopy from a male child of African descent. Note in the center of the image a corkscrew hair: a broken hair presenting with multiple twists. There are also several comma hairs in the image. This image was taken with immersion fluid to cancel out reflection from scales.

Comma hairs and corkscrew hairs

Comma hairs and corkscrew hairs are both broken hairs, but their shape is very characteristic and indicative of the diagnosis of tinea capitis. Comma hairs are short broken hairs that are bent, possibly because of partial damage of hair shafts caused by fungal invasion, resembling a comma (Fig. 3.35).[44] Corkscrew hairs differ from comma hairs for having multiple twists. It has been suggested that corkscrew hairs are typically seen in cases of tinea capitis in African patients because of the helical shape of African hair.[45] (Fig. 3.36). Comma and corkscrew hairs can be found in both endo- and

ectothrix infections. Other trichoscopic features of tinea capitis include morse code and zigzag hairs. Even though trichoscopy may indicate the diagnosis of tinea capitis, it is not able to point the causative agent.

Hair shafts in congenital syndromes

Trichoscopy is useful in diagnosing most hair shaft disorders.

Monilethrix is a genetic hair shaft disorder characterized by hair fragility with alopecia due to hair breakage. Breakage and, consequently, alopecia will be more intense in areas of friction, such as the occipital scalp. Trichoscopy reveals typical hair beading, showing elliptical nodes separated by constrictions at regular intervals (Fig. 3.37).[46] Shafts will break at the

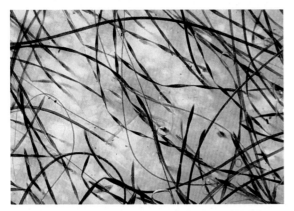

FIG. 3.37 Trichoscopy from a female child presenting with severe alopecia. Note hair beading with constrictions seen at regular intervals. Some shafts are bent at the point of constrictions and will eventually break with friction.

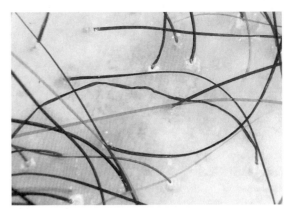

FIG. 3.39 Trichoscopy from a patient with lichen planopilaris. Note a hair shaft presenting multiple twists. Perifollicular scaling indicates that the disease is active.

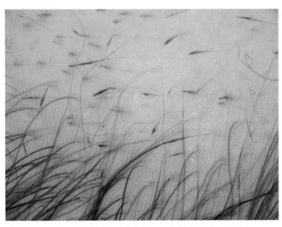

FIG. 3.38 Monilethrix-like hairs in a patient with alopecia areata.

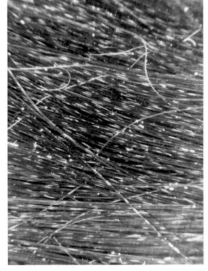

FIG. 3.40 Pili annulati. The presence of cavities filled with air causes alternating of light and dark bands on the hair shafts.

constrictions where the medulla of the hair is absent. In AA, successive periods of disease activity may cause a series of constrictions along the hair shaft, producing monilethrix-like hairs (Fig. 3.38). Chemotherapy cycles also produce a similar finding, in which case they are known as Pohl-Pinkus constrictions.

Pili torti are flattened hair shafts that twist 180 degrees at irregular intervals. They may be present in a variety of congenital and also in acquired conditions, usually in association with other features. They are a characteristic feature of Menkes and Bjornstad syndromes. In patients with acquired hair loss presenting pili torti, one should always consider a scarring condition among the differentials (Fig. 3.39).

Trichorrhexis Invaginata is said to be pathognomonic of Netherton syndrome, which is characterized by the triad of bamboo hair, ichthyosis, and atopic dermatitis. Trichoscopy reveals multiple knots along the hair shafts; the knots consist of a proximal invaginated cup-shaped portion and a distal ball-shaped end. After breakage, only the proximal portion is left, resembling a golf tee.[47]

Pili annulati is an autosomal dominant hair shaft abnormality characterized by shafts with air-filled cavities. Trichoscopy reveals alternating light and dark bands that result in a particularly shiny hair (Fig. 3.40).

In pili trianguli et canaliculi, also known as uncombable hair syndrome, hair shafts have longitudinal grooves that prevent them from settling on the scalp or getting organized in bundles of hair. Cross sections of hair shafts reveal hairs with impressions and of triangular shape, which give name to the syndrome. Usually, scanning electron microscopy is necessary for diagnosis, but trichoscopy may suggest the present of longitudinal grooves.

REFERENCES

1. Miteva M, Tosti A. Hair and scalp dermatoscopy. *J Am Acad Dermatol*. 2012;67(5):1040–1048. https://doi.org/10.1016/j.jaad.2012.02.013.
2. Olszewska M, Rudnicka L, Rakowska A, Kowalska-Oledzka E, Slowinska M. Trichoscopy. *Arch Dermatol*. 2008;144(8):1007. https://doi.org/10.1001/archderm.144.8.1007.
3. Miteva M, Tosti A. Dermoscopy guided scalp biopsy in cicatricial alopecia. *J Eur Acad Dermatol Venereol*. 2013;27(10):1299–1303. https://doi.org/10.1111/j.1468-3083.2012.04530.x.
4. Mubki T, Rudnicka L, Olszewska M, Shapiro J. Evaluation and diagnosis of the hair loss patient: part II. Trichoscopic and laboratory evaluations. *J Am Acad Dermatol*. 2014;71(3):431.e1–431.e11. https://doi.org/10.1016/j.jaad.2014.05.008.
5. Inui S, Nakajima T, Nakagawa K, Itami S. Clinical significance of dermoscopy in alopecia areata: analysis of 300 cases. *Int J Dermatol*. 2008;47(7):688–693. https://doi.org/10.1111/j.1365-4632.2008.03692.x.
6. Seo J, Lee JW, Choi MJ, Cho S, Kim DY. Serial trichoscopy vs. modified hair pull test for monitoring the disease activity and treatment response of localized alopecia areata. *J Eur Acad Dermatol Venereol*. 2017;31(3):e149–e150. https://doi.org/10.1111/jdv.13942.
7. Tosti A, Torres F, Misciali C, et al. Follicular red dots: a novel dermoscopic pattern observed in scalp discoid lupus erythematosus. *Arch Dermatol*. 2009;145(12):1406–1409. https://doi.org/10.1001/archdermatol.2009.277.
8. Pirmez R. Acantholytic hair casts: a dermoscopic sign of pemphigus vulgaris of the scalp. *Int J Trichology*. 2012;4(3):172–173. https://doi.org/10.4103/0974-7753.100087.
9. Sar-Pomian M, Kurzeja M, Rudnicka L, Olszewska M. *An Bras Dermatol*. 2014;89(6):1007–1012.
10. Piraccini BM, Broccoli A, Starace M, et al. Hair and scalp manifestations in secondary syphilis: epidemiology, clinical features and trichoscopy. *Dermatology*. 2015;231(2):171–176. https://doi.org/10.1159/000431314.
11. Miteva M, Wei E, Milikowski C, Tosti A. Alopecia in systemic amyloidosis: trichoscopic-pathologic correlation. *Int J Trichol*. 2015;7(4):176–178. https://doi.org/10.4103/0974-7753.171585.
12. Panchaprateep R, Tanus A, Tosti A. Clinical, dermoscopic, and histopathologic features of body hair disorders. *J Am Acad Dermatol*. 2015;72(5):890–900. https://doi.org/10.1016/j.jaad.2015.01.024.
13. Vendramini DL, Silveira BR, Duque-Estrada B, Boff AL, Sodré CT, Pirmez R. Isolated body hair loss: an unusual presentation of lichen planopilaris. *Skin Appendage Disord*. 2017;2(3–4):97–99. https://doi.org/10.1159/000449229.
14. Zalaudek I, Schmid K, Niederkorn A, et al. Proposal for a clinical-dermoscopic classification of scalp naevi. *Br J Dermatol*. 2014;170(5):1065–1072. https://doi.org/10.1111/bjd.12722.
15. Rudnicka L, Rusek M, Borkowska B. Introduction. In: Rudnicka L, Olszewska M, Rakowska A, eds. *Atlas of Trichoscopy – Dermoscopy in Hair and Scalp Disease*. 1st ed. London: Springer-Verlag; 2012:3–8.
16. Verzì AE, Lacarrubba F, Micali G. Use of low-cost videomicroscopy versus standard videodermatoscopy in trichoscopy: a controlled, blinded noninferiority trial. *Skin Appendage Disord*. 2016;1(4):172–174. https://doi.org/10.1159/000442993.
17. Vicenzi C, Tosti A. Instruments for scalp dermoscopy. In: Tosti A, ed. *Dermoscopy of the Hair and Nails*. 2nd ed. Boca Raton: CRC Press; 2016:25–28.
18. Rudnicka L, Rakowska A, Kerzeja M, Olszewska M. Hair shafts in trichoscopy: clues for diagnosis of hair and scalp diseases. *Dermatol Clin*. 2013;31(4):695–708. https://doi.org/10.1016/j.det.2013.06.007.
19. Rudnicka L, Olszewska M, Rakowska A, Slowinska M. Trichoscopy update 2011. *J Dermatol Case Rep*. 2011;5(4):82–88. https://doi.org/10.3315/jdcr.2011.1083.
20. de Moura LH, Duque-Estrada B, Abraham LS, Barcaui CB, Sodre CT. Dermoscopy findings of alopecia areata in an African-American patient. *J Dermatol Case Rep*. 2008;2(4):52–54. https://doi.org/10.3315/jdcr.2008.1020.
21. Lanuti E, Miteva M, Romanelli P, Tosti A. Trichoscopy and histopathology of follicular keratotic plugs in scalp discoid lupus erythematosus. *Int J Trichol*. 2012;4(1):36–38. https://doi.org/10.4103/0974-7753.96087.
22. Ross EK, Vincenzi C, Tosti A. Videodermoscopy in the evaluation of hair and scalp disorders. *Am Acad Dermatol*. 2006;55(5):799–806.
23. Pirmez R, Piñeiro-Maceira J, Sodré CT. Exclamation marks and other trichoscopic signs of chemotherapy-induced alopecia. *Australas J Dermatol*. 2013;54(2):129–132. https://doi.org/10.1111/j.1440-0960.2012.00946.x.
24. Papaiordanou F, da Silveira BR, Piñeiro-Maceira J, Pirmez R. Trichoscopy of noncicatricial pressure-induced alopecia resembling alopecia areata. *Int J Trichol*. 2016;8(2):89–90. https://doi.org/10.4103/0974-7753.188043.
25. Tosti A, Torres F, Miteva M. Dermoscopy of early dissecting cellulitis of the scalp simulates alopecia areata. *Actas Dermosifiliogr*. 2013;104(1):92–93. https://doi.org/10.1016/j.ad.2012.05.008.

26. Pirmez R, Piñeiro-Maceira J, Almeida BC, Sodré CT. Follicular red dots: a normal trichoscopy feature in patients with pigmentary disorders? *An Bras Dermatol.* 2013;88(3):459–461. https://doi.org/10.1590/abd1806-4841.20132555.

27. Kossard S, Zagarella S. Spotted cicatricial alopecia in dark skin. A dermoscopic clue to fibrous tracts. *Australas J Dermatol.* 1993;34(2):49–51.

28. Abraham LS, Piñeiro-Maceira J, Duque-Estrada B, Barcaui CB, Sodré CT. Pinpoint white dots in the scalp: dermoscopic and histopathologic correlation. *J Am Acad Dermatol.* 2010;63(4):721–722. https://doi.org/10.1016/j.jaad.2009.12.011.

29. Deloche C, de Lacharrière O, Misciali C, et al. Histological features of peripilar signs associated with androgenetic alopecia. *Arch Dermatol Res.* 2004;295(10):422–428.

30. Duque-Estrada B, Tamler C, Sodré CT, Barcaui CB, Pereira FB. Dermoscopy patterns of cicatricial alopecia resulting from discoid lupus erythematosus and lichen planopilaris. *An Bras Dermatol.* 2010;85(2):179–183.

31. Miteva M, Tosti A. Dermatoscopic features of central centrifugal cicatricial alopecia. *J Am Acad Dermatol.* 2014;71 (3):443–449. https://doi.org/10.1016/j.jaad.2014.04.069.

32. Pirmez R, Abraham LS, Duque-Estrada B, et al. Trichoscopy of steroid-induced atrophy. *Skin Appendage Disord.* 2017;3:171–174. https://doi.org/10.1159/000471771.

33. Vicenzi C, Tosti A. Trichoscopy patterns. In: Tosti A, ed. *Dermoscopy of the Hair and Nails.* 2nd ed. Boca Raton: CRC Press; 2016:1–20.

34. de Lacharrière O, Deloche C, Misciali C, et al. Hair diameter diversity: a clinical sign reflecting the follicle miniaturization. *Arch Dermatol.* 2001;137(5):641–646.

35. Herskovitz I, de Sousa IC, Tosti A. Vellus hairs in the frontal scalp in early female pattern hair loss. *Int J Trichol.* 2013;5 (3):118–120. https://doi.org/10.4103/0974-7753.125601.

36. Tosti A, Whiting D, Iorizzo M, Pazzaglia M, Misciali C, Vincenzi C, Micali G. The role of scalp dermoscopy in the diagnosis of alopecia areata incognita. *J Am Acad Dermatol.* 2008;59(1):64-67. doi: 10.1016/j.jaad.2008.03.031.

37. Rudnicka L, Rakowska A, Olszewska M, et al. Hair shafts. In: Rudnicka L, Olszewska M, Rakowska A, eds. *Atlas of Trichoscopy – Dermoscopy in Hair and Scalp Disease.* 1st ed. London: Springer-Verlag; 2012:11–46.

38. Quaresma MV, Martinez Velasco MA, Tosti A. Hair breakage in patients of African descent: role of dermoscopy. *Skin Appendage Disord.* 2015;1(2):99–104. https://doi.org/10.1159/000436981.

39. Rakowska A, Slowinska M, Olsz ewska M, Rudnicka L. New trichoscopy findings in trichotillomania: flame hairs, V-sign, hook hairs, hair powder, tulip hairs. *Acta Derm Venereol.* 2014;94(3):303–306. https://doi.org/10.2340/00015555-1674.

40. Miteva M, Tosti A. Flame hair. *Skin Appendage Disord.* 2015;1(2):105–109. https://doi.org/10.1159/000438995.

41. Quaresma MV, Mariño Alvarez AM, Miteva M. Dermatoscopic-pathologic correlation of lichen simplex chronicus on the scalp: 'broom fibres, gear wheels and hamburgers'. *J Eur Acad Dermatol Venereol.* 2016;30(2):343–345. https://doi.org/10.1111/jdv.12748.

42. Alkhalifah A, Alsantali A, Wang E, et al. Alopecia areata update: part I. Clinical picture, histopathology, and pathogenesis. *J Am Acad Dermatol.* 2010;62:177–188.

43. Pirmez R. Revisiting coudability hairs in alopecia areata: the story behind the name. *Skin Appendage Disord.* 2016; 2(1–2):76–78.

44. Slowinska M, Rudnicka L, Schwartz RA, et al. Comma hairs: a dermatoscopic marker for tinea capitis: a rapid diagnostic method. *J Am Acad Dermatol.* 2008;59(5 suppl): S77–S79. https://doi.org/10.1016/j.jaad.2008.07.009.

45. Hughes R, Chiaverini C, Bahadoran P, Lacour JP. Corkscrew hair: a new dermoscopic sign for diagnosis of tinea capitis in black children. *Arch Dermatol.* 2011;147(3): 355–356. https://doi.org/10.1001/archdermatol.2011.31.

46. Sharma VK, Chiramel MJ, Rao A. Dermoscopy: a rapid bedside tool to assess monilethrix. *Indian J Dermatol Venereol Leprol.* 2016;82:73–74.

47. Rakowska A, Kowalska-Oledzka E, Slowinska M, Rosinska D, Rudnicka L. Hair shaft videodermoscopy in netherton syndrome. *Pediatr Dermatol.* 2009;26(3):320–322. https://doi.org/10.1111/j.1525-1470.2008.00778.x.

FURTHER READING

1. Abraham LS, Torres FN, Azulay-Abulafia L. Dermoscopic clues to distinguish trichotillomania from patchy alopecia areata. *An Bras Dermatol.* 2010;85(5):723–726.

Alopecia Areata and Alopecia Areata Incognita

MATILDE IORIZZO, MD, PHD • ANTONELLA TOSTI, MD

INTRODUCTION

Alopecia areata (AA) is a common form of nonscarring alopecia characterized by acute hair loss in the absence of cutaneous inflammatory signs. The disease usually starts abruptly with one or multiple patches that enlarge in a centrifugal way. The entire scalp (AA totalis [AAT]) and body (AA universalis [AAU]) may be affected.

The disease occurs in all ethnic groups, ages, and sexes, with an estimated lifetime risk of 1.7% among the general population.[1] Pediatric AA has been estimated around 20% of all patients with AA and more than 50% of patients present their first episode before the age of 20 years.[2]

The psychologic impact of AA is very severe because of the acute onset and the unpredictable course. In fact, the prognosis of this disorder is very difficult to predict due to the unknown etiology and the influence of several negative factors (Table 4.1).[3]

ETIOPATHOGENESIS

The etiology of AA is still not completely understood, although there is much evidence that argues for an autoimmune disorder with a genetic predisposition.[4,5] Genome Wide Association Studies (GWAS)[5] revealed, in eight regions of the Genome, 139 single nucleotide polymorphisms linked to AA and provided evidence that both innate and acquired immunity play a role in the pathogenesis of AA. For unknown reasons, the immune privilege (the nonexpression of major histocompatibility complex I and II that usually bind pathogens to present to the immune system) of the anagen hair follicles is lost and the peribulbar area is infiltrated by cytotoxic CD8+ T lymphocytes. The anagen growth is then interrupted and the hair sheds. The bulge area (the region where the stem cells are situated) is spared by the T-cell infiltrate, explaining why this form of alopecia is not cicatricial. The hair follicles always retain the potential for recovery despite a persistent hair loss for many years, but, unfortunately, it is not always possible to remove the lymphocytic infiltrate to obtain hair regrowth. At present there is no treatment that can induce a permanent remission of AA and there is no drug approved for the treatment of this disorder.[6] However, particularly in patchy AA, the inflammatory infiltrate may resolve spontaneously and hair can regrow without any treatment.

CLINICAL FEATURES

AA may involve any hairy body area, but the scalp is the most commonly affected site (>90%) (Fig. 4.1). Usually AA starts abruptly and symptomless, even if some patients report a slight itch preceding the hair shedding and subsequently affecting the alopecic area. The affected skin is however normal, without signs of inflammation. The presence of itching should not be underevaluated because it could explain a possible role of the neurogenic inflammation in the pathogenesis of AA.[7,8]

A patch of acute and active AA (Fig. 4.2) is characterized, at the naked eye, by the presence of the following:

1. Cadaverized hairs that are hair shafts retained within the hair follicles due to a breakage at the scalp surface. They present as black dots only in patients with dark hair; for obvious reasons in other patients they are less visible.

2. "Exclamation mark" hairs are hairs with a frayed tip and tapered proximal end. They represent the telogen hair shafts retained within the follicle and expelled later. These can be easily extracted with a gentle pulling. They are most commonly seen at the border of the patch. Sometimes patients and untrained clinicians misdiagnose exclamation mark hairs as regrowing hairs that are instead tightly attached to the scalp and need a pluck and not a pull to be removed.

Chronic AA presents instead with a smooth patch totally devoid of hair (Fig. 4.3) or covered by very fine, short vellus hairs.

TABLE 4.1
Negative Prognostic Factors Linked Up With Alopecia Areata

Ophiasis (hair loss in the occipital scalp)
Onset before puberty
Association with atopy/autoimmune
   disorders/trisomy 21
Nail involvement (regular pitting/trachyonychia)
Positive family history
Longstanding disease

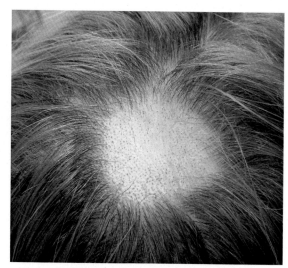

FIG. 4.2 Acute alopecia areata of the scalp showing cadaverized hair and exclamation mark hair.

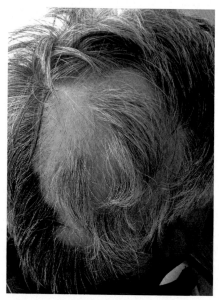

FIG. 4.1 Typical patches of alopecia areata that enlarges in a centrifugal way.

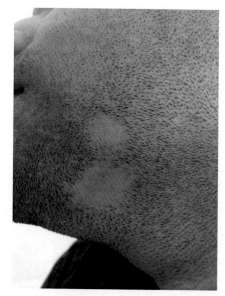

FIG. 4.3 Chronic alopecia areata of the beard.

Other presentations of AA include the following:

Ophiasis and Sisaipho: the first case, which is more common, is when the alopecic area involves the hairline of the parietal and occipital scalp in toto. The second case, which is more rare, is when the alopecic area involves the frontal hairline and the central scalp.

Sudden whitening of the hair: when the hair turns white in a few days. In this case, the disease causes a selective involvement of pigmented hairs that shed, whereas white hairs are spared and remain on the scalp.

Alopecia areata incognito/incognita: this condition is characterized by acute diffuse and symptomless shedding of hairs in the absence of typical patches and by a much more favorable prognosis. According to Rebora,[9] it occurs when AA affects individuals with high percentages of telogen hairs on the scalp and scarce early anagen VI hairs, the ones with the highest mitotic rate and,

therefore, more affected by the disease. This results in a diffuse hair loss rather than patches. Diagnosis always requires a scalp biopsy. Clinically it might resemble not only telogen effluvium but also androgenetic alopecia because of a diffuse thinning more severe on androgen-dependent scalp. In patients with this variety of AA, the pull test is strongly positive with easy extraction of tufts of hair. Microscopic examination of the extracted hairs reveals telogen roots at different degrees of maturation with a high prevalence of early telogen roots.

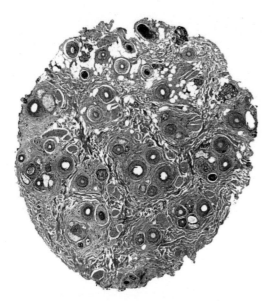

FIG. 4.4 Alopecia areata incognita: This is a horizontal section at the level of the isthmus showing decreased follicular density (35 follicles) with increased telogen count (29%) and follicular miniaturization of 1.3:1. Some vellus follicles show features of nanogen (Hematoxylin and Eosin, x2). (Image courtesy of Mariya Miteva.)

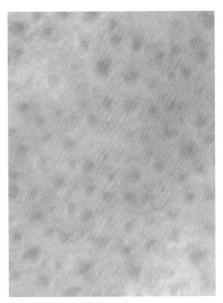

FIG. 4.5 Dermoscopy of an acute patch of alopecia areata showing *yellow dots*.

Dermoscopy examination of the scalp shows diffusely distributed yellow dots and a large number of short regrowing hairs. The areas with numerous yellow dots are the best places to take a biopsy.[10] The pathologic diagnosis of alopecia areata incognita (AAI) requires horizontal sections (Fig. 4.4) that demonstrate decreased follicular density with increased number of telogen follicles (more than 30% telogen counts) and follicular miniaturization (terminal:vellus ratio of 3.3:1 or lower). Telogen germinal units and/or small telogen follicles may be present, and the follicular infundibula are dilated. Subtle peribulbar lymphocytic infiltrate is rarely seen only around vellus anagen hair follicles in the dermis.[11] Recently it has been reported that 36 biopsy specimens from AAI, when studied by real-time polymerase chain reaction, showed statistically significant increase in the ULBP3 levels compared with biopsies from patients with telogen effluvium or androgenetic alopecia.[12] The finding of this marker, which represents a cell surface glycoprotein normally turned off in the healthy hair follicle, may act as a further confirmatory test in the diagnosis of AAI.

DIAGNOSIS
The diagnosis of AA is clinical, and biopsy is required only in doubtful cases.

No routine test is indicated in these patients but an autoimmunity check could be performed to detect an associated disease that otherwise should be overlooked.

The pull test is useful to establish if the disease is slowly or rapidly progressing. In the latter, case tufts of hairs are easily extracted. Examination under the light microscopy shows telogen and dystrophic hairs. Examination with the dermoscope reveals instead more useful informations, even if not all are truly specific for AA[13-15]:

1. Yellow dots—round or polycyclic dots around the hair follicles that may be devoid of hairs or contain miniaturized or dystrophic hairs (Fig. 4.5). Yellow dots are visible in most Caucasian and Asian patients but not in patients with dark skin and children. They correspond on pathology to the dilated infundibular ostia filled with sebum and degenerated follicular keratinocytes. They are the most sensitive marker of AA, being present in all patients with this disorder, independent from its clinical presentation and activity.
2. Black dots—as stated earlier, they represent the cadaverized hairs (Fig. 4.6). They correlate with disease severity and activity.
3. Exclamation mark hairs—much more evident than the tapered and poorly pigmented proximal end is the pigmented and frayed distal end (Fig. 4.7). They also correlate with disease severity and activity.

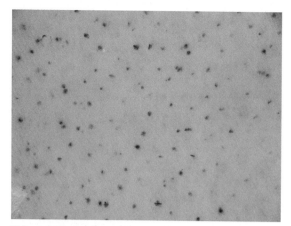

FIG. 4.6 Dermoscopy of an acute patch of alopecia areata showing *black dots*.

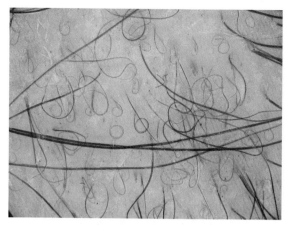

FIG. 4.8 Circle hairs.

6. Pseudo-monilethrix hairs—hair with constrictions along the shaft similar to those observed in monilethrix (hair shafts with a beaded appearance).
7. Broken hairs/flame hairs—these last ones are, in particular, broken hairs resulting from an anagen arrest.
8. Short regrowing hairs—they may appear as circle hairs (Fig. 4.8) when resulting from a hair follicle not completely recovered.

Examining the patch of AA with the dermoscope most of the time helps the clinician in performing a correct diagnosis. When a biopsy is required, this device is also useful because it helps in identifying the best biopsy site to punch.

The classic histopathologic features of acute AA include peribulbar lymphocytic infiltrate (*swarm of bees*), dilated follicular infundibula (*Swiss cheese* pattern),[16] and increased percentage of telogen hairs. However, the pathology changes according to the stage of the disease with increased telogen counts in the subacute stage (Fig. 4.9) and increased number of vellus follicles and nanogen hairs, with absence of *swarm-of-bees* infiltrate in the chronic stage.[17]

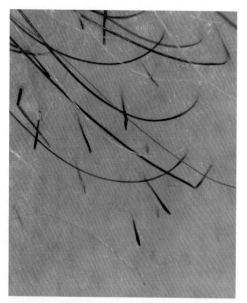

FIG. 4.7 Dermoscopy of an acute patch of alopecia areata showing *yellow dots*, exclamation mark hair, elbow hair, and broken hair.

4. Coudability hairs—hair with a proximal tapering probably because of a less severe insult that leaves the hair in anagen without fracturing the shaft or shifting it to telogen.
5. Elbow hairs—hair with one or more constrictions along the shaft. These constrictions correspond to the insults the hair has suffered and are also called Pohl-Pinkus constrictions.

DIFFERENTIAL DIAGNOSIS

Trichotillomania: this is probably the most difficult disorder to be distinguished from AA, also because the two disorders may coexist. Broken hairs at different levels, flame hairs, hairs with trichoptilosis, black dots, and yellow dots are usually seen at dermoscopy in trichotillomania. Coiled hairs, comma hairs, and corkscrew hairs are also typical but they are not present in all cases.[18] The patches with broken or no hairs

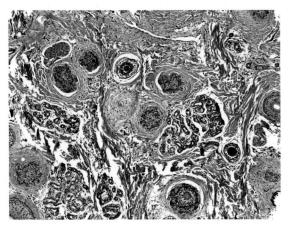

FIG. 4.9 Alopecia areata, subacute stage: This is a horizontal section at the low follicular level. There is predominant number of telogen follicles (vs. only one terminal anagen follicle). One follicle shows features of nanogen (at the bottom) (hematoxylin and eosin, ×10). (Image courtesy of Mariya Miteva.)

are usually more irregular in shape compared to those of AA.

Tinea capitis: it should always be suspected in children, but adults can also be affected. Scalp scaling is generally present. Broken hairs, comma hairs, and corkscrew hairs are a typical dermoscopic finding.[19]

Congenital triangular alopecia: this alopecia also is typical of children and usually present in the frontotemporal area even if atypical locations in the parietal areas may occur. Dermoscopy is helpful in avoiding a biopsy; diversity of hair diameter, empty follicles, and normal follicular openings containing long thin vellus hairs have been reported.[20,21]

Atrichia with papular lesions: this form of congenital alopecia should always be considered when facing a child with alopecia totalis/alopecia universalis. Patients with a mutation in the hairless gene may present with scalp alopecia alone and develop the keratin-filled epithelial cysts only after years. The lack of these characteristic cysts may confuse even an expert eye.

ASSOCIATED DISEASES

AA may be associated with other autoimmune disorders, such as thyroiditis, atopy, celiac disease, rheumatoid arthritis, vitiligo, type-1 diabetes, and pernicious anemia, among others.[22] GWAS reported a number of risk loci in common between AA and other autoimmune disorders.[5] When AA presented in association with other autoimmune disorders, the formation of organ-specific autoantibodies that played a pathogenic role in both disorders was observed. Up to 60% of AA patients, particularly children, present with nail abnormalities. Regular pitting, trachyonychia, punctate leukonychia, and mottled erythema of the lunula are the most common findings and are associated, usually, with severe forms of AA and poor prognosis.

Ocular abnormalities have also been reported in patients affected by AA and, in particular, iris color changes, lens alterations, and retinal changes. These associations are still under discussion and are not required to perform an ophthalmologic evaluation in patients with AA. No relationship has been detected between these changes and duration of illness, patient's age and, eventually, previous steroid therapy.

TREATMENT

No drug is currently approved for AA and all available treatments are considered "off label." No treatment, in fact, has been proved to induce and sustain remissions and, at the same time, spontaneous remissions make sometimes difficult to assess efficacy of treatments. Moreover, many trials have been limited to patients with severe and/or long-standing AA that tend to be resistant to all forms of treatment, and the failure in this setting does not exclude efficacy in mild forms of the disease.

Topical steroids: their efficacy is influenced by the potency of the active ingredient and the penetration of the vehicle. Clobetasol propionate, 0.05% ointment or foam, is usually the drug of choice. Patchy AA and AAT/AAU, either active or stable, respond better to treatment if this is applied under occlusion.[23] Daily dosage should not exceed 2.5 g, and scalp folliculitis is a frequent side effect.

Intralesional steroids: they are effective in stable patchy AA but, despite their common use, there are no randomized controlled trials or studies about their efficacy.[24] Triamcinolone acetonide is the drug generally used, and it should be diluted in saline solution before being injected within the patch (0.1 mL per injection at 1 cm interval with a 30 G needle, 12 mm long in the upper dermis). Maximum dosage should not exceed 20 mg for session. Dilution of 2.5 mg/mL is as effective as 10 mg/mL according to a recent study.[25] Treatment should be repeated monthly for at least 6 months but not prolonged over if no efficacy is reported. The major side effect is skin atrophy in the injection site.

Systemic steroids: high-dose pulse corticosteroids therapy is 60% effective in the acute forms of AA, but not in ophiasis alopecia and chronic AAT/AAU. A continuous treatment is often required to maintain hair regrowth and this means more side effects over time (osteoporosis, diabetes, weight gain, suppression of the adrenocorticotropic axes). Relapses are very common after stopping treatment, and several studies show that long-term results in children are very poor.[26] However, available options include the following:

- Methylprednisolone, 500 mg/day intravenously for 3 days a month (10 mg/kg in children).[27,28]
- Oral prednisolone, 300 mg/month (5 mg/kg in children).[29]
- Oral dexamethasone, 0.1 mg/kg/day for two consecutive days every week.[30]

All these options are difficult to compare because treatment protocols and patient selection are too different. However, patchy AA seems the one that responds better.

Topical immunotherapy: this is the best-documented treatment for AA. Before starting treatment, it is necessary to sensitize patients with a 2% solution of squaric acid dibutylester (SADBE) or diphenylcyclopropenone (DPCP) under closed patch applied on the alopecic scalp for 48 h.[31] After 3 weeks, treatment can start with a weekly application of SADBE or DPCP diluted in acetone at a concentration chosen according to the severity of the dermatitis obtained with the sensitization. These concentrations considerably vary among patients and even in the same patient during the treatment period. The objective of the application is to induce a mild scalp contact dermatitis and shift the inflammatory infiltrate localized around the hair follicle towards the dermatitis. Mechanisms of action are still not completely understood: a study showed change in the CD4:CD8 lymphocyte ratio from 4:1 to 1:1 in perifollicular tissue[32] and a modification in the cytokine profile has also been proposed. Topical immunotherapy is not effective in acute, rapidly expanding disease. It is useful for longstanding AA and in children (50% of cases).[33] Side effects are urticarial reactions, cervical lymphadenopathy, and dyschromias.

Anthralin (Dithranol): the cream must be applied at a high-enough concentration (0.5%–1%) to induce mild erythema of the scalp. The application in the alopecic site starts for 10–20 min a day, then the contact time is increased by 5 min weekly up to 1–2 h maximum. Anthralin acts as an immunomodulator targeting the cytokine expression. No side effects are reported

with its use except for black staining of the scalp and mild pruritus. Cosmetically acceptable hair regrowth is achieved in 25% of cases, but studies proving its efficacy are still lacking.[34]

Phototherapy: an option for patients with stable AAT/AAU because the absence of hair permits UV penetration, but after hair regrowth is achieved it is difficult to maintain the results. Moreover, the continuous treatment (3 times/week for several months) necessary for long-term results implies a UV cumulative dose too high. Usually psoralen and ultraviolet A radiation (PUVA) is performed with oral psoralen but the PUVA turban with 0.0001% 8-MOP solution is another good option, especially because it is devoid of the side effects related to systemic psoralens.[35]

Laser therapy: excimer laser therapy is administered 2 times a week for at least 6 months. Initial fluence should be 50 mJ/cm^2, increased by 50 mJ every two sessions. At present results of studies seem controversial and long-term data are still lacking.[36]

Other treatments: oral cyclosporine, 5 mg/kg/day, is an option because of its immunosuppressive action, but the side effects related to its use (high blood pressure and kidney dysfunction) are not worth the risk compared with the results obtained. Methotrexate, sulfasalazine, and azathioprine have been utilized in association with systemic steroids with variable results. The combination simvastatin-ezetimibe, 40 mg/10 mg, has been reported with some success in acute but not in longstanding severe AA.[37] Subcutaneous administration of low-dose IL2 in patients with longstanding AAU showed improvement of the disease in 80% of cases after 6 months. The rationale of IL2 use is based on the activation of regulatory T lymphocytes.[38]

Future treatments: the class of drugs, Janus Kinase (JAK) inhibitors, seem to be the future for AA treatment. Tofacitinib, ruxolitinib, and baricitinib have already been evaluated and other JAK inhibitors are on trials, for adults and adolescents, with promising results. They are very expensive drugs, approved for disorders different from AA, but they seem effective in this disorder too. They have been shown to prevent the disease development in animal models and to promote hair regrowth reversing established disease both in animal and human models.[39] JAK inhibitors interfere with the JAK pathway, reducing the production of IL-15, an inflammatory cytokine increased in AA and produced by IFNγ with the intent of supporting the activity of CD8+ T lymphocytes. At present there is no validated dosage for AA, and the problem still remains when to stop with the treatment and the possible relapses after cessation. The side effects related to these drugs may limit their systemic use, and this is the reason why they are becoming more and more interesting as topicals. Assuming there is no systemic absorption, the vehicle also becomes very important.[40] Clinical studies evaluated tofacitinib, ruxolitinib, and baricitinib in the following dosages:

- Tofacitinib: dosage higher than 5 mg/twice a day is often necessary[41]
- Ruxolitinib: 20 mg/twice a day[42]
- Baricitinib: 7 mg/day for 6 months and then 7 mg/ morning and 4 mg/evening.[43]

Ruxolitinib has been evaluated also as a 0.6% cream to be applied twice a day on the alopecic areas. It has been a complete success for the eyebrows and less for the scalp.[44]

REFERENCES

1. McDonagh AJ, Tazi-Ahnini R. Epidemiology and genetics of alopecia areata. *Clin Exp Dermatol.* 2002;27(5):405–409.
2. Alkhalifah A, Alsantali A, Wang E, McElwee KJ, Shapiro J. Alopecia areata update: part I. Clinical picture, histopathology and pathogenesis. *J Am Acad Dermatol.* 2010;62(2):177–188.
3. Tosti A, Bellavista S, Iorizzo M. Alopecia areata: a long term follow-up study of 191 patients. *J Am Acad Dermatol.* 2006;55(3):438–441.
4. Gilhar A, Etzioni A, Paus R. Alopecia areata. *N Engl J Med.* 2012;366(16):1515–1525.
5. Petukhova L, Duvic M, Hordinsky M, et al. Genome-wide association study in alopecia areata implicates both innate and adaptive immunity. *Nature.* 2010;466(7302):113–117.
6. Messenger AG, McKillop J, Farrant P, McDonagh AJ, Sladden M. British Association of Dermatologists' guidelines for the management of alopecia areata. *Br J Dermatol.* 2012;166(5):916–926.
7. Siebenhaar F, Sharov AA, Peters EM, et al. Substance P as an immunomodulatory neuropeptide in a mouse model for autoimmune hair loss (alopecia areata). *J Invest Dermatol.* 2007;127(6):1489–1497.
8. Daly TJ. Alopecia areata has low plasma levels of the vasodilator/immunomodulatory calcitonin gene related peptide. *Arch Dermatol.* 1998;134(9):1164–1165.
9. Rebora A. Alopecia areata incognita: a hypothesis. *Dermatologica.* 1987;174(5):214–218.
10. Tosti A, Whiting D, Iorizzo M, et al. The role of scalp dermoscopy in the diagnosis of alopecia areata incognita. *J Am Acad Dermatol.* 2008;59(1):64–67.
11. Miteva M, Misciali C, Fanti PA, Tosti A. Histopathologic features of alopecia areata incognito: a review of 46 cases. *J Cutan Pathol.* 2012;39(6):596–602.
12. Moftah NH, El-Barbary RA, Rashed L, Said M. ULBP3: a marker for alopecia areata incognita. *Arch Dermatol Res.* 2016;308(6):415–421.
13. Miteva M, Tosti A. Hair and scalp dermatoscopy. *J Am Acad Dermatol.* 2012;67(5):1040–1048.
14. Inui S, Nakajima T, Nakagawa K, Itami S. Clinical significance of dermoscopy in alopecia areata: analysis of 300 cases. *Int J Dermatol.* 2008;47(7):688–693.
15. Pirmez R. Revisiting coudability hairs in alopecia areata: the story behind the name. *Skin Appendage Disord.* 2016;2(1–2):76–78.
16. Müller CS, El Shabrawi-Caelen L. 'Follicular Swiss cheese' pattern–another histopathologic clue to alopecia areata. *J Cutan Pathol.* 2011;38(2):185–189.
17. Whiting DA. Histopathologic features of alopecia areata: a new look. *Arch Dermatol.* 2003;139(12):1555–1559.
18. Rakowska A, Slowinska M, Olszewska M, Rudnika L. New trichoscopy findings in trichotillomania: flame hairs, V-sign, hook hairs, hair powder, tulip hairs. *Acta Derm Venereol.* 2014;94(3):303–306.
19. Bourezane Y, Bourezane Y. Analysis of trichoscopic signs observed in 24 patients presenting tinea capitis: hypotheses based on physiopathology and proposed new classification. *Ann Dermatol Venereol.* 2017;144(8–9):490–496.
20. Iorizzo M, Pazzaglia M, Starace M, et al. Videodermoscopy: a useful tool for diagnosing congenital triangular alopecia. *Pediatr Dermatol.* 2008;25(6):652–654.
21. Fernandez-Crehuet P, Vano-Galvan S, Martorell-Calatayud A, Arias-Santiago S, Grimalt R, Camacho-Martinez FM. Clinical and trichoscopic characteristics of temporal triangular alopecia: a multicenter study. *J Am Acad Dermatol.* 2016;75(3):634–637.
22. Hordinsky M, Junqueira AL. Alopecia areata update. *Semin Cutan Med Surg.* 2015;34(2):72–75.
23. Tosti A, Piraccini BM, Pazzaglia M, Vincenzi C. Clobetasol propionate 0.05% under occlusion in the treatment of alopecia totalis/universalis. *J Am Acad Dermatol.* 2003;49(1):96–98.
24. Chang KH, Rojhirunsakool S, Goldberg LJ. Treatment of severe alopecia areata with intralesional steroid injections. *J Drugs Dermatol.* 2009;8(10):909–912.
25. Chu TW, Al Jasser M, Alharbi A, Abahussein O, McElwee K, Shapiro J. Benefit of different concentrations of intralesional triamcinolone acetonide in alopecia areata: an intrasubject pilot study. *J Am Acad Dermatol.* 2015;73(2):338–340.
26. Hubiche T, Léauté-Labrèze C, Taïeb A, Boralevi F. Poor long term outcome of severe alopecia areata in children treated with high dose pulse corticosteroid therapy. *Br J Dermatol.* 2008;158(5):1136–1137.
27. Friedli A, Labarthe MP, Engelhardt E, Feldmann R, Salomon D, Saurat JH. Pulse methylprednisolone therapy for severe alopecia areata: an open prospective study of 45 patients. *J Am Acad Dermatol.* 1998;39(4 Pt 1):597–602.
28. Smith A, Trueb RM, Theiler M, Hauser V, Weibel L. High relapse rates despite early intervention with intravenous methylprednisolone pulse therapy for severe childhood alopecia areata. *Pediatr Dermatol.* 2015;32(4):481–487.

29. Sharma VK. Pulsed administration of corticosteroids in the treatment of alopecia areata. *Int J Dermatol.* 1996;35(2):133–136.

30. Vañó-Galván S, Hermosa-Gelbard Á, Sánchez-Neila N, et al. Pulse corticosteroid therapy with oral dexamethasone for the treatment of adult alopecia totalis and universalis. *J Am Acad Dermatol.* 2016;74(5):1005–1007.

31. Happle R, Hausen BM, Wiesner-Menzel L. Diphencyprone in the treatment of alopecia areata. *Acta Derm Venereol.* 1983;63(1):49–52.

32. Singh G, Lavanya M. Topical immunotherapy in alopecia areata. *Int J Trichol.* 2010;2(1):36–39.

33. Rokhsar CK, Shupack JL, Vafai JJ, Washenik K. Efficacy of topical sensitizers in the treatment of alopecia areata. *J Am Acad Dermatol.* 1998;39(5 Pt 1):751–761.

34. Schmoeckel C, Weissmann I, Plewig G, Braun-Falco O. Treatment of alopecia areata by anthralin induced dermatitis. *Arch Dermatol.* 1979;115(10):1254–1255.

35. Taylor CR, Hawk JL. PUVA treatment of alopecia areata partialis, totalis and universalis: audit of 10 years' experience at St John's Institute of Dermatology. *Br J Dermatol.* 1995;133(6):914–918.

36. McMichael AJ. Excimer laser: a module of the alopecia areata common protocol. *J Invest Dermatol Symp Proc.* 2013;16(1):S77–S79.

37. Cervantes J, Jimenez JJ, Del Canto GM, Tosti A. NAAF symposium: role of statins in the treatment of alopecia areata. *J Investig Dermatol Symp Proc.* 2018;19(1):S25–S31.

38. Castela E, Le Duff F, Butori C, et al. Effects of low-dose recombinant interleukin 2 to promote T-regulatory cells in alopecia areata. *JAMA Dermatol.* 2014;150(7):748–751.

39. Xing L, Dai Z, Jabbari A, et al. Alopecia areata is driven by cytotoxic lymphocytes and is reversed by JAK inhibitors. *Nat Med.* 2014;20(9):1043–1049.

40. Sherberk-Hassidim R, Ramot Y, Zlotogorski A. Janus kinase inhibitors in dermatology: a systematic review. *J Am Acad Dermatol.* 2017;76(4):745–753.

41. Liu LY, Craiglow BG, Dai F, King BA. Tofacitinib for the treatment of severe alopecia areata and variants: a study of 90 patients. *J Am Acad Dermatol.* 2017;76(1):22–28.

42. MacKay-Wiggan J, Jabbari A, Nguyen N, et al. Oral ruxolitinib induces hair regrowth in patients with moderate-to-severe alopecia areata. *JCI Insight.* 2016;1(15):e89790.

43. Jabbari A, Dai Z, Xing L, et al. Reversal of alopecia areata following treatment with the JAK1/2 inhibitor baricitinib. *EBioMedicine.* 2015;2(4):351–355.

44. Craiglow BG, Tavares D, King BA. Topical ruxolitinib for the treatment of alopecia universalis. *JAMA Dermatol.* 2016;152(4):490–491.

CHAPTER 5

Androgenetic Alopecia

RACHEL SENNETT, MD, PHD • LUIS GARZA, MD, PHD

INTRODUCTION

Androgenetic alopecia (AGA) is the most common cause of hair loss in both men and women, with an increasing prevalence with age. As the population grows older, dermatology clinic appointments booked to evaluate hair loss will likely increasingly herald patients presenting with AGA. Many more patients with AGA will never come to the clinic; as the condition is so common, some consider it an inevitability and do not seek a professional opinion. Although AGA is nonfatal, it can become a significant source of stress for those not resigned to baldness, or for those who first see symptoms at an unusually young age. In addition to the immense general public interest that would follow the discovery of a cure for baldness, the problem of stunted hair follicle production represents a fascinating model system with which to improve our understanding of adult stem cell niches and long-term tissue homeostasis and repair.

In terms of nomenclature, patients might be more familiar with the synonymous terms "male-" or "female pattern hair loss" (MPHL/FPHL) for men and women, respectively. Although MPHL, FPHL, and AGA are often used interchangeably, the presenting features of this alopecia are stereotypically different in men and women, and there are some inconsistencies in the field about their shared and distinct molecular drivers. In general, although the precise molecular mechanisms underlying AGA susceptibility and initiation remain unknown, two factors are considered driving forces in disease progression for both men and women: heredity and hormones. These dual forces have long been considered equally important since methodic physicians in the mid-twentieth century formulated their initial hypotheses based on careful history taking and observation of individuals with unconventional hormonal status. But despite the long-standing understanding that androgens drive MPHL, targeted therapeutics were only recently developed. And as miraculous as these medications may have seemed at their advent, they can only stave off disease progression; as of yet, no cure to reverse

androgenetic hair loss exists. Current research is still seeking to understand the precise cellular targets and genetic underpinnings of disease progression, with the ultimate goal to reveal other relevant signaling pathways or cell types that might be manipulated to one day reverse a bald phenotype.

This review aims to summarize the most common elements of a patient's history and examination suggestive of an AGA diagnosis, in addition to outlining the current standard pharmacologic and procedural approaches to treatment. Finally, we highlight the most exciting ongoing areas of research and speculate how this might translate to a paradigm shift for AGA treatment in the near future.

CLINICAL AND HISTOLOGIC PRESENTATION

The hallmark for androgen-mediated alopecia is gradual hair loss in a characteristic pattern distinct by gender. Men typically present with hair loss from the frontotemporal and vertex scalp, whereas in women hair thinning is most pronounced around the midline part, respectively depicted in the graduated Hamilton–Norwood and Ludwig scales[1-4] (Figs. 5.1 and 5.2). Diffuse hair thinning in target areas can occur early, and only trichoscopic inspection with magnification will reveal the loss of individual hairs from grouped follicular units, well before macroscopic hair loss is appreciated.[4] Below the surface of the skin, hair follicles affected by AGA are miniaturized with smaller matrix/transit-amplifying cell compartments that produce correspondingly thinner and less-pigmented vellus hair shafts; this is compared with robust terminal hairs produced by healthy follicles elsewhere on the scalp.[5,6]

Histologic classification defines early AGA as a nonscarring alopecia, which entails intact follicular stem cell compartments and the theoretical potential for disease reversal before extensive follicular damage ensures. Importantly, sustained AGA eventually progresses to permanent, irreversible follicle loss—a

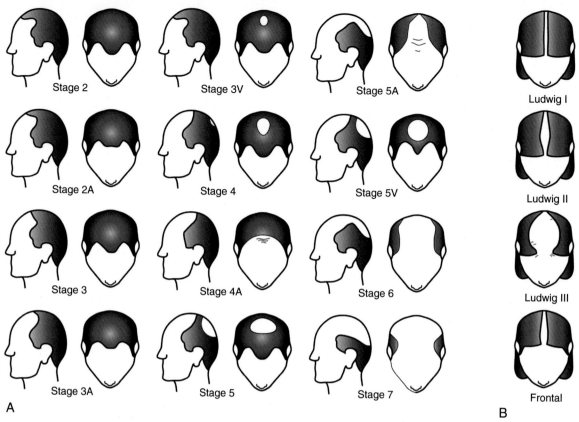

FIG. 5.1 Hamilton–Norwood **(A)** and Ludwig **(B)** scales calibrate the phenotypic progression of typical male pattern and female pattern hair loss, respectively.

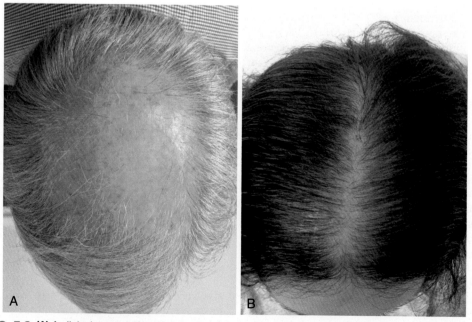

FIG. 5.2 **(A)** A clinical presentation of male pattern hair loss, with frank balding over the vertex and frontal hair thinning compared to the lateral edges. **(B)** A clinical presentation of female pattern hair loss, in a Christmas tree pattern with frontal accentuation.

natural progression that is not uncommon for other types of nonscarring alopecias as well.[7] This pattern contrasts with primary scarring alopecias (e.g., hair loss related to discoid lupus erythematous, lichen planopilaris, or central centrifugal cicatricial alopecia, and others) in which follicles are targeted by lymphocytic infiltrates that cause irreparable follicular destruction and permanent cessation of hair growth from the onset of disease. Perhaps counterintuitively, select histologic studies of AGA biopsies have reported the presence of activated T cells surrounding the hair follicle infundibulum and/or monocytic perivascular infiltrates, but their role in initiating or propagating AGA progression is unclear.[8,9] Follicles in AGA scalp can additionally display thickened follicular sheaths, suggesting the presence of smoldering activated fibroblasts that might gradually induce fibrosis and subsequently cause AGA to evolve from nonscarring to ultimately irreversible.

In horizontal sections of 4-mm punch biopsies from AGA, the classic finding is follicular miniaturization (terminal:vellus ratio of less than 4:1 according to some studies or less than 2.2:1 according to others).[10-12] Besides miniaturization, other histologic changes in AGA-affected scalp include an increased fraction of follicles in the telogen resting phase rather than the anagen growth phase. Healthy hair follicles cyclically and asynchronously degenerate and regrow, reflected by periods of hair growth and shedding. At any given time, 80%–90% of follicles in the healthy human scalp are in the anagen growth phase, with a minority of follicles in the transient degenerative phase of catagen, or the telogen resting phase from which a hair shaft could also be expelled or shed naturally during exogen.[13,14] This distribution changes as follicles are affected by AGA and begin to miniaturize; in balding scalp follicles will spend increasing lengths of time in the resting telogen stage so that only 60%–80% of total hair is in anagen.[15,16]

EPIDEMIOLOGY

AGA is the most common cause of hair loss in men and women, affecting 50% of Caucasian men by age 50 years and 80% by age 80 years.[17,18] The disease commonly affects older women as well, with as many as 40% of women over age 70 years who experience some degree of FPHL.[17,19,20] Although AGA is less prevalent in Asian men and women or African-American men, the prevalence in all ethnicities increases with advancing age.[21-26]

ETIOLOGY AND PATHOGENESIS

There is a general consensus that the etiology of AGA is multifactorial, with unknown hereditary factors and hormones playing central roles in driving initiation and progression. Evidence for the role of genetics in AGA progression comes most convincingly from twin studies comparing the significant concurrence of baldness in monozygotic versus dizygotic twins—an observation that holds true regardless of subject age or degree of balding.[27,28] Other studies note a significant percentage of bald men who report a history of baldness in their fathers, a correlation that is particularly robust when the balding patients in question are young. Not only is the family history of hair loss predictive of future balding generations, but the distinct pattern (primary frontotemporal vs. vertex hair loss) is thought to be inherited as well.[29] Conversely, elderly men with notable hair retention are significantly more likely to report a family history of nonbaldness.[30] The role of family history and genetics in specifically predicting progression of FPHL is murkier, because limited data are available.

Although the idea of baldness as a family trait is intuitive, and has been scientifically validated in numerous studies, research has been slow to identify specific genes directly linked to progression of disease. Early, and more recent, analyses debunked a long-standing hypothesis that AGA in men was driven by the inheritance of a single dominant allele and asserted the modern belief of polygenic inheritance.[30,31] More recently, studies have probed the hereditary tendencies of AGA with either forward or reverse genetic screening methods, either by examining specific genes with functions relevant to hair growth or with a genome-wide association study (GWAS) to identify polymorphisms in the genomes of bald versus nonbald patients and subsequently implicate nearby genes. In one example, aware of the established link between androgen levels, AGA progression, and the utility of the 5-alpha-reductase inhibitor finasteride to combat progressive hair loss (to be discussed later in detail), one research team assumed the target enzyme of this medication would be differentially expressed in bald versus haired scalp. However, a detailed genetic examination of the 5-alpha-reductase gene *SRD5A2* failed to uncover any difference in gene expression or activity in bald cases versus haired controls.[32] On the other hand, an in-depth analysis of the androgen receptor (AR) did reveal genetic polymorphisms significantly associated with balding scalp, a finding confirmed by multiple GWAS as well.[33,34] Other genes linked to polymorphisms significantly associated with AGA include *EDA2R* and *WNT10B*, which are particularly notable for their known roles in coordinating hair morphogenesis during embryogenesis.[35-37] Exactly how, or even if, these minute genomic changes affect gene expression or protein function, or if they are necessarily conserved in affected family members, is not yet known.

As alluded to already, although the role of specific genetic alterations in coordinating AGA phenotypes remains unclear, there is an obvious role for hormones in orchestrating disease onset and progression. The earliest evidence stems from work conducted in the 1940s, with the observation that castrated men deprived of testosterone rarely developed AGA.[38,39] More recent studies clarified the specific role of testosterone derivative dihydrotestosterone (DHT) and subsequently the utility of finasteride as therapy, which blocks the manufacture of DHT and slows disease progression.[40-42] Additional studies support a link between hormones and AGA by noting a decreased incidence of AGA in male patients with AR mutations that limit receptor functionality and an increased incidence of AGA in female patients with androgen-secreting tumors or in women exposed to extraneous testosterone.[43-45] Of note, patterned hair loss is infrequently a presenting symptom of polycystic ovarian syndrome (PCOS) despite the role of hyperandrogenism in PCOS pathogenesis; together with one case report of a female patient with androgen insensitivity syndrome who did develop AGA, these few studies suggest that FPHL at least is not always androgen-dependent.[46,47]

Finally, aside from the established power of inheritance and hormones, a number of studies have identified putative risk factors that appear to increase the likelihood of AGA development in patients not inherently predisposed to baldness. Identified and modifiable factors include smoking, hyperlipidemia, excessive alcohol consumption, increased body mass, and decreased serum ferritin.[48-51] Although the associations between these activities and hair loss are not yet robustly proved or widely accepted, a conscientious healthcare provider could offer risk reduction of AGA progression as a possible incentive for patients to consider managing these otherwise harmful behaviors.

As many common dermatologic presentations reflect systemic disease, a controversial idea in AGA literature proposes that MPHL is associated with other conditions related to hormonal imbalances.

For example, discrete studies have independently found that heart disease, hypertension, prostate cancer, diabetes, and metabolic syndrome are associated with an increased incidence of AGA.[24,48,52-57] If these associations are valid and significant, providers might think to screen balding male patients earlier for any of these common diseases. It is equally important to consider how any of these conditions could be affected by systemic medication that men take for their hair loss. Notably, a recent large-scale GWAS that incorporated data from over 50,000 European men failed to find any correlation between symptoms of AGA and other systemic diseases, so these questionable associations are still open to investigation.[58]

MANAGEMENT: DIAGNOSIS AND DIFFERENTIAL

A diagnosis of AGA is usually made based on a patient's history and appearance. Typical symptoms include pattern hair loss that is slowly progressive, starting for many patients around or after age 30 years. In addition, a patient's history should lack specific details that would indicate a more inflammatory nature to the hair loss, notably, a sudden loss of many hairs, ongoing scalp pain, itching, or redness. A history of habitual hair plucking or hair trauma, such as restrictive and/or chemically damaging styling practices, should be assessed and absent. A family history of baldness is likely to be positive for patients with AGA but is generally a common finding and unlikely to sway any differential.

In classic cases of AGA (Fig. 5.2)—the majority of presenting patients—a diagnosis can be made with history and physical examination alone, and no additional laboratory testing is needed. However, in select cases additional tests could be warranted to rule out underlying, modifiable, or other reversible causes of hair loss. For example, additional workup could be justified for an exceptionally young patient presenting with a stereotypical pattern of hair loss but without a strong family history of premature baldness or for a patient describing a relatively rapid and/or diffuse decrease in hair density. Screening tests to assess for iron stores or other vitamin deficiencies are important, along with an assessment of hormonal ratios and thyroid function (Table 5.1). Additional tests for syphilis or autoimmune disease are important for at-risk patients.[59] Finally, a thorough medication history is crucial to

TABLE 5.1
Screening Tests to Order in a Patient Presenting With Alopecia and Features Atypical for Androgenetic Alopecia

Irregularity	Tests to Order
Iron status	Iron, ferritin, TIBC
Hormone balance	Testosterone, DHEAS, FSH, LH
Vitamin deficiency	B6, B12, vitamin D
Thyroid dysfunction	TSH, T3, T4
Syphilis	VDRL
SLE	ANA, anti-dsDNA/Sm, C3/C4

ANA, antinuclear antibody; *DHEAS*, dehydroepiandrosterone sulphate; *FSH*, follicle stimulating hormone; *LH*, luteinizing hormone; *SLE*, systemic lupus erythematosus; *TIBC*, total iron-binding capacity; *TSH*, thyroid stimulating hormone; *VDRL*, venereal disease research laboratory.

TABLE 5.2
Common Medications With Alopecia as a Potential Side Effect

Medications That Can Cause Alopecia	Medication Indication
Valproic acid, Phenytoin, Carbamazepine	Seizure Disorder
Chemotherapy	Cancer
Retinoids (acitretin, isotretinoin)	Acne
β-blockers (i.e., propranolol)	Hypertension
Anticoagulants (i.e., heparin)	Clotting prophylaxis

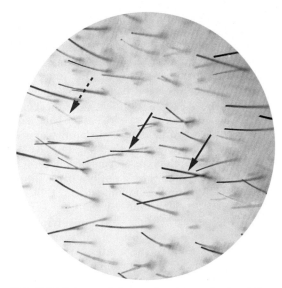

FIG. 5.3 Trichoscopic image of androgenetic alopecia scalp demonstrating hair shaft diameter diversity (*arrows*), including the presence of thin, less-pigmented vellus hairs (*dotted arrow*).

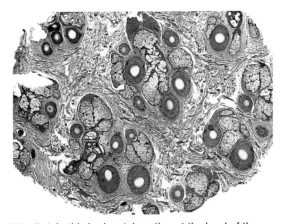

FIG. 5.4 In this horizontal section at the level of the isthmus, there is preserved follicular architecture (10 follicular units) with decreased follicular density (total of 25 follicles) and decreased terminal:vellus ratio of 1.4:1. The vellus follicles are the ones with thin hair shafts (thinner than 0.03 mm) compared with the terminal follicles (hematoxylin and eosin ×4). (Image courtesy of Mariya Miteva.)

ensure new-onset alopecia is not secondary to drug exposure (Table 5.2).

Other modalities for assessing hair loss include the hair pull test, which is generally negative in patients with AGA.[59] Trichoscopy will reveal hair diameter diversity and fewer hair shafts per follicular unit (Fig. 5.3).[60] Although a scalp biopsy is generally not necessary for a patient with classic AGA, histopathologic analysis is contributory for more subtle cases and would reveal a normal number of follicular units, but with an increased presence of small, miniaturized vellus hairs and increased telogen resting hairs (Fig. 5.4).[10,61] Other specific observations include the presence of "fibrous streamers" trailing from follicle bulbs, which is distinct from the extensive fibrosis that might be seen in biopsies from scarring alopecia.[62]

As mentioned before, although AGA is considered a noninflammatory alopecia, perifollicular immune infiltrates are not uncommon in affected scalp.[10] However, this infiltrate is mild, periinfundibular, and greatly diminished when compared with that seen in a classic autoimmune-mediated disease, such as alopecia areata (AA).

A differential diagnosis for patients with suspected AGA must include diffuse AA, another common cause of nonscarring hair loss. However, AA is typically characterized by more rapid hair loss in either discrete, annular patches or diffusely over the entire scalp. "Exclamation point" or short, broken hair shafts might be detected. Symptoms of scalp burning or itching might precede appreciable shedding, as is typical for an inflammatory alopecia. AA patients subjected to additional testing will display a positive hair pull test result and robust perifollicular infiltrates upon biopsy inspection. Telogen effluvium, yet another common cause of nonscarring hair loss, will similarly present with rapid and diffuse hair loss but will typically follow an inciting stressful event or disease. Unlike AGA, patients with acute telogen effluvium will have a positive hair pull test result. Biopsies reveal an increased percentage of hairs in telogen, as in AGA, but without evidence of follicular miniaturization or inflammatory infiltrates. Thyroid dysfunction commonly incurs changes in hair density and texture; once again, the changes are more likely to be diffuse than patterned, and a patient is likely to describe additional symptoms, such as changes in subjective temperature regulation or weight. Finally, in women presenting with early FPHL and no family history, it might be warranted to rule out an underlying virilizing disorder. However, these patients are much more likely to present with other manifestations of hyperandrogenism, such as menstrual irregularities, acne, or hirsutism, before reporting patterned baldness.

MANAGEMENT: PREVENTION, TREATMENT, MECHANISMS OF ACTION, AND PROGNOSIS

For both men and women patients with AGA, the first-line pharmacologic recommendation is topical **minoxidil**, proved by numerous randomized, double-blind, and case-control studies, to slow hair loss in AGA compared with a placebo treatment.[63–66] Originally developed as an antihypertensive medication, the mechanism of action behind its hair growth–stimulating effect is still unknown (Table 5.3). Some have suggested vasodilatory effects promote hair retention, whereas others have demonstrated an increased percentage of anagen follicles in treated AGA scalp (possibly also secondary to scalp vessel vasodilation).[67] Careful analysis failed to demonstrate that regular minoxidil application converts vellus hairs back into terminal hairs, indicating that the medication is most helpful in staving off additional hair loss after AGA is diagnosed.[68] Besides its widespread and long-standing use with notably few adverse effects, the greatest advantage of minoxidil is its topical availability. Currently available formulations include 2% and 5% solutions, in addition to 5% foam, and specific formulations have been approved

TABLE 5.3
Commonly Prescribed Therapies for AGA

Medication	Route	Dose	MOA	Adverse Effects
Minoxidil	Topical	2% or 5% solution; 5% foam BID	Unknown; vasodilation	Dermatitis, hypertrichosis
Finasteride	Oral	1 mg once daily	5-Alpha-reductase II inhibition	Decreased libido, erectile dysfunction
Dutasteride	Oral	0.5 mg once daily (off-label)	5-Alpha-reductase I/II inhibition	Sexual dysfunction
Spironolactone	Oral	50–200 mg daily (off-label)	Testosterone antagonism	Hyperkalemia, teratogenicity
Hair transplant	Procedure	n/a	Follicle relocation	Expense, disease progression
LLLT	Procedure	Variable	Unknown	Minimal; dermatitis
PRP	Procedure	Variable	Unknown; platelet secreted factors	Injection site irritation

AGA, androgenetic alopecia; *LLLT,* low-level light therapy; *MOA,* mechanism of action; *PRP,* platelet-rich plasma.

by Food and Drug Administration (FDA) for treatment of both MPHL and FPHL since 1991. The rare adverse events that occur with topical minoxidil are typically dry, peeling, or itchy skin; most often indicating dermatitis related to the solution vehicle rather than the active ingredient. Besides the caveat that minoxidil must be used indefinitely to maintain an effect, the only other substantial downside is the potential for off-target effects. It is prudent to warn patients that the applied solution could inadvertently move to an area of the face or neck where one does not desire hair growth and promote the development of unwanted terminal hairs. This is particularly possible when patients apply the solution just prior to sleeping. Patients might also appreciate a warning that a transitory increase in hair shedding upon drug initiation is to be expected and that it will resolve after a few weeks of consistent use.

Since the late 1990s, **finasteride** has been an equally popular FDA-approved solution to treat AGA in men (Table 5.3). The medication is taken as 1 mg orally daily and works as a 5-alpha-reductase type II inhibitor to decrease the conversion of testosterone to its potent metabolite DHT. This medication must also be taken continuously and works best when started early to prevent progressive hair loss, although some studies have rigorously shown an increase in hair follicle diameter and percentage of scalp hairs in anagen after drug initiation, suggesting affected follicles can be restored to a slight degree.[16,40,69] Studies have alternatingly reported more impressive results in patients using either minoxidil or finasteride, without a clear winner, with all outcomes consistently better in treatment arms versus placebo.[70–72] The most feared side effect is the risk of sexual dysfunction, which was notably irreversible despite drug discontinuation in a few alarming yet contested reports.[73–75] In this regard, postfinasteride syndrome (PFS) is a term recently coined to characterize a constellation of reported undesirable side effects described in postmarketing reports and small uncontrolled studies that developed during or after stopping finasteride treatment and persisted after drug discontinuation.[76] The syndrome was included in the National Institute of Health's Genetic and Rare Diseases Information Center (GARD) even though inclusion in the GARD is not an official recognition of PFS by the NIH as explained in the website disclaimer.[76] Symptoms include decreased libido, erectile dysfunction, sexual anhedonia, decreased sperm count, gynecomastia, skin changes, cognitive impairment, fatigue, anxiety, depression, and suicidal ideation. Decreased libido, ejaculatory failure, and erectile dysfunction were also shown in

a meta-analysis of over 3500 patients to be significantly more frequent in patients on finasteride, with an estimated 1 in 80 patients reporting erectile dysfunction.[69] However, patients informed of the potential sexual side effects of the drug reported a significant higher proportion of sexual side effects (43.6%) as compared to those who were not informed (15.3%).[77] As per current evidence, persistent sexual and psychiatric side effects after using 5-alpha-reductase inhibitors are not documented by high-quality studies, and prospective studies to establish true incidence and frequency are needed. In addition, a controversial perspective warns about an increased risk of delayed detection of high-grade prostate cancer in patients taking finasteride, although a causal link has not been definitively established.[78] Finasteride treatment for FPHL is similarly controversial, with literature suggesting both its utility and futility in select subpopulations of female patients; additional well-designed trials are warranted to reveal its true efficacy or relevance.[79–81] Specific adverse side effects in women include the established teratogenicity of finasteride—women of childbearing age must use birth control concomitantly—and a theoretical increased risk of breast cancer.[67]

Dutasteride is another 5-alpha-reductase inhibitor that uniquely blocks both type I and II isoforms of the target enzyme and has a long half-life of 4 weeks (Table 5.3). Although several small randomized clinical trials have proved that dutasteride effectively prevents disease progression in AGA scalp by increasing hair counts or thickness, at a degree similar to or slightly better than finasteride, it has only been approved for treatment of MPHL in a few countries. Its effectiveness has been demonstrated in a dose-dependent fashion with high dosage (up to 2.5 mg daily) and the standard dose used to treat benign prostatic hyperplasia (0.5 mg daily); adverse effects are notably similar to those for finasteride, including sexual dysfunction and decreased libido, the risk of which also increases along with dose.[82–84] It is not approved by the FDA for treatment of AGA.

Spironolactone is another hormone modulator and off-label option to address hair loss, prescribed most frequently to female patients at 50–200 mg once daily (Table 5.3). In off-target effects, it inhibits signaling through the AR and decreases testosterone levels with minimal side effects; although physicians reflexively regularly monitor for the rare potential side effects of hyperkalemia, recent evidence suggests the practice is overzealous.[11,85] Spironolactone does not seem to work for all women, with only 40% reporting improved hair regrowth in an open-label study,[11] but represents a low-risk option to try in willing and patient patients; experts recommend starting with a low dose and gradually increasing up to 200 mg daily for at least a 6-month trial before determining efficacy.[86] Because of its broad antitestosterone activity, it is a teratogen and must also be taken with strict contraception.

Aside from the most popular pharmacologic treatments for AGA, several advanced procedural techniques are gaining popularity for both MPHL and FPHL as methods become increasingly refined. Hair transplantation performed using individual follicular unit transplantation has greatly improved cosmetic outcomes compared to earlier en bloc haired skin relocation surgeries.[87] Although the results following hair transplantation can be sudden and impressive, not all patients are appropriate candidates and it is important to establish realistic patient expectations prior to surgery; for example, following transplantation there is a risk of reoccurring hair loss, because follicles continue to be affected by unchanged genetic or hormonal forces. The frustration of ongoing AGA progression is compounded by the great out-of-pocket expense this procedure presents for most patients. Patients are typically counseled not to expect a surgery that restores a head of hair from their youth; rather the goal is merely to improve their hairline to a realistic extent. Patients are also frequently counseled to use minoxidil or finasteride as adjuvants to slow additional disease progression in the peri- and post-operative time.

Low-level light therapy (LLLT) is another alternative modality for addressing AGA and while clinical trials are in process, several devices are commercially available and some even already FDA-approved for home use.[67,88] Light stimulation was proposed as a treatment for alopecia years ago, but only recent studies have been conducted to support its use. It involves the application of specific wavelengths of light to the scalp for various amounts of time and/or numbers of sessions per week; the specifics vary by trial. One benefit of LLLT is that it causes very few side effects. In addition, although the cost to obtain a device could at first seem prohibitive, a one-time purchase might actually be economical compared to the life-long refills needed to sustain a scalp dependent on minoxidil or finasteride. Although randomized controlled studies and comprehensive meta-analyses have determined that use of LLLT devices can increase the amount and thickness of hair in a patient with AGA to a statistically significant extent, the mechanism of action behind its efficacy remains a mystery. Proposed explanations include vasodilation, cytokine release, and stimulation of follicles to reenter or spend more time in the anagen growth phase. Given the relatively modest treatment effects, potentially the best way to use this device for now is as an adjuvant to other systemic therapies.

A more experimental new therapy gaining traction is the injection of platelet-rich plasma into AGA scalp, which randomized, case-controlled studies have revealed to be partially effective in treating symptoms of hair loss through an unclear mechanism.[89,90] The therapy entails intradermal injections of plasma enriched with a patient's own platelets at superphysiologic concentrations. In vitro, activated platelets make and release a cocktail of cytokines and growth factors, which in turn have been implicated in promoting hair stem cell growth and/or sustaining the hair follicle stem cell niche, including mesenchymal and immune cells. Whether a single injection is enough or multiple injections would be needed as part of an extended treatment plan remains to be determined. Additional studies to establish the exact contents of platelet-rich plasma, which are currently unregulated and differ between clinical trials, are important before this therapy could be considered ready for mainstream use.

RESEARCH RELATED TO AGA PATHOGENESIS, MECHANISMS OF DISEASE, AND PROPOSED AREAS OF TREATMENT

Genetic/Genomic Targets

Many different approaches have attempted to untangle the polygenic mechanisms of hair loss. Nonhypothesis-driven studies, such as the microarray or GWASs, provide insight into transcriptional or genomic differences, respectively, between balding and nonbalding scalp as a first step to unveiling molecular differences that could be functionally significant. The GWAS method involves interrogating DNA for minute coding differences (single nucleotide polymorphisms [SNPs]) at established loci and associating specific base-pair patterns with externally recognizable phenotypes, such as degree of baldness.

One meta-analysis of early GWAS data was the first to recognize that genomic changes in the vicinity of the AR gene were consistently flagged in multiple studies assessing differences between genomes of balding and fully haired individuals.[91] This meta-study drew power from the number of primary studies analyzed; seven studies, inclusive of over 12,000 patients of European ancestry, were incorporated into the final data. A separate recent study procured original samples and used previously generated GWAS data to ask which of the formerly identified SNPs were significantly associated with baldness in their newly sampled population.[92] Of 50 SNPs investigated, 29 remained associated in a population of over 600 healthy male European donors, and a subset was used to construct a model of phenotype prediction from genotypic input. More recently, primary studies have been incorporating increasing numbers of subjects into their analyses; a GWAS published in 2016 incorporated data from over 6000 Latin American subjects.[93] Although the purpose of this study was to broadly identify genomic loci associated with a variety of hair traits, it managed to highlight again the significance of genomic changes near the *AR* gene associated with baldness in addition to recognizing *GRID1*, a new potential gene of interest tied to a hair loss phenotype. Finally, an enormous primary GWAS published in 2017 incorporated data from over 50,000 European patients and subsequently found over 200 loci significantly associated with baldness.[58] These data were also used to build a polygenic prediction score that was particularly sensitive to identifying patients likely to suffer severe hair loss.

Other studies have used methods such as microarray or RNA-sequencing to assess genetic differences between case and control scalp on a transcriptional level. Investigations of the *AR* gene relationship to AGA progression found that the receptor is expressed in the dermal papilla (DP) of hair follicles and differentially expressed between DP cells from balding versus nonbalding scalp. Furthermore, immortalized DP cell lines from case and control scalp differentially respond to DHT stimulation as assessed by microarray.[94,95] In one example utilizing next-generation sequencing, hair follicle bulbs from balding and nonbalding vertex and occipital scalp were isolated to simultaneously assess gene expression differences between cases and controls, based on scalp position.[96] Antioxidant genes were distinctly upregulated in balding vertex follicles, suggesting oxidative stress as a potential underlying mechanism of disease. Although this study represents major progress in the goal to understand the molecular basis of balding, and does notably isolate the bulb region of microdissected follicles, future studies will likely improve analysis further by follicle dissociation and cell sorting to analyze cell type–specific gene changes in bald scalp.

Signaling Targets

Fewer studies have taken evidence from these initial, large-scale genetic screening studies to explore the mechanisms by which specific signaling pathways or proteins promote or mitigate AGA progression. Notably, investigations of prostaglandins and hair growth are relatively new and exciting in that the work presents a potential area for therapeutic intervention. Comparing gene expression in balding versus haired scalp of individual patients revealed upregulation of prostaglandin synthase concomitantly with increased production of prostaglandin D2 (*PGD2*).[97] Subsequent animal studies recognized physiologic PGD2 upregulation immediately before the destructive phase of murine hair cycle, providing evidence for its role as an antigrowth signal, and further demonstrated the importance of the GPR44 receptor in mediating the effects of PGD2. Furthermore, exogenous PGD2 impeded wound healing and hair follicle neogenesis in mice.[98] Specific investigations of human hair from other groups later verified that factors related to this pathway are genetically distinct in bald compared with haired scalp.[96,99,100] The logical next hurdle is to develop an antagonist that reduces PGD2 signaling in human scalp and test its ability to prevent hair loss in AGA; and indeed, clinical trials for PGD2 receptor antagonist setipiprant are currently in progress. Of note, the prostaglandin PGF2A analog bimatoprost, which works by increasing the time follicles spend in the anagen growth phase, is widely used for promoting eyelash growth but has yet to be established as a terminal hair promoter in the scalp although clinical trials are also currently underway.

Wnt signaling has been extensively studied as a key player in the context of hair development, growth, and cycling, and recent studies have questioned if signaling through this conserved pathway could be relevant for human hair loss and AGA as well. One early study found *DKK1*, a Wnt signaling inhibitor, upregulated in bald compared with control scalp.[101] The secreted factor was specifically expressed from DP cells after treatment with DHT and inhibited growth of hair follicle epithelial cells in vitro. A separate study confirmed that an SNP genotype associated with *WNT10A* conferred increased AGA risk, potentially by decreasing production of this Wnt ligand.[36] There is additional evidence for a reciprocal interaction between androgen and Wnt signaling in both human and mouse tissue, as downstream components of both pathways compete for similar nuclear response elements.[102] The key to reversing AGA progression could thus lie in simultaneous androgen inhibition and Wnt stimulation. Notably, topical application of Wnt signaling activator, methyl vanillate, did increase hair count and scalp *WNT10B* mRNA in women with AGA (who were not permitted to simultaneously use androgen- or progesterone-modifying therapies over the duration of the trial).[103]

Independent studies have assessed a potential role of oxidative stress in hampering robust hair follicle maintenance. At least in culture, exposing DP cells to conditions with increased oxidative stress significantly decreases cell viability, increases senescence, and induces secretion of antigrowth factors; meanwhile, investigation of human biopsies revealed increased oxidative stress in balding compared with occipital scalp.[96,104] Finally, fascinating studies of fibroblast growth factor FGF5 have firmly implicated FGF signaling in controlling onset and duration of the anagen stage of the hair cycle; families with inherited inactivating mutations have individuals with markedly long terminal hairs.[105] Congruently, multiple animal species with impaired FGF5 expression or activity display an angora or long-haired phenotype. Although a relation to AGA onset or progression has yet to be determined, inhibiting FGF5 signaling certainly represents an attractive target to enhance anagen proclivity in hair follicles susceptible to AGA progression.

Finally, very exciting new data and opportunities for therapeutic intervention stem from the recent discovery that JAK-STAT inhibitors revitalize hair growth in patients with AA, presumably by interfering with immune cell–mediated follicular destruction and possibly by directly stimulating follicle regeneration and promoting anagen progression.[103,104] The results in AA patients are dramatic, and although immune cell infiltrates in AGA scalp are scant, these medications will likely be tested in MPHL once safety and dosage guidelines are clearly established.

Cell Therapy

Epithelial stem cells are crucial for hair follicle formation and maintenance and represent a fascinating model system for understanding adult stem cell organization and activation. In mature follicles, stem cells reside in a protected "bulge" area. They are periodically activated to proliferate and generate transit amplifying progenitors, which subsequently differentiate into the molecularly and functionally distinct layers comprising a complete hair follicle capable of producing a terminal hair shaft. In AGA, when follicles are no longer able to produce robust hair shafts, it seems logical to wonder if the all-important stem cells might be functionally compromised.

Importantly, histologic and fluorescence-activated cell sorting analysis of follicles within balding scalp revealed intact stem cell numbers, localization, and relatively unchanged signature gene expression.[106,107] However, the same reassuring observations could not be made for their progeny, the transit amplifying progenitor cells, whose presence was markedly decreased in balding scalp. This concludes that although stem cells are present in AGA-affected follicles, deficiencies in their activation and downstream differentiation likely contribute to a bald phenotype. The potential for therapeutic intervention is clear, as follicles in AGA scalp retaining their dormant stem cells could be rejuvenated once the appropriate activating signals are elucidated.

In addition to the warranted concern for stem cell viability in preserving hair follicle functionality, many studies focus on DP cells as another key target for follicle rejuvenation. These mesenchymal cells reside toward the bottom of the hair follicle bulb and interact with neighboring epithelial progenitor cells to promote follicle growth, maintenance, and hair shaft production. As DP cells are considered a crucial part of the equation to establish and maintain healthy follicles, the observation that follicles in AGA-affected scalp contain fewer DP and related dermal sheath cells could represent either a notable cause or an effect of follicle deterioration.[6] In addition, the remaining DP cells in balding scalp display distinct protein expression profiles and respond differently to secreted signal stimuli (as discussed earlier), but the question of how to reverse these genetic alterations is less clear. Several studies have noted improved DP cell survival, signature gene expression, and hair inducibility when these cells are grown in spheroid cultures.[108] Attempts to "reprogram" ailing DP cells by reintroducing lost signature transcription factors are also ongoing and very exciting as genomic manipulation becomes increasingly facile.

Morphologically, haired and bald scalp differ in that AGA scalp contains follicles with degenerating arrector pili muscles and sebaceous gland enlargement and multilobulation, changes that are not necessarily observed in histologic sections from patients suffering from different causes of alopecia.[109,110] Although the significance of these observations is unclear, especially whether changes occur as a cause or an effect of AGA progression, they present other cellular targets for putative future therapeutic intervention.[111,112] Exciting ongoing clinical trials are separately harvesting epithelial, dermal, or adipose progenitor cells and testing the effects of their transplantation or implantation on reviving stalled hair growth and/or prompting new follicle generation.

Animal Models of Human Androgenetic Alopecia

Although it is most relevant to examine samples from human scalp in efforts to understand AGA pathogenesis, it is not always easy to obtain samples from otherwise relatively healthy individuals or to account for the many confounding conditions or medications that human subjects are exposed to with unknown effects on hair loss. To rigorously study AGA progression in a more controlled setting, a few laboratories have turned to animal models of disease.[113] So far, the stump-tailed macaque is the only animal noted to suffer hair loss in a similar pattern and time frame as humans and was used in the earliest trials of pharmacologic intervention for AGA progression.[114] Now, one engineered mouse model harnesses the power of excessive androgen signaling to impede hair regrowth. When the human *AR* gene is transgenically overexpressed in mouse epithelial cells and animals exposed to exogenous DHT, hair regrowth is inhibited, following depilation.[115]

Another mouse model used to study molecular mechanisms of hair regrowth in general entails wound-induced hair neogenesis (WIHN). This method follows from the observation that large-enough wounds incurred in mouse back skin will heal and sprout new hair follicles, seemingly recapitulating what occurs during skin and hair morphogenesis.[116] The promise of WIHN as a technique to revive follicle activity or create nascent active follicles has yet to be explored in the human scalp, but studies are ongoing to understand the molecular forces behind the phenomenon; notably, Wnt/beta-catenin signaling has been implicated in animal studies.[117] Interestingly, applying PGD2 (the prostaglandin overrepresented in AGA scalp discussed earlier) impeded hair neogenesis in this model system, suggesting the applicability of WIHN for testing other signals capable of inhibiting or promoting follicular regrowth.[98]

CONCLUSIONS

It is remarkable that the pathogenesis and progression of AGA remains such a conundrum in light of how many patients are affected and the massive public and commercial interest in developing a cure. Although the role of hormone involvement is undeniable and the most popular medications used to treat progressive hair loss have been successful as long-term therapy, they are minimally effective in reversing the disease. Ongoing efforts to clarify the molecular and cellular aberrancies

in AGA-affected scalp are crucial for the development of new and improved treatment options, especially as therapeutic genetic manipulation becomes a reality. Going forward, progress is likely to depend on increasing the precision of tissue collection and analysis, as skin is a uniquely heterogeneous organ and sample collection in the form of a punch biopsy encompasses a diverse mix of epithelial, dermal, vascular, and immune cells, among others. Aberrant gene expression in only one cell type could be the culprit behind an AGA phenotype but has so far been undetectable because of a high noise-to-signal ratio when gene expression of the tissue is interrogated as a whole. Isolating and separately analyzing cell types from control versus affected tissue will be one key to uncovering new targets for focused pharmacologic intervention. Furthermore, a diagnosis of AGA encompasses a range of phenotypes with variable progression. Parsing out the molecular changes unique to distinct patterns of balding—temporal, vertex, frontal, male, female—could be more straightforward than the hunt for a single gene mediating all androgenetic forms of hair loss. Finally, studies are specifically needed to understand balding in discrete patient populations, as we face a dearth of data regarding AGA in individuals other than males of European descent. And ultimately, translating the powerful insights gained from such large-scale and inclusive population studies to something relevant for personalized medicine—for example, being able to predict an individual's disease progression or response to a certain therapeutic approach—will be crucial for delivering the most effective patient care.

REFERENCES

1. Norwood OT. Male pattern baldness: classification and incidence. *South Med J*. 1975.
2. Hamilton JB. Patterned loss of hair in man; types and incidence. *Ann N Y Acad Sci*. 1951;53(3):708–728.
3. Ludwig E. Classification of the types of androgenetic alopecia (common baldness) occurring in the female sex. *Br J Dermatol*. 1977;97(3):247–254.
4. Sinclair R, Torkamani N, Jones L. Androgenetic alopecia: new insights into the pathogenesis and mechanism of hair loss. *F1000research*. 2015;4(F1000 Faculty Rev).
5. Rebora A. Pathogenesis of androgenetic alopecia. *J Am Acad Dermatol*. 2004;50(5):777–779.
6. Whiting D. Possible mechanisms of miniaturization during androgenetic alopecia or pattern hair loss. *J Am Acad Dermatol*. 2001;45(3):S81–S86.
7. Templeton SF, Solomon AR. Scarring alopecia: a classification based on microscopic criteria. *J Cutan Pathol*. 1994;21(2):97–109.

8. Jaworsky C, Kligman AM, Murphy GF. Characterization of inflammatory infiltrates in male pattern alopecia: implications for pathogenesis. *Br J Dermatol.* 1992;127(3):239–246.

9. Lattanand A, Johnson WC. Male pattern alopecia a histopathologic and histochemical study. *J Cutan Pathol.* 1975;2(2):58–70.

10. Whiting D. Diagnostic and predictive value of horizontal sections of scalp biopsy specimens in male pattern androgenetic alopecia. *J Am Acad Dermatol.* 1993;28(5 Pt 1):755–763.

11. Sinclair R, Wewerinke M, Jolley D. Treatment of female pattern hair loss with oral antiandrogens. *Br J Dermatol.* 2005;152(3):466–473.

12. Whiting DA. Scalp biopsy as a diagnostic and prognostic tool in androgenetic alopecia. *Dermatol Ther.* 1998;8: 24–33.

13. Oh J, Kloepper J, Langan E, et al. A guide to studying human hair follicle cycling in vivo. *J Invest Dermatol.* 2016;136(1):34–44.

14. Shapiro J. Clinical practice. Hair loss in women. *N Engl J Med.* 2007;357(16):1620–1630.

15. Courtois M, Loussouarn G, Hourseau C, Grollier JF. Hair cycle and alopecia. *Skin Pharmacol.* 1994;7(1–2):84–89.

16. Neste D, Fuh V, Sanchez-Pedreno P, et al. Finasteride increases anagen hair in men with androgenetic alopecia. *Br J Dermatol.* 2000;143(4):804–810.

17. Gan DCC, Sinclair RD. Prevalence of male and female pattern hair loss in Maryborough. *J Investig Dermatol Symp Proc.* 2005;10(3):184–189.

18. Rhodes T, Girman CJ, Savin RC, et al. Prevalence of male pattern hair loss in 18–49 year old men. *Dermatol Surg.* 1998;24(12):1330–1332.

19. Norwood O. Incidence of female androgenetic alopecia (female pattern alopecia). *Dermatol Surg.* 2001;27(1): 53–54.

20. Birch MP, Messenger JF, Messenger AG. Hair density, hair diameter and the prevalence of female pattern hair loss. *Br J Dermatol.* 2001;144(2):297–304.

21. Wang TL, Zhou C, Shen YW, et al. Prevalence of androgenetic alopecia in China: a community-based study in six cities. *Br J Dermatol.* 2010;162(4):843–847.

22. Paik J, Yoon J, Sim W, Kim B, Kim N. The prevalence and types of androgenetic alopecia in Korean men and women. *Br J Dermatol.* 2001;145(1):95–99.

23. Setty LR. Hair patterns of scalp of white and Negro males. *Am J Phys Anthropol.* 1970;33(1):49–55.

24. Zeigler-Johnson C, Morales KH, Spangler E, Chang B-LL, Rebbeck TR. Relationship of early-onset baldness to prostate cancer in African-American men. *Cancer Epidemiol Biomarkers Prev.* 2013;22(4):589–596.

25. Lee W-S, Lee H-J. Characteristics of androgenetic alopecia in asian. *Ann Dermatol.* 2012;24(3):243–252.

26. Bas Y, Seckin HY, Kalkan G, et al. Prevalence and types of androgenetic alopecia in north Anatolian population: a community-based study. *J Pak Med Assoc.* 2015; 65(8):806–809.

27. Nyholt DR, Gillespie NA, Heath AC, Martin NG. Genetic basis of male pattern baldness. *J Invest Dermatol.* 2003;121(6):1561–1564.

28. Rexbye H, Petersen I, Iachina M, et al. Hair loss among elderly men: etiology and impact on perceived age. *J Gerontol Biol Sci Med Sci.* 2005;60(8):1077–1082.

29. Lee W-S, Oh Y, Ji J, et al. Analysis of familial factors using the basic and specific (BASP) classification in Korean patients with androgenetic alopecia. *J Am Acad Dermatol.* 2011;65(1):40–47.

30. Birch MP, Messenger AG. Genetic factors predispose to balding and non-balding in men. *Eur J Dermatol.* 2001.

31. Küster W, Happle R. The inheritance of common baldness: two B or not two B? *J Am Acad Dermatol.* 1984.

32. Ellis JA, Stebbing M, Harrap SB. Genetic analysis of male pattern baldness and the 5alpha-reductase genes. *J Invest Dermatol.* 1998;110(6):849–853.

33. Ellis JA, Stebbing M, Harrap SB. Polymorphism of the androgen receptor gene is associated with male pattern baldness. *J Invest Dermatol.* 2001;116(3):452–455.

34. Hillmer A, Hanneken S, Ritzmann S, et al. Genetic variation in the human androgen receptor gene is the major determinant of common early-onset androgenetic alopecia. *Am J Hum Genet.* 2007;77(1):140–148.

35. Prodi D, Pirastu N, Maninchedda G, et al. EDA2R is associated with androgenetic alopecia. *J Invest Dermatol.* 2008;128(9):2268–2270.

36. Heilmann S, Kiefer A, Fricker N, et al. Androgenetic alopecia: identification of four genetic risk loci and evidence for the contribution of WNT signaling to its etiology. *J Invest Dermatol.* 2013;133(6):1489–1496.

37. Sennett R, Rendl M. Mesenchymal–epithelial interactions during hair follicle morphogenesis and cycling. *Semin Cell Dev Biol.* 2012;23(8):917–927.

38. Hamilton J. Male hormone stimulation is prerequisite and an incitant in common baldness. *Am J Anat.* 1942.

39. Ayob S, Messenger A. Androgens, hair loss and eugenics: a tale of discovery and American social history. *Exp Dermatol.* 2015;24(6):412–413.

40. Kaufman KD, Olsen EA, Whiting D, et al. Finasteride in the treatment of men with androgenetic alopecia. Finasteride male pattern hair loss study group. *J Am Acad Dermatol.* 1998;39(4 Pt 1):578–589.

41. Dallob AL, Sadick NS, Unger W, et al. The effect of finasteride, a 5 alpha-reductase inhibitor, on scalp skin testosterone and dihydrotestosterone concentrations in patients with male pattern baldness. *J Clin Endocrinol Metab.* 1994;79(3):703–706.

42. Ellis J, Sinclair R, Harrap S. Androgenetic alopecia: pathogenesis and potential for therapy. *Expert Rev Mol Med.* 2002;4(22):1–11.

43. Sinclair R, Greenland KJ, Egmond S, Hoedemaker C, Chapman A, Zajac JD. Men with Kennedy disease have a reduced risk of androgenetic alopecia. *Br J Dermatol.* 2007;157(2):290–294.

44. Rivera-Arkoncel M, Pacquing-Songco D, Lantion-Ang F. Virilising ovarian tumour in a woman with an adrenal nodule. *BMJ Case Rep.* 2010;2010:bcr0720103139.

45. Lattouf C, Miteva M, Tosti A. Connubial androgenetic alopecia. *Arch Dermatol.* 2011;147(11):1329–1330.

46. Carmina E, Rosato F, Jannì A, Rizzo M, Longo RA. Relative prevalence of different androgen excess disorders in 950 women referred because of clinical hyperandrogenism. *J Clin Endocrinol Metab.* 2006;91(1):2–6.

47. Cousen P, Messenger A. Female pattern hair loss in complete androgen insensitivity syndrome. *Br J Dermatol.* 2010;162(5):1135–1137.

48. Su L, Chen TH. Association of androgenetic alopecia with metabolic syndrome in men: a community-based survey. *Br J Dermatol.* 2010;163(2):371–377.

49. Su L-HH, Chen TH. Association of androgenetic alopecia with smoking and its prevalence among Asian men: a community-based survey. *Arch Dermatol.* 2007;143(11):1401–1406.

50. Severi G, Sinclair R, Hopper JL, et al. Androgenetic alopecia in men aged 40–69 years: prevalence and risk factors. *Br J Dermatol.* 2003;149(6):1207–1213.

51. Kantor J, Kessler LJ, Brooks DG, Cotsarelis G. Decreased serum ferritin is associated with alopecia in women. *J Invest Dermatol.* 2003.

52. Su L-H, Chen L-S, Lin S-C, Chen H-H. Association of androgenetic alopecia with mortality from diabetes mellitus and heart disease. *JAMA Dermatol.* 2013;149(5):601–606.

53. Matilainen VA, Mäkinen PK, Keinänen-Kiukaanniemi SM. Early onset of androgenetic alopecia associated with early severe coronary heart disease: a population-based, case-control study. *J Cardiovasc Risk.* 2001;8(3):147–151.

54. Ahouansou S, Le Toumelin P, Crickx B, Descamps V. Association of androgenetic alopecia and hypertension. *Eur J Dermatol.* 2007;17(3):220–222.

55. Arias-Santiago S, Gutiérrez-Salmerón M, Castellote-Caballero L, Buendía-Eisman A, Naranjo-Sintes R. Androgenetic alopecia and cardiovascular risk factors in men and women: a comparative study. *J Am Acad Dermatol.* 2010;63(3):420–429.

56. Rebora A. Baldness and coronary artery disease: the dermatologic point of view of a controversial issue. *Arch Dermatol.* 2001;137(7):943–947.

57. Matilainen V, Koskela P, Keinänen-Kiukaanniemi S. Early androgenetic alopecia as a marker of insulin resistance. *Lancet.* 2000;356(9236):1165–1166.

58. Hagenaars S, Hill W, Harris S, et al. Genetic prediction of male pattern baldness. *PLoS Genet.* 2017;13(2):e1006594.

59. Shapiro J, Wiseman M, Lui H. Practical management of hair loss. *Can Fam Physician Médecin De Fam Can.* 2000;46:1469–1477.

60. De Lacharrière O, Deloche C, Misciali C, et al. Hair diameter diversity: a clinical sign reflecting the follicle miniaturization. *Arch Dermatol.* 2001;137(5):641–646.

61. Aslani F, Dastgheib L, Banihashemi B. Hair counts in scalp biopsy of males and females with androgenetic alopecia compared with normal subjects. *J Cutan Pathol.* 2009;36(7):734–739.

62. Horenstein M, Jacob J. Follicular streamers (stelae) in scarring and non-scarring alopecia. *J Cutan Pathol.* 2008;35(12):1115–1120.

63. Van Zuuren EJ, Fedorowicz Z, Schoones J. Interventions for female pattern hair loss. *Cochrane Database Syst Rev.* 2016;(5):CD007628.

64. Blumeyer A, Tosti A, Messenger A, et al. Evidence-based (S3) guideline for the treatment of androgenetic alopecia in women and in men. *JDDG J der Deutschen Dermatologischen Gesellschaft.* 2011;9(s6):S1–S57.

65. Olsen EA, Whiting D, Bergfeld W, et al. A multicenter, randomized, placebo-controlled, double-blind clinical trial of a novel formulation of 5% minoxidil topical foam versus placebo in the treatment of androgenetic alopecia in men. *J Am Acad Dermatol.* 2007;57(5):767–774.

66. Olsen E, Dunlap F, Funicella T, et al. A randomized clinical trial of 5% topical minoxidil versus 2% topical minoxidil and placebo in the treatment of androgenetic alopecia in men. *J Am Acad Dermatol.* 2002;47(3):377–385.

67. Kelly Y, Blanco A, Tosti A. Androgenetic alopecia: an update of treatment options. *Drugs.* 2016;76(14):1349–1364.

68. Rushton H, Norris M, Neste D. Hair regrowth in male and female pattern hair loss does not involve the conversion of vellus hair to terminal hair. *Exp Dermatol.* 2016;25(6):482–484.

69. Mella JMM, Perret MCC, Manzotti M, Catalano HN, Guyatt G. Efficacy and safety of finasteride therapy for androgenetic alopecia: a systematic review. *Arch Dermatol.* 2010;146(10):1141–1150.

70. Arca E, Açıkgöz G, Taştan HB, Köse O, Kurumlu Z. An open, randomized, comparative study of oral finasteride and 5% topical minoxidil in male androgenetic alopecia. *Dermatology.* 2004;209(2):117–125.

71. Saraswat A, Kumar B. Minoxidil vs finasteride in the treatment of men with androgenetic alopecia. *Arch Dermatol.* 2003;139(9):1219–1221.

72. Khandpur S, Suman M, Reddy B. Comparative efficacy of various treatment regimens for androgenetic alopecia in men. *J Dermatol.* 2002;29(8):489–498.

73. Irwig MS. Androgen levels and semen parameters among former users of finasteride with persistent sexual adverse effects. *JAMA Dermatol.* 2014;150(12):1361–1363.

74. Guo M, Heran B, Flannigan R, Kezouh A, Etminan M. Persistent sexual dysfunction with finasteride 1 mg taken for hair loss. *Pharmacother J Hum Pharmacol Drug Ther.* 2016;36(11):1180–1184.

75. Irwig MS, Kolukula S. Persistent sexual side effects of finasteride for male pattern hair loss. *J Sex Med.* 2011;8(6):1747–1753.

76. Fertig R, Shapiro J, Bergfeld W, Tosti A. Investigation of the plausibility of 5-alpha-reductase inhibitor syndrome. *Ski Appendage Disord.* 2016;2(3–4):120–129.

77. Mondaini N, Gontero P, Giubilei G, et al. Finasteride 5 mg and sexual side effects: how many of these are related to a nocebo phenomenon? *J Sex Med.* 2007;4(6):1708–1712.

78. D'Amico A, Roehrborn C. Effect of 1 mg/day finasteride on concentrations of serum prostate-specific antigen in men with androgenic alopecia: a randomised controlled trial. *Lancet Oncol.* 2007;8(1):21–25.

79. Karimkhani C, Boyers L, Prescott L, et al. Global burden of skin disease as reflected in cochrane database of systematic reviews. *JAMA Dermatol.* 2014;150(9):945–951.

80. Price VH, Roberts JL, Hordinsky M, et al. Lack of efficacy of finasteride in postmenopausal women with androgenetic alopecia. *J Am Acad Dermatol.* 2000;43(5 Pt 1):768–776.

81. Whiting DA, Waldstreicher J, Sanchez M, Kaufman KD. Measuring reversal of hair miniaturization in androgenetic alopecia by follicular counts in horizontal sections of serial scalp biopsies: results of finasteride 1 mg treatment of men and postmenopausal women. *J Invest Dermatol Symp Proc.* 1999;4(3):282–284.

82. Harcha W, Martínez J, Tsai T-F, et al. A randomized, active- and placebo-controlled study of the efficacy and safety of different doses of dutasteride versus placebo and finasteride in the treatment of male subjects with androgenetic alopecia. *J Am Acad Dermatol.* 2014;70(3): 489–498.e3.

83. Olsen EA, Hordinsky M, Whiting D, et al. The importance of dual 5alpha-reductase inhibition in the treatment of male pattern hair loss: results of a randomized placebo-controlled study of dutasteride versus finasteride. *J Am Acad Dermatol.* 2006;55(6):1014–1023.

84. Eun HC, Kwon OS, Yeon JH, et al. Efficacy, safety, and tolerability of dutasteride 0.5 mg once daily in male patients with male pattern hair loss: a randomized, double-blind, placebo-controlled, phase III study. *J Am Acad Dermatol.* 2010;63(2):252–258.

85. Plovanich M, Weng Q, Mostaghimi A. Low usefulness of potassium monitoring among healthy young women taking spironolactone for acne. *JAMA Dermatol.* 2015;151(9):941–944.

86. Camacho-Martínez FM. Hair loss in women. *Semin Cutan Med Surg.* 2009.

87. Avram M, Rogers N. Contemporary hair transplantation. *Dermatol Surg.* 2009;35(11):1705.

88. Afifi L, Maranda EL, Zarei M, et al. Low-level laser therapy as a treatment for androgenetic alopecia. *Lasers Surg Med.* 2017;49(1):27–39.

89. Schiavone G, Raskovic D, Greco J, Abeni D. Platelet-rich plasma for androgenetic alopecia: a pilot study. *Dermatol Surg.* 2014;40(9):1010.

90. Alves R, Grimalt R. Randomized placebo-controlled, double-blind, half-head study to assess the efficacy of platelet-rich plasma on the treatment of androgenetic alopecia. *Dermatol Surg.* 2016;42(4):491.

91. Li R, Brockschmidt F, Kiefer A, et al. Six novel susceptibility loci for early-onset androgenetic alopecia and their unexpected association with common diseases. *PLoS Genet.* 2012;8(5):e1002746.

92. Marcińska M, Pośpiech E, Abidi S, et al. Evaluation of DNA variants associated with androgenetic alopecia and their potential to predict male pattern baldness. *PLoS One.* 2015;10(5):e0127852.

93. Adhikari K, Fontanil T, Cal S, et al. A genome-wide association scan in admixed Latin Americans identifies loci influencing facial and scalp hair features. *Nat Commun.* 2016;7:10815.

94. Chew E, Tan J, Bahta A, et al. Differential expression between human dermal papilla cells from balding and non-balding scalps reveals new candidate genes for androgenetic alopecia. *J Invest Dermatol.* 2016;136(8):1559–1567.

95. Inui S, Itami S. Molecular basis of androgenetic alopecia: from androgen to paracrine mediators through dermal papilla. *J Dermatol Sci.* 2011;61(1):1–6.

96. Chew EGY, Ho BS-Y, Ramasamy, et al. Comparative transcriptome profiling provides new insights into mechanisms of androgenetic alopecia progression. *Br J Dermatol.* 2017;176(1):265–269.

97. Garza LA, Liu Y, Yang Z, et al. Prostaglandin D2 inhibits hair growth and is elevated in bald scalp of men with androgenetic alopecia. *Sci Transl Med.* 2012;4(126): 126–134.

98. Nelson A, Loy D, Lawson J, Katseff A, FitzGerald G, Garza L. Prostaglandin D2 inhibits wound-induced hair follicle neogenesis through the receptor, GPR44. *J Invest Dermatol.* 2012;133(4):881–889.

99. Heilmann S, Nyholt DR, Brockschmidt FF, et al. No genetic support for a contribution of prostaglandins to the aetiology of androgenetic alopecia. *Br J Dermatol.* 2013;169(1):222–224.

100. Nieves A, Garza L. Does prostaglandin D2 hold the cure to male pattern baldness? *Exp Dermatol.* 2014;23(4):224–227.

101. Kwack M, Sung Y, Chung E, et al. Dihydrotestosterone-inducible dickkopf 1 from balding dermal papilla cells causes apoptosis in follicular keratinocytes. *J Invest Dermatol.* 2007;128(2):262–269.

102. Kretzschmar K, Cottle D, Schweiger P, Watt F. The androgen receptor antagonizes WNT/β-catenin signaling in epidermal stem cells. *J Invest Dermatol.* 2015;135(11): 2753–2763.

103. Tosti A, Zaiac M, Canazza A, et al. Topical application of the WNT/β-catenin activator methyl vanillate increases hair count and hair mass index in women with androgenetic alopecia. *J Cosmet Dermatol.* 2016;15(4): 469–474.

104. Upton J, Hannen R, Bahta A, Farjo N, Farjo B, Philpott M. Oxidative stress–associated senescence in dermal papilla cells of men with androgenetic alopecia. *J Invest Dermatol.* 2015;135(5):1244–1252.

105. Higgins C, Petukhova L, Harel S, et al. FGF5 is a crucial regulator of hair length in humans. *Proc Natl Acad Sci.* 2014;111(29):10648–10653.

106. Garza L, Yang C-C, Zhao T, et al. Bald scalp in men with androgenetic alopecia retains hair follicle stem cells but lacks CD200-rich and CD34-positive hair follicle progenitor cells. *J Clin Invest.* 2011;121(2):613–622.

107. Rittié L, Stoll SW, Kang S, Voorhees JJ, Fisher GJ. Hedgehog signaling maintains hair follicle stem cell phenotype in young and aged human skin. *Aging Cell.* 2009;8(6):738–751.

108. Higgins C, Chen J, Cerise J, Jahoda C, Christiano A. Microenvironmental reprogramming by three-dimensional culture enables dermal papilla cells to induce de novo human hair-follicle growth. *Proc Natl Acad Sci.* 2013;110(49):19679–19688.

109. Torkamani N, Rufaut NW, Jones L, Sinclair R. Destruction of the arrector pili muscle and fat infiltration in androgenic alopecia. *Br J Dermatol.* 2014;170(6):1291–1298.

110. Kure K, Isago T, Hirayama T. Changes in the sebaceous gland in patients with male pattern hair loss (androgenic alopecia). *J Cosmet Dermatol.* 2015;14(3):178–184.

111. Torkamani N, Rufaut N, Jones L, Sinclair R. The arrector pili muscle, the bridge between the follicular stem cell niche and the interfollicular epidermis. *Anat Sci Int.* 2016;92(1):151–158.

112. Torkamani N, Rufaut NW, Jones L, Sinclair RD. Beyond goosebumps: does the arrector pili muscle have a role in hair loss? *Int J Trichol.* 2014;6(3):88–94.

113. Sundberg JP, King LE, Bascom C. Animal models for male pattern (androgenetic) alopecia. *Eur J Dermatol.* 2001.

114. Diani AR, Mulholland MJ, Shull KL, et al. Hair growth effects of oral administration of finasteride, a steroid 5 alpha-reductase inhibitor, alone and in combination with topical minoxidil in the balding stumptail macaque. *J Clin Endocrinol Metab.* 1992;74(2):345–350.

115. Crabtree J, Kilbourne E, Peano B, et al. A mouse model of androgenetic alopecia. *Endocrinology.* 2010;151(5):2373–2380.

116. Ito M, Yang Z, Andl T, et al. Wnt-dependent de novo hair follicle regeneration in adult mouse skin after wounding. *Nature.* 2007;447(7142):316–320.

117. Bae J, Jung H, Goo B, Park Y. Hair regrowth through wound healing process after ablative fractional laser treatment in a murine model. *Lasers Surg Med.* 2015;47(5):433–440.

CHAPTER 6

Telogen Effluvium

WILLIAM C. CRANWELL, MBBS(HONS), BMEDSC(HONS), MPH&TM •
RODNEY SINCLAIR, MBBS, MD, FACD

INTRODUCTION

Telogen effluvium (TE) is a form of diffuse, nonscarring alopecia, which is a delayed consequence of a shift in the hair cycle from anagen through catagen and then telogen. This shift in the hair cycle leads to an abnormal shift in the follicular cycling that leads to premature shedding of hair at the end of the telogen phase approximately two to three months after the inciting event. Although some degree of telogen hair shedding is normal, TE is characterized by a greater proportion of hairs on the scalp in the telogen phase. This results in widespread hair shedding or diffuse loss of hair volume. TE may be acute or chronic, depending on the timing of onset and duration of hair loss.

Various endogenous and exogenous factors are implicated in the induction of TE. In approximately one-third of patients, an inciting factor is not identified. Common causes include major surgery, childbirth, serious illness, malnutrition, and medications. The cause of chronic TE is usually difficult to determine.

TE is usually a reactive and self-limiting condition. Removal of the inciting factor will usually lead to spontaneous improvement. Therefore, the prognosis is dependent on the ability to identify and remove the inciting factor. Chronic TE in which the underlying cause cannot be identified may persist for many years. Cosmetic measures and psychologic support are important components of treatment. Topical minoxidil and nutritional supplements have been trialed, but their efficacy remains unclear.

EPIDEMIOLOGY

Data on the epidemiology of TE are limited, with the incidence and prevalence unclear.[1,2] TE is one of the most common forms of noncicatricial alopecia seen in clinical practice, along with male androgenetic alopecia and alopecia areata.[3] A retrospective study investigating prevalence and factors associated with TE in women found an incidence of 1.7%.[4] More robust epidemiologic studies are needed to determine the true prevalence and incidence.

TE may present as either acute or chronic variants. TE does not appear to have a predilection for any racial or ethnic populations. Acute TE may occur at any age, including infanthood and childhood.[5,6] Women are more affected by TE of all variants.[1] Chronic TE is less common than acute TE, most commonly affecting women aged between 30 and 60 years.[7,8] There is no known genetic cause for TE.[9]

PATHOGENESIS
Physiology of Hair Shedding

Hair is lost and replaced cyclically. The hair cycle is traditionally divided into the growth phase (anagen), regression phase (catagen), and resting phase (telogen). Hair follicles undergo repetitive growth and resting phases, growing continuously during anagen by 0.3 mm/day.[10] The duration of anagen greatly depends on the body region. On the face, anagen lasts 4–14 weeks, on the arms 6–12 weeks, on the legs 19–26 weeks, and on the scalp 3–5 years.[11] As hair elongation is relatively constant, the duration of the anagen phase is the primary determinant of the final hair length in each body area. At the end of anagen, the hair fiber is retained without further hair growth before being shed and replaced.

At the beginning of the catagen phase, apoptosis of the keratinocytes in the bulb leads to involution of the transient portion of the follicle below the insertion of the arrector pili muscle over a two-week period.[10] The telogen phase is characterized by the presence of a "club" hair (a fully keratinized hair with a club-shaped proximal end).[12] The follicle appears to remain dormant for approximately 2 months, before a new anagen phase is initiated. The dead hair is released from the follicle (exogen) at either the end of the telogen phase or the commencement of the next anagen phase. Follicular activity is asynchronous in each body region after childhood so that hair shedding occurs continuously. Normal shedding does not produce visible alopecia. Many animals routinely molt most hair at specific times of the year. In comparison, human scalps normally shed between 50 to 150 telogen hairs each day.[13]

The normal scalp has a constant number of follicles, with approximately 86% of hairs in anagen, 1% in catagen, and 13% in telogen.[14] The duration of telogen remains constant (2–3 months).[15] Therefore, the duration of anagen determines the number of hair follicles in telogen. The biologic factors affecting the termination of the anagen phase are complex and are influenced by various metabolic factors.[16]

A complex network of sequential activation of autocrine, paracrine, and endocrine signaling pathways controls the "autonomous clock" driving the hair cycle.[10] Signaling molecules of the Wnt pathway, fibroblast growth factor (FGF), transforming growth factor β (TGF-β), and Hedgehog pathways regulate the hair cycle.[17,18] Key inducers of anagen include Wnt family proteins, β-catenin pathway, noggin, and the transcription factor Stat3.[17,18] Sonic hedgehog proteins and hepatic growth factor (HGF) promote anagen development. The duration of anagen phase is prolonged by insulin growth factor-1 (IGF-1), vascular endothelial growth factor, and thyrotropin-releasing hormone. IGF-1 and IGF-2 are hair follicle growth stimulators that prevent entry of the follicle into catagen. Polyamine-spermidine is a key anagen prolongator and catagen inhibitor.[18]

Anagen is terminated by concurrent decrease in anagen prolonging factors (IGF-1, HGF, FGF-5S) and increase in hair growth inhibitors (TGF-β1, TGF-β2, and FGF). Dickkopf-1–related protein is implicated in the transition from anagen to catagen by regulating the activity of follicular keratinocytes.[10,18]

Bone morphogenetic protein 4 and 17-β estradiol arrest the follicle in the telogen phase.[10,18] The cyclic epithelial FGF18 also regulates the resting phase.

Shedding of the hair follicle (exogen) has its own regulators, with protease cathepsin L and Msx-2 implicated.[19]

Pathophysiology of Telogen Effluvium

TE occurs if a significant proportion of hair follicles in the anagen phase are triggered to stop growing prematurely. This increases the proportion of hairs entering the catagen phase, followed by the telogen phase. Approximately two to three months after the initial insult, there is excessive hair shedding. It is estimated that 7%–35% of the follicles would normally have been in anagen phase shift to telogen phase.[20] Excessive loss of these telogen hairs manifests as increased hair shedding or diffuse loss of hair volume.

The direct mechanism of hair loss in TE is not clearly understood. Headington describes five functional alterations in the hair cycle that may lead to increased telogen hair shedding.[21] These mechanisms include immediate anagen release, delayed anagen release, short anagen syndrome, immediate telogen release, and delayed telogen release. Immediate anagen release and delayed anagen release are the two most commonly cited theories.

Immediate anagen release is a short-onset effluvium characterized by a large number of anagen fibers stimulated to enter telogen prematurely. Follicles enter catagen and then telogen, with increased hair shedding approximately 2–3 months later.[10] Triggers include high fever, medications, and stress. Immediate anagen release is associated with premature exogen. This is seen in alopecia areata, with telogen follicle shed on the periphery of patches 2–3 weeks after first appearance.[10]

Delayed anagen release occurs when anagen follicles are maintained in anagen for longer than normal. The anagen fibers are then released into telogen at the same time and shed simultaneously. Delayed anagen release is the cause of postpartum hair loss. It occurs due to the high level of circulating placental estrogen, which prolongs anagen.[16] Withdrawal of this circulating estrogen at once causes all overdue anagen hair to enter catagen phase together.[16]

Short anagen syndrome is an idiopathic shortening of the duration of anagen. A 50% decrease in anagen duration leads to double the amount of hair shedding. This results in resistant TE and an inability to grow long hair. This also occurs in loose anagen syndrome.

Immediate telogen release results from shortening of the normal telogen phase. Hairs that would normally remain in telogen for weeks are cycled into anagen within a few days. Drugs such as minoxidil, which promote anagen-phase follicles, can precipitate immediate telogen release.

Delayed telogen release occurs after prolonged telogen followed by transition to anagen. There is increased synchronicity in follicle cycling, leading to a greater proportion of shedding simultaneously. This occurs naturally in animals with synchronous hair cycles during shedding of their winter coats.

Inciting Factors

A number of factors have been associated with the induction of TE. Data concerning the actual risk of each factor are lacking. An inciting factor cannot be identified in approximately one-third of cases.[1] Inciting factors can be classified according to physiologic causes, febrile states, stress, drugs, endocrine, organ dysfunction, hair cycle disorder, nutritional factors, local cause, and others (Table 6.1).[16]

The relationship between TE and serum ferritin and Vitamin D is controversial. Results have not consistently

TABLE 6.1
Causes of Telogen Effluvium

Physiologic causes	Postpartum effluvium (telogen gravidarum)
	Physiologic effluvium of newborn
Febrile states	Typhoid
	Malaria
	Tuberculosis
	HIV infection
Stress	Severe febrile illness
	Emotional stress
	Serious injuries
	Major surgery
	Difficult labor
	Hemorrhage
	Starvation
	Crash diet
Drugs	Oral retinoids (etretinate and acitretin)
	Oral contraceptives
	Antithyroid drugs
	Anticonvulsants
	Hypolipidemic drugs
	Heavy metals
	Beta blockers
	Captopril
	Amphetamines
Endocrine	Hyperthyroidism
	Hypothyroidism
Organ dysfunction	Renal failure
	Hepatic failure
Hair cycle disorder	Short anagen syndrome
Nutritional factors	Iron deficiency anemia
	Acrodermatitis enteropathica
	Acquired zinc deficiency
	Malnutrition
Local cause	Hair dye application
Others	Syphilis
	Systemic lupus erythematosus

Taken from Shashikant M. Telogen effluvium: a review. *J Clin Diagn Res*. 2015;9:WE01–WE03.

proved an association.[22–29] Additional studies are required to confirm a relationship between ferritin or Vitamin D and alopecia and whether supplementation in nonanemic patients is beneficial.

Identified causes of chronic diffuse telogen hair loss are thyroid disease, profound iron deficiency anemia, acrodermatitis enteropathica, and malnutrition.[30] Both hypothyroidism and hyperthyroidism can produce diffuse hair loss in 33% and 50% of patients, respectively.[10] Drug-induced hypothyroidism is also implicated. Hypothyroidism inhibits cell division in the epidermis and the skin appendages. The role of iron deficiency anemia in diffuse hair loss is controversial. In 20% of cases, the iron deficiency occurs in the absence of clinical anemia, with a serum ferritin less than 20 µg/L.[10] Acrodermatitis enteropathica and acquired zinc deficiency can lead to severe TE. Subclinical zinc deficiency does not cause diffuse hair shedding. Therefore, alternative causes of hair loss should be excluded in cases of subclinical zinc deficiency.

CLINICAL FEATURES

The major clinical feature of TE is an acute or chronic increase in hair shedding. This can be quantified using a validated clinical grading scale (Fig. 6.1). In cases of acute and chronic TE, patients present with stage 5 or 6 hair shedding. Some, but not all patients with acute TE notice an associated reduction in scalp hair density. Loss of hair volume invariably presents with a reduction in the thickness of the ponytail in those with long hair; however, midfrontal scalp hair density is invariably normal in chronic TE despite the persistent increased hair shedding (>6 months). Bitemporal recession is common in both acute and chronic TE (Fig. 6.2).[16] The hair pull test result is invariably positive in acute TE but may be negative in chronic TE (Fig. 6.3A and B). Examination of the bulbs of the hairs extracted on hair pull shows club ends (Fig. 6.4). Patients are often concerned that they may shed all hair. Loss is not usually more than 50% of scalp hair.[31] Therefore, progression to complete baldness does not occur.[7]

In isolated cases of TE, the scalp and hair shafts appear normal, and TE may affect other hair-bearing areas.[20,32] Hair thinning due to TE may lead to recognition of other concomitant hair loss disorders not previously identified. Early male or female androgenetic alopecia or central centrifugal cicatricial alopecia may be marked in the presence of TE.

Acute Telogen Effluvium

Dramatic diffuse telogen hair loss develops 2–3 months after the inciting factor. This produces marked thinning of the hair. Patients often do not relate hair loss to the inciting event.

Chronic Telogen Effluvium

Diffuse shedding of telogen hairs persists beyond four to six months. It is characterized by an abrupt diffuse shedding of hair that runs a fluctuating course over

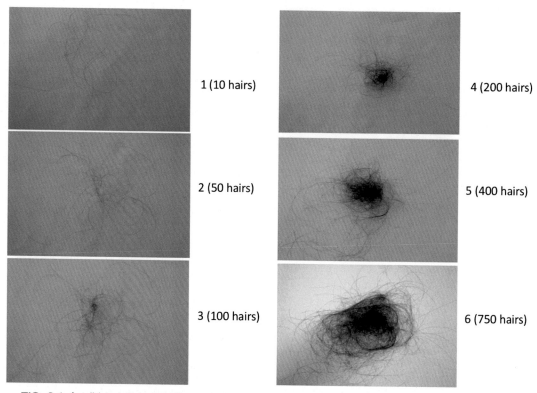

1 (10 hairs)

2 (50 hairs)

3 (100 hairs)

4 (200 hairs)

5 (400 hairs)

6 (750 hairs)

FIG. 6.1 A validated clinical grading scale for hair shedding. Patients are asked to identify the photograph that best correlates with the amount of hair shed on a wash day and the photo that correlated best with the amount shed on a nonwash day. Hair loss of severity 1–3 is considered normal. Stage 5 and 6 is always abnormal. Stage 4 can be normal for a woman with very long hair but is excessive for women with short hair.

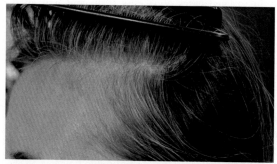

FIG. 6.2 Bitemporal recession in acute telogen effluvium. This patient presented with increased hair shedding, reduction in the thickness hair by 50%, mild bitemporal recession but without any widening of the midline part line. Scalp biopsy was normal with no increase in the ratio of terminal:vellus hairs.

several years,[33] and may be primary chronic TE (idiopathic) or due to an inciting factor listed in Table 6.1. Some patients develop a chronic-repetitive pattern of TE, in which chronic thinning is punctuated by additional episodes of acute hair loss. The baseline hair volume is lower than premorbid hair volume.

HISTOPATHOLOGY
The key histologic finding in TE is an increased proportion of telogen follicles.[34] In normal controls the mean terminal:vellus ratio is 7:1, compared with a mean terminal:vellus ratio of 9:1 in chronic TE (Fig. 6.5A and B).[8] Unlike in androgenetic alopecia, the proportion of vellus hair follicles is not increased (Fig. 6.6).[8] Inflammatory changes are not demonstrated, unless TE is induced by inflammatory disorders that affect the scalp. Patients with TE induced by inflammatory conditions of the scalp, including seborrheic dermatitis or

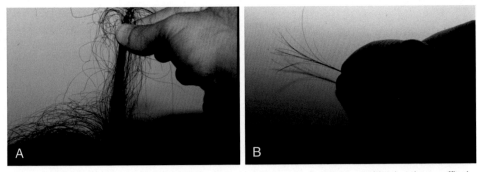

FIG. 6.3 **(A)** The hair pull test identifies active hair shedding and is invariably positive in telogen effluvium. To perform the test, 50–60 hairs are pulled with constant force close to the skin surface from the proximal to distal ends. **(B)** The hair pull test result is positive if greater than 6–10 hairs are extracted from the scalp. Examination using light microscopy identifies telogen hairs.

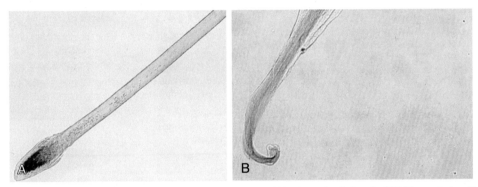

FIG. 6.4 Following a hair pull test, the extracted hairs should be inspected visually. **(A)** Telogen hair, with a club-shaped proximal end and usually not pigmented. **(B)** Anagen hair, with a tapered end and usually pigmented.

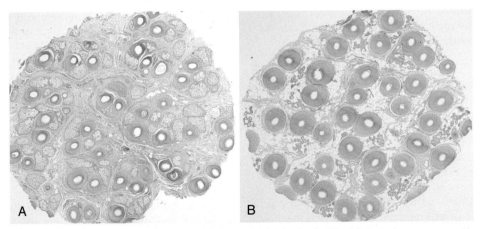

FIG. 6.5 **(A)** Chronic telogen effluvium: horizontal section at the level of the isthmus shows preserved follicular architecture with normal follicular density of 47 follicles. The terminal:vellus ratio is 8.4:1 and the telogen count is 5% (hematoxylin and eosin, 4×). **(B)** Chronic Telogen Effluvium: the same specimen at the bulbar level shows normal follicular density (busy fat) as compared to androgenetic alopecia in which less follicular density is appreciated at the bulbar level because of follicular miniaturization (hematoxylin and eosin, 4×). (Courtesy of Mariya Miteva.)

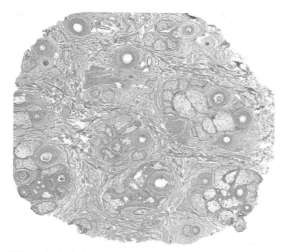

FIG. 6.6 Androgenetic alopecia: horizontal section at the level of the isthmus shows preserved follicular architecture with decreased follicular density of 22 follicles. The terminal:vellus ratio is 1.3:1 and the telogen count is 8% (hematoxylin and eosin, 4×). (Courtesy of Mariya Miteva.)

TABLE 6.2 Key Inquiries of the Patient History	
Course of hair loss	Date of onset Duration of shedding Apparent triggers and temporal relationship
Characteristics of hair loss	Estimated hair loss daily Appearance of shed hair (intact versus broken)
Medical history	Recent acute or chronic illness Major surgeries Rapid weight loss Dietary restrictions Recent childbirth or miscarriage Iron deficiency anemia and thyroid disorder Review of systems
Psychologic history	Recent significant psychologic stressors Grief or other serious loss
Drug and nutritional supplement history	See Table 6.1 list of inciting medications Known iron deficiency anemia
History of toxin exposure	

syphilis, demonstrate an increased proportion of telogen hair follicles and histologic features of the underlying inflammatory disorder (e.g., perivascular and perifollicular lymphocytic infiltrates).[35]

DIAGNOSIS

The diagnosis of TE can usually be made based on the patient history, physical examination, hair pull test, and basic investigations. TE should be considered in any case of diffuse, noninflammatory, nonscarring alopecia, particularly if preceded by a physiologic or psychologic stressor.

History

Thorough patient history focuses on the course and pattern of hair loss, potential underlying cause of TE, and ruling out of other causes of diffuse hair loss. Patients report an abrupt onset of hair shedding often sufficient to block their shower drain, along with general hair shedding. A history of difficulty in growing hair long is suggestive of chronic TE. Other aspects of the history include features of other forms of alopecia. Inquiring about menstrual and reproductive history may elucidate features of androgenetic alopecia. Inquiry about family history of alopecia may increase suspicion for hereditable hair loss disorders.

Key components of the patient history are listed in Table 6.2.

Physical Examination

Examination of the scalp and scalp skin typically finds no inflammation, scarring, scale, or pustules. The detection of these signs suggests a concomitant or alternative scalp disorder. Broken hair fibers are visualized in patients with heat or chemical-related damage to the hair shaft, trichotillomania, and structural hair disorders.

Chronic starvation (particularly marasmus) may result in lusterless, dry, fine, and straight hair that is sparse and easily plucked from the scalp. Kwashiorkor results in periods of interrupted hair growth that sends the hair into telogen phase if severe. Hair color change is a prominent feature of Kwashiorkor. Dark hair becomes brown or red, whereas brown hair changes to blond. This color change along with periodic constrictions produces the so-called "flag sign" of Kwashiorkor.[16]

Examination of the entire skin surface characterizes additional body hair loss and detects features of other hair and skin disorders. Examination of the nails may aid identification of inciting factors. For example, Beau lines suggest recent significant medical illness, and koilonychias suggests iron deficiency anemia.

Serial clinical photography assesses progress between consultations and provides an objective measure of progress.

Hair Pull Test

In acute TE, the hair pull test result is strongly positive. Clumps of telogen hairs are extracted from the vertex and scalp margin with ease. The hair pull test is performed by grasping 40–60 closely grouped scalp hairs between the thumb and index finger, then quickly and gently pulling the hairs from proximal to distal ends. The extraction of more than 6–10 fibers is abnormal.[36] The trichogram from a hair pull sample in TE is abnormal, with greater than 25% telogen hairs. Inspection with the naked eye can distinguish anagen from telogen hair. The collected hairs can be examined with a light microscope to confirm that the hairs are telogen hairs. Telogen hairs have depigmented bulbs and absence of an inner root sheath (Fig. 6.4).

A false-negative hair pull test result can occur if a patient has washed his/her hair with shampoo or vigorously groomed their hair on the day of examination. Conversely, a false-positive result is likely if the patient has not used shampoo or combed their hair for several days.

Dermoscopy

Trichoscopy (Fig. 6.7) can be useful for differentiating chronic TE and female androgenetic alopecia. Acute TE may show a decreased hair density with the presence of empty follicles and numerous short regrowing hairs.[10,37] Unlike TE, androgenetic alopecia demonstrates hair shaft diameter variation and peripilar halo.[37]

Wood's Lamp Examination

Wood's lamp examination is not routinely used in the diagnosis of TE. Wood's lamp may be useful for confirming a diagnosis of seborrheic dermatitis if greasy scale and erythema are seen on the scalp. In addition, *Malassezia* yeasts, implicated in seborrheic dermatitis, can fluoresce under ultraviolet lamp.[38]

Investigations

Routine laboratory investigations are useful for identifying potential underlying causes. There are no serologic tests that definitively diagnose TE. A full blood count with red blood cell indices, complete metabolic panel, iron studies, thyroid function test, syphilis serology, serum zinc, and antinuclear antibody should be performed to identify an underlying cause.[13] The selection of additional laboratory investigations is guided by the clinical situation and

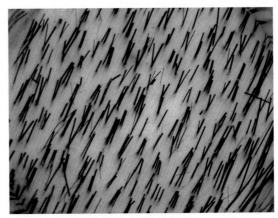

FIG. 6.7 Dermoscopy in telogen effluvium reveals normal hair density with multiple compound follicles. Multiple hair fibers are seen exiting from a single pore.

the need to rule out additional underlying disease or differentials.

Scalp biopsies are usually not required in cases of acute TE, but are the most definitive method of confirming the diagnosis. This may provide reassuring prognostic information to particularly anxious patients. Scalp biopsy can also rule out female pattern hair loss, diffuse alopecia areata, secondary syphilis, systemic lupus erythematosis, and dermatomyositis, which can all present with diffuse hair loss. The diagnosis of chronic TE can usually be made based on clinical features, but a scalp biopsy is required to differentiate chronic TE from alopecia areata and androgenetic alopecia.[10]

The optimal scalp biopsy includes two 4-mm punch biopsies taken from the vertex of the scalp. One specimen is sectioned horizontally and the second is sectioned vertically. The vertex is the chosen site as androgenetic alopecia is a patterned disease that preferentially affects the vertex of the scalp, making diagnostic yield greatest.[10]

DIFFERENTIAL DIAGNOSES

A number of diffuse nonscarring hair and scalp disorders share clinical characteristics with TE. Table 6.3 outlines the relevant clinical features that differentiate TE and the differential diagnoses.

MANAGEMENT

Given that TE is generally a reactive and self-limiting condition, few treatment options exist. Many patients

---

TABLE 6.3
Differentiating Features of Telogen Effluvium and Differential Diagnoses

Anagen effluvium	Anagen effluvium is the acute loss of anagen hair secondary to chemotherapy or toxin exposure. Anagen effluvium typically involves more than 80% hair loss. Examination findings of anagen effluvium include exclamation point hairs. Microscopic examination of shed hair is characterized by dystrophic anagen hairs, rather than telogen hairs.
Androgenetic alopecia	Androgenetic alopecia occurs in a highly reproducible pattern that preferentially affects the temples, vertex, and midfrontal scalp. Miniaturized hairs are commonly seen in androgenetic alopecia. Telogen effluvium and androgenetic alopecia may coexist, particularly in the early stages when diffuse shedding reveals characteristic patterns.
Diffuse alopecia areata	Diffuse alopecia areata has two distinct presentations. Patients may present with acute diffuse hair loss or a chronic form. Patients may present with dramatic active hair loss, with positive hair pull test result for hundreds of hairs. The chronic form is rare, presenting with profound hair loss but no active shedding. One or two patches of alopecia may also be present. Exclamation point hairs may be present. Microscopy may reveal dystrophic anagen hairs. A biopsy will reveal an inflammatory infiltrate consistent with alopecia areata.
Loose anagen syndrome	A rare, nonscarring alopecia characterized by easy extraction of anagen hairs from the scalp. Young children, particularly blonde females, are particularly affected. Examination of pulled hair fibers reveals anagen hair, rather than telogen in telogen effluvium.
Structural hair disorder	Structural hair disorders cause weakened hair fibers that are prone to fracturing. Fibers are broken, rather than shed from the follicle. Trichoscopy reveals hair fibers broken at the shaft.

are reassured that complete baldness is not possible (unless concomitant hair disorder exists), TE is temporary, and regrowth is likely. The management approach for TE includes identification and removal of the inciting factor, camouflaging hair loss, and psychologic support. It is unclear whether topical therapy and iron supplementation are beneficial for altering the disease course. Serial scalp photography can be used to demonstrate that there is no progressive baldness developing (Fig. 6.8).

Removal of the Inciting Factor

Most patients with an isolated event (e.g., pregnancy) will experience spontaneous resolution. Patients with an inciting factor that is prolonged or requires treatment should have the cause eliminated or treated if possible. In cases of suspected drug-induced TE, the responsible drug should be discontinued for at least 3 months if possible to assess improvement in hair loss.[1] Concomitant scalp and hair loss disorders should be treated accordingly.

Cosmetic Treatments

Some patients may require a wig while awaiting regrowth.[13] Involving a hairdresser or stylist experienced in alopecia may minimize the cosmetic effects of hair loss and thinning. Patients may benefit from

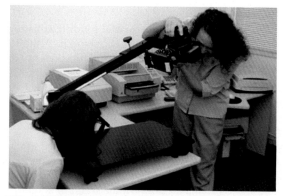

FIG. 6.8 Stereotactic photographic device used for serial monitoring of hair density.

particular hair styling and hair coloring. Hair transplantation is not an appropriate treatment for TE.

Psychologic Support

Hair is an essential aspect of an individual's self-image and the profound psychologic effect may be out of keeping with the degree of hair loss.[39,40] Therefore, the main consequence of TE is predominantly psychologic. It is important for the physician to address the possible emotional responses to alopecia, including anger, anxiety, and depression.[41] Education about the hair growth cycle and the expected time-frame for hair shedding and regrowth may set realistic expectations and reassure the patient. Early referral of patients to a clinical psychologist benefits those who require further evaluation and those with persistent TE.

Topical Minoxidil

The efficacy of topical minoxidil in TE is unclear. Theoretically, minoxidil should hasten resolution of hair growth by prolonging anagen and stimulating telogen hairs to reenter anagen. The drug also enlarges miniaturized hair follicles.[1]

Topical minoxidil is unlikely to hasten regrowth in cases of acute TE that is because of an isolated or treatable inciting factor. However, many specialists prescribe topical minoxidil in cases of chronic TE in an attempt to maintain hair density and encourage new hair regrowth. Minoxidil topical preparations are available in 2% and 5% solutions. Minoxidil 2% is applied twice daily to the entire scalp, and 5% is applied once daily. Any positive effect may be delayed, and treatment should continue for at least 12 months before deemed ineffective.

Prior to initiating topical minoxidil, inform patients that increased hair shedding is common within 2–8 weeks of initiating treatment. This is because of dormant telogen follicles stimulated to reenter anagen and push out old club hair.[3,42] This is often perceived by patients as worsening of their condition and often leads to cessation of treatment.

Nutritional Supplementation

Iron deficiency with or without anemia is a common finding in the investigation of diffuse alopecia.[13] The supplementation of iron for the treatment of TE in the absence of iron deficiency or iron deficiency anemia is controversial. This uncertainty has contributed to disagreement among experts, with no universal recommendation for optimal ferritin levels. This is complicated by the fact that ferritin reference ranges are assay-specific. Nonetheless, many clinicians recommend that treatment for hair loss is optimized by greater serum ferritin levels.[3,22,26,43]

The benefit of other supplements, including zinc (in the absence of symptomatic zinc deficiency), vitamin D, and biotin are also unclear.

Emerging Treatments

A number of novel cosmetic treatments for TE have been reported. However, none of the treatments below are proved to improve the cosmetic outcome in TE.

A leave-on technology combination of caffeine, niacin amide, panthenol, dimethicone, and an acrylate polymer (CNPDA) reportedly increases hair diameter by 2–3 μm.[46] This increase in diameter yields an overall increased cross-sectional area of scalp hair of 10%. CNPDA-treated hair fibers also have increased strength, reducing hair breakage and additional loss. Efficacy in TE has not been established.[44]

Nioxin is a scalp cleanser and serum that is based on bionutrient actives and protectives.[10] Nioxin enhances hair moisture and provides vitamin nourishment. This includes vitamins and minerals including copper, iron, biotin, and caffeine, and herbal supplements including ginseng, ginkgo, and saw palmetto.[10,45]

Stemoxydine is a potent prolyl-4-hydroxylase inhibitor theoretically beneficial in TE. Stemoxydine is a novel approach to sustain hair growth and cycling through induction of hypoxialike signaling. It is hypothesized from in vitro studies that hypoxia signaling may be important in maintaining hair follicle stem cell functioning.[10] An in vivo study found that daily topical treatment with 5% solution for three months resulted in increased hair follicle density compared with placebo.[46]

PROGNOSIS

The prognosis of acute TE depends greatly on the ability to identify and remove the inciting factor. The condition is generally self-limiting if the inciting factor spontaneously resolves or is treated. Patients tend to experience hair shedding for 2–3 months. This is followed by a period of stability and regrowth of hair. Significant cosmetic improvement generally takes 6–12 months, with most women experiencing full restoration of their hair.[13] In a small proportion of patients, hair can remain thin. This may be because of underlying androgenetic alopecia, and a biopsy will further delineate the expected prognosis.[13]

The prognosis for patients with chronic TE is more variable. The course of the disease is variable, with general hair thinning punctuated by periods of increased shedding. The condition usually resolves spontaneously within 3–4 years. The condition can be persistent, lasting greater than 10 years.

Given that approximately 50% of hairs are affected in TE, complete baldness does not occur in either the acute or the chronic variants.[8,13]

REFERENCES

1. Harrison S, Sinclair R. Telogen effluvium. *Clin Exp Dermatol.* 2002;27:389–395.
2. Sinclair RD, Banfield CC, Dawber RP. Diffuse hair loss. In: Sinclair RD, Banfield CC, Dawber RP, eds. *Handbook of Diseases of the Hair and Scalp.* UK: Blackwell Science Ltd; 1999:64–74.

3. Hordinsky MK. Medical treatment of noncicatricial alopecia. *Semin Cutan Med Surg.* 2006;25(1):51–55.
4. Fatani MI, Mahdi AH, Alafif KA, Hussain WA, Khan AS, Banjar AA. Prevalence and factors associated with telogen effluvium in adult females at Makkah region, Saudi Arabia: a retrospective study. *J Dermatol Dermatol Surg.* 2015;19(1):27–30.
5. Atton AV, Tunnessen Jr WW. Alopecia in children: the most common causes. *Pediat Rev Am Acad Pediat.* 1990;12(1):25–30.
6. Nnoruka EN, Obiagboso I, Maduechesi C. Hair loss in children in South-East Nigeria: common and uncommon cases. *Int J Dermatol.* 2007;46(s1):18–22.
7. Trüeb RM. Systematic approach to hair loss in women. *JDDG: Journal der Deutschen Dermatologischen Gesellschaft.* 2010;8(4):284–297.
8. Whiting DA. Chronic telogen effluvium: increased scalp hair shedding in middle-aged women. *J Am Acad Dermatol.* 1996;35(6):899–906.
9. Chartier MB, Hoss DM, Grant-Kels JM. Approach to the adult female patient with diffuse nonscarring alopecia. *J Am Acad Dermatol.* 2002;47:818–820.
10. Liyanage D, Sinclair R. Telogen effluvium. *Cosmetics.* 2016;3(2):13.
11. Sinclair RD, Banfield CC, Dawber RP. *Handbook of Diseases of the Hair and Scalp.* Oxford, UK: Blackwell Science Ltd; 1999:64–74.
12. Paus R, Cotsarelis G. The biology of hair follicles. *N Engl J Med.* 1999;341(7):491–497.
13. Sinclair R. Diffuse hair loss. *Int J Dermatol.* 1999;38(suppl 1):8–18.
14. Kligman AM. The human hair cycle. *J Invest Dermatol.* 1959;33:307–316.
15. Price VH. Treatment of hair loss. *N Engl J Med.* 1999; 341(13):964–973.
16. Shashikant M. Telogen effluvium: a review. *J Clin Diagn Res.* 2015;9:WE01–WE03.
17. Krause K, Foitzik K. Biology of the hair follicle: the basics. *Semin Cutan Med Surg.* 2006;25:2–10.
18. Brajac L, Vícíc M, Periša D, Kaštelan M. Human hair follicle: an update on biology and perspectives in hair growth disorders treatment. *Hair Ther Transplant.* 2014;4.
19. Schneider MR, Schmidt-Ullrich R, Paus R. The hair follicle as a dynamic miniorgan. *Curr Biol.* 2009;19: R132–R142.
20. Bergfeld WF. Telogen effluvium. In: McMichael A, Hordinsky M, eds. *Hair and Scalp Diseases: Medical, Surgical and Cosmetic Treatments.* Informa Health Care; 2008:119.
21. Headington JT. Telogen effluvium: new concepts and review. *Arch Dermatol.* 1993;129:356–363.
22. Trost LB, Bergfeld WF, Calogeras E. The diagnosis and treatment of iron deficiency and its potential relationship to hair loss. *J Am Acad Dermatol.* 2006;54(5):824–844.
23. Olsen EA, Reed KB, Cacchio PB, Caudill L. Iron deficiency in female pattern hair loss, chronic telogen effluvium, and control groups. *J Am Acad Dermatol.* 2010;63(6): 991–999.
24. Kantor J, Kessler LJ, Brooks DG, Cotsarelis G. Decreased serum ferritin is associated with alopecia in women. *J Invest Dermatol.* 2003;121(5):985–988.
25. Sinclair R. There is no clear association between low serum ferritin and chronic diffuse telogen hair loss. *Br J Dermatol.* 2002;147(5):982–984.
26. Rushton DH. Nutritional factors and hair loss. *Clin Exp Dermatol.* 2002;27(5):396–404.
27. Bregy A, Trüeb RM. No association between serum ferritin levels >10 µg/l and hair loss activity in women. *Dermatology.* 2008;217(1):1–6.
28. Rasheed H, Mahgoub D, Hegazy R, et al. Serum ferritin and vitamin D in female hair loss: do they play a role? *Skin Pharmacol Physiol.* 2013;26(2):101–107.
29. Du X, She E, Gelbart T, et al. The serine protease TMPRSS6 is required to sense iron deficiency. *Science.* 2008;320(5879):1088–1092.
30. Dawber RPR, Simpson NB, Barth JH. Diffuse alopecia: endocrine, metabolic and chemical influences on the follicular cycle. In: Dawber RPR, ed. *Diseases of the Hair and Scalp.* Oxford, UK: Blackwell Science; 1997:123–150.
31. Trueb RM. Hair growth and disorders. In: Blume-Peytavi U, Tosti A, Whiting DA, Trueb R, eds. *Diffuse Hair Loss.* 1st ed. Berlin: Springer; 2008:259–272.
32. Bergfeld WF, Mulinari-Brenner F. Shedding: how to manage a common cause of hair loss. *Cleveland Clin J Med.* 2001;68(3):256–261.
33. Messenger AG, Berker DA, Sinclair RD. Rook's text book of dermatology. In: Burns T, Breathnach S, Cox N, Griffiths C, eds. *Disorders of Hair.* 8th ed. Oxford: Blackwell Publishing; 2010:66.1–66.100.
34. Weedon D. Diseases of cutaneous appendages. In: *Weedon's Skin Pathology.* 3rd ed. Edinburgh: Elsevier Limited; 2010:397.
35. Jordaan HF, Louw M. The moth-eaten alopecia of secondary syphilis a histopathological study of 12 patients. *Am J Dermatopathol.* 1995;17(2):158–168.
36. Hillmann K, Blume-Peytavi U. Diagnosis of hair disorders. *Semin Cutan Med Surg.* 2009;28(1):33–38. Frontline Medical Communications.
37. Miteva M, Tosti A. Hair and scalp dermatoscopy. *J Am Acad Dermatol.* 2012;67(5):1040–1048.
38. Mayser P, Stapelkamp H, Krämer HJ, et al. Pityrialactone-a new fluorochrome from the tryptophan metabolism of *M. alassezia* Furfur. *Antonie van Leeuwenhoek.* 2003;84(3):185–191.
39. Hadshiew IM, Foitzik K, Arck PC, Paus R. Burden of hair loss: stress and the underestimated psychosocial impact of telogen effluvium and androgenetic alopecia. *J Invest Dermatol.* 2004;123:455.
40. Reid EE, Haley AC, Borovicka JH, et al. Clinical severity does not reliably predict quality of life in women with alopecia areata, telogen effluvium, or androgenic alopecia. *J Am Acad Dermatol.* 2012;66:e97.
41. Tabolli S, Sampogna F, di Pietro C, Mannooranparampil TJ, Ribuffo M, Albeni D. Health status, coping strategies, and alexithymia in subjects with androgenetic alopecia a questionnaire study. *Am J Clin Dermatol.* 2013;14:139–145.

42. Blumeyer A, Tosti A, Messenger A, et al. Evidence-based (S3) guideline for the treatment of androgenetic alopecia in women and in men. *J Dtsch Dermatol Ges.* 2011;9 (suppl 6):S1.
43. Tosti A, Piraccini BM, Sisti A, Duque-Estrada B. Hair loss in women. *Minerva Ginecol.* 2009;61:445.
44. Davis MG, Thomas JH, van de Velde S, et al. A novel cosmetic approach to treat thinning hair. *Br J Dermatol.* 2011;165:24–30.
45. Matt L, Leavitt MD. Hair loss treatments: a word of caution. *Dermatol.* 2003;11:3.
46. Rathman-Josserand M, Bernard BA, Misra N. Hair density recovery: new insights in hair growth biology—L'Oreal research: O 10: the niche of human hair follicle stem cells: a specific environment. *Int J Trichol.* 2014;6:113–139.

CHAPTER 7

Trichotillomania

AISLEEN A. DIAZ, BS • MARIYA MITEVA, MD

INTRODUCTION

Definition

Trichotillomania (TT) is a compulsive desire or habit to pluck hair, either consciously or unconsciously. Psychiatric classification, *Diagnostic and Statistical Manual of Mental Disorders, Fifth Edition* (*DSM-5*), lists TT under obsessive-compulsive and related disorders. The diagnostic criteria for TT include the following[1]:

1. recurrent pulling out of one's hair, resulting in noticeable hair loss;
2. repeated attempts to decrease or stop hair pulling;
3. disturbance causes clinically significant distress or impairment in social, occupational, or other important areas of functioning;
4. the hair pulling or hair loss is not attributable to another medical condition; and
5. the hair pulling is not better explained by the symptoms of another mental disorder.

General Concepts

TT is seen in both children and adults.[2] Typically there are two populations: those who present early in childhood, with an initial mean age of onset of 12 years and two peaks at 5–8 and 13 years of age.[2] Children as young as 1 year have been diagnosed. Also, there are chronic cases presenting in adults who have continued hair pulling activity from adolescence or who developed the disorder in early adult life. In children it is usually benign and self-limited, but in adults it usually accompanies other psychopathologies and requires psychologic intervention.[3] Patients with TT frequently will not admit their habit, and parents of affected children may be recalcitrant to accept the diagnosis.

TT is more common among women. One possible explanation is the fact that women are more inclined to seek help, and that men may blame male pattern baldness, or that men have the advantage of shaving their heads with minimal social stigma.[4] There is also a difference in terms of the hair pulling site, with men pulling hair from the stomach, back, mustache, and beard areas, whereas women typically pull from the scalp.[5]

TT usually involves the scalp but can also affect any hair-bearing region of the body.

Patients with TT typically have a high rate of *psychiatric comorbidity.*[6]

ETIOLOGY

TT is a complex disorder involving biologic, psychologic, genetic, and social factors. Family studies report higher-than-expected rates of TT among relatives of affected individuals, but few twin concordance studies have been completed to estimate heritability rates.[7] A twin study was conducted in which 34 twin pairs were identified, 24 were monozygotic (MZ) and 10 were dizygotic (DZ). Respective concordance rates for MZ and DZ twin pairs were significantly different at 38.1% and 0% for *DSM-IV* TT criteria and 58.3% and 20% for noticeable noncosmetic hair pulling, leading to a heritability estimate of 76.2%. These findings suggest that genetic factors play a significant role in the etiology of TT.[7] Several gene candidates were reported as contributing to disease development. Rare variations in *SLITRK1* were associated with disorders of the obsessive-compulsive spectrum, including TT.[8] However, the genetic component of TT is complex and still not well understood.[3]

The onset of TT and worsening of hair pulling symptoms are often precipitated by stressful or traumatic life events. Stressors may involve school problems, sibling rivalry, moving to a new house, hospitalization of a parent, or a disturbed parent-child relationship. Research indicates that 86% of patients report instances of violence occurring just before the onset of TT.[9] Other studies have found that patients with TT report relatively high rates of lifetime traumatic experiences, have higher scores than healthy individuals on self-report scales measuring lifetime trauma severity, and show abnormally high rates of lifetime posttraumatic stress disorder.[9,10] Thus, it has been suggested that hair pulling in TT may evolve as a maladaptive coping strategy for the negative affective experiences caused by trauma.

Apart from TT, a number of other *"tricho-"*factitious disorders characterized by hair loss exist.

Trichoteiromania

The term trichoteiromania refers to a type of artificial hair loss, which results from perpetual rubbing of the scalp with fracturing of the hair shafts. In contrast to TT, trichoteiromania has no diagnostic histopathologic features and has a normal trichogram. Traumatic changes to the hair shaft are more conspicuous, with splitting at the ends of the hairs, giving the impression of white tips.[11] The underlying mental disorders represent a more heterogeneous group.

Trichotemnomania

Trichotemnomania is an obsessive-compulsive habit to deliberately cut the hair with scissors or with a razor and is less frequent. One case reported a female patient who presented with a complete hairless scalp initially misdiagnosed as alopecia areata (AA) totalis. However, histopathologic findings revealed normal hair follicles with an absence of inflammatory infiltrates.[12]

Trichodaganomania

Trichodaganomania is characterized by the compulsive habit of biting one's own hair during times of stress or anxiety. A case was reported of a young male with localized areas of hair loss on the dorsal surfaces of his forearms with a history of anxiety and depression.[13] As with classic TT, the patient reported irresistible urge to bite his forearm hair, followed by a sense of relief. Microscopic findings revealed a fraction of vellus hair with a smooth, blunted shaft at the bitten end and a natural tapered end distally. In contrast to TT, an attached root sheath or hair bulb was absent.[13]

Trichophagia and Trichobezoar

Reports have indicated that TT patients indulge in trichophagia, in which they consume their hair to the extent that a gastrointestinal hair ball forms, also known as a trichobezoar.[14] Children with TT who present with episodes of obscure abdominal pain, weight loss, nausea, vomiting, anorexia, and foul breath should be investigated. Gastric trichobezoars have a high morbidity, and complications can be fatal. They may lead to intestinal bleeding, pancreatitis, obstructive symptoms, or vitamin deficiencies and thus require surgical removal.[14]

CLINICAL PRESENTATION

Clinically, a patient with TT exhibits patches of alopecia with broken hairs at varying lengths.[15] The scalp is the most frequent hair pulling site, followed by the eyebrows, eyelashes, pubic area, trunk, and extremities. Hair pulling usually occurs daily, or nearly daily, and can occupy several hours or more. A common location for pulling hair is the crown of the head, leading some patients to develop a *tonsure pattern* also referred to as the "Friar Tuck" sign (Fig. 7.1A).[16] It is characterized by areas of hair loss with broken hairs

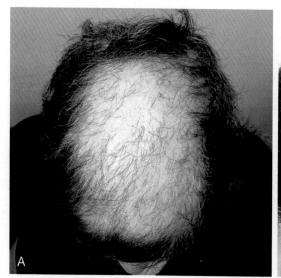
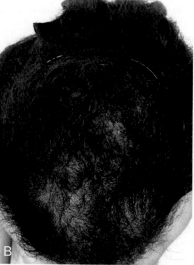

FIG. 7.1 **(A)** A young woman with trichotillomania: tonsure pattern, Friar Tuck sign. **(B)** Another young woman with trichotillomania: Hair is broken at different levels.

of varying lengths arranged in a circular pattern surrounded by unaffected hair. There is no inflammation of the scalp, and during the regrowing phase, patients exhibit signs of variable lengths of hair shafts (Fig. 7.1B). Some hairs may be broken midshaft or appear as uneven stubble, whereas others appear as small black dots on the surface of the scalp. Overall hair density is normal, and a *hair pull test is negative*.[16] There is usually no scaling on the scalp, but excoriations may be noted. Many find the resultant hair loss embarrassing, and efforts are often made to camouflage the loss with hairstyles, scarves, wigs, makeup, or clothing.[15] Others find it difficult to admit to the hair pulling when asked or may attribute pulling to other skin disorders that cause pruritus. Patients often feel ashamed and will hide their behavior from family, friends, and healthcare providers.[15]

TRICHOSCOPY

Description of common trichoscopic findings are summarized in Table 7.1.

Trichoscopy is a quick, noninvasive method that has proven to be a useful tool for differential diagnosis of TT. Findings show decreased hair density, short vellus hair, broken hairs with different shaft lengths, coiled hairs, trichoptilosis, sparse yellow dots, and black dots (Fig. 7.2A).[17] Several common trichoscopic features characteristic for TT have been described, including flame hairs, the "v-sign," tulip hairs, hook hairs, and hair powder.[18]

Flame hairs are a trichoscopic feature described as hair residue from traumatic pulling of anagen hairs in TT. They are a type of broken hair that may be seen in various hair loss disorders, including radiotherapy- and chemotherapy-induced alopecia, AA and, occasionally, traction alopecia and central centrifugal cicatricial alopecia.[19] Flame hairs are defined as very short (<1 mm) pigmented hairs with a thin, wavy, distal tip, resembling the flame on a match point[19] (Fig. 7.2B). In TT, flame hairs occur due to mechanical injury to anagen hairs, which results in the thin and irregular proximal remnant of the traumatized hair shaft. On pathology, this feature corresponds to a distorted hair shaft. The flame hairs differ from a hair powder by the presence of a hair shaft. The *"hair powder'"* (Fig. 7.2A) sign is commonly seen in patients with TT. It occurs when hair shafts are almost completely damaged by mechanical manipulation and solely a sprinkled hair residue is visible.[18] Although not exclusive to TT, when present it is a helpful clue to the diagnosis.

TABLE 7.1
Common Trichoscopic Findings Identified in Patients With Trichotillomania

Trichoscopic Findings	Description
Flame hairs	Short (<1 mm) pigmented hairs with a thin, wavy, distal tip Proximal hair residue that remains attached to the scalp after pulling anagen hairs Develops as a result of severe mechanical hair pulling and shredding
Tulip hairs	Short hairs with darker, tulip flower–shaped ends Develops when a hair shaft fractures diagonally
Coiled hairs	Manifestation of proximal hair parts remaining attached to the scalp after distal portion has been pulled and hair shaft fractured Irregular in shape with a jagged end Partially coiled hairs have a hook-like appearance
Exclamation mark hairs	Rare in trichotillomania Flat distal end and a pigmented proximal end
Hair powder sign	Result of damage to the hair shaft by mechanical manipulation and only a sprinkled hair residue is visible
V-sign	When two or more hairs emerge from one follicular unit pulled simultaneously and break at the same length above the scalp surface Surrounded by long terminal hairs
Burnt matchstick sign	Dark bulbar proximal tip with a linear stem of variable length Linear in morphology, nonwavy, longer in length, conical tip absent

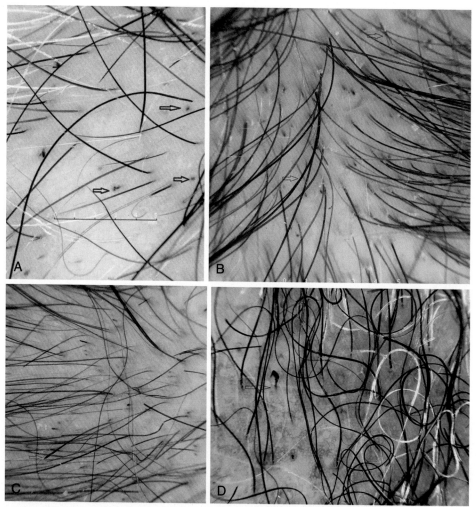

FIG. 7.2 **(A)** Black dots and broken hairs in trichotillomania. Note the hair powder (*red arrows*) (Handyscope 10x). **(B)** V-sign in trichotillomania (*red arrows*), note also the presence of broken hairs at different lengths (Handyscope, 10x). **(C)** Tulip hair in trichotillomania (*red arrow*) (Handyscope, x10). **(D)** Coiled hair in tricho-tillomania (partially coiled hairs have a question mark like appearance) (*red arrow*) (Handyscope 10x).

A "v-sign" is created when two or more hairs emerging from one follicular unit are pulled simultaneously and break at the same length above the scalp surface (Fig. 7.2B). This feature may be distinguished from a pair of healthy regrowing terminal hairs in a person with a shaved scalp in that all hairs in the field of view will have similar length, whereas in a patient with TT, the v-sign is surrounded by long terminal hairs.[18] *Tulip hairs* are short hairs with darker, tulip flower–shaped ends that develop when a hair shaft fractures diagonally. They are characteristic for TT but may also be observed in other diseases

(Fig. 7.2C).[18] *Coiled hairs* represent another manifestation of proximal hair parts remaining attached to the scalp after the distal part has been pulled (Fig. 7.2D). They may have diverse trichoscopic appearance depending on the hair thickness, mechanical force, and angle of hair tearing. Partially coiled hairs, also termed "hook hairs," may have a question mark or hooklike appearance.[18] Coiled hairs should be differentiated from regrowing pigtail hairs, circle hairs, by their irregular appearance and frayed end. The pigtail hairs are regular, circular or oval, and with a pointed end, characteristic of regrowing hairs.[18]

Exclamation mark hairs are rare in TT,[20] and their presence usually favors a diagnosis of AA. In TT, exclamation mark hairs more often tend to have a flat distal end and a pigmented proximal end. In AA, exclamation mark hairs more commonly have an uneven, ragged, distal end and a hypopigmented proximal end. However, both types of exclamation mark hairs have been observed in both diseases.[18] Of note, AA may be the initial trigger for TT and these two conditions may coexist,[21] making trichoscopic differential diagnosis challenging in the presence of exclamation mark hairs. Yellow dots are generally not observed in TT.[22] Studies have shown that yellow dots in patients with TT contain a black dot or fine black hair residues. Unlike most cases of AA, in TT yellow dots may be sparse and not regularly distributed. Also, black dots tend to be uniform in size and shape in AA, whereas in TT there is a high variability in the diameter and shape.[18]

A case report recently described a novel trichoscopic finding in two different cases named the *"burnt matchstick"* sign that is considered to be specific for TT. The appearance is described as a dark bulbar proximal tip with a linear stem of variable length.[23] It may be differentiated from a flame hair by being linear in morphology, nonwavy, and longer in length and with an absent conical tip. This trichoscopic feature may be helpful in differentiating TT from trichotemnomania and trichoteiromania because the latter two do not have traction involved, which is the essence for development of this particular sign.[23]

PATHOLOGY

The most relevant histologic feature of TT is the presence of normally growing hairs among empty hair follicles in a noninflammatory dermis.[24] These features are due to the mechanical traction on the hair. Often, in the same biopsy, it is possible to observe alternating damaged and intact follicles, even very close to one another, and this finding correlates with the clinical observation of incomplete hair loss in the patches of alopecia. Follicular plugging with keratin debris can be prominent.[24]

There is increased numbers of catagen and telogen hairs without evidence of inflammation.[25] As a response to the forcible injury, the follicle may enter the catagen phase, increasing the catagen/telogen count up to 70%. Thus, increase in the percentage of catagen/telogen, though not diagnostic, is a frequent feature of TT.[26] The damaged follicles fail to form normal hair shafts, resulting in trichomalacia. *Trichomalacia* is the most characteristic histopathologic finding of TT and refers to shafts with a smaller diameter and abnormal

shape and pigmentation.[27] Because of trauma, the individual damaged follicles demonstrate intra- and perifollicular hemorrhage.[27] Perifollicular hemorrhage near the hair bulb, or between the outer root sheath and connective tissue sheath, is diagnostic.[25] In TT, *pigmented casts* consist of matrical or cortex cells containing melanin that are removed from the follicle by plucking.[28] These cells are displaced in the upper hair canal, where they shrink forming a black mass.[28] In most follicles with pigmented casts, there may be an increased number of apoptotic cells in the outer root sheath as a feature of early conversion to catagen.[29] In some follicles, minor repeated pulling forces result in disruption of the cortex, in which melanin granules will aggregate in a linear arrangement with a *zip shape* in the center or closer to the periphery (Fig. 7.3A).[29] Other studies included biopsy findings of individual follicles revealing features of pigmented casts, centrally located inside the hair canal (Fig. 7.3B and C). When the hair shaft is plucked, melanin granules aggregate in a button shape surrounded by the collapsed inner root sheath. This *"black button"* sign is a common finding in TT.[28] A biopsy with the hair shafts conserved may exhibit the characteristic *"hamburger sign,"* resulting from longitudinal breakage of the hair shaft in a vertical orientation with accumulation of proteinaceous material and erythrocytes in the resulting intermediate space.[30] Recognition of these various signs provides additional tools in the diagnosis of TT.

In conclusion, the increased number of catagen follicles and presence of pigmented casts are a feature of both AA and TT and can therefore lead to a misdiagnosis.[31] In TT, however, the vellus hairs are spared and do not form pigmented casts. Signs of follicular injury in the biopsy will also help in the differential diagnosis for TT. Histology indicative of traumatic hair injury are the characteristic "hamburger sign" and the zip- and button-shaped pigmented casts.[29]

DIFFERENTIAL DIAGNOSIS

When assessing a patient with possible TT, it is important to assess for comorbid skin disorders that may trigger hair pulling. Thyroid function tests and serum ferritin levels should be routinely assessed in all women with hair loss to rule out monosymptomatic hypothyroidism or iron deficiency, respectively.[32] Typically, TT hair loss is patchy, nonscarring, and features broken hairs of different length. Linear excoriations may also be present. The most common differential diagnoses are AA, tinea capitis, pressure-induced alopecia, and traction alopecia (see Table 7.2).[18,22,33–38]

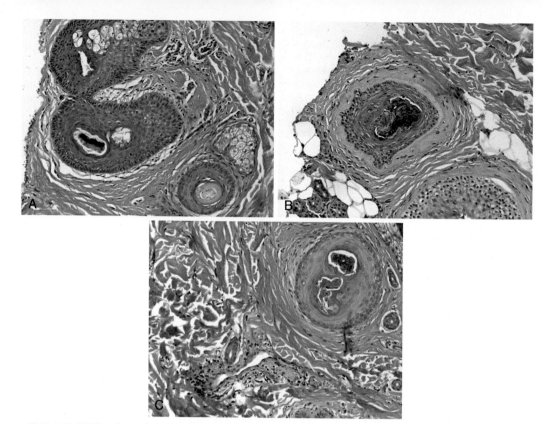

FIG. 7.3 **(A)** Histology of trichotillomania shows trichomalacia with pigmented casts (zip-like pigment cast in the hair canal of a terminal anagen follicle). The vellus follicle is unaffected (hematoxylin and eosin, 20×). **(B)** Histology of trichotillomania shows disrupted matrix at the level of the bulb (hematoxylin and eosin, 20×). **(C)** Histology of trichotillomania: In this example there is trichomalacia at the level of the isthmus. Note the presence of eosinophils in perivascular distribution (hematoxylin and eosin, 20×).

TABLE 7.2
Differential Diagnoses of Trichotillomania

Diagnosis	Dermoscopy	Pathology
Trichotillomania	Broken hair shafts of varying morphology and lengths: coiled hairs, trichoptilosis, black dots, flame hairs, tulip hairs, v-sign, hair powder	Increased number of catagen follicles Distorted hair shafts and pigment cats (trichomalacia and pigment casts) at all follicular levels
Alopecia areata	Exclamation mark hairs, black dots, coiled hairs, yellow dots, circle hairs	Increased telogen count, peribulbar lymphocytic infiltrates (swarm of bees) and nanogen follicles Individual hair follicles with trichomalacia at the infundibular level
Traction alopecia	Empty follicular ostia Increased number of vellus follicles Cylindrical hair casts	Absence of terminal follicles/follicular units Vellus follicles outnumber terminal follicles Preserved sebaceous glands
Pressure induced alopecia	Black dots, broken hairs Absent yellow dots Absent tapering hairs	Increased number of catagen/telogen follicles
Tinea capitis	Comma hairs, corkscrew hairs, Bar-code like hairs Scale usually present	Fungal spores within hair shafts (endothrix) or within hair follicle (ectothrix) Abscess like inflammation in kerion

TABLE 7.3
Patchy Alopecia in Children

Diagnosis	Pull test	Dermoscopy	Pathology
Alopecia areata	Positive	Black dots Yellow dots Broken hairs Exclamation mark hairs	Acute (swarm of bees infiltrate) Subacute (increased telogen count) Chronic (vellus follicles and nanogen follicles)
Trichotillomania	Negative	Black dots Yellow dots Broken hairs at different lengths and distorted hair shafts	Increased catagen count up to 70% Trichomalacia Pigmented casts
Congenital triangular alopecia	Negative	Upright regrowing hairs Vellus hairs Regrowing pigtail hairs Terminal hairs on outskirts of lesion	Miniaturized hair follicles Increased proportion of vellus hairs Rare terminal follicles

Cases have been reported in which AA may appear in conjunction with TT,[39] thus making it difficult for the clinician to distinguish the two types of hair loss. Trichoscopic features that differentiate AA from TT in children are summarized in Table 7.3.

MANAGEMENT

Currently there are no treatments for TT approved by the U.S. Food and Drug Administration, which poses a challenge for physicians. However, *N*-acetylcysteine (NAC) is effective in treating TT patients, but its mechanism of action is unknown. In a double-blind placebo trial, 56% of patients with TT received NAC for 12 weeks (dosing range, 1200–2400 mg/day) and results revealed a reduction in hair pulling symptoms compared with 16% of patients taking placebo.[40]

In children, TT is usually self-limited and parents should be reassured. Psychotherapeutic interventions

are helpful. In adolescents and adults, the first-line treatment is group cognitive behavioral therapy, in particular habit reversal therapy.[15] This treatment requires considerable commitment to monitor symptoms, practice coping skills, and tolerate urges and discomfort while working to reduce hair pulling symptoms. It is also important to refer patients with TT for psychiatric evaluation for comorbid conditions, which should be treated aggressively. In the absence of clear guidance about the choice of appropriate drugs, selection of medication should take into consideration factors such as the severity of the disorder, psychiatric comorbidity, and timing of the onset of TT.

REFERENCES

1. American Psychiatric Association. *Diagnostic and Statistical Manual of Mental Disorders*. 5th ed. Washington, DC: American Psychiatric Association; 2013.
2. Kuhn H, Mennella C, Magid M, et al. Psychocutaneous disease: clinical perspectives. *J Am Acad Dermatol.* 2017;76:779–791.
3. Ramot Y, Maly A, Horev L, Zlotogorski A. Familial trichotillomania in three generations. *Int J Trichol.* 2013;5:86–87.
4. Duke DC, Keeley ML, Geffken GR, Stroch EA. Trichotillomania: a current review. *Clin Psychol Rev.* 2010;30:181–193.
5. Lochner C, Seedat S, Stein DJ. Chronic hair-pulling: phenomenology-based subtypes. *J Anxiety Disord.* 2010;24(2):196–202.
6. Woods D, Flessner C, Franklin M, et al. The trichotillomania impact: exploring phenomenology, functional impairment, and treatment utilization. *J Clin Psychiat.* 2006;67:1877–1888.
7. Novak CE, Keuthen NJ, Stewart SE, Pauls DL. A twin concordance study of trichotillomania. *Am J Med Genet B Neuropsychiatr Genet.* 2009;150B(7):944–949.
8. Zuchner S, Cuccaro ML, Tran-Viet KN, et al. SLITRK1 mutations in trichotillomania. *Mol Psychiat.* 2006;11:887–889.
9. Boughn S, Holdom JJ. The relationship of violence and trichotillomania. *J Nurs Scholarsh.* 2003;35:165–170.
10. Houghton DC, Compton SN, Twohig MP, et al. Measuring the role of psychological inflexibility in trichotillomania. *Psychiat Res.* 2014;220(1–2):356–361.
11. Reich S, Trüeb RM. Trichoteiromania. *J Dtsch Dermatol Ges.* 2003;1:22–28.
12. Happle R. Trichotemnomania: obsessive-compulsive habit of cutting or shaving the hair. *J Am Acad Dermatol.* 2005;52(1):157–159.
13. Jafferany M, Feng J, Hornung RL. Trichodaganomania: the compulsive habit of biting one's own hair. *J Am Acad Dermatol.* 2009;60(4):689–691.
14. Frey A, McKee M, King R, Martin A. Hair apparent: rapunzel syndrome. *Am J Psychiat.* 2005;162:242–248.

15. Walsh K, McDougle C. Trichotillomania: presentation, etiology, diagnosis and therapy. *Am J Clin Dermatol.* 2001;2:327–333.

16. Dimino-Emme L, Camisa C. Trichotillomania associated with the "Friar Tuck sign" and nail-biting. *Cutis.* 1991;47:107–110.

17. Ross EK, Vincenzi C, Tosti A. Videodermoscopy in the evaluation of hair and scalp disorders. *J Am Acad Dermatol.* 2006;55:799–806.

18. Rakowska A, Slowinska M, Olszewska M, Rudnicka L. New trichoscopy findings in trichotillomania: flame hairs, V-sign, hook hairs, hair powder, tulip hairs. *Acta Derm Venereol.* 2014;94:303–306.

19. Miteva M, Tosti A. Flame hair. *Skin Appendage Disord.* 2015;1(2):105–109.

20. Rudnicka L, Olszewska M, Rakowska A, Slowinska M. Trichoscopy update. *J Dermatol Case Rep.* 2011;5:82–88.

21. Sah DE, Koo J, Price VH. Trichotillomania. *Dermatol Ther.* 2008;21:13–21.

22. Abraham LS, Torres FN, Azulay-Abulafia L. Dermoscopic clues to distinguish trichotillomania from patchy alopecia areata. *An Bras Dermatol.* 2010;85:723–726.

23. Malakar S, Mukherjee SS. Burnt matchstick sign – a new trichoscopic finding in trichotillomania. *Int J Trichol.* 2017;9(1):44–46.

24. Bergfeld W, Mulinari-Brenner F, McCarron K, Embi C. The combined utilization of clinical and histological findings in the diagnosis of trichotillomania. *J Cutan Pathol.* 2002;29:207–214.

25. Muller SA. Trichotillomania: a histopathologic study in 66 patients. *J Am Acad Dermatol.* 1990;23:56–62.

26. Sperling LC, Lupton GP. Histopathology of non-scarring alopecia. *J Cutan Pathol.* 1995;22:97–114.

27. Lachapelle JM, Pierard GE. Traumatic alopecia in trichotillomania: a pathogenic interpretation of histologic lesions in the pilosebaceous unit. *J Cutan Pathol.* 1977;4:51–67.

28. Sperling LC, ed. *An Atlas of Hair Pathology with Clinical Correlations.* vol. 1. New York, NY: The Parthenon Publishing Group; 2003:58–63.

29. Miteva M, Romanelli P, Tosti A. Pigmented casts. *Am J Dermatopathol.* 2014;36:58–63.

30. Royer M, Sperling L. Splitting hairs: the 'hamburger sign' in trichotillomania. *J Cutan Pathol.* 2006;33:63–64.

31. Bernárdez C, Molina-Ruiz AM, Requena L. Histopatología de las alopecias. Parte I: alopecias no cicatriciales. *Actas Dermosifiliogr.* 2015;106:158–167.

32. Peckham SJ, Sloan SB, Elston DM. Histologic features of alopecia areata other than peribulbar lymphocytic infiltrates. *J Am Acad Dermatol.* 2011;65:615–620.

33. Hautmann G, Hercogova J, Lotti T. Trichotillomania. *J Am Acad Dermatol.* 2002;46(6):807–826.

34. Inui S, Nakajima T, Nakagawa K, Itami S. Clinical significance of dermoscopy in alopecia areata: analysis of 300 cases. *Int J Dermatol.* 2008;47:688–693.

35. Tangjaturonrusamee C, Piraccini BM, Vincenzi C, Starace M, Tosti A. Tinea capitis mimicking folliculitis decalvans. *Mycoses.* 2011;54:87–88.

36. Slowinska M, Rudnicka L, Schwartz RA, et al. Comma hairs: a dermatoscopic marker for tinea capitis: a rapid diagnostic method. *J Am Acad Dermatol.* 2008;59(5 suppl):S77–S79.

37. Lacarrubba F, Verzi AE, Micali G. Newly described features resulting from high-magnification dermoscopy of tinea capitis. *JAMA Dermatol.* 2015;151:308–310.

38. Hanly AJ, Jorda M, Badiavas E, et al. Postoperative pressure-induced alopecia: report of a case and discussion of the role of apoptosis in non-scarring alopecia. *J Cutan Pathol.* 1999;26:357–361.

39. Brzezinski P, Cywinska E, Chiriac A. Report of a rare case of alopecia aerate coexisting with trichotillomania. *Int J Trichol.* 2016;8:32–34.

40. Grant JE, Odlaug BL, Kim SW. N-Acetylcysteine, a glutamate modulator, in the treatment of trichotillomania. *Arch Gen Psychiat.* 2009;66:756–763.

CHAPTER 8

Frontal Fibrosing Alopecia

RODRIGO PIRMEZ, MD • YANNA KELLY, MD

INTRODUCTION

Frontal fibrosing alopecia (FFA) is a distinctive form of primary lymphocytic cicatricial alopecia that has been considered as a variant of lichen planopilaris (LPP) because of the histopathologic similarity between both diseases. Since the first description by Kossard in 1994, FFA has evolved from a "recently described disease" to the status of "a growing epidemic."[1,2] A number of case series clearly demonstrate that the incidence of FFA has markedly increased over the last years.

In 2005, a case series comprising 16 patients already highlighted that Kossard's postmenopausal FFA had been increasing.[3] In 2009, Tan et al. reported the features of 18 patients, and in 2010, 36 more cases were described.[4,5] In the same year, Chew et al. demonstrated that involvement in FFA was generalized rather than localized only to the frontal scalp and eyebrows.[6] In 2012, a new case series of 60 patients was published, once again drawing attention to the increasing number of cases.[7] Finally, in 2014, the larger multicenter case series since the first description of FFA was published with 355 patients.[8] Even though there are no population-based studies with reliable information about the incidence of FFA, currently almost every dermatologist has seen at least one case of FFA and many specialists in the field of hair disorders agree that there is indeed an epidemic growth of the disease.

EPIDEMIOLOGY

FFA mostly affects postmenopausal women, but it is also described in premenopausal women and men. The larger series published so far confirmed these data, showing that 83% of the patients were postmenopausal women, whereas 14% were premenopausal, and men represented only 3% of the cases. An exception was found in one study where the majority of patients were premenopausal women (65.2%). However, the earlier age of onset in this study was attributed to the possible follicular damage caused by traction, as most patients were Africans.[9] Most studies report data from Caucasians, but, as mentioned, there are publications on African-Americans and also on Asian patients.[10–12]

Population based studies are needed to establish the true distribution of FFA among different ethnicities.

PATHOGENESIS

FFA's exact etiology is not as clearly elucidated as some of the pathways involved. Nevertheless, several possible factors have been implicated since its first description.

Autoimmune Etiology

Autoimmune disorders have been reported in association with FFA, such as collagen diseases, hypo- and hyperthyroidism, and vitiligo.[7,13–15] In the large multicentric study from Spain, Vañó-Galván et al. reported that 15% of patients presented with associated hypothyroidism, a substantial percentage when compared with Spanish overall prevalence.[8] Within the skin, the hair follicle is a site of relative immune privilege, which serves as a protective strategy against autoimmune injury. Therefore, it has been suggested that an autoimmune mechanism could be involved in the pathogenesis of FFA and other primary cicatricial alopecias, such as collapse of the immune privilege at the level of the bulge and a subsequent cell-mediated immune reaction against follicular keratinocytes.[16]

Hormonal Etiology

FFA is known to almost exclusively affect women of postmenopausal age. Its postmenopausal occurrence led to the speculation of a hormone-related triggering mechanism. Estrogen has been found to have antifibrotic effects in vivo and act as a potent immunomodulator, and postmenopausal estrogen decline could act as one of the possible culprits in disease pathogenesis. Additionally, 5α-reductase inhibitors such as finasteride and dutasteride have been used with positive results, although it has been argued that the beneficial effect of these may be on any concomitant androgenetic element of hair loss.[3,8,17-20] It is still uncertain how hormonal changes after menopause could act as a trigger to the inflammatory cicatricial reaction in FFA patients.

Lipid Metabolism Dysfunction

In 2009, Karnik et al. described disturbed lipid metabolism in the pilosebaceous unit of patients with LPP.[21] The authors suggested that the initial trigger of inflammation in LPP is an abnormal functioning of the peroxisome proliferator–activated receptor γ (PPAR-γ), which leads to aberrant lipid metabolism in the sebaceous gland, a toxic buildup of lipids, and a subsequent inflammatory response. Based on these findings, LPP and FFA patients have been treated with the PPAR-γ agonist pioglitazone with variable results.[22–24]

Neurogenic Inflammation

One hypothesis for the pathogenesis of scarring alopecias encompasses neurogenic cutaneous inflammation. Evidence for this comes from animal models where stressed mice show increased expression of neuropeptides, increased degranulation of mast cells, and loss of hair follicle (HF) immune privilege.[25,26] Recent data examining nerve fiber density and expression of substance P and calcitonin gene–related peptide in FFA patients show variability in the expression of these neuropeptides between lesional and nonlesional scalp skin, as well as differences between LPP and FFA groups.[27]

Genetics

In recent years, familial cases of FFA have been reported. Despite the discrete evidence, they suggest that genetic factors may be implicated in disease development.[28–31] It is true that a number of relatives affected by the same condition could merely point to exposure to common environmental triggers. However, it is known that susceptibility of an individual to toxic substances may be genetically determined.[32]

Environmental Factors

The recent onset of FFA as well as its increasing incidence argues in favor of a possible role of environmental factors in disease pathogenesis. In this regard, a questionnaire-based study by Aldoori et al. inquired FFA patients and controls about exposure to a wide range of lifestyle, social, and medical factors and found that the use of sunscreens was significantly greater in the FFA group compared with controls. The authors also found that FFA patients tested positive for the use of fragrances (namely, linalool and balsam of Peru) more frequently than the overall patch-tested population.[33] A number of considerations were drawn in response to these observations. According to Callender et al.,[34] the frequent use of sunscreen chemicals in both leave-in and wash-off hair care products could explain why

FFA often progresses to wider scalp involvement. On the other hand, Seegobin et al. questioned the methodology of the Aldoori et al. study and replied that "there is no statistically significant association with leave-on facial skin care products and sunscreens."[35] Dhana et al. raised possible bias of the study, including selection and recall bias. Importantly, the study by Aldoori et al. does not allow one to conclude whether regular sunscreen use preceded the onset of disease or was a newly adopted behavior as a consequence of disease diagnosis.[36]

CLINICAL FEATURES

A frontal or frontotemporal band of scarring alopecia with eyebrow involvement is the classic feature of FFA. Since the first report by Kossard,[1] additional characteristics and variants not contemplated in the original description have been incorporated to the clinical picture, and FFA is now considered a generalized skin condition with a wide range of manifestations.[6]

It has been noted that hairline recession is not uniform in every patient, and Moreno-Arrones et al.[37] have recently proposed a clinical classification based on the pattern of hairline recession:
1. **Pattern I or "linear pattern":** Patients present with a band of uniform frontal hairline recession in the absence of loss of hair density behind the hairline (Fig. 8.1A).
2. **Pattern II or "diffuse pattern":** Patients present with a diffuse or zigzag bandlike alopecia affecting the frontal hairline with significant loss of hair density behind it (Fig. 8.1B).
3. **Pattern III or "pseudo 'fringe sign' pattern":** It is defined as an FFA presenting with a frontal or temporal unaffected primitive hairline, forming the *pseudo* "fringe sign" (Fig. 8.1C).

The *pseudo* "fringe sign" refers to the peculiar sparing of the hairline observed in some patients, and its name is a reminder of the original sign described in traction alopecia, one of the major differential diagnoses with FFA.[38] Even though it seems to be the least common pattern of presentation (6.2%), patients with the *pseudo* "fringe sign" had the best prognosis in this study, whereas patients with the "diffuse pattern" presented with the worst.

Hairline recession in FFA may not be limited to the frontotemporal area and may extend behind the ears, involving the occipital region (Fig. 8.2).[8] FFA may also be associated with patches of classical LPP in a small percentage of individuals.[39] Therefore, the entire scalp should be checked at every consultation.

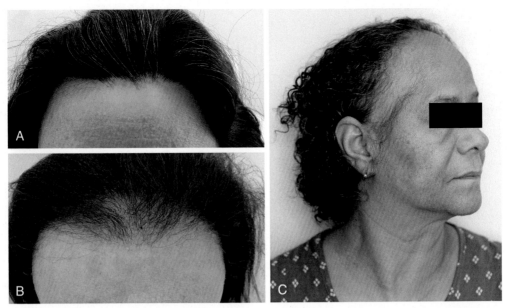

FIG. 8.1 Patterns of presentation in patients with frontal fibrosing alopecia: **(A)** linear pattern; **(B)** diffuse pattern; and **(C)** pseudo "fringe sign" pattern. Note sparing of the original hairline, specially in the temporal scalp.

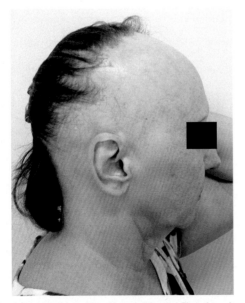

FIG. 8.2 A patient with advanced frontal fibrosing alopecia showing involvement of the entire hairline, including occipital scalp.

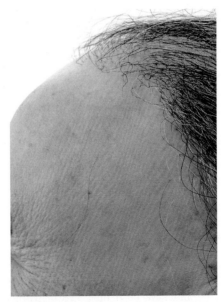

FIG. 8.3 The "lonely hair" sign: a clue to the diagnosis of frontal fibrosing alopecia.

An interesting feature of FFA is that as disease progresses, it may "leave behind" some unaffected terminal hairs (Fig. 8.3). The "lonely hairs," as they were named, are an important clue in the differential diagnosis with other alopecias that also affect the hairline, such as alopecia areata and traction alopecia.[40]

The skin in between the old and new hairline in FFA is usually referred as atrophic and sometimes

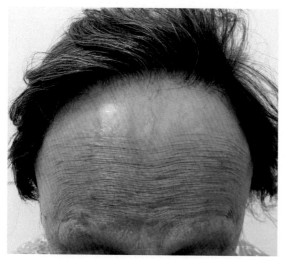

FIG. 8.4 The skin between the old and new hairlines is atrophic.

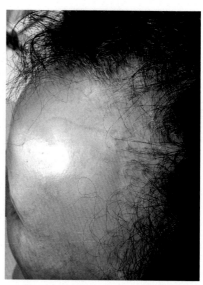

FIG. 8.5 Frontal fibrosing alopecia in a patient presenting with depression of the frontal veins. Perifollicular erythema may be clinically seen and may indicate that the disease is active.

as hypopigmented, even in patients who were never exposed to topical or intralesional corticosteroids (Fig. 8.4). The mechanisms underlying such findings have not been explored, but in a small case series, Lin et al. have documented that the epidermis of FFA patients is indeed thinner when compared with that in controls and with lower melanocyte counts.[41] Such cutaneous atrophy may be responsible for the depression of the frontal veins, a clinical feature described in some patients (Fig. 8.5).[42]

Reports of hair loss at areas other than the scalp and eyebrows, such as limbs and axillary and pubic regions, have expanded the spectrum of the disease.[43] Body hair loss is usually silent but may affect up to 38% of patients.[3,12] When noticed, patients tend to associate it with age and postmenopausal status. For this reason, patients do not usually report body hair involvement spontaneously, and they should always be inquired about it at their first visit.

Involvement of facial vellus hairs, on the other hand, has been associated with characteristic cutaneous changes. Facial papules are skin-colored follicular papules (Fig. 8.6) that may be noted in 14%–18% of patients[8,37] and have been linked to lichenoid perifollicular inflammation of facial vellus hairs.[44,45] In most cases, they are discrete and may go unnoticed by patients, as some of them believe changes to their skin surface are age-related or a consequence of chronic sun damage. Some individuals, however, present with prominent facial papules, which can be a source of distress and even be the primary reason for consulting a

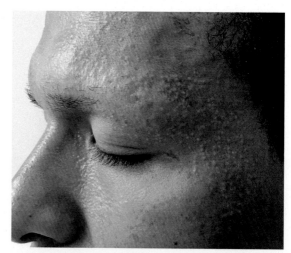

FIG. 8.6 Prominent facial papules in a young male patient with frontal fibrosing alopecia.

dermatologist. Our group recently observed that histopathologic features of facial papules might not be limited to perifollicular inflammation, as previously described, and that structural changes involving elastic fibers and sebaceous glands could be responsible for their clinical formation. According to our findings, we proposed that an abnormal elastic framework could be responsible for remodeling the shape of sebaceous

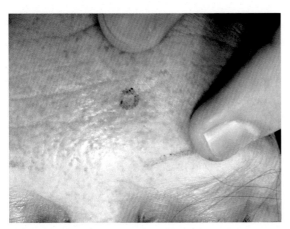

FIG. 8.7 Glabellar *red dots* in frontal fibrosing alopecia.

lobules and ducts, leading to the "pop out" of sebaceous glands and the formation of facial papules in
individuals with FFA.[46] Corroborating this model,
prominent sebaceous glands in biopsy specimens from
facial papules were also reported by another study.[47]

Another sign associated with facial vellus involvement are follicular red dots at the glabellar region
(Fig. 8.7).[48] They were present in 28% of patients in
a large case series,[37] but their prevalence in a given
population is possibly influenced by patient skin type
because they are more easily observed in patients of
lighter complexion. After the initial description, later
reports have found similar red dots also on the cheeks
and hips of patients, so it is likely that this sign is not
restricted to the facial skin.[49,50]

Lichen planus pigmentosus (LPPigm), a macu-
lar variant of lichen planus, may be seen in association with FFA, especially in dark-skinned patients.[9] In
reported FFA patients, LPPigm is characterized by gray
or bluish gray macules affecting mainly facial skin and
occasionally the neck and cleavage area. At least three
patterns of pigmentation have been reported: (1) diffuse, (2) reticulated, and (3) composed of multiple
pigmented macules.[51] (Fig. 8.8). In the original description, LPPigm preceded hair loss in all subjects and was
therefore suggested as a herald sign of FFA.

Men are a minority among FFA patients, and currently there are only two small case series focusing on
this population.[52,53] Apparently, male patients seem
to be affected with FFA at younger ages than female
patients and to present with higher rates of facial papules. However, these data need to be corroborated in
larger case series.

Disease activity may be monitored through signs
of inflammation in the affected hairline, which may

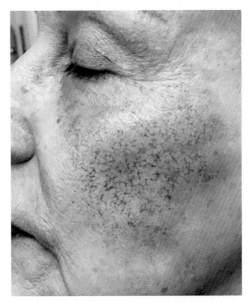

FIG. 8.8 Frontal fibrosing alopecia in a patient presenting
with associated lichen planus pigmentosus with a reticulated pattern of pigmentation.

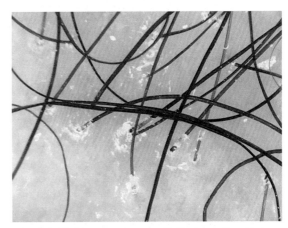

FIG. 8.9 Trichoscopy shows perifollicular scaling. Note
that scaling in frontal fibrosing alopecia may have a tubular
shape. Once scales detach from the scalp, they form hair
casts.

be better appreciated through trichoscopy. Perifollicular erythema and scaling are typically seen in FFA
patients and traditionally considered as signs of ongoing follicular damage (Fig. 8.9). The value of perifollicular erythema as an indicative of disease activity has
been questioned by some authors, who argue that it
may persist even in patients who do not present further progression of the hairline recession.[7] Severity

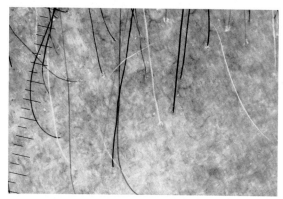

FIG. 8.10 Loss of vellus hairs in the hairline. Perifollicular scaling indicates that the disease is still active.

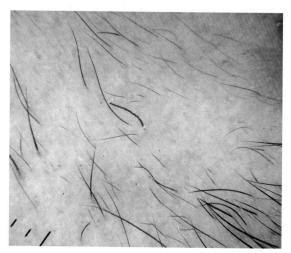

FIG. 8.11 Trichoscopy of the eyebrows from a patient with early disease shows a dystrophic hair (in the center) and *black dots*.

of perifollicular scaling, on the other hand, has been shown to correlate with the degree of lymphocytic infiltration in scalp biopsies and may be, therefore, a more accurate parameter to be used in clinical practice.[54] In trichoscopy, scaling in FFA is generally subtler than in LPP, especially if performed in the sideburns area. An additional feature that may suggest FFA in this particular location is the presence of translucent skin surrounding the emergence of shafts.[55] In both FFA and LPP, scales may embrace the proximal hair shaft forming characteristic tubular structures. Once these structures detach from the scalp, they form *hair casts*, which can move freely along hair shafts and are sometimes mistaken for nits. Symptoms such as pain, pruritus, or a burning sensation are also indicative of disease activity. A trichoscopic hallmark of FFA is the loss of vellus hairs in the affected hairline[56] (Fig. 8.10). This sign is particularly useful in early cases and also when other features such as erythema and scaling are absent. It is also a clue in the differential diagnosis with other alopecias that may also affect the hairline. Trichoscopy of the alopecic band will reveal loss of follicular openings, a common feature of all end-stage scarring alopecias.

Trichoscopy of the eyebrows can be particularly useful in cases of isolated eyebrow loss, which can be the first sign of FFA in some patients, allowing early diagnosis and treatment (Fig. 8.11).[57]

FFA is generally considered to have a slow progression, and even though prospective studies are scarce, spontaneous remission is the most frequently reported outcome.[4,17]

DIAGNOSIS

Generally, FFA diagnosis is made based on the clinical and trichoscopic findings previously discussed.

However, in doubtful cases, it is reasonable to perform a dermoscopy-guided scalp biopsy. FFA histopathologic features include the typical lichenoid lymphocytic infiltrate at isthmus and infundibulum, perifollicular fibrosis, and, in advances cases, loss of hair follicles, which are replaced by follicular scars (follicular dropout) (Fig. 8.12). Sebaceous glands are generally absent or only focally present.[58] Although most authors agree that these findings are indistinguishable from those seen in LPP, Poblet et al. have suggested that FFA cases would normally present with less inflammation and more apoptotic cells when compared with LPP cases.[59] Another study evaluated the use of direct immunofluorescence, and authors concluded that direct immunofluorescence (DIF) is likely to be negative in FFA cases. They rarely observed typical LPP (9%) or lupus erythematosus (7%) patterns in FFA, suggesting that the same value that DIF may have for differentiating pathologically ambiguous cases of LPP from lupus erythematosus (LE) is not present for FFA.[60]

TREATMENT

There is no current consensus on the best treatment option for FFA. Moreover, no therapeutic modality seems to be consistently effective in every patient. Although several treatments have been reported in the literature, their effect on hair loss progression remains uncertain.

FFA therapeutic modalities include topical, intralesional, and systemic drugs, but the quality of evidence available is poor and outcome measures are not standardized, with no randomized controlled trials

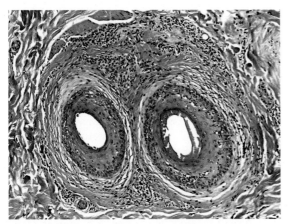

FIG. 8.12 In this horizontal section at the level of the isthmus, two terminal anagen follicles, devoid of sebaceous glands, form a compound follicular structure (eyes sign). There are perifollicular fibrosis and lichenoid inflammation. Note the presence of apoptotic cells in the outer root sheaths (hematoxylin and eosin, 20×).

available so far. In addition, long-term results could be attributed to spontaneous stabilization.

Because FFA is currently considered a generalized condition, the use of systemic drugs as a first therapeutic choice seems reasonable. Despite different authors reporting contrasting results, a common first approach is trying to diminish disease inflammation using antimalarials, such as hydroxychloroquine.[61,62] Doxycycline (or another tetracycline) is also commonly used in the same context.

Association with antiandrogen therapy, namely 5α-reductase inhibitors, may also be helpful. Even though studies have suggested that improvement in these patients may be due to coexistent androgenetic alopecia, others have shown improvement of FFA clinical features.[20,63,64] Finasteride (type 1 5α-reductase inhibitor) and dutasteride (type 1 and 2 5α-reductase inhibitor) are known teratogenic drugs. Women of childbearing age should take these drugs under strict birth control measures, as they can cause feminization of the male fetus.[65] Another concern regarding 5α-reductase inhibitor use in women is that conditions resulting in relative estrogen excess or lack of androgen are associated with an increased risk of breast cancer.[66] During finasteride and dutasteride use, estrogen excess may occur as the inhibition of Dihydrotestosterone (DHT) production alters the estrogen:androgen ratio, with slightly increased estrogen levels because of the conversion of testosterone to estradiol by aromatase. The possible effects of the increased estrogen levels in women taking

5α-reductase inhibitors have not been addressed in any study to date. For this reason, it is recommended not to use these drugs in women with a family or personal history of breast cancer. Considering the abovementioned precautions, finasteride 2.5–5.0 mg/day or dutasteride 0.5 mg/day is commonly used by the authors to treat FFA in association with either hydroxychloroquine 400 mg/day or doxycycline 100–200 mg/day.

Another therapeutic option that gained attention a few years ago was the antidiabetic drug pioglitazone, a PPAR-γ agonist. The work by Karnik et al. suggested that anomalous PPAR-γ functioning with consequent disturbance in sebaceous gland lipid metabolism could play a role in the pathogenesis of primary cicatricial alopecias.[21] Results of pioglitazone in LPP and FFA have been variable with positive results ranging between 20% and 70% and adverse effects occurring in up to 50% of patients. The authors have tried to use this drug to treat LPP/FFA patients. However, the achieved results have not been as satisfactory as expected, in our experience. Moreover, patients frequently complained about side effects, remarkably lower limb edema, which was often a reason to abandon treatment.[24]

Recently, a small retrospective study by Rakowska et al.[67] assessed the efficacy of retinoids in treating FFA. Arrest of disease progression was observed in 76% of patients using oral isotretinoin (20 mg/day) and in 73% of patients treated with acitretin (20 mg/day). These results were superior to those of the control group, who were treated with finasteride 5 mg/day (arrest of disease progression in 43%). Importantly, there was no further progression of disease following the discontinuation of systemic retinoids in most patients.

Other systemic drugs have been used to treat FFA, usually with anecdotal reports. These include cyclosporine[5] and methotrexate.[68] Despite reports of successful treatment, further studies with greater number of patients are needed to evaluate efficacy and safety of these drugs in the treatment of FFA patients.

Topical treatments are also used. The authors generally use them in association with systemic drugs or in isolation if the patient is already improving and therapy is being tapered down. High-potency topical steroids (e.g., clobetasol) have shown efficacy and can be used in patients with prominent inflammatory signs. Because the frontal skin in FFA patients is usually atrophic, we keep close monitoring to withdraw the drug as soon as inflammatory activity has ceased or diminished. Despite limited evidence on topical calcineurin inhibitors (e.g., tacrolimus and pimecrolimus) in FFA, they are another option of topical treatment. Personally, we use tacrolimus once a day in patients with discrete inflammatory signs or when skin atrophy is present. The ointment vehicle of tacrolimus may be inconvenient, and we usually compound it in cream or soap-free cleansing lotion. Topical minoxidil can be considered as an adjuvant therapy, helping to increase hair density in FFA patients, especially in those presenting with associated female pattern hair loss.

Intralesional corticosteroids may be carefully used in patients with prominent inflammatory signs and ongoing hair loss. In addition, Donovan et al. reported eyebrow hair regrowth after the use of 10 mg/mL triamcinolone acetonide in eyebrow injections.[69] In our experience, steroid injections are the only treatment with potential of reverting hair loss in the eyebrows in patients with early disease (Fig. 8.13). However, because of the risk of skin atrophy, we use triamcinolone acetonide in concentrations up to 2.5 mg/mL both for scalp and eyebrows.

Excimer laser (308 nm) has also been used as a therapeutic option for LPP and FFA. Navarini et al. demonstrated that low-dose excimer was able to decrease inflammatory activity in 13 patients with LPP and variants.[70] Recently, Fertig and Tosti also published their clinical experience using the excimer laser in FFA patients, reporting decreased inflammation and reduction of peripilar casts after treatment.[71]

Hair transplantation has been considered in cases of cicatricial alopecias, usually after a remission period of 1–2 years. To date, there are few studies demonstrating variable results. In most reported cases, grafts grow normally during the first years but are destroyed after an average of 4 years.[72-74] For such reason, eligible patients should be clearly warned about the possibility of failure in the long term.

Finally, facial papules may be a source of distress for some FFA patients. Pirmez et al. successfully treated facial papules with oral isotretinoin.[75] The dosage used was 20 mg/day during the first month, followed by 40 mg/day for another 2 months. At the end of treatment, papules had completed disappeared or were considered minimal. A subsequent study by Pedrosa et al.[47] proposed the use of 10 mg every other day. In the study by Pirmez et al. patients reported improvement by the second week of treatment; However, in the latter, patients noticed improvement of skin roughness only after a median time of 2 months. For such, it seems that the choice of therapeutic regimen may affect the time to response of oral isotretinoin, and further studies are necessary to better evaluate dosage and treatment duration.

FOLLOW-UP

The natural history of FFA is variable. Slow progression with subsequent spontaneous remission is the most frequent outcome reported in the literature.[1,7] Some authors have reported different methods to assess disease progression and therapeutic response in an attempt to better guide treatment decisions.[5,54]

The Lichen Planopilaris Activity Index (LPPAI) is a numerical clinical score that was introduced to compare pre- and posttreatment response in patients with LPP and FFA.[61] It includes both objective signs (perifollicular and diffuse erythema, perifollicular scaling, and progression of hair loss) and subject symptoms

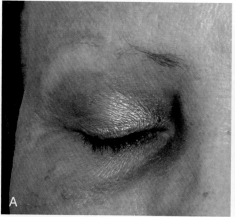 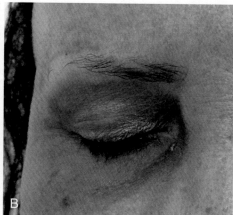

FIG. 8.13 A patient with frontal fibrosing alopecia: **(A)** before and **(B)** after one session of intralesional triamcinolone acetonide, showing partial hair regrowth.

(itching, burning, and pain). This index has been questioned by Donati et al. who monitored LPP patients under treatment with hydroxychloroquine using hair count assessment.[62] They noted that after 6 months, patients presented with decreased hair counts despite therapy, which contrasted with the Chiang et al. study. Overestimation of subjective parameters in LPPAI, such as symptoms reported by the patients, may account for the discrepancy observed. In addition, Donati et al. hypothesized that, possibly, reduction of inflammatory signs would not be enough to halt disease progression. Posteriorly, another scoring system was proposed, the Frontal Fibrosing Alopecia Severity Index (FFASI). In FFASI, hairline recession comprises the greatest proportion of the assessment, but other clinical features are also considered.[76] However, this scoring system has received criticism from different authors.[77,78] Recently, Saceda-Corralo et al. published and validated the FFASS, providing a global severity score that includes the extent of alopecia, signs of local inflammation, and patients' symptoms. This score separates features related to the extent of alopecia from those linked with inflammation, making it possible to perform distinct analyses and to study the relationship between them.[79] Of note, in FFASS, inflammatory signs are analyzed without using trichoscopy, which can detect perifollicular signs of inflammation with higher sensibility. A consensual grading score for FFA is still in need.

A less elaborate but reasonable way to follow up patients in the clinic is through recording clinical and trichoscopic signs of disease activity. Martinez et al. have recently demonstrated correlation between severity of hair casts observed under trichoscopy and degree of inflammation seen in pathology, confirming reliability of the method.[53]

REFERENCES

1. Kossard S. Postmenopausal frontal fibrosing alopecia: scarring alopecia in a pattern distribution. *Arch Dermatol.* 1994;130:770–774.
2. Kossard S, Lee MS, Wilkinson B. Postmenopausal frontal fibrosing alopecia: a frontal variant of lichen planopilaris. *J Am Acad Dermatol.* 1997;36:59–66.
3. Moreno-Ramirez D, Camacho Martinez F. Frontal fibrosing alopecia: a survey in 16 patients. *J Eur Acad Dermatol Venereol.* 2005;19:700–705.
4. Tan KT, Messenger AG. Frontal fibrosing alopecia: clinical presentations and prognosis. *Br J Dermatol.* 2009;160:75–79.
5. Samrao A, Chew AL, Price V. Frontal fibrosing alopecia: a clinical review of 36 patients. *Br J Dermatol.* 2010;163:1296–1300.
6. Chew AL, Bashir SJ, Wain EM, Fenton DA, Stefanato CM. Expanding the spectrum of frontal fibrosing alopecia: a unifying concept. *J Am Acad Dermatol.* 2010;63:653–660.
7. MacDonald A, Clark C, Holmes S. Frontal fibrosing alopecia: a review of 60 cases. *J Am Acad Dermatol.* 2012; 67:955–961.
8. Vañó-Galván S, Molina-Ruiz AM, Serrano-Falcón C, et al. Frontal fibrosing alopecia: a multicenter review of 355 patients. *J Am Acad Dermatol.* 2014;70:670–678.
9. Dlova NC. Frontal fibrosing alopecia and lichen planus pigmentosus: is there a link? *Br J Dermatol.* 2013;168:439–442.
10. Inui S, Nakajima T, Shono F, Itami S. Dermoscopic findings in frontal fibrosing alopecia: report of four cases. *Int J Dermatol.* 2008;47:796–799.
11. Miteva M, Whiting D, Harries M, Bernardes A, Tosti A. Frontal fibrosing alopecia in black patients. *Br J Dermatol.* 2012;167:208–210.
12. Dlova NC, Jordaan HF, Skenjane A, Khoza N, Tosti A. Frontal fibrosing alopecia: a clinical review of 20 black patients from South Africa. *Br J Dermatol.* 2013;169:939–941.
13. Banka N, Mubki T, Bunagan MJ, McElwee K, Shapiro J. Frontal fibrosing alopecia: a retrospective clinical review of 62 patients with treatment outcome and long-term follow-up. *Int J Dermatol.* 2014;53(11):1324–1330.
14. del Rei M, Pirmez R, Sodré CT, Tosti A. Coexistence of frontal fibrosing alopecia and discoid lupus erythematosus of the scalp in 7 patients: just a coincidence? *J Eur Acad Dermatol Venereol.* 2016;30(1):151–153.
15. Miteva M, Aber C, Torres F, et al. Frontal fibrosing alopecia occurring on scalp vitiligo: report of four cases. *Br J Dermatol.* 2011;165:445–447.
16. Tziotzios C, Stefanato CM, Fenton DA, Simpson MA, McGrath JA. Frontal fibrosing alopecia: reflections and hypotheses on aetiology and pathogenesis. *Exp Dermatol.* 2016;25(11):847–852. https://doi.org/10.1111/exd.13071.
17. Tosti A, Piraccini BM, Iorizzo M, Misciali C. Frontal fibrosing alopecia in postmenopausal women. *J Am Acad Dermatol.* 2005;52:55–60.
18. Racz E, Gho C, Moorman PW, Noordhoek Hegt V, Neumann HA. Treatment of frontal fibrosing alopecia and lichen planopilaris: a systematic review. *J Eur Acad Dermatol Venereol.* 2013;27:1461–1470.
19. Donovan JC. Finasteride-mediated hair regrowth and reversal of atrophy in a patient with frontal fibrosing alopecia. *JAAD Case Rep.* 2015;1(6):353–355. https://doi.org/10.1016/j.jdcr.2015.08.003.
20. Tziotzios C, Fenton DA, Stefanato CM, McGrath JA. Finasteride is of uncertain utility in treating frontal fibrosing alopecia. *J Am Acad Dermatol.* 2016;74(4):e73–e74. https://doi.org/10.1016/j.jaad.2015.09.076.
21. Karnik P, Tekeste Z, McCormick TS, et al. Hair follicle stem cell-specific PPAR gamma deletion causes scarring alopecia. *J Invest Dermatol.* 2009;129:1243–1257.
22. Mirmirani P, Karnik P. Lichen planopilaris treated with a peroxisome proliferator-activated receptor gamma agonist. *Arch Dermatol.* 2009;145:1363–1366.

23. Mesinkovska NA, Tellez A, Dawes D, Piliang M, Bergfeld W. The use of oral pioglitazone in the treatment of lichen planopilaris. *J Am Acad Dermatol.* 2015;72:355–356.

24. a. Márquez-García A, Camacho FM. Tratamiento de la alopecia frontal fibrosante: pioglitazonas. *Monogr Dermatol.* 2016;29:66–76.
b. Apud Vañó-Galván S, Camacho F. New treatments for hair loss. *Actas Dermosifiliogr.* 2017;108(3):221–228. https://doi.org/10.1016/j.ad.2016.11.010.

25. Peters EM, Kuhlmei A, Tobin DJ, Muller-Rover S, Klapp BF, Arck PC. Stress exposure modulates peptidergic innervation and degranulates mast cells in murine skin. *Brain Behav Immun.* 2005;19:252–262.

26. Peters EM, Liotiri S, Bodo E, et al. Probing the effects of stress mediators on the human hair follicle: substance P holds central position. *Am J Pathol.* 2007;171:1872–1886.

27. Hordinsky M, Doche I. Nerves and scarring alopecia disorders: a novel treatment approach. In: *Cicatricial Alopecia Workshop – 23rd World Congress of Dermatology 2015. Vancouver*; June 2015.

28. Junqueira Ribeiro Pereira AF, Vincenzi C, Tosti A. Frontal fibrosing alopecia in two sisters. *Br J Dermatol.* 2010;162:1154–1155.

29. Roche M, Walsh MY, Armstrong DKB. Frontal fibrosing alopecia – occurrence in male and female siblings. *J Am Acad Dermatol.* 2008;58(suppl 2):AB91.

30. Dlova N, Goh CL, Tosti A. Familial frontal fibrosing alopecia. *Br J Dermatol.* 2013;168:220–222.

31. Navarro-Belmonte MR, Navarro-López V, Ramírez-Boscà A, et al. Case series of familial frontal fibrosing alopecia and a review of the literature. *J Cosmet Dermatol.* 2015;14(1):64–69.

32. Thier R, Bruning T, Roos PH, et al. Markers of genetic susceptibility in human environmental hygiene and toxicology: the role of selected CYP, NAT and GST genes. *Int J Hyg Environ Health.* 2003;206:149–171.

33. Aldoori N, Dobson K, Holden CR, et al. Frontal fibrosing alopecia: possible association with leave-on facial skin care products and sunscreens; a questionnaire study. *Br J Dermatol.* 2016;175:762–767.

34. Callander J, Frost J, Stone N. Ultraviolet filters in hair-care products: a possible link with frontal fibrosing alopecia and lichen planopilaris. *Clin Exp Dermatol.* October 10, 2017. https://doi.org/10.1111/ced.13273. [Epub ahead of print].

35. Seegobin SD, Tziotzios C, Stefanato CM, et al. Frontal fibrosing alopecia: there is no statistically significant association with leave-on facial skin care products and sunscreens. *Br J Dermatol.* 2016. https://doi.org/10.1111/bjd.15054.

36. Dhana A, Gumedze F, Khumalo NP. Regarding 'Frontal fibrosing alopecia: possible association with leave-on facial skincare products and sunscreens; a questionnaire study. *Br J Dermatol.* 2017;176(3):836–837.

37. Moreno-Arrones OM, Saceda-Corralo D, Fonda-Pascual P, et al. Frontal fibrosing alopecia: clinical and prognostic classification. *J Eur Acad Dermatol Venereol.* 2017. https://doi.org/10.1111/jdv.14287. [Epub ahead of print].

38. Pirmez R, Duque-Estrada B, Abraham LS, et al. It's not all traction: the pseudo "fringe sign" in frontal fibrosing alopecia. *Br J Dermatol.* 2015;173:1336–1338.

39. Saceda-Corralo D, Fernández-Crehuet P, Fonda-Pascual P, et al. Clinical description of frontal fibrosing alopecia with concomitant lichen planopilaris. *Skin Appendage Disord.* 2018;4:105–107. https://doi.org/10.1159/000479799.

40. Tosti A, Miteva M, Torres F. Lonely hair: a clue to the diagnosis of frontal fibrosing alopecia. *Arch Dermatol.* 2011;147(10):1240.

41. Lin J, Valdebran M, Bergfeld W, Conic RZ, Piliang M, Atanaskova Mesinkovska N. Hypopigmentation in frontal fibrosing alopecia. *J Am Acad Dermatol.* 2017;76(6):1184–1186. https://doi.org/10.1016/j.jaad.2017.01.001.

42. Vañó-Galván S, Rodrigues-Barata AR, Urech M, et al. Depression of the frontal veins: a new clinical sign of frontal fibrosing alopecia. *J Am Acad Dermatol.* 2015;72:1087–1088.

43. Miteva M, Camacho I, Romanelli P, Tosti A. Acute hair loss on the limbs in frontal fibrosing alopecia: a clinicopathological study of two cases. *Br J Dermatol.* 2010;163:426–428.

44. Abbas O, Chedraoui A, Ghosn S. Frontal fibrosing alopecia presenting with components of Piccardi-Lassueur-Graham-Little syndrome. *J Am Acad Dermatol.* 2007;57:S15–S18.

45. Donati A, Molina L, Doche I, et al. Facial papules in frontal fibrosing alopecia: evidence of vellus follicle involvement. *Arch Dermatol.* 2011;147:1424–1427.

46. Pirmez R, Barreto T, Duque-Estrada B, Quintella DC, Cuzzi T. Facial papules in frontal fibrosing alopecia: beyond vellus hair follicle involvement. *Skin Appendage Disord.* 2018;4:145–149. https://doi.org/10.1159/000481695.

47. Pedrosa AF, Duarte AF, Haneke E, Correia O. Yellow facial papules associated with frontal fibrosing alopecia: a distinct histologic pattern and response to isotretinoin. *J Am Acad Dermatol.* 2017;77(4):764–766. https://doi.org/10.1016/j.jaad.2017.04.1118.

48. Pirmez R, Donati A, Valente NS, et al. Glabellar red dots in frontal fibrosing alopecia: a further clinical sign of vellus follicle involvement. *Br J Dermatol.* 2014;170:745–746.

49. López-Pestaña A, Tuneu A, Lobo C, et al. Facial lesions in frontal fibrosing alopecia (FFA): clinicopathological features in a series of 12 cases. *J Am Acad Dermatol.* 2015;73(6): 987.e1-6.

50. Meyer V, Sachse M, Rose C, Wagner G. Follicular red dots of the hip in frontal fibrosing alopecia - do we have to look twice? *J Dtsch Dermatol Ges.* 2017;15(3):327–328. https://doi.org/10.1111/ddg.13193.

51. Pirmez R, Duque-Estrada B, Donati A, et al. Clinical and dermoscopic features of lichen planus pigmentosus in 37 patients with frontal fibrosing alopecia. *Br J Dermatol.* 2016;175(6):1387–1390. https://doi.org/10.1111/bjd.14722.

52. Alegre-Sánchez A, Saceda-Corralo D, Bernárdez C, et al. Frontal fibrosing alopecia in male patients: a report of 12 cases. *J Eur Acad Dermatol Venereol.* 2017;31(2):e112–e114. https://doi.org/10.1111/jdv.13855.

53. Ormaechea-Pérez N, López-Pestaña A, Zubizarreta-Salvador J, et al. Frontal fibrosing alopecia in men: presentations in 12 cases and a review of the literature. *Actas Dermosifiliogr.* 2016;107(10):836–844. https://doi.org/10.1016/j.ad.2016.07.004.

54. Martinez Velasco MA. Dermoscopic activity index in FFA. In: *Hair and Scalp Dermoscopy-American Academy of Dermatology Annual Meeting 2017.* Orlando; March 2017.

55. Cervantes J, Miteva M. Distinct trichoscopic features of the sideburns in frontal fibrosing alopecia compared to the frontotemporal scalp. *Skin Appendage Disord.* 2018;4:50–54. https://doi.org/10.1159/000479116.

56. Lacarrubba F, Micali G, Tosti A. Absence of vellus hair in the hairline: a videodermatoscopic feature of frontal fibrosing alopecia. *Br J Dermatol.* 2013;169(2):473–474. https://doi.org/10.1111/bjd.12316.

57. Anzai A, Donati A, Valente NY, Romiti R, Tosti A. Isolated eyebrow loss in frontal fibrosing alopecia: relevance of early diagnosis and treatment. *Br J Dermatol.* 2016;175(5):1099–1101. https://doi.org/10.1111/bjd.14750.

58. Miteva M, Tosti A. The follicular triad: a pathological clue to the diagnosis of early frontal fibrosing alopecia. *Br J Dermatol.* 2012;166:440–442.

59. Poblet E, Jimenez F, Pascual A, Pique E. Frontal fibrosing alopecia versus lichen planopilaris: a clinicopathological study. *Int J Dermatol.* 2006;45:375–380.

60. Donati A, Gupta AK, Jacob C, Cavelier-Balloy B, Reygagne P. The use of direct immunofluorescence in frontal fibrosing alopecia. *Skin Appendage Disord.* 2017;3:125–128.

61. Chiang C, Sah D, Cho B, et al. Hydroxychloroquine and lichen planopilaris: efficacy and introduction of Lichen Planopilaris Activity Index scoring system. *J Am Acad Dermatol.* 2010;62:387–392.

62. Donati A, Assouly P, Matard B, Jouanique C, Reygagne P. Clinical and photographic assessment of lichen planopilaris treatment efficacy. *J Am Acad Dermatol.* 2011;64(3):597–598. https://doi.org/10.1016/j.jaad.2010.04.045; author reply 598–9.

63. Danesh M, Murase JE. Increasing utility of finasteride for frontal fibrosing alopecia. *J Am Acad Dermatol.* 2015;72(6):e157. https://doi.org/10.1016/j.jaad.2015.02.1101.

64. Katoulis A, Georgala, Bozi E, Papadavid E, Kalogeromitros D, Stavrianeas N. Frontal fibrosing alopecia: treatment with oral dutasteride and topical pimecrolimus. *J Eur Acad Dermatol Venereol.* 2009;23:580–582.

65. Bowman CJ, Barlow NJ, Turner KJ, Wallace DG, Foster PM. Effects of in utero exposure to finasteride on androgen-dependent reproductive development in the male rat. *Toxicol Sci.* 2003;74:393–406.

66. Roussouw JE, Anderson GL, Prentice RL, et al. Risks and benefits of estrogen plus progestin in healthy postmenopausal women: principal results from the Women's Health Initiative randomized controlled trial. *JAMA.* 2002;288:321–333.

67. Rakowska A, Gradzińska A, Olszewska M, Rudnicka L. Efficacy of isotretinoin and acitretin in treatment of frontal fibrosing alopecia: retrospective analysis of 54 cases. *J Drugs Dermatol.* 2017;16(10):988–992.

68. Ladizinski B, Bazakas A, Selim MA, Olsen EA. Frontal fibrosing alopecia: a retrospective review of 19 patients seen at Duke University. *J Am Acad Dermatol.* 2013;68:749–755.

69. Donovan JC, Samrao A, Ruben BS, Price VH. Eyebrow regrowth in patients with frontal fibrosing alopecia treated with intralesional triamcinolone acetonide. *Br J Dermatol.* 2010;163(5):1142–1144.

70. Navarini AA, Kolios AG, Prinz-Vavricka BM, Haug S, Trüeb RM. Low-dose excimer 308-nm laser for treatment of lichen planopilaris. *Arch Dermatol.* 2011;147:1325–1326.

71. Fertig R, Tosti A. Frontal fibrosing alopecia treatment options. *Intractable Rare Dis Res.* 2016;5(4):314–315.

72. Nusbaum B, Nusbaum AG. Frontal fibrosing alopecia in a man: results of follicular unit test grafting. *Dermatol Surg.* 2010;36:959–962.

73. Gurfinkiel A, Garcia H, Casas J, Kaminsky A. Trasplante capilar en una paciente con alopecia fibrosante frontal asociada con liquen escleroatrofico de vulva. *Dermatol Argent.* 2011;17:110–115.

74. Jiménez F, Poblet E. Is hair transplantation indicated in frontal fibrosing alopecia? The results of test grafting in three patients. *Dermatol Surg.* 2013;39(7):1115–1118.

75. Pirmez R, Duque-Estrada B, Barreto T, Quintella DC, Cuzzi T. Successful treatment of facial papules in frontal fibrosing alopecia with oral isotretinoin. *Skin Appendage Disord.* 2017;3(2):111–113.

76. Holmes S, Ryan T, Young D, Harries M. Frontal Fibrosing Alopecia Severity Index (FFASI): a validated scoring system for assessing frontal fibrosing alopecia. *Br J Dermatol.* 2016;175:203–207.

77. Saceda-Corralo D, Moreno-Arrones OM, Fonda-Pascual P, Alegre-Sánchez A, Vañó-Galván S. Reply to: 'Frontal Fibrosing Alopecia Severity Index (FFASI): a validated scoring system for assessing frontal fibrosing alopecia'. *Br J Dermatol.* 2016;175(3):648. https://doi.org/10.1111/bjd.14670.

78. Dlova NC, Dadzie OE. Frontal fibrosing alopecia severity index (FFASI): a call for a more inclusive and globally relevant severity index for frontal fibrosing alopecia. *Br J Dermatol.* June 6, 2017. https://doi.org/10.1111/bjd.15694. [Epub ahead of print].

79. Saceda-Corralo D, Moreno-Arrones OM, Fonda-Pascual P, et al. Development and validation of the frontal fibrosing alopecia severity score. *J Am Acad Dermatol.* September 22, 2017. https://doi.org/10.1016/j.jaad.2017.09.034. [Epub ahead of print].

CHAPTER 9

Fibrosing Alopecia in a Pattern Distribution

RALPH M. TRÜEB, MD • MARIA FERNANDA REIS GAVAZZONI DIAS, MD, PHD

PATTERNED HAIR LOSS

Patterned hair loss or androgenetic alopecia (AGA) is generally understood to represent a hereditary, androgen-sensitive, progressive thinning of the scalp hair with sex-dependent differences in frequency, age of onset, and pattern of alopecia. The male pattern, as originally classified by Hamilton and Norwood,[1,2] is characterized by its typical symmetrical bitemporal or frontal recession of the hairline and balding vertex, whereas the female pattern, as later reported by Ludwig,[3] is set apart by a more diffuse thinning of the crown area, while the frontal hairline remains intact.

Its pathogenesis is traditionally related to a polygenic hereditary background and peculiarities of androgen metabolism, resulting in androgen-dependent, progressive thinning of hair associated with a decrease of anagen duration in the hair cycle, miniaturization of the hair follicle, and gradual transformation of terminal to vellus hair in the affected areas.[4]

Therefore, diversity of hair shaft diameter[5] or anisotrichosis[6] is a diagnostic dermoscopic feature of AGA (Fig. 9.1A). It is best appreciated in a central hair part at low magnification and is very useful to detect the condition, particularly in women.[7]

Treatment aims at either blocking the effect of androgens with antiandrogens, such as cyproterone acetate and spironolactone, or 5α-reductase inhibitors, such as finasteride and dutasteride, or at increasing the duration of anagen with the hair growth–promoting agent minoxidil.[8]

The limited success rate of treatment with these agents means that additional pathogenic factors may be considered. The implication of follicular inflammation and fibrosis associated with patterned hair loss has emerged from several independent studies: An early study referred to an inflammatory infiltrate of activated T cells and macrophages in the upper third region of the hair follicles, associated with an enlargement of the follicular dermal sheath composed of collagen bundles (perifollicular fibrosis) in regions of actively progressing alopecia.[9] The significance of this finding was at first controversial. However, Whiting soon demonstrated in morphometric studies in patients with male pattern AGA treated with minoxidil that 55% of patients with microinflammation had regrowth in response to treatment in comparison with 77% of those without inflammation and fibrosis.[10] Whiting's horizontal section studies of scalp biopsies indicated that the perifollicular fibrosis is generally mild, consisting of loose, concentric layers of collagen that must be distinguished from cicatricial alopecia.[10] Therefore, Mahé et al. subsequently proposed the term microinflammation, inasmuch as the process involves a slow, subtle, and indolent course in contrast to the inflammatory and destructive process in the classical inflammatory scarring alopecias.[11] With introduction of the dermoscope for the evaluation of hair loss, peripilar cupular atrophy or peripilar signs (Fig. 9.1B) were soon reported in AGA and have been linked to histopathologic evidence of perifollicular inflammation.[12]

Nevertheless, the inflammatory component has so far not been included in treatment protocols for male and female pattern hair loss. The use or addition of either topical corticosteroids or systemic anti-inflammatory agents, such as oral hydroxychloroquine or doxycycline, in the treatment plan of AGA with microinflammation and fibrosis has so far not been systematically evaluated. For now, we can only deduce a putative added benefit by analogy from their successful use in selected cases of inflammatory scarring alopecia, such as lichen planopilaris (LPP).

CICATRICIAL PATTERN HAIR LOSS

Ultimately, Zinkernagel and Trüeb reported a peculiar type of cicatricial pattern hair loss with histopathologic features consistent with LPP and named it fibrosing alopecia in a pattern distribution (FAPD)[13] (Fig. 9.2A–D).

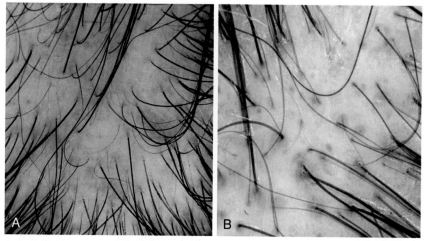

FIG. 9.1 Dermoscopy in androgenetic alopecia: **(A)** diversity of hair shaft diameters or anisotrichosis and **(B)** peripilar signs are characterized by presence of a brown halo, roughly 1 mm in diameter, at the follicular ostium around the emerging hair shaft.

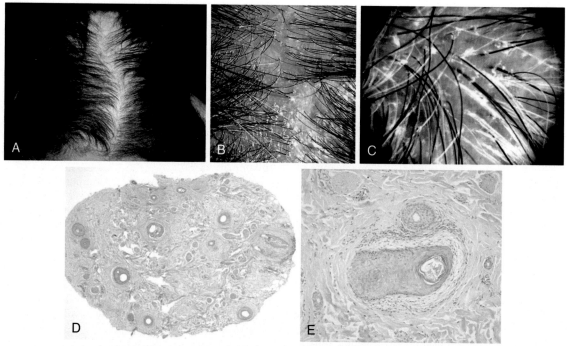

FIG. 9.2 Fibrosing alopecia in a pattern distribution. **(A)** Patterned hair loss with evidence of scarring hair loss in the vertex, **(B)** evidence of perifollicular erythema and keratosis, and **(C)** respective dermoscopic findings of perifollicular erythema and perifollicular keratosis. Histopathology with hematoxylin and eosin stain: **(D)** Horizontal section from a scalp biopsy reveals decreased follicular density with areas of follicular dropout and absent sebaceous glands, and there is increased number of miniaturized follicles, some of which show perifollicular fibrosis and mild lichenoid infiltrate (original magnification 4×). **(E)** Horizontal section from another case reveals the perifollicular lamellar fibrosis associated with lymphocytic lichenoid infiltrate at the isthmus (original magnification, 20×). (Images D and E courtesy of Mariya Miteva)

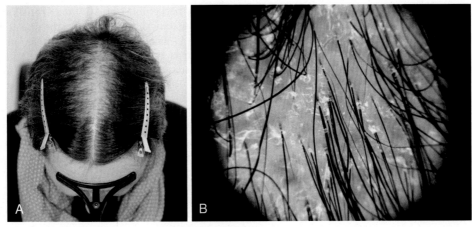

FIG. 9.3 Chronic graft-versus-host disease: **(A)** Cicatricial pattern hair loss, **(B)** with respective dermoscopic finding of perifollicular erythema, keratosis, and fibrosis.

The original report triggered a controversial discussion with regard to its nosologic classification as a distinctive entity within the spectrum of scarring alopecia.[14] The authors themselves discussed whether FAPD is AGA with a lichenoid tissue reaction pattern or patterned LPP. In any case, there exists a striking analogy to LPP and to yet another form of patterned cicatricial hair loss, frontal fibrosing alopecia (FFA), originally reported by Kossard in postmenopausal women.[15] Both, FAPD and FFA, share distinctive patterns of cicatricial alopecia with the histopathology of LPP and may coexist in the same patient. And yet, they bear significant differences.

With regard to its pathogenesis, LPP is considered to be a T cell–mediated autoimmune reaction that triggers apoptosis of follicular epithelial cells. This autoimmune process is thought to be in response to some antigenic challenge, but a specific antigen has not yet been identified. Harries et al. provide the first evidence that LPP may result from an immune privilege collapse of the hair follicle's epithelial stem cell niche.[16] When a causal or triggering agent is identified, this is termed a lichenoid reaction rather than lichen planus. This may include drug reactions, viral hepatitis, and cutaneous graft-versus-host disease (GvHD).

GvHD is a common complication following allogeneic tissue transplantation and is induced and maintained by immunocompetent cells from the donor tissue (graft) that particularly attack epithelia of fast proliferating tissues of the recipient (host), such as those from the gastrointestinal tract, liver, and skin. The skin is the most common organ involved. Although the cutaneous, mucosal, and nail manifestations of chronic GvHD are well recognized, involvement of the hair follicle has so far found lesser attention. Miyazaki et al. reported the first case of GvHD with follicular involvement.[17] Because of its analogies with lichen planus, GvHD constitutes a model that may lead to a better understanding of the pathophysiologic features of lichen planus and LPP. Notably, chronic GvHD may present on the scalp as FAPD (personal observation, Fig. 9.3A and B), as originally reported by Basilio et al. as permanent alopecia after bone marrow transplantation.[18]

The *clinical characteristics* of FAPD are alopecia in the distribution of typical male or female pattern hair loss with perifollicular erythema and hyperkeratosis and eventually loss of follicular openings (Fig. 9.2A and B).

Dermoscopic features of FAPD include perifollicular erythema and keratosis (Fig. 9.2C), whitish perifollicular halo, loss of follicular ostia, and small white patches replacing the follicular openings, in association with hair diameter diversity.

Histopathologic features are miniaturization of hair folilcles and perifollicular lamellar fibrosis, associated with a lymphocytic infiltration around the isthmus and infundibular area of the hair follicles (vacuolar interface alteration of the upper portion of the follicular epithelium), fibrotic tract replacing the portion of the orginal follicular infundibulum, and decrease in sebaceous glands (Fig. 9.2D and E). In advanced stages, there are concentric perifollicular lamellar fibrosis and fibrosed follicular tracts. The histology of FAPD therefore shares histologic features with other scarring alopecias, but the androgenetic pattern of distribution suggests a possible common background and pathogenic mechanisms in both conditions.

FFA represents yet another peculiar condition with a distinctive pattern of scarring alopecia. Steven Kossard is credited with the original description of the condition in 1994,[15] when he reported six postmenopausal women with progressive frontal hairline recession that was associated with perifollicular erythema within the marginal hairline, producing a FFA extending to the temporal and parietal hair margins. Scalp biopsy specimens revealed histologic features that were indistinguishable from those seen in LPP. Eventually, Kossard interpreted this type of alopecia as a frontal variant of LPP on the basis of extended immunohistochemical studies.[19]

Originally considered to be an uncommon condition, the number of cases of FFA has exploded exponentially worldwide, whereas its etiology has remained obscure. A recent questionnaire-based study suggested a possible association between FFA and the use of facial skin care products, particularly sunscreens,[20,21] but the causality of this relationship remains to be confirmed because the study may have been biased through patient and question selection, as well as confounding factors that had not been included in the questionnaire. Finally, there is compelling evidence that FFA existed well before 1994 from physician Axel Munthe's (1857–1948) description of Mamsell Agata in his account of *The Story of San Michele* (1929): "*An exceptionally high and narrow forehead, no eyebrows…*".[22] For this reason, the eponym Axel Munthe's syndrome has been proposed for FFA in recognition of the legacy of Munthe's reminiscences and medical observations recorded in his timeless book for posterity.[23]

FFA has meanwhile also been described in premenopausal women and in men[24–28] though with a significantly lesser frequency. Moreover, it has been recognized to represent a more generalized rather than localized process of inflammatory scarring alopecia, with extension well beyond the frontotemporal hairline to include the parietooccipital hairline, involving peculiar facial papules as evidence of facial vellus hair involvement[29] and hair loss of peripheral body.[30,31] More recently, lichen planus–type nail involvement has also been reported,[32] again pointing to a close relationship of FFA to lichen planus.

Ultimately, cutaneous lupus erythematosus is capable of presenting as FFA,[33] suggesting that the pattern of clinical disease presentation might be more specific for the syndrome than the underlying inflammatory autoimmune reaction. It may be speculated to what extent a background of AGA may contribute to this particular clinical presentation of the disease; nevertheless, the localization of FFA in androgen-independent areas, the lack of evidence of associated AGA (diversity of hair shaft diameters) in some cases of FFA, and a limited success rate of antiandrogen therapy, including 5α-reductase inhibitors, all point to the fact that AGA represents only a facultative comorbidity of FFA, setting the condition apart from FAPD.

In contrast to FFA, FAPD represents by definition the combination of patterned hair loss with evidence of a lichenoid follicular inflammation within the androgenetic area.

An important question to be addressed in further studies is how the lichenoid tissue reaction pattern is generated around the individual androgenetic hair follicle. Follicles with some form of damage or malfunction might express cytokine profiles that attract inflammatory cells to assist in damage repair or in the initiation of apoptosis-mediated organ deletion (Fig. 9.4). Alternatively, an as-yet-unknown antigenic stimulus from the damaged or malfunctioning hair follicle might initiate a lichenoid tissue reaction in the immunogenetically susceptible individual. Remarkably, in healthy murine skin, clusters of perifollicular macrophages have been described as perhaps indicating the existence of a physiologic program of immunologically controlled hair follicle degeneration by which malfunctioning follicles are removed by programmed organ deletion.[35]

Various forms of clinically perceptible, permanent alopecia might represent pathologic exaggeration of this type of programmed organ deletion,[35] resulting in a lichenoid tissue reaction pattern and true scarring alopecia. Further studies are required to elucidate a presumable role of androgenetic factors in addition to that of the lymphohistiocytic infiltrate, perifollicular lamellar fibrosis, and apoptosis-mediated follicular regression in the patterned scarring alopecias, including central centrifugal cicatricial alopecia (CCCA).

CCCA was originally titled "hot comb alopecia" in 1968[36] and considered to be associated with excessive use of hot combs, as well as oil pomades and other hair care chemicals in African-Americans. It was thought that the oils applied to the hair and heated by the hot comb would travel down the hair shaft into the hair follicular unit opening and cause inflammation around upper follicles. However, it was later recognized that although hot combing might elicit the condition in some individuals, CCCA can also present in the absence of any cosmetic procedure. With this additional discovery, the condition was retitled "follicular

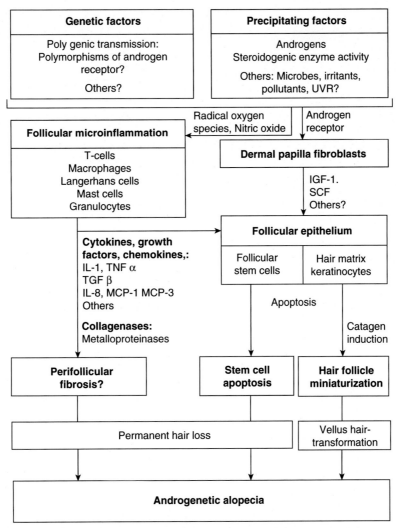

FIG. 9.4 Scheme of events, including follicular inflammation and fibrosis, resulting in patterned hair loss. *UVR*, ultraviolat radiation; *IGF-1*, insulin like growth factor-1; *SCF*, stem cell factor; *IL-1*, interleukin-1; *TNFalpha*, tumor necrosis factor alpha; *TGF beta*, transforming growth factor beta; *IL- 8*, interleukin-8; *MCP-1*, monocyte chemoattractant-1; *MCP-3*, monocyte chemoattractant-3. (Modified from Trüeb RM. Molecular mechanisms of androgenetic alopecia. *Exp Gerontol.* 2002;37(8–9):981–990.)

degeneration syndrome" by Sperling and Sau in 1992[37] who suggested that premature desquamation of the inner hair root sheath, only recognizable on a transverse section of hair, was diagnostic of the condition until 1995 when Ackerman challenged CCCA to represent a discrete entity and regarded the premature desquamation of the inner hair root sheath to be an unspecific finding and nothing more than a fixation artifact.[38] Nevertheless, the condition was again retitled "CCCA" and included within the lymphocytic group of primary scarring alopecia by the North American Hair Research Society in 2003 in their respective working classification.[39]

The condition presents again with a quasisymmetrical alopecia centered on the crown/vertex of the scalp and gradually progresses centrifugally. It tends to begin in the 20s and progresses over the following 20–30 years. Tenderness, itching, or burning sensation may be present but is usually mild. A considerable amount of hair is often lost before the alopecia and scarring are recognized. Therefore, it has been recommended to consider the possibility of CCCA in

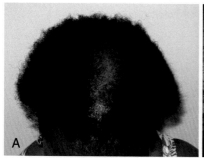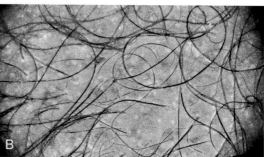

FIG. 9.5 Central centrifugal cicatricial alopecia/fibrosing alopecia in a pattern distribution in a woman of African origin: **(A)** quasisymmetrical alopecia centered on the crown/vertex of the scalp with gradual centrifugal progression and **(B)** respective dermoscopic findings of perifollicular erythema, perifollicular keratosis, whitish perifollicular halo, loss of follicular ostia, and small white patches replacing the follicular openings, in association with hair diameter diversity.

female patients of African origin with what appears to be female pattern hair loss.[40]

The etiopathogenesis of CCCA has so far also remained elusive and is probably multifactorial and heterogeneous. However, one hypothesis involves excessive pressure exerted by the curled hair shaft on the internal root sheath leading to damage and recruitment of inflammatory cells with the end result of scarring. To investigate medical and environmental risk factors for CCCA, Kyei et al.[41] performed a population study involving a quantitative cross-sectional survey of risk factors. Diabetes mellitus type 2 was significantly higher in those with CCCA, as were bacterial scalp infections, and hair styles associated with traction.

Histopathologic features of CCCA include again a perifollicular lymphocytic infiltrate, concentric lamellar fibrosis, and sebaceous gland loss. Also, granulomatous inflammation secondary to follicular rupture may be noted. Ultimately, Miteva and Tosti found, in their samples of CCCA, evidence of a high proportion of hair follicle miniaturization on histopathology[42] and hair shaft variability together with peripilar white halo on dermoscopy,[43] similar to the findings in FAPD. This ultimately raises the question whether CCCA may, at least in part, not represent cicatricial pattern hair loss or FAPD in patients of African origin (Fig. 9.5A and B), whereas Zinkernagel and Trüeb's original observations on FAPD involved exclusively Caucasians.

CONCLUSION

As with the epidemiologic considerations on FFA, the concept of CCCA in African-American women is reminiscent of the conflict originally appreciated by

French philosopher Michel Foucault (1926–84) in his *Archaeology of Medical Perception* (1963): "*A medicine of epidemics is opposed at every point to a medicine of classes, just as the collective perception of a phenomenon that is widespread but unique and unrepeatable may be opposed to the individual perception of the identity of an essence as constantly revealed in the multiplicity of phenomena.*"[44]

Ultimately, dissecting the molecular controls of immune-mediated hair follicle degeneration by apoptosis-mediated organ deletion, specifically in AGA with histologic evidence of follicular inflammation and fibrosis, in FAPD and CCCA, could provide insights into how progression of some forms of permanent alopecia might be halted, which can be suppressed with only limited success by current treatment modalities for AGA.

We strongly suggest recognition of FAPD, and possibly also of CCCA in women of African origin, as a subtype of AGA or complicated AGA, and therefore that the presence of dermoscopic (diversity of hair shaft diameters) and histologic features (hair follicle miniaturization) of AGA along with a follicular lichenoid infiltrate or lamellar fibrosis is prerequisite for the diagnosis, otherwise we are dealing with LPP.

In conclusion, FAPD represents a unique entity that is by definition related to AGA but with a perifollicular lichenoid inflammatory infiltrate that, in late stages, evolves to lamellar fibrosis. Genetic, environmental, and hormonal factors may explain the clinical pattern and the efficacy of combined treatments with antiandrogens, hair growth–promoting agents, autologous hair transplantation, and anti-inflammatory modalities (Figs. 9.6–9.9).

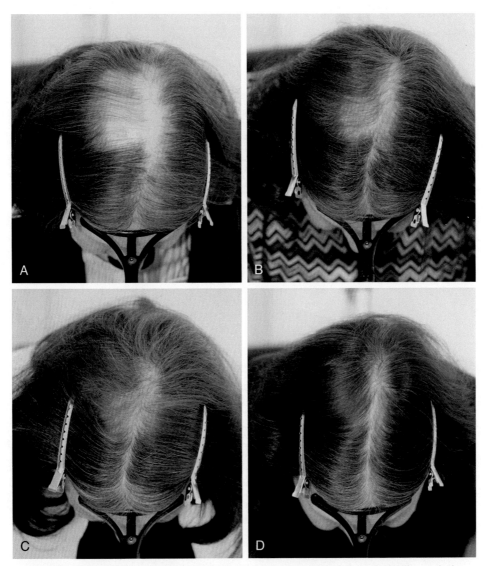

FIG. 9.6 Fibrosing alopecia in a pattern distribution in a woman successfully treated with a topical compound of 5% minoxidil and 0.2% triamcinolone acetonide solution b.i.d. and oral hydroxychloroquine 200 mg daily: **(A)** before and after **(B)** 3 months, **(C)** 6 months, and **(D)** 12 months of treatment.

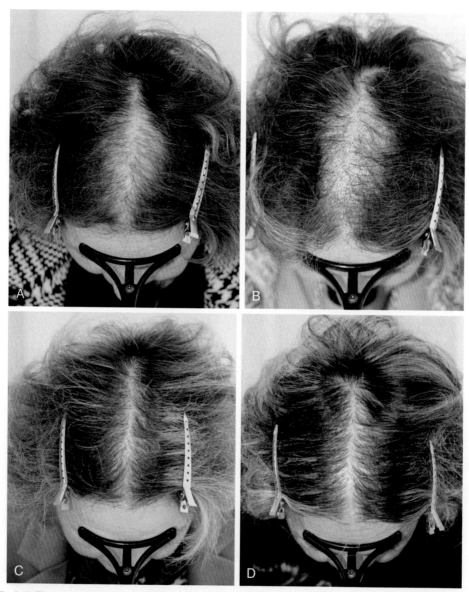

FIG. 9.7 Fibrosing alopecia in a pattern distribution in a woman successfully treated with 0.5 mg oral dutasteride, a compound of 3% topical minoxidil and 0.2% triamcinolone acetonide solution b.i.d., and autologous hair transplantation: **(A)** before, **(B)** 1 month and **(C)** 9 months after autologous hair transplantation, and **(D)** with sustained result after 2 years.

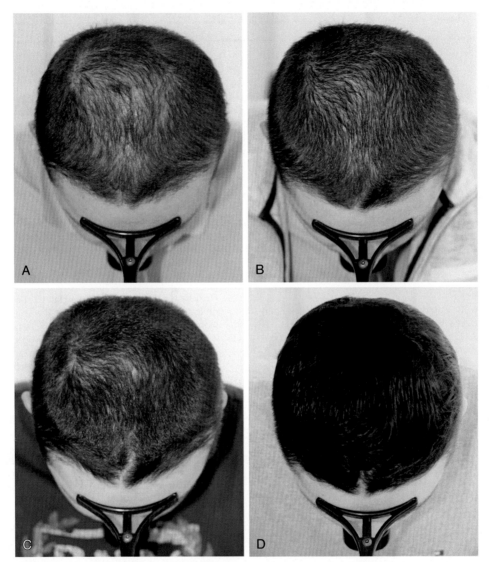

FIG. 9.8 Fibrosing alopecia in a pattern distribution in a man successfully treated with 1 mg oral finasteride and 100 mg oral doxycycline in combination with a compound of 3% minoxidil and 0.2% triamcinolone acetonide and witch hazel–based shampoo. For the last 3 months, 1 mg oral finasteride was switched to 0.5 mg oral dutasteride: (**A**) before and after (**B**) 3 months, (**C**) 6 months, and (**D**) 12 months of treatment.

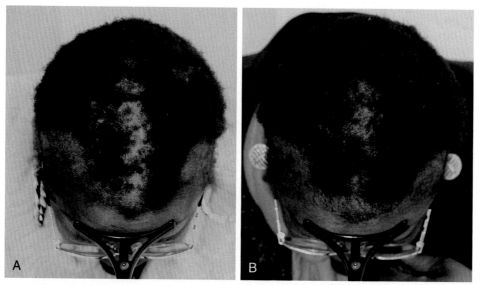

FIG. 9.9 Central centrifugal cicatricial alopecia/fibrosing alopecia in a pattern distribution in a woman of African origin successfully treated with 100 mg oral doxycycline and a compound of topical 5% minoxidil and 0.2% triamcinolone acetonide, avoiding traction, chemicals, and heat: **(A)** before and **(B)** after 2 months of treatment.

REFERENCES

1. Hamilton JB. Patterned loss of hair in men; types and incidence. *Ann N Y Acad Sci.* 1951;53:708–728.
2. Norwood OT. Male patten baldness: classification and incidence. *South Med J.* 1975;68:1359–1365.
3. Ludwig E. Classification of the types of androgenetic alopecia (common baldness) occurring in the female sex. *Br J Dermatol.* 1977;97:247–254.
4. Paus R, Cotsarelis G. The biology of hair follicles. *N Engl J Med.* 1999;341:491–497.
5. de Lacharrière O, Deloche C, Misciali C, et al. Hair diameter diversity: a clinical sign reflecting the follicle miniaturization. *Arch Dermatol.* 2001;137:641–646.
6. Sewell LD, Elston DM, Dorion RP. "Anisotrichosis": a novel term to describe pattern alopecia. *J Am Acad Dermatol.* 2007;56:856.
7. Galliker NA, Trüeb RM. Value of trichoscopy versus trichogram for diagnosis of female androgenetic alopecia. *Int J Trichology.* 2012;4:19–22.
8. Price VH. Treatment of hair loss. *N Engl J Med.* 1999;341:964–973.
9. Jaworsky C, Kligman AM, Murphy GF. Characterisation of inflammatory infiltrates in male pattern alopecia: implication for pathogenesis. *Br J Dermatol.* 1992;127:239–246.
10. Whiting DA. Diagnostic and predictive value of horizontal sections of scalp biopsy specimens in male pattern androgenetic alopecia. *J Am Acad Dermatol.* 1993;28:755–763.
11. Mahé YF, Michelet JF, Billoni N, et al. Androgenetic alopecia and microinflammation. *Int J Dermatol.* 2000;39:576–584.
12. Deloche C, de Lacharrière O, Misciali C, et al. Histological features of peripilar signs associated with androgenetic alopecia. *Arch Dermatol Res.* 2004;295:422–428.
13. Zinkernagel MS, Trüeb RM. Fibrosing alopecia in a pattern distribution. Patterned lichen planopilaris or androgenetic alopecia with a lichenoid tissue reaction pattern? *Arch Dermatol.* 2000;136:205–211.
14. Sperling LC, Solomon AR, Whiting DA. A new look at scarring alopecia. *Arch Dermatol.* 2000;136:235–242.
15. Kossard S. Postmenopausal frontal fibrosing alopecia: scarring alopecia in a pattern distribution. *Arch Dermatol.* 1994;130:770–774.
16. Harries MJ, Meyer K, Chaudhry I, et al. Lichen planopilaris is characterized by immune privilege collapse of the hair follicle's epithelial stem cell niche. *J Pathol.* 2013;231(2):236–247.
17. Miyazaki K, Higaki S, Maruyama T, Takahashi S, Morohashi M, Ito K. Chronic graft-versus-host disease with follicular involvement. *J Dermatol.* 1993;20(4):242–246.
18. Basilio FM, Brenner FM, Werner B, Rastelli GJ. Clinical and histological study of permanent alopecia after bone marrow transplantation. *An Bras Dermatol.* 2015;90(6):814–821.
19. Kossard S, Lee MS, Wilkinson B. Postmenopausal frontal fibrosing alopecia: a frontal variant of lichen planopilaris. *J Am Acad Dermatol.* 1997;36:59–66.
20. Aldoori N, Dobson K, Holden CR, McDonagh AJ, Harries M, Messenger AG. Frontal fibrosing alopecia: possible association with leave-on facial skin care products and sunscreens; a questionnaire study. *Br J Dermatol.* 2016;175(4):762–767.

21. Debroy-Kidambi A, Dobson K, Holmes S, et al. Frontal fibrosing alopecia in men - an association with facial moisturisers and sunscreens. *Br J Dermatol.* January 23, 2017. https://doi.org/10.1111/bjd.15311. [Epub ahead of print].

22. Munthe Axel. *The Story of San Michele.* London, UK: John Murray Publishers Ltd; 2004. Chapter XIII (Mamsell Agata), page 157.

23. Trüeb RM. A comment on frontal fibrosing alopecia (Axel Munthe's syndrome). *Int J Trichol.* 2016;8(4):203–205.

24. Samrao A, Chew AL, Price V. Frontal fibrosing alopecia: a clinical review of 36 patients. *Br J Dermatol.* 2010;163(6):1296–1300.

25. MacDonald A, Clark C, Holmes S. Frontal fibrosing alopecia: a review of 60 cases. *J Am Acad Dermatol.* 2012;67(5):955–961.

26. Ladizinski B, Bazakas A, Selim MA, Olsen EA. Frontal fibrosing alopecia: a retrospective review of 19 patients seen at Duke University. *J Am Acad Dermatol.* 2013;68(5):749–755.

27. Banka N, Mubki T, Bunagan MJ, McElwee K, Shapiro J. Frontal fibrosing alopecia: a retrospective clinical review of 62 patients with treatment outcome and long-term follow-up. *Int J Dermatol.* 2014;53(11):1324–1330.

28. Vañó-Galván S, Molina-Ruiz AM, Serrano-Falcón C, et al. Frontal fibrosing alopecia: a multicenter review of 355 patients. *J Am Acad Dermatol.* 2014;70(4):670–678.

29. Donati A, Molina L, Doche I, Valente NS, Romiti R. Facial papules in frontal fibrosing alopecia: evidence of vellus follicle involvement. *Arch Dermatol.* 2011;147:1424–1427.

30. Armenores P, Shirato K, Reid C, Sidhu S. Frontal fibrosing alopecia associated with generalized hair loss. *Australas J Dermatol.* 2010;51:183–185.

31. Chew AL, Bashir SJ, Wain EM, et al. Expanding the spectrum of frontal fibrosing alopecia: a unifying concept. *J Am Acad Dermatol.* 2010;63:653–660.

32. Macpherson M, Hohendorf-Ansari P, Trüeb RM. Nail involvement in frontal fibrosing alopecia. *Int J Trichol.* 2015;7(2):64–66.

33. Trüeb RM, El Shabrawi L, Kempf W. Cutaneous lupus erythematosus presenting as frontal fibrosing alopecia: report of 2 patients. *Skin Appendage Disord.* 2017;3:205–210.

34. Trüeb RM. Molecular mechanisms of androgenetic alopecia. *Exp Gerontol.* 2002;37(8–9):981–990.

35. Eichmüller S, van der Veen C, Mill I, et al. Clusters of perifollicular macrophages in normal murine skin: physiological degeneration of selected hair follicles by programmed organ deletion. *J Histochem Cytochem.* 1998; 46:361–370.

36. LoPresti P, Papa CM, Kligman AM. Hot comb alopecia. *Arch Dermatol.* 1968;98(3):234–238.

37. Sperling LC, Sau P. The follicular degeneration syndrome in black patients. 'Hot comb alopecia' revisited and revised. *Arch Dermatol.* 1992;128(1):68–74.

38. Gibbons G, Ackerman. Resolving quandaries: follicular degeneration syndrome? *Dermatol Dermatopathol Pathol Pract Concept.* 1995;1:197–200.

39. Olsen EA, Bergfeld WF, Cotsarelis G, et al. Summary of North American Hair Research Society (NAHRS)-sponsored workshop on cicatricial alopecia, Duke University Medical Center, February 10 and 11, 2001. *J Am Acad Dermatol.* 2003;48:103–110.

40. Khumalo NP. Grooming and central centrifugal cicatricial alopecia. *J Am Acad Dermatol.* 2010;62(3):507–508.

41. Kyei A, Bergfeld WF, Piliang M, Summers P. Medical and environmental risk factors for the development of central centrifugal cicatricial alopecia: a population study. *Arch Dermatol.* 2011;147(8):909–914.

42. Miteva M, Tosti A. Pathologic diagnosis of central centrifugal cicatricial alopecia on horizontal sections. *Am J Dermatopathol.* 2014;36(11):859–864.

43. Miteva M, Tosti A. Dermatoscopic features of central centrifugal cicatricial alopecia. *J Am Acad Dermatol.* 2014;71:443–449.

44. Foucault M. *The Birth of the Clinic. An Archaeology of Medical Perception.* New York: Vintage Books; 1994:26.

CHAPTER 10

Central Centrifugal Cicatricial Alopecia

KIASHA GOVENDER, MBCHB (UKZN), FCDERM (SA) • NCOZA C. DLOVA, MBCHB (UKZN), FCDERM (SA), PHD (UKZN)

INTRODUCTION

Central centrifugal cicatricial alopecia (CCCA) is a common form of lymphocyte-mediated scarring alopecia mostly seen in females of African descent and rarely in men. Alopecia represents one of the five top conditions for African Americans and Africans to consult a dermatologist.[1-5]

Cicatricial alopecia is characterized by destruction of the hair follicle and its replacement by fibrous tissue. CCCA is the commonest subtype after traction alopecia that is seen in both African and African-American middle-aged females[2] and is distinguished from other scarring alopecias by a gradually progressive hair loss that originates at the vertex of the scalp and expands centrifugally.[6]

Despite its prevalence, there remains minimal data regarding its exact incidence, etiology, inheritance pattern, and evidence-based treatments.

HAIR MORPHOLOGY AND PRACTICES AMONGST AFRICAN PATIENTS

The increased prevalence of CCCA amongst Black females is a direct result of unique morphologic features of African hair and hair care practices. Transverse sectioning of African hair depicts an elliptical shape; irregular diameter; multiple twists and random, abrupt reversals in direction, as well as being more opaque and curlier with more knots.[7-11] There is a decreased amount of integral hair lipids and sebum coating the hair, leading to dryer, less shiny appearance with less tensile strength[12] and easy breakage. Less elastic fibers anchor the hair follicles[13,14] as well as an overall decrease in hair density compared with Caucasians.[12] All of these features contribute to weakness of African hair along its length and increased fragility.[15]

Hair care practices have for decades been implicated as eliciting[16,17] or aggravating factors[16-19] in the etiopathogenesis of CCCA; hence an understanding of the common styling methods used is crucial. Hair straightening is the commonest styling method in patients of African descent worldwide.[20] This is achieved by thermal methods, such as hot combing or pressing, or the use of flat irons or chemical straightening with the use of relaxers. The latter rearranges disulphide bonds in the hair depleting cysteine and making it more brittle.[21] Styling practices in the way of braids, weaves, and dreadlocks or application of extensions glued onto the scalp exert traction on the hair root.[19,22] It has been shown that African-American women cleanse the scalp less frequently than Caucasians to maintain the longevity of specific hairstyles.[9,23] Whether this contributes to overgrowth of scalp microorganisms precipitating CCCA is currently unknown.

HISTORY AND TERMINOLOGY

Initially the entity was termed "hot comb alopecia" by LoPresti et al.[17] In 1987, Price suggested abandoning the term as it was shown that the use of hot combs was not essential in the development of the disorder.[24] Sperling and Sau revisited alopecia in 1992 and greatly expanded on our understanding of the disease. They suggested a primary defect of premature desquamation of the internal root sheath (IRS) and subsequent influence by mechanical factors and hair grooming practices in its pathogenesis. The term "follicular degeneration syndrome" was thus coined.[18] Headington et al. reviewed the literature and shunned the term as he argued that premature desquamation of the IRS may be seen in a variety of other scarring alopecias.[25] He favored the term "scarring alopecia in African Americans." In 2000, the name was once again changed to central centrifugal scarring alopecia by Sperling et al.[26] This term included hair loss patterns with the following characteristics:

1. Crown or vertex hair loss
2. Chronic, progressive disease with ultimate burnout
3. Symmetric disease activity with peripheral active disease
4. Clinical and histologic evidence of inflammation in the active peripheral zone

This includes other forms of scarring alopecia. The current disease terminology was adopted by the North American Hair Research Society in 2001.[27] They encompassed the previous hot comb alopecia and follicular degeneration syndrome under the term "central centrifugal cicatricial alopecia."

EPIDEMIOLOGY

Large epidemiologic studies on CCCA are lacking. It occurs predominantly in Black females, being the commonest cause of scarring alopecia in this population.[17,18,27] Isolated case reports and small case series of disease occurrence in males[28] and Caucasians[17] exist. Prevalence ranges from 2.7%[29] to 5.6%[30] with the average age of onset being 36 years[1] and has been rarely described in childhood.[31]

ETIOPATHOGENESIS

Several etiologic agents have been implicated in the pathogenesis of the disorder but none have been conclusively proved. Studies suggest that there may be a genetic defect in the IRS in some patients of African descent[32] inherited in an autosomal dominant pattern with variable penetrance.[33] Triggering of the disease or aggravation may then occur secondary to traumatic hair care practices, such as braids, weaves, relaxers, and thermal straighteners.[7,32,34] Other postulates suggest that CCCA may originate as female pattern hair loss (FPHL), which progresses to classic features of CCCA secondary to hair care practices.[35,36]

Infection leading to chronic inflammation within lower portions of the hair follicle has been suggested with some authors reporting increased incidence of tinea capitis[30] and bacterial infections[37] in CCCA patients, although other studies have dispelled this finding.[19] It is possible that comorbid medical conditions may be associated with CCCA. An increased prevalence of type II diabetes mellitus[37] was found in one study, but the relevance of this very low prevalence is at this stage uncertain.

CLINICAL PRESENTATION

The classic clinical presentation of CCCA, as originally described, has remained consistent over the years. Patients present with chronic progressive hair loss commencing centrally at the crown or scalp vertex (Fig. 10.1) before expanding peripherally in a centrifugal and symmetric manner (Figs. 10.2–10.5). An unusual variant presenting with multiple irregular patches of hair loss on the lateral, posterior, and central scalp was described in a series of 14 patients.[38]

In the early stages of disease, patients display thinning of hair, similar to androgenetic alopecia. Hair breakage has been described as an early sign in some patients.[39] The relevance of this finding requires more research as it has not been universally found in all CCCA patients. Also hair breakage is found in a number of other conditions and is especially associated with traumatic hair practices. So whether this finding is a feature of the CCCA itself or from the hair care practices, seen in this group of patients that may only affect secondarily the disease, remains to be elucidated.

Patients typically present late in the course of disease when a considerable amount of hair loss has already

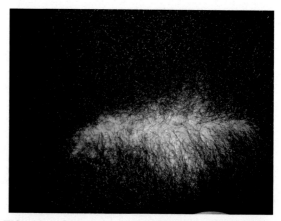

FIG. 10.1 Central centrifugal cicatricial alopecia grade 1 (according to the validated photographic severity scale[42]).

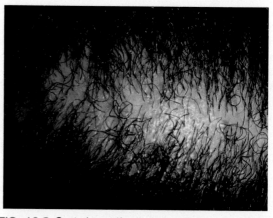

FIG. 10.2 Central centrifugal cicatricial alopecia grade 2 with painful erythema and papules.

occurred.[19] In later stages the scalp demonstrates a shiny, smooth appearance with significant absence of follicular ostia (follicular dropout). Within these alopecic areas, a few isolated strands of hair may remain and polytrichia has also been described.[1,40] Erythema, seborrheic-type scale, follicular papules, and pustules may occasionally occur, but this is not typical and when present is not as impressive as seen in the traditional inflammatory scarring alopecias.

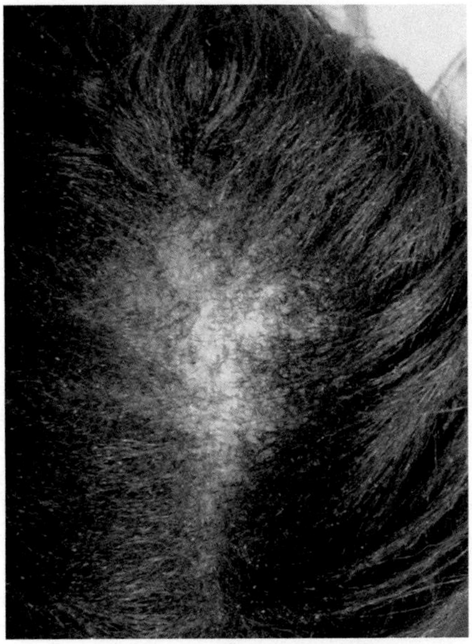

The disease progresses slowly if not treated and may proceed to involve the entire central scalp. Patients with CCCA may be completely asymptomatic, hence the often late presentation. Symptoms, when present, range from mild to disabling and may include tenderness, burning, dysesthesia, or pruritus,[16,19] the latter being implicated through stimulation of protease-activated receptor 2 in the skin.[41] There are no data available regarding frequency of these symptoms in patients with CCCA.[16] A previously validated photographic scale ranging from 0 to 5 is used to classify the disease severity; the more severely affected anatomic area is subclassified as A subtype (the frontal scalp) or B subtype (the vertex)[42] (see Figs. 10.1–10.5).

DERMOSCOPY

Dermoscopy is a useful noninvasive tool in the diagnosis of multiple cutaneous disorders, including those involving the hair and scalp.[33] Trichoscopy (hair dermoscopy) assists in the visualization and analysis of scalp and hair structures and patterns.[34] Besides contributing significantly to the clinical diagnosis, in CCCA it has been shown that dermoscopically selected biopsy sites yield higher diagnostic results on histology.[34]

FIG. 10.3 Central centrifugal cicatricial alopecia grade 3.

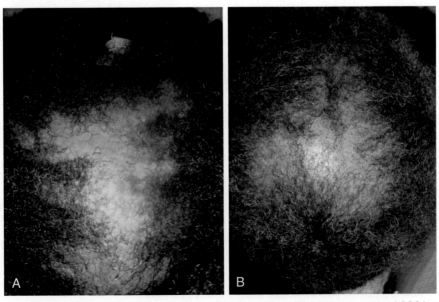

FIG. 10.4 **(A)** Central centrifugal cicatricial alopecia (CCCA) grade 4. **(B)** Another example of CCCA grade 4.

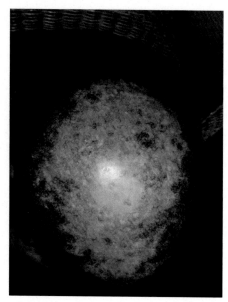

FIG. 10.5 Central centrifugal cicatricial alopecia grade 5.

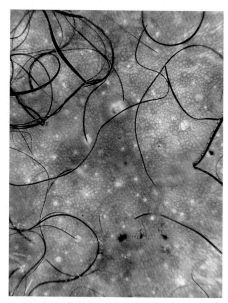

FIG. 10.6 Dermoscopy shows disrupted pigmented network with focal white patches, peripilar white halos (*white gray circles* surrounding the emergences of the hair shafts), irregularly distributed pint-point *white dots*, and two broken hairs. (Image courtesy of Mariya Miteva.)

The most sensitive and specific dermoscopic sign for CCCA is the presence of peripilar white or grey halos, which corresponds to concentric peripilar fibrosis in the affected follicles[43] (Fig. 10.6). Broken hairs, visualized as black dots inside the follicular openings, is also another important feature.[43] These two areas are the optimal sites for cutaneous biopsy.[44] Other dermoscopic findings include pinpoint white dots, a honey-comb–pigmented network, white patches, perifollicular erythema, concentric white scales, and interfollicular stellate brown macules.[43,45]

HISTOLOGY

The most specific diagnostic feature seen in CCCA is the premature desquamation of the IRS below the level of the isthmus in affected and unaffected hair follicles.[28,46] It is however not a sensitive finding as it is not always present in a single biopsy specimen. Inflammatory cells are usually few or absent altogether. In early stages, a lichenoid perifollicular lymphocytic infiltrate from the lower infundibulum to the isthmus may be seen, which is later replaced by perifollicular fibrosis.[44] Similar to other scarring alopecias, there is an altered architecture of the follicle with decreased follicular density and eventual follicular dropout[44,46] (Fig 10.7). Sebaceous glands are absent or decreased in number with remnants usually seen in a "hugging pattern" surrounding vellus

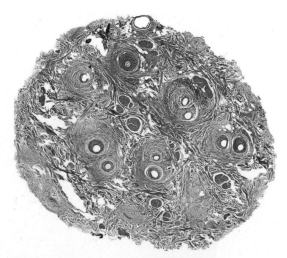

FIG. 10.7 Histopathology (hematoxylin and eosin stain) at the midfollicular level shows disrupted follicular architecture with absence of sebaceous glands and areas of follicular drop out. There are compound follicular structures forming "gogglelike" structures surrounded by perifollicular fibrosis and mild lichenoid inflammation. Note the absence of the inner root sheath. (Image courtesy of Mariya Miteva.)

hairs.[44,46] Other histologic findings include naked dermal hair shafts, follicular miniaturization, and lamellar hyper or parakeratosis within the hair follicle.[44,46]

Premature desquamation of the IRS coupled with other features described earlier is diagnostic for CCCA.[39] However, histologic confirmation is not always easy because premature desquamation of the IRS is not always seen in the region sampled and all other findings are not specific for CCCA,[16] being seen in other forms of scarring alopecia as well.[25] Clinicopathologic correlation is therefore often required to make a definitive diagnosis.

DIFFERENTIAL DIAGNOSIS

CCCA is most often a clinical diagnosis; depending on the stage of diagnosis, it may be confused with other hair disorders.

In early stages, the distribution of hair loss may closely resemble that of androgenetic alopecia (FPHL).[19] Because FPHL is a noncicatricial alopecia, the presence of follicular openings argues in its favor when trying to distinguish it from early CCCA.

Hair breakage, whilst described in CCCA, is often seen in *traction alopecia* of the scalp.[19] The problem of distinguishing between the two conditions is compounded by the fact that they may often occur concurrently. In pure traction alopecia, hair loss is mainly present at hair margins, behind the frontal hairline or temporal scalp.

Clinically, inflammatory changes in CCCA are mild, if at all present, and easily distinguished from the other lymphocytic and neutrophilic scarring alopecias. In active disease, histologic differentiation from the other cicatricial lymphocytic alopecias, such as lichen planopilaris (LPP) and discoid lupus erythematosus (DLE), may be challenging. In full-blown end-stage CCCA, differentiation from end-stage LPP, DLE, folliculitis decalvans, keratosis follicularis spinulosa decalvans, or classic pseudopelade of Brocq is usually impossible, both clinically and histologically.[47,48]

MANAGEMENT

Like all scarring alopecias, management is notoriously challenging. Because of the late presentation in most cases, a significant amount of hair is already irreversibly lost at initial diagnosis. There are currently no published randomized control trials on the treatment of CCCA, so management recommendations are based largely on anecdotal treatment successes reported from case reports or small case series. The goal of treatment is to halt the inflammatory process to preserve the remaining hair and avoid disease progression and further scarring.

GENERAL MEASURES

- The psychologic impact of the disease should not be underestimated. CCCA, like most scarring alopecias, is associated with a dramatic decline in quality of life (QOL)[49] because of the psychologic ramifications of the permanent hair loss. It is essential to counsel patients early on regarding the permanent nature of the alopecia and to identify realistic management expectations. Formulating strategies to mitigate mental anguish to improve QOL may include suggesting disease-specific support groups as well as referral to a mental healthcare practitioner if necessary.
- Although there is no evidence to suggest that hair styling practices are the primary cause of disease, it has been shown to aggravate hair loss.[7,34] Most authors therefore concur that thermal/chemical straightening and traction inducing hairstyles should be avoided to diminish further damage to hair. For those patients who are unwilling to stop these practices, they should be encouraged to have styling performed less frequently and only by a professional hair stylist in an attempt to protect the scalp and hair as much as possible with the use of heat/chemical protectors applied to the hair prior to straightening or the application of looser weaves and braids.[16,19]

MEDICAL TREATMENT

- Corticosteroids in the form of daily potent or superpotent topical formulations or monthly intralesional steroid injections (5–10 mg/mL) for 7–8 months are usually used as first-line treatment. These are targeted at the active peripheral spreading margins to prevent disease progression and alleviate symptoms. Once controlled, they are tapered to topical steroid application 3× weekly.[50] Injections are usually discontinued only after at least 6 months or so. Use of antiseborrheic shampoos help to alleviate pruritus and scale sometimes associated with disease.[51]

Other topical treatments described in the literature include topical calcineurin inhibitors[52] and minoxidil.[53]

- In severe active inflammation or when topical treatment is proved unsuccessful, systemic agents, such as tetracyclines, antimalarials, thalidomide, antiandrogens, 5α reductase inhibitors, and immunosuppressants, such as mycophenolate mofetil and cyclosporine, have shown some success in the literature.[52-56] These are usually used for a 6–9 month period until disease progression has been aborted.

SURGICAL TREATMENT

- Surgical intervention in the form of hair transplant grafts is reserved for those patients with histologically proven stable disease, without inflammation for at least 9–12 months.[19] The procedure unfortunately comes with a high risk of failure as the limited blood supply in the scarred area may decrease graft survival rate.[51] A test area is therefore necessary prior to full hair transplant. If successful, it offers patients a permanent solution to hair loss. The procedure is however time consuming, costly, and only performed in specialized centers, with most patients not having access to the treatment. In these patients, options are limited to camouflage techniques in the form of wigs and scalp micropigmentation.

CONCLUSION

Almost 50 years since its initial description, CCCA remains an enigmatic scalp disorder with incompletely understood etiology, pathogenesis, and genetics. Very few epidemiologic and management studies have been reported in the literature. Further studies are required in various aspects of the disease to elucidate the exact role played by genetic factors, hair care practices, infection, and comorbid disorders in the pathogenesis of disease. Large epidemiologic studies and QOL research needs to be conducted to determine exact incidence and burden of the disease.

Randomized controlled trials examining efficacy of treatment are essential to explore the most effective treatment and to establish clear management guidelines in CCCA.

REFERENCES

1. Whiting DA, Olsen EA. Central centrifugal cicatricial alopecia. *Dermatol Ther.* 2008;21(4):268–278.
2. Halder RM, Grimes PE, McLaurin CI, et al. Incidence of common dermatoses in a predominantly black dermatologic practice. *Cutis.* 1983;32(4):388–390.
3. Rodney IJ, Onwudiwe OC, Callender VD, et al. Hair and scalp disorders in ethnic populations. *J Drugs Dermatol.* 2013;12(4):420–427.
4. Alexis AF, Sergay AB, Taylor SC. Common dermatologic disorders in skin of colour: a comparative practice survey. *Cutis.* 2007;80(5):387–394.
5. Dlova NC, Mankahla A, Madala N, Grobler A, Tsoka-Gwegweni J, Hift RJ. The spectrum of skin diseases in a black population in Durban, KwaZulu-Natal, South Africa. *Int J Dermatol.* 2015;54(3):279–285.
6. Ross EK, Tan E, Shapiro J. Update on primary cicatricial alopecias. *J Am Acad Dermatol.* 2005;53:1–40.
7. Lawson CN, Hollinger J, Sethi S, et al. Updates in the understanding and treatments of skin and hair disorders in women of color. *Int J Womens Dermatol.* 2015;1:59–75.
8. Franbourg A, Hallegot P, Baitenneck F, et al. Current research on ethnic hair. *J Am Acad Dermatol.* 2003;48(suppl 6):S115–S119.
9. McMichael AJ. Ethnic hair update: past and present. *J Am Acad Dermatol.* 2003;48(suppl 6):S127–S133.
10. Khumalo NP, Doe PT, Dawber RP, et al. What is normal black African hair? A light and scanning electron-microscopic study. *J Am Acad Dermatol.* 2000;43(5 Pt 1):814–820.
11. Johnson BA. Requirements in cosmetics for black skin. *Dermatol Clin.* 1988;6(3):489–492.
12. Ji JH, Park TS, Lee HJ, et al. The ethnic differences of the damage of hair and integral hair lipid after ultra violet radiation. *Ann Dermatol.* 2013;25:54–60.
13. Taylor S. Practical tips for managing hair disorders in African-American females. *Przegl Dermatol.* 2006;3(7):25–27.
14. Richards GM, Oresajo CO, Halder RM. Structure and function of ethnic skin and hair. *Dermatol Clin.* 2003;21(4):595–600.
15. Bernard BA. Hair shape of curly hair. *J Am Acad Dermatol.* 2003;48(6):S120–S126.
16. Herskovitz I, Miteva M. Central centrifugal cicatricial alopecia: challenges and solutions. *Clin Cosmet Invest Dermatol.* 2016;9:175–181.
17. LoPresti P, Papa CM, Kligman AM. Hot comb alopecia. *Arch Dermatol.* 1968;98(3):234–236.
18. Sperling LC, Sau P. The follicular degeneration syndrome in black patients. "Hot comb alopecia" revisited and revised. *Arch Dermatol.* 1992;128(1):68–74.
19. Ogunleye TA, McMichael A, Olsen EA. Central centrifugal cicatricial alopecia. What has been achieved, current clues for future research. *Dermatol Clin.* 2014;32:173–181.
20. Callender V. African-American scalp disorders and treatment considerations. *Skin Aging.* 2002;10(suppl):12–14.
21. Khumalo NP, Stone J, Gumedze F, et al. 'Relaxers' damage hair: evidence from amino acid analysis. *J Am Acad Dermatol.* 2010;62(3):402–408.
22. Grimes PE. Skin and hair cosmetic issues in women of color. *Dermatol Clin.* 2000;18(4):659–665.
23. Hall RR, Francis S, Whitt-Glover M, et al. Hair care practices as a barrier to physical activity in African American women. *JAMA Dermatol.* 2013;149(3):310–314.

24. Price V. Hair loss in cutaneous disease. In: Baden HP, ed. *Symposium on Alopecia.* New York: HP Publishing Co; 1987.

25. Headington JT. Cicatricial alopecia. *Dermatol Clin.* 1996;14(4):773–782.

26. Sperling LC, Solomon AR, Whiting DA. A new look at scarring alopecia. *Arch Dermatol.* 2000;136(2):235–242.

27. Olsen EA, Bergfield WF, Cotsarelis G, et al. Summary of North American hair research society (NAHRS) - sponsored workshop on cicatricial alopecia, Duke University Medical center, February 10 and 11, 2001. *J Am Acad Dermatol.* 2003;48(1):103–110.

28. Sperling LT, Skelton 3rd HG, Smith KJ, et al. Follicular degeneration syndrome in men. *Arch Dermatol.* 1994; 130(6):763–769.

29. Khumalo NP, Jessop S, Gumedze F, et al. Hairdressing and the prevalence of scalp disease in African adults. *Br J Dermatol.* 2007;157(5):981–988.

30. Olsen EC, Callender V, McMichael A, et al. Central hair loss in African American women: incidence and potential risk factors. *J Am Acad Dermatol.* 2011;64(2):245–252.

31. Eginli AN, Dlova NC, McMichael A. Central centrifugal cicatricial alopecia in the pediatric population: a case series and review of the literature. *Paed Dermatol.* 2017;34:133–137.

32. Dlova NC, Forder M. Central centrifugal cicatricial alopecia: possible familial aetiology in two African families from South Africa. *Int J Dermatol.* 2012;51(suppl 1): 17–20.

33. Dlova NC, Jordaan FH, Sarig O, et al. Autosomal dominant inheritance of central centrifugal cicatricial alopecia in black South Africans. *J Am Acad Dermatol.* 2014;70(4):679–682.

34. Suchonwanit P, Hector CE, Bin Saif GA, et al. Factors affecting the severity of central centrifugal cicatricial alopecia. *Int J Dermatol.* 2016;55(6):338–343.

35. Olsen E. Pattern hair loss. In: Olsen EA, ed. *Disorders of Hair Growth: Diagnosis and Treatment.* New York: McGraw-Hill; 2003:326.

36. Olsen EA. Female pattern hair loss and its relationship to permanent/cicatricial alopecia: a new perspective. *J Invest Dermatol Symp Proc.* 2005;10(3):217–221.

37. Kyei A. Medical and environmental risk factors for the development of central centrifugal cicatricial alopecia. *Arch Dermatol.* 2011;147(8):909.

38. Miteva M, Tosti A. Central centrifugal cicatricial alopecia presenting with irregular patchy alopecia on the lateral and posterior scalp. *Skin Appendage Disord.* 2015;1(1): 1–5.

39. Callender VD, Wright DR, Davis EC, et al. Hair breakage as a presenting of early or occult central centrifugal cicatricial alopecia: clinicopathological findings in 9 patients. *Arch Dermatol.* 2012;148(9):1047–1052.

40. Gathers RC, Jankowski M, Eide M, et al. Hair grooming practices and central centrifugal cicatricial alopecia. *J Am Acad Dermatol.* 2009;60(4):574–578.

41. Bin Saif GA, McMichael A, Kwatra SG, et al. Central centrifugal cicatricial alopecia severity is associated with cowhage-induced itch. *Br J Dermatol.* 2013;168(2):253–256.

42. Olsen E, Callender V, Sperling L, et al. Central scalp alopecia photographic scale in African American women. *Dermat Ther.* 2008;21(4):264–267.

43. Miteva M, Tosti A. Dermatoscopic features of central centrifugal cicatricial alopecia. *J Am Acad Dermatol.* 2014;71(3):443–449.

44. Miteva M, Tosti A. Pathologic diagnosis of central centrifugal cicatricial alopecia on horizontal sections. *Am J Dermatopathol.* 2014;36(11):859–864.

45. Miteva M, Tosti A. Hair and scalp dermatoscopy. *J Am Acad Dermatol.* 2012;67(5):1040–1048.

46. Sperling LC. *J Cutan Pathol.* 2001;28:333–342.

47. Sperling L. Broqc's alopecia (pseudopelade of Broqc) and "burn out" scarring alopecia. In: Sperling LC, ed. *An Atlas of Hair Pathology with Clinical Correlations.* New York: The Parthenon Publishing Group; 2003:115–118.

48. Alzolibani AA, Kang H, Otberg N, et al. Pseudopelade of Broqc. *Dermatol Ther.* 2008;21(4):257–263.

49. Dlova NC, Fabbrocini G, Lauro C, et al. Quality of life in South African Black women with alopecia: a pilot study. *Int J Dermatol.* 2016;55:875–881.

50. Gathers RC, Lim HW. Central centrifugal cicatricial alopecia: past, present and future. *J Am Acad Dermatol.* 2009;60(4):660–668.

51. Callender VD, McMichael AJ, Cohen GF. Medical and surgical therapies for alopecias in black women. *Dermatol Ther.* 2004;17(2):164–176.

52. Semble A, McMichael A. Hair loss in patients with skin of color. *Semin Cutan Med Surg.* 2015;34(2):99–103.

53. Scott DA. Disorders of the hair and scalp in blacks. *Dermatol Clin.* 1988;6(3):387–395.

54. McMichael AJ. Hair and scalp disorders in ethnic populations. *Dermatol Clin.* 2003;21(4):629–644.

55. Bulengo-Ransby SM, Bergfeld WF. Chemical and traumatic alopecia from thioglycolate in a black woman: a case report with unusual clinical and histologic findings. *Cutis.* 1992;49(2):99–103.

56. Price VH. The medical treatment of cicatricial alopecia. *Semin Cutan Med Surg.* 2006;25(1):56–59.

CHAPTER 11

Traction Alopecia

RENÉE A. BEACH, MD, FRCPC • NONHLANHLA P. KHUMALO, MBCHB, FCDERM, PHD

INTRODUCTION

Traction alopecia (TA) is form thought to develop because of pulling of hair or high-tension hairstyles. It generally predominates in women, particularly in women with Afro-textured hair. This chapter details clinical presentations of TA and a validated method of TA severity grading, as well as histopathologic and trichoscopic findings of TA. Variable presentations of TA include reversible, nonscarring alopecia that will respond to behavioral modification and more chronic, scarred, irreversible alopecia. Primary TA treatment is discontinuation of the source of traction or pulling. Eliminating hairstyles that are associated with pain as well as avoidance of traction hairstyles installed on chemically straightened hair has a significantly decreased risk of TA.

DEMOGRAPHIC FACTORS

TA can occur in both men and women but predominates in women, particularly in women with Afro-textured hair. In epidemiologic literature, the prevalence of TA in high school girls and adult South African women was found to be 17% and 32%, respectively.[1] Similarly, prevalence data from the United States reported an 18% prevalence among young African-American women.[2] In contrast, there was no TA in South African school boys and only a 3% prevalence in men who wore their hair in cornrows and dreadlocks.[1,3] Women with Afro-textured hair may wear their hair in its natural or a chemically processed state; both states are susceptible to traction-based hair loss when tension or traction styles are worn. Women who wear chemically relaxed hair and add hair extensions or hair weave; who wear natural hair and add braid extensions; or who admit to specific symptoms (pain, pimplelike lesions, stinging, and crust formation on chemical relaxer application)[4] with hairstyling are at greatest risk to be diagnosed with TA. Oftentimes, hairstyles that include added hair are applied with greater tension and remain installed for several weeks, which provide a sustained traction effect. Other demographic groups identified as being at risk for developing TA include Sikh men and Turkish women who wear turbans[5,6]; ballerinas wearing buns[7]; and nurses using a pin to secure the nursing cap into the hair.[8]

Despite consistent evidence of certain hair textures and demographic groups exhibiting TA, the adaptation of various hairstyling and accessorizing options by nontraditional demographic groups, such as those with Caucasian or Asian hair textures, also puts them at risk of developing this form of hair loss. The strongest predictor of TA is the type and frequency of hairstyle worn. Therefore, the most important information to establish with the patient is the hairstyle worn most consistently and/or the use of accompanying hair accessories that have a pulling effect.

CLINICAL PRESENTATION

TA can be divided into marginal and nonmarginal presentations.

In patients with **marginal TA**, alopecia occurs along the perimeter of the scalp, especially the frontotemporal scalp and the temples[4] (Fig. 11.1A and B). This presentation would typically occur in a ballerina pulling her hair into a bun or a Sikh man pulling his hair up to fit underneath a turban.[6] It is also seen in dreadlock styles formed from tight twisting of dreadlocks at the hairline or when the frontal hairline locks are consistently pulled back. Patients with marginal alopecia also display the "fringe sign." This clinical feature presents as hair loss framed by fine vellus hair; the vellus hairs are retained at the very edge of the frontotemporal hairlines and mimic a bang or "fringe" style.[9] This is a key clinical feature of TA that exists in both acute and chronic presentations (Fig. 11.2). The Marginal Traction Alopecia Severity Score (M-TAS Score) was developed to provide an objective, validated assessment of this form of TA.[10] The patient is examined at a total of six sites along the frontal and posterior hairlines. Assessors then match the patient's perimeter hair loss to photos that score the TA severity from 1 (mild) to 4 (severe). A score of 0 denotes normal, non-TA hair. A score of 24 over the six areas would indicate severe TA at both the frontal and

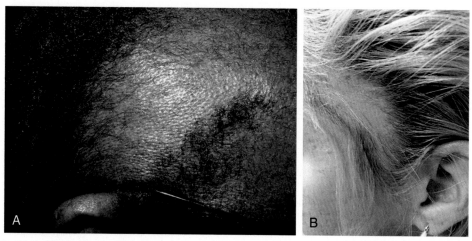

FIG. 11.1 **(A)** Marginal traction alopecia in a woman with Afro-textured hair. **(B)** Marginal traction alopecia in a Hispanic female patient who has been wearing a tight bun at least 3 days a week for 20 years. (Image courtesy of Mariya Miteva, MD.)

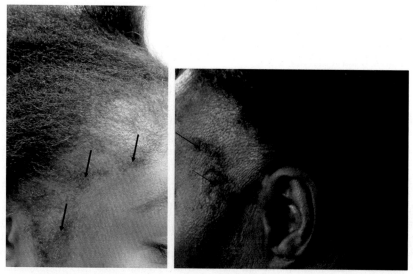

FIG. 11.2 Marginal traction alopecia displaying the fringe sign (*arrows*).

posterior hairlines (Fig. 11.3). This tool enables TA progression to be tracked serially in the clinical setting and allows for interobserver reliability of assessments within research.

Although the marginal presentation is the most clinically apparent presentation of TA, this form of hair loss can also occur at other sites on the scalp, in a **nonmarginal** distribution. For example, women who wear their hair in tight cornrows, box-braids, or microbraids could exhibit this presentation throughout the scalp, as tension forms at the root of each of the braids installed

(Fig. 11.4). Patients with hair extensions glued throughout the scalp also display TA at the site of extension application. Oftentimes, these patients have TA that is not only clinically less apparent but also asymptomatic.[11] Given these characteristics, it is critical to examine the scalp interior to avoid missing this diagnosis.

Physical examination of the scalp should take note of the patient's hairstyle; certain hairstyles are particularly prone to traction and more commonly result in TA. Pulling the hair back into a bun or tight ponytail or "one" is a commonly recognizable style

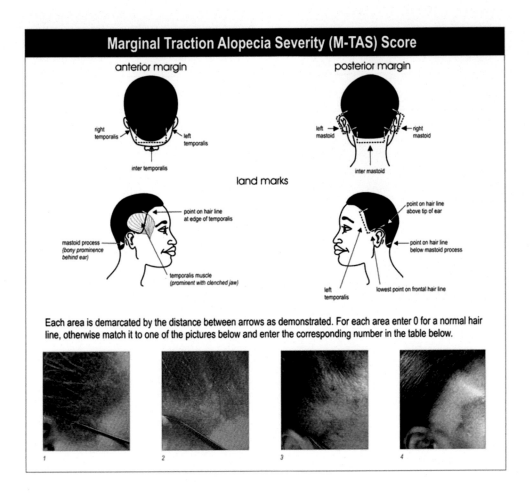

Marginal Traction Alopecia Severity (M-TAS) Score

anterior margin

posterior margin

right temporalis

left temporalis

inter temporalis

left mastoid

right mastoid

inter mastoid

land marks

point on hair line at edge of temporalis

mastoid process (bony prominence behind ear)

temporalis muscle (prominent with clenched jaw)

point on hair line above tip of ear

point on hair line below mastoid process

left temporalis

lowest point on frontal hair line

Each area is demarcated by the distance between arrows as demonstrated. For each area enter 0 for a normal hair line, otherwise match it to one of the pictures below and enter the corresponding number in the table below.

1

2

3

4

Patient name: Folder number:

Date										
Right temporalis										
Inter temporalis										
Left temporalis										
Total anterior score										
Right mastoid										
Inter mastoid										
Left mastoid										
Total posterior score										

FIG. 11.3 Marginal Traction Alopecia Severity (M-TAS) Score. (Copyrighted material is owned by or exclusively licensed to John Wiley & Sons, Inc. Permission granted for reprint.)

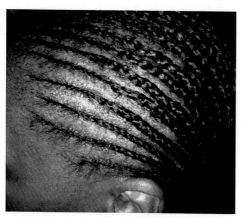

FIG. 11.4 Nonmarginal traction alopecia in a patient with cornrow braid hairstyle.

TABLE 11.1
Risk Factors for Traction Alopecia

Factor	Example
• Hairstyles with tension	• Buns, ponytails
• Added hair	• Extensions • Weaves • "box-braids" • microbraids • cornrow braids • twists
• Hairstyles with added hair installed on relaxed/chemically processed hair	–
• Styling wet hair with tension	–
• Tightly fit head gear	• Turbans • head scarves • head bands • wigs

associated with TA (Table 11.1). Other less commonly known TA-producing hairstyles would include single box-braids or microbraids, cornrow braids, and twists. The occurrence of TA is especially high when these hairstyles are installed with hair extensions in patients with chemically processed hair.[4] Hair that is styled when it is wet has increased extensibility. This increased extensibility can result in greater pull applied to the hair during styling and can cause TA. TA due to pulling of wet, extensible hair may not be clinically apparent or even symptomatic until the hairstyle dries.

TABLE 11.2
Differential Diagnosis of Traction Alopecia

• Nonscarring alopecia	• Trichotillomania • Scalp folliculitis • Alopecia areata • Congenital triangular alopecia
• Scarring alopecia	• Frontal fibrosing alopecia

The diagnosis of TA is largely made by clinical examination; however, the patient history for hairstyles and the existence of TA risk factors are still paramount. In addition to an extensive inventory of hairstyles and hair accessories worn such as dreadlocks, twists, cornrows, box-braids, microbraids, hair extensions, and buns/ponytails, other key questions include pain or headache forming during or shortly after installation of a hairstyle or hair accessory. Other patients may report noting scalp erythema or pustules or pimple-like lesions after a traction-based hairstyle.[4] Use of analgesia to "ease the pain" of the newly installed hairstyle can also convey that a history of severe traction is present. Patients may admit to patting or tapping the scalp repeatedly to provide momentary relief of tightness. Some patients may wet the hairstyle to provide comfort; the process of wetting the hair increases its elasticity and can ease scalp tension. It is uncommon for patients to remove the hairstyle given the time spent and the cost incurred in its installation.

DIFFERENTIAL DIAGNOSIS

Other diagnostic considerations include forms of nonscarring and scarring alopecia. For example, trichotillomania (TM) is a consideration, particularly in a pediatric patient or a patient with anxiety or obsessive-compulsive tendencies.[12] Although TM also occurs due to repetitive actions, it differs from TA in that it occurs at sites not necessarily subjected to tension. It tends to display hairs broken along the hair shaft rather than hairs pulled out by the hair bulb. In the acute stage of TA, with erythema and follicular pustules, another diagnosis to contemplate is folliculitis of the scalp.[4] Alopecia areata is yet another diagnostic consideration[13]; the ophiasis pattern for patients with frontal hairline loss or occipital hairline loss mimics presentations of marginal TA (Table 11.2).

Among the scarring alopecias, the lichen planopilaris variant frontal fibrosing alopecia (FFA) is included in the differential diagnosis. Evidence suggests that the two diagnoses can even coexist.[14]

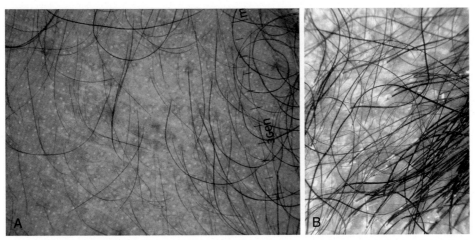

FIG. 11.5 **(A)** Trichoscopy of traction alopecia showing pinpoint *white dots* and vellus hairs. **(B)** Trichoscopy of acute traction alopecia showing hair casts. (Image courtesy of Antonella Tosti, MD.)

However, FFA contains key contrasting features such as the presence of "lonely hairs"; perifollicular erythema or hyperpigmentation; deterioration of skin to an atrophic, sclerotic state (at the margin of the receding hairline); and oftentimes loss of eyebrows.[15] An uncommon but plausible differential diagnosis would also include temporal triangular alopecia/congenital triangular alopecia. This can be differentiated from true TA in its early childhood clinical presentation and in that it fails to respond to traction-free hairstyle modification.

DIAGNOSTIC WORKUP

Trichoscopy

As dermoscopy has emerged as a prominent diagnostic tool in dermatology, the branch of trichoscopy has emerged as an effective, noninvasive method of hair and scalp evaluation. Chief trichoscopic features of TA include broken hairs and black dots, seen in 100% and 92% of TA patients, respectively. Despite being the most common features of TA trichoscopy, they are not unique to TA. Broken hairs can also be viewed in 100% of patients with TM.[5] Black dots have also been reported in approximately 40% of trichoscopic evaluation of patients with TM, alopecia areata, and tinea capitis.[16] Secondary dermoscopic features found in TA are clustered, short vellus hairs (Fig. 11.5A) and yellow dots; these findings are documented less frequently than the features noted earlier.

Hair casts can also be viewed in the trichoscopy of TA (Fig. 11.5B). Casts are white or brown cylinders present along the proximal hair shaft. They are mobile and represent the inner and/or outer root sheath. This

TABLE 11.3 Histopathologic Features of Traction Alopecia	
• Acute/subacute presentations	• Trichomalacia • (Pigmented) hair casts • Perifollicular and intrafollicular hemorrhage
• Chronic presentations	• Follicular dropout • Fibrous tracts • Empty hair shafts • Preservation of sebaceous glands

finding is unique to TA and represents early and ongoing moderate traction.[17]

When differentiating between recent onset and chronic TA, trichoscopy findings differ. There is a significantly higher incidence of loss of follicular openings in chronic TA cases, which supports a transition of TA toward scarring alopecia. Correspondingly, there is an absence of hair casts in these patients.[5] The lack of hair casts indicates both the absence of ongoing traction in longer-term TA as well as loss of the actual hairs (i.e., reduced density seen as spaces between hairs). Neither of these features are present in TA cases of recent onset.

Histology

Biopsy findings in TA may be distinguished between subacute, short-term cases and chronic, long-standing cases (Table 11.3). Biopsied cases of TA that develop over weeks or months can show an increase in the catagen to telogen count on horizontal sections as well as pigment casts and pigment incontinence in the hair

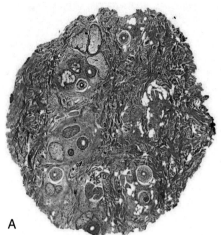 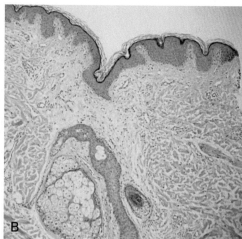

FIG. 11.6 **(A)** Horizontal section of traction alopecia: There is aberrant follicular architecture with areas of follicular dropout. There are no terminal follicles but only vellus follicles (n = 8). Note the focal preservation of the sebaceous glands (hematoxylin and eosin, 2×). **(B)** Vertical section of traction alopecia demonstrates preserved sebaceous glands adjacent to a vellus follicle (hematoxylin and eosin, 4×). ((A) Image courtesy of Mariya Miteva, MD.)

shaft on vertical sections. Trichomalacia, known as distortion of the hair shaft, is also a noted feature. TA viewed on horizontal sectioning will show a decrease in terminal hairs, whereas the amount of vellus hairs is relatively consistent[18] (Fig. 11.6A).

Alternatively, although long-standing TA cases can have some of the same histologic findings as those seen in shorter-term cases, there can also be follicular dropout, fibrous tracts at the pilosebaceous unit isthmus, and preservation of sebaceous glands (Fig. 11.6B).[13,19]

Overall, histopathologic findings of early TA share similarities with those exhibited in TM.[13,18,19] They both exhibit a lack of inflammatory infiltrate, hemorrhage both within and surrounding the hair follicle, hair pigment incontinence in the upper portions of the pilosebaceous unit, and the previously noted trichomalacia. Distinctively, these features are generally less severe and less diffusely distributed in TA than in TM.

TREATMENT, EDUCATION, AND PROGNOSIS

The foremost treatment for TA is an adjustment in behavior with adoption of non-traction-based, low-tension hairstyles. Patients should be encouraged to diversify hairstyle selection and loosen their existing hairstyles. Hairstyle diversification includes stoppage of repetitive braids or buns or ponytails that put traction on the same areas of the scalp and introduction

of alternate ways of parting and arranging the hair, which provide the desired function or aesthetic effect. For patients who, for religious or stylistic reasons, are not amenable to removal of hair accessories or hairstyles, loosening the source of traction is paramount. For example, patients who wear turbans should be encouraged to apply a traction-free covering before wrapping the turban around the scalp itself. For patients who wear their hair in dreadlocks, the frequency of loc tightening and the tension applied by the loctician can be decreased. More recently, various young men and women with AT hair who consistently wear their hair in dreadlock or microbraid styles shave the frontal 1–2 cm hairline down and begin the hairstyle further into the scalp to help remove tension and thus preserve the hairline. This adjustment may only redistribute the tension and therefore, the traction slightly posteriorly.

Successful regrowth of diagnosed TA with minoxidil has been reported.[20,21] Patients diagnosed with TA used this concentration of minoxidil faithfully for a minimum period of 6 months and displayed hair regrowth at sites previously void of hair.[20] To avoid providing the patient with conflicting medical management, it is prudent to emphasize that application of minoxidil is only a secondary, supplemental measure to the primary measure of hairstyle modification. Patients who continue traction-based hairstyling and concurrent use of minoxidil therapy may grow vellus hairs that are still vulnerable to the ongoing, daily traction. A cycle of hair regrowth followed by mechanical hair loss could develop.

In chronic TA, where there is no ability to stimulate hair regrowth, surgical methods of management can yield success. There is mention of hair transplantation having been performed in the form of punch grafting, minigrafting, micrografting, and follicular unit transplantation methods for patients with TA.[21] A more detailed account of a young woman who underwent micro- and minigrafts in a single hair transplantation session indicates the potential for successful hair transplantation after 5 years with TA.[22] Although possible, surgical methods of treatment are an invasive, costly form of therapy for a condition that is amenable to simple behavioral modification.

TA is an avoidable form of alopecia and, as such, falls within the realm of disease prevention in dermatology. Given that dermatologists are more knowledgeable of the condition, the at-risk demographic groups, and the clinical signs consistent with traction, it is of utmost importance that clinicians inform patients and those who style their patients' hair of the factors leading to TA. When initial signs of TA are identified, a dermatologist has the professional credibility to warn of its potential permanent effects. Motivated dermatologists may even consider educating primary care physicians and hairdressers within their practice catchment area via a bulletin or an in-person information session. In today's digital age, both primary care and dermatology office websites and social media pages can graphically display examples of TA and tips to avoid it, such as avoidance of pain with braiding; removal of hairstyles if pustules or pimplelike lesions form; rejection of heavy extensions; and rotation of hairstyles with different parting patterns at least every 6–8 weeks. Such an approach has the potential to reach a younger, under-18 demographic, the demographic currently noted to be most at risk of mild TA. This generation may then learn appropriate styling practices and incorporate measures to circumvent TA, thus avoiding the higher prevalence currently seen in 26- to 50-year-old women.[4] It is crucial that dermatologists communicate techniques that decrease traction and allow patients to enjoy popular hairstyles safely without associated TA.

Patient prognosis in TA is variable and is based on expediency of diagnosis and, in turn, patient adherence to traction avoidance. Clinicians may use both trichoscopy and histology as diagnostic clues that will also indicate the progression of TA, in large part by the presence of persistent follicles. If these are present, reasonable behavioral and therapeutic efforts can be used to preserve traction-free hairs. As a matter of public education, dermatologists and other clinicians must take it upon themselves to be proactive in the counseling process, so that traction-promoting practices are corrected at the first sign of the condition.

REFERENCES

1. Khumalo NP, Jessop S, Gumedze F, Ehrlich R. Hairdressing and the prevalence of scalp disease in African adults. *Br J Dermatol.* 2007;157(5):981–988.
2. Rucker Wright D, Gathers R, Kapke A, Johnson D, Joseph CL. Hair care practices and their association with scalp and hair disorders in African American girls. *J Am Acad Dermatol.* 2011;64(2):253–262.
3. Khumalo NP, Jessop S, Gumedze F, Ehrlich R. Hairdressing is associated with scalp disease in African schoolchildren. *Br J Dermatol.* 2007;157(1):106–110.
4. Khumalo NP, Jessop S, Gumedze F, Ehrlich R. Determinants of marginal traction alopecia in African girls and women. *J Am Acad Dermatol.* 2008;59(3):432–438.
5. Polat M. Evaluation of clinical signs and early and late trichoscopy findings in traction alopecia patients with Fitzpatrick skin type II and III: a single-center, clinical study. *Int J Dermatol.* 2017.
6. James J, Saladi RN, Fox JL. Traction alopecia in Sikh male patients. *J Am Board Fam Med JABFM.* 2007;20(5):497–498.
7. Samrao A, Chen C, Zedek D, Price VH. Traction alopecia in a ballerina: clinicopathologic features. *Arch Dermatol.* 2010;146(8):930–931.
8. Hwang SM, Lee WS, Choi EH, Lee SH, Ahn SK. Nurse's cap alopecia. *Int J Dermatol.* 1999;38(3):187–191.
9. Samrao A, Price VH, Zedek D, Mirmirani P. The "Fringe Sign" – a useful clinical finding in traction alopecia of the marginal hair line. *Dermatol Online J.* 2011;17(11):1.
10. Khumalo NP, Ngwanya RM, Jessop S, Gumedze F, Ehrlich R. Marginal traction alopecia severity score: development and test of reliability. *J Cosmetic Dermatol.* 2007;6(4):262–269.
11. Yang A, Iorizzo M, Vincenzi C, Tosti A. Hair extensions: a concerning cause of hair disorders. *Br J Dermatol.* 2009;160(1):207–209.
12. Chandran NS, Novak J, Iorizzo M, Grimalt R, Oranje AP. Trichotillomania in children. *Skin Appendage Disord.* 2015;1(1):18–24.
13. Barbosa AB, Donati A, Valente NS, Romiti R. Patchy traction alopecia mimicking areata. *Int J Trichol.* 2015;7(4):184–186.
14. Callender VD, Reid SD, Obayan O, McClellan L, Sperling L. Diagnostic clues to frontal fibrosing alopecia in patients of African descent. *J Clini Aesthetic Dermatol.* 2016;9(4):45–51.
15. Mirmirani P, Khumalo NP. Traction alopecia: how to translate study data for public education–closing the KAP gap? *Dermatol Clin.* 2014;32(2):153–161.

16. Shim WH, Jwa SW, Song M, et al. Dermoscopic approach to a small round to oval hairless patch on the scalp. *Ann Dermatol.* 2014;26(2):214–220.

17. Tosti A, Miteva M, Torres F, Vincenzi C, Romanelli P. Hair casts are a dermoscopic clue for the diagnosis of traction alopecia. *Br J Dermatol.* 2010;163(6):1353–1355.

18. Bernardez C, Molina-Ruiz AM, Requena L. Histologic features of alopecias-part I: nonscarring alopecias. *Actas Dermo-sifiliograficas.* 2015;106(3):158–167.

19. Stefanato CM. Histopathology of alopecia: a clinicopathological approach to diagnosis. *Histopathology.* 2010;56(1):24–38.

20. Khumalo NP, Ngwanya RM. Traction alopecia: 2% topical minoxidil shows promise. Report of two cases. *J Eur Acad Dermatol Venereol JEADV.* 2007;21(3):433–434.

21. Callender VD, McMichael AJ, Cohen GF. Medical and surgical therapies for alopecias in black women. *Dermatol Therapy.* 2004;17(2):164–176.

22. Ozcelik D. Extensive traction alopecia attributable to ponytail hairstyle and its treatment with hair transplantation. *Aesthetic Plastic Surg.* 2005;29(4):325–327.

CHAPTER 12

Lichen Planopilaris

NISHA S. DESAI, MD • PARADI MIRMIRANI, MD

INTRODUCTION

Lichen planopilaris (LPP) (also known as follicular lichen planus) was initially described by Pringle in 1895.[1] LPP belongs to a group of disorders called cicatricial or scarring alopecias. LPP is further subclassified as a primary lymphocytic cicatricial alopecia, based upon the type of inflammation (lymphocytes) seen on routine biopsies in the early stages of the disease.[2] Common to all primary cicatricial alopecias, the pilosebaceous unit is the target of the inflammatory attack, which eventually results in replacement of the hair follicle with fibrous tissue. The end result is progressive scarring and permanent hair loss. LPP can be subdivided into three groups, including classic LPP, frontal fibrosing alopecia (FFA), and Graham-Little-Piccardi-Lasseur syndrome.[3] This chapter will focus mostly on classic LPP. Extracranial variants and Graham-Little syndrome will be briefly discussed. The frontal fibrosing variant is discussed in another chapter of this book.

EPIDEMIOLOGY

LPP typically affects Caucasian middle-aged adult females, but it can also affect men and individuals as young as teenagers. The female to male ratio is reported to be 4.9:1–8:1.[4,5] The annual incidence rate of LPP in the United States is on the rise and varies from 1.15% to 7.59% when measured in four tertiary referral centers for hair loss.[6]

ETIOLOGY

Many studies suggest that LPP has an autoimmune pathogenesis, but no clear association between LPP and autoimmunity has been made (nor entirely excluded).[7] Therefore, LPP likely results from a combination of genetic susceptibility and other factors (environmental, medical comorbidities, medications, etc). Familial cases are rare, but have been reported.[8] A recent study has shown that HLA DRB1*11 and DQB1*03 alleles were expressed with higher frequency in patients diagnosed with LPP, also supporting a genetic link.[9]

Depending on the study, between 17% and 28% of LPP patients may have other forms of lichen planus.[10,11] In addition, LPP has been associated with other dermatologic diseases, including psoriasis, epidermolysis bullosa pruriginosa, dermatitis herpetiformis, scleroderma (en coup de sabre), and erythema dyschromicum perstans.[12-16] More recently, in two separate retrospective studies performed at the Cleveland Clinic Foundation, hypothyroidism was found in 29% of patients with LPP, and androgen excess/polycystic ovarian syndrome was found in 28% of patients with LPP.[17,18]

The onset of LPP has been described after starting several medications, including tumor necrosis factor (TNF)-α inhibitors (etanercept and infliximab) and topical imiquimod.[12,19-21] The role of infection in the development of lichen planus and LPP has been postulated and include hepatitis C virus, human immunodeficiency virus, herpes simplex virus 2, *Helicobacter pylori*, human papillomavirus, and syphilis.[3] LPP has been reported to develop to the scalp after traumas, including hair restoration surgery, face-lift surgeries, and whole brain irradiation.[22] Although the mechanism is unclear, it is thought that after scalp trauma, there is exposure of hair follicle antigens to the immune system, which is normally an immunoprivileged site.

PATHOGENESIS

Understanding of the pathogenesis of LPP remains an evolving process. Murine models with mutations of genes expressed in the sebaceous gland, specifically the asebia mouse (stearyl-coenzyme A desaturase gene) and defolliculation (gasdermin 3, a transcription factor), have a clinical and histologic picture similar to cicatricial alopecia seen in humans.[23-28] These observations suggest that the sebaceous gland may be central to the pathogenesis of all forms of cicatricial alopecias. The role of the sebaceous gland, in addition to secreting sebum and lipid metabolic products, is to facilitate the coordinated breakdown of the inner root sheath during normal hair cycling.[24] This step may be critical for follicular regeneration, and absence of the normal gland may lead to obstructed outflow of the hair shaft. This in turn may lead to inflammation in the sebaceous gland and subsequent destruction of the pilosebaceous unit.

Histopathologic studies of cicatricial alopecias in humans have consistently shown that the sebaceous gland is lost, even in early stages of the disease.[29] Furthermore, biopsies of clinically unaffected scalp in patients with LPP have shown early sebaceous gland atrophy.[30] This suggests that the sebaceous gland dysfunction and eventual loss may play a central role not only in LPP but also in all cicatricial alopecias.

More recent studies using microarray technique has shown that there is a defect in a "master regulator" protein called the peroxisome proliferator-activated receptor γ (PPAR-γ).[31] PPAR-γ is a transcription factor responsible for the regulating peroxisome biogenesis and lipid metabolism. PPAR-γ also has antiinflammatory effects and modulates inflammatory responses. Karnik et al. have shown through microarray studies that the expression of PPAR-γ is significantly decreased in LPP.[31] This suppression may be caused by genetics, environment, toxins, infection, metabolic, immunologic, or dietary changes. Loss of PPAR-γ leads to sebaceous gland dysfunction, which causes abnormal processing and buildup of proinflammatory "toxic" lipids. This abnormal buildup of lipids is what is thought to trigger inflammation and subsequently destroy the sebaceous gland and the nearby stem cells, leading to permanent hair loss and scarring in LPP.

CLINICAL FEATURES

Classic LPP of the scalp can be subdivided into three clinical forms: patchy LPP, diffuse LPP, and the more recently described, patterned LPP. In *patchy LPP*, hair loss occurs in small patches, which may enlarge and slowly merge with other patches to form larger scarred areas (Fig. 12.1). In a typical scarred area, the center is smooth and devoid of follicular markings. Also depending on the skin type, the scarred area may be hypopigmented or hyperpigmented. Hair follicles at the margins of the scarred areas show varying degrees of perifollicular erythema and perifollicular scale, depending on disease activity. A positive hair pull test result of anagen hairs may indicate areas of high disease activity. In *diffuse LPP*, often the top or crown of the scalp is initially affected, but lesions can occur anywhere. Hair loss is difficult to appreciate in early disease, but over time focal scarring can transform into diffuse hair thinning and patchy scarring (Fig. 12.2). Recently a new variant of LPP has been suggested, termed patterned

LPP or fibrosing alopecia in a pattern distribution.[32–34] In *patterned LPP*, clinical features overlap between diffuse LPP and androgenetic alopecia, and the inflammatory findings of perifollicular erythema and follicular hyperkeratosis are only found in the areas of androgenetic alopecia[32] (Fig. 12.3). Histologically this form is identical to LPP; miniaturized hairs as well as terminal hairs appear to be targeted by inflammation.[33] It is unclear whether patterned LPP is a distinct form of LPP or whether it is patterned hair loss with a lichenoid host reaction.

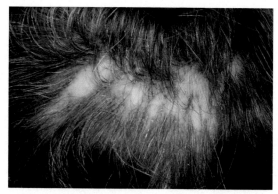

FIG. 12.1 Lichen planopilaris with patchy areas of alopecia showing loss of follicular markings. At the active edge there is evidence of perifollicular erythema and scaling.

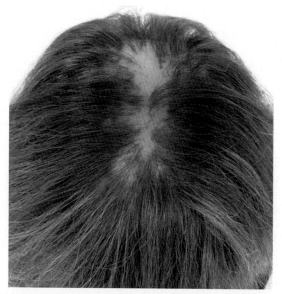

FIG. 12.2 Lichen planopilaris with central scalp patchy alopecia.

In Graham-Little-Picardi-Lasseur syndrome, there is a triad of cicatricial alopecia of the scalp, lichen planus of the skin with widespread follicular papules (lichen planus spinulosus), and nonscarring hair loss of axillary and pubic area.[10] Other forms of LPP of the scalp include linear LPP, in which a small linear segment of the scalp is involved. This form of LPP is rare and only one case has been reported in the literature.[35] Extracranial forms of LPP have been reported and include linear LPP of the face and linear LPP of the trunk.[36–40] LPP has also been reported to occur on the extremities and vulvar area.[41,42] LPP can also overlap with its other variant FFA.

LPP can be very symptomatic with intense burning, itching, tingling, or pain, or it may be largely asymptomatic. Sometimes heavy shedding can be accompanied with periods of high symptom activity. The course of LPP is variable and the natural history of the disease is unknown. It may evolve slowly with a few patches of hair loss or mild thinning, which slowly progresses over many years. In other cases, the course is rapid, and within a few months many patches of hair loss or widespread thinning spreads over large areas of the scalp. Although uncommon, some patients will have periods of time when the disease is not active (remissions).

DERMOSCOPY

Dermoscopy is a helpful tool when considering the diagnosis of LPP (Fig. 12.4). Perifollicular erythema and follicular hyperkeratosis, as well as early scarring can be seen with dermoscopy, which may be missed when looking at the scalp with the naked eye. Other dermatoscopic features include keratotic plugs, elongated concentric blood vessels, violaceous blue interfollicular areas, and big irregular white dots.[43] The use of dermoscopy can also be instrumental in guiding where to take a scalp biopsy from to confirm the diagnosis.[44]

HISTOPATHOLOGY

A biopsy is warranted in the diagnosis of all cicatricial alopecias to establish the correct diagnosis and to quantify the degree of inflammation and scarring, which can help guide the provider's choice of treatment.[45] The biopsy should be taken from the active border of hair loss where some hairs still remain. A 4-mm punch biopsy is the standardized size for scalp biopsies, and the depth should include the subcutaneous fat to ensure that the entire pilosebaceous unit is available for examination. The biopsies may be sectioned horizontally and vertically or both (HoVert technique).[46]

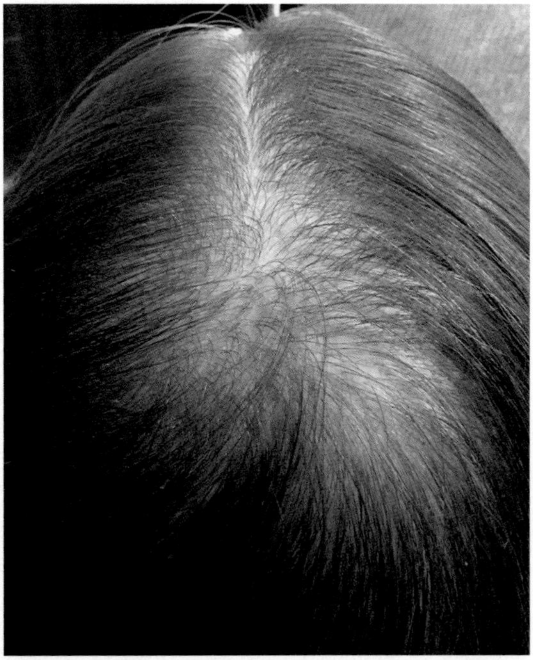

FIG. 12.3 Lichen planopilaris with a patterned distribution of alopecia.

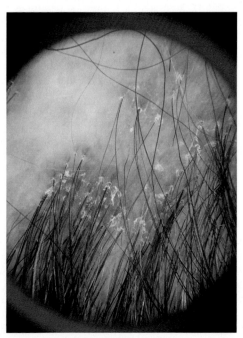

FIG. 12.4 Dermoscopy of lichen planopilaris: perifollicular erythema and follicular hyperkeratosis, as well as scarring are seen.

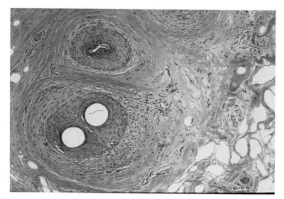

FIG. 12.5 Lichen planopilaris histopathology showing perifollicular lymphocytic inflammation and compound follicles.

Depending on the preference of the histopathologist, either one or two scalp biopsies may be requested. Vertical sections are useful for giving information about the epidermis; however, only a fraction of the hair follicles can be examined in each section. Horizontal sections are becoming the method of choice as they offer the advantage of evaluating large numbers of follicles simultaneously, determining hair density, telogen/vellus ratio, anagen to telogen ratio, and location of inflammatory infiltrate.[47–49] Routine staining with hematoxylin and eosin is recommended as a standard evaluation. Histopathologic findings of LPP include a lichenoid interface perifolliculitis, consisting of lymphocytes distributed around the infundibulum and isthmus of the hair follicle. Low follicular density, sebaceous gland atrophy, and/or loss of sebaceous glands are routinely seen features. One can also find lamellar perifollicular fibrosis, fibrous tract formation, and the presence of compound follicles ("owl eyes or goggles"), which is a finding in later stage disease, representing the fusion of multiple hair follicles from the scarring process[50] (Fig. 12.5).

MANAGEMENT

Management of LPP is complex. Treatment is case-dependent, based on the severity of symptoms and signs (itching and inflammation), findings on histopathology, and the extent and progression of hair loss. Response to treatment varies from individual to individual. Once the disease is stabilized or in remission, treatment may be continued for another 6–12 months at which time treatment may be discontinued. However, recurrences are common. Documentation of symptoms and signs of inflammation and use of photography to

TABLE 12.1 Treatment Options for Lichen Planopilaris	
Disease Severity (As Measured by Signs and Symptoms, Degree of Inflammation on Biopsy and Progression of Hair Loss)	Treatment Options
Mild	Topical corticosteroids Topical calcineurin inhibitors Intralesional corticosteroids
Moderate	All treatments listed in mild along with one or more of the following: Tetracycline antibiotics Antimalarials Thiazolidinediones Retinoids
Severe	All treatments listed in mild along with the following: Mycophenolate mofetil Cyclosporine Prednisone

document extent of hair loss can be useful in assessing response to treatment. The LPP activity index is one objective measure for assessing disease activity and response to treatment.[51]

The treatment options are summarized in Table 12.1.

Topical/Intralesional Therapies

In general, mild disease or localized disease may be managed by topical corticosteroids (TCs). Initially ultrapotent TCs may be used daily to twice daily for 4–6 weeks. As the disease improves, transitioning the ultrapotent TCS to 2–3 times per week, or switching to midpotency TCs will help prevent tachyphylaxis as well as steroid atrophy. TCs come in many vehicles suitable for patients depending on their preferences, including solutions, foams, sprays, and gels. Oils and ointments are available formulations that work well for patients with afro-textured hair. Potential side effects of TCs include steroid acne/folliculitis, steroid atrophy, and rarely short-term hypothalamic–pituitary–adrenal axis supression.[52] The clinician should be closely monitoring for these side effects.

Topical calcineurin inhibitors (TCIs) offer a great alternative or adjunctive to TCs for treatment of LPP. They are available commercially as in tacrolimus ointment and pimecrolimus cream, but they can be compounded into topical solutions and lotions for ease of use on the scalp. The recently approved crisaborole ointment (phosphodiesterase 4 inhibitor) is another nonsteroidal antiinflammatory agent currently approved by Food and Drug Administration (FDA) to treat atopic dermatitis, which may be of benefit to treat LPP. Antiinflammatory shampoos (such as corticosteroid shampoos, antidandruff shampoos, or those containing tea tree oil) can also be used adjunctively with TCS and TCIs to treat LPP. In the case topical therapy alone is not effective for small or localized areas, the next step could be the addition of intralesional corticosteroid injections (triamcinolone acetonide) to the involved areas in concentrations ranging from 2.5 to 10 mg/mL every 4–12 weeks. They can provide dramatic relief of symptoms and are often used as a "bridge" treatment for a few months until the full effect of other treatments has taken effect.

Systemic Therapies

For more diffuse or severe cases, oral antiinflammatory and immunosuppressive medications can be used. Tetracycline antibiotics, such doxycycline or minocycline, can be used as first-line and long-term antibiotics for their antiinflammatory properties, either in standard dosing (100 mg twice daily) or more preferably in low or submicrobial dosing (20–40 mg daily) to reduce the chance of antibiotic resistance. According to a review article by Racz et al., 57% of patients showed a partial or good response to the tetracycline class of antibiotics for treatment of LPP.[53]

Antimalarials such as hydroxychloroquine (HCQ), chloroquine, and quinacrine are established steroid-sparing antilymphocytic medications. Given its safety and low side-effect profile and efficacy, HCQ is considered to be the gold-standard systemic treatment for lymphocytic-mediated cicatricial alopecias. The usual starting dose of HCQ is 5 mg/kg/day based on actual body weight, daily or divided twice daily. Because of the long half-life of HCQ (~40 days), the medication may not start to take effect until 10–12 weeks. In fact, stable blood concentration of HCQ may not be reached until after 6 months of treatment.[45] The efficacy of HCQ (partial and complete responders) is reported to be between 53% and 83% based on several retrospective studies.[51,53,54] A comprehensive ophthalmologic examination is recommended at baseline and yearly after 5 years.[55] Complete blood count and liver function tests are also screened at baseline and every 6–12 months. Adverse reactions are very rare, but include gastrointestinal upset, myalgia, skin hyperpigmentation, hematologic changes, and ophthalmologic damage. HCQ should be used with caution in the elderly,

preexisting maculopathy, renal/liver disease, patients taking tamoxifen, and after 7 years of use.

The thiazolidinediones (pioglitazone and rosiglitazone) are PPAR-γ agonists currently available in the United States and are FDA-approved for the treatment of type 2 diabetes mellitus. These medications can be safely used in nondiabetic patients. Potential side effects include fluid retention, secondary peripheral edema, and weight gain (which may pose a cardiovascular risk in patients with congestive heart failure). The risk of bladder cancer in patients taking pioglitazone long term is controversial but has been reported to be increased after 2 years of exposure to the drug.[56-58] As far as efficacy is concerned, in several case series there has been a response rate ranging from 20% to 70%, with response being defined as decreased symptoms, inflammation, and progression of hair loss.[59-61] The onset of action can be seen as early as several weeks to several months; however, long-lasting efficacy is still not well documented.[61]

The use of oral retinoids, including acitretin at low doses (10 mg) as well as low-dose isotretinoin has been advocated for patients with LPP because of their efficacy for treating cutaneous lichen planus.[62,63] In one retrospective review, oral retinoid therapy was found to be a helpful adjunctive treatment for resistant cases; 5 of 21 (24%) patients with LPP had a benefit.[64] Therefore, oral retinoids may be a reasonable strategy for patients with LPP; however, they may cause telogen effluvium (which in turn will exacerbate hair loss) and thus limit their use. In addition, the use of oral retinoids in women of childbearing potential must be done with extreme caution because of its known teratogenic side effects. Baseline and monthly laboratory tests include liver function, lipid panel, and urine or serum human chorionic gonadotropin (in women of childbearing potential).

Mycophenolate mofetil (MMF) is an antimetabolite that inhibits activated lymphocytes. It is FDA approved for treatment and prevention of organ rejection in transplant recipients. Given its effectiveness, tolerability, and safety profile, it has been advocated as the preferred second-line treatment for LPP patients with persistent symptoms and hair loss after a 6-month trial of HCQ.[45] In a series of 16 patients, MMF (dose ranges from 500 mg twice daily to 1000 mg twice daily) was effective in achieving either complete or partial response in 83% of patients, who had failed multiple prior treatments after at least 6 months of treatment.[65] Baseline and monthly laboratory tests include liver function and complete blood counts. MMF is associated with increased risk of congenital malformations and first-trimester pregnancy loss and therefore should be used with caution in females of childbearing potential. In a study comparing long-term safety of MMF with cyclosporine (CsA), it was concluded that MMF has less long-term risk for cancer or end-organ damage.[66]

CsA is a calcineurin inhibitor that acts by suppressing T-cell activation and proliferation and also inhibits T-cell secretion of proinflammatory cytokines, such as interferon-γ, which is responsible for macrophage activation.[67] Beneficial effects of short-term CsA therapy (2–5 months) in patients with LPP[68] have been reported in dosages of 3–5 mg/kg/day. Patient monitoring includes documentation of blood pressure, kidney function, complete blood count, liver function tests, and urinalysis at baseline, every 2 weeks for 1 month, then monthly for the duration of therapy.[69] Because of its cumulative nephrotoxic side effects, CsA is also not appropriate for long-term use and should be used only as a temporary or bridge treatment for 3–6 months.

Oral prednisone can be used to rapidly diminish the inflammatory signs and symptoms; however given the side-effect profile, it is not appropriate for long-term use and is used only as a temporary or bridge treatment. A dosage of 0.5–1 mg/kg oral prednisone tapered over several weeks to months can be considered.

CONCLUSION

LPP is a chronic lymphocytic cicatricial alopecia likely caused by genetic susceptibility and environmental factors. It is characterized by perifollicular erythema and scaling and eventual patchy or diffuse loss with scarring. Establishing the diagnosis early and beginning treatment as soon as the diagnosis is made is essential to prevent widespread involvement and permanent loss. Treatment options depend on age, gender, symptom, and disease severity (clinically and histopathologically). TCs and nonsteroidal agents, intralesional corticosteroids, and a variety of systemic antiinflammatory or immunosuppressive therapies may be used singly or in combination to adequately control the disease.

REFERENCES

1. Adamson, HG. Lichen pilaris, seu spinulosus. *Br J Dermatol.* 1905;17(2):39–54.
2. Olsen EA, Bergfeld WF, Cotsarelis G, et al. Summary of North American Hair Research Society (NAHRS)-sponsored workshop on cicatricial alopecia, Duke University Medical Center, February 10 and 11, 2001. *J Am Acad Dermatol.* 2003;48(1):103–110.
3. Kang H, Alzolibani AA, Otberg N, Shapiro J. Lichen planopilaris. *Dermatol Ther.* 2008;21(4):249–256.
4. Meinhard J, Stroux A, Lünnemann L, Vogt A, Blume-Peytavi U. Lichen planopilaris: epidemiology and prevalence of subtypes - a retrospective analysis in 104 patients. *J Dtsch Dermatol Ges.* 2014;12(3):229–235, 229–236.
5. Soares VC, Mulinari-Brenner F, Souza TE. Lichen planopilaris epidemiology: a retrospective study of 80 cases. *An Bras Dermatol.* 2015;90(5):666–670.
6. Ochoa BE, King LE, Price VH. Lichen planopilaris: annual incidence in four hair referral centers in the United States. *J Am Acad Dermatol.* 2008;58(2):352–353.
7. Karnik P, Stenn K. Cicatricial alopecia symposium 2011: lipids, inflammation and stem cells. *J Invest Dermatol.* 2012;132(6):1529–1531.
8. Misiak-Galazka M, Olszewska M, Rudnicka L. Lichen planopilaris in three generations: grandmother, mother, and daughter - a genetic link? *Int J Dermatol.* 2016;55(8):913–915.
9. Pavlovsky L, Israeli M, Sagy E, et al. Lichen planopilaris is associated with HLA DRB1*11 and DQB1*03 alleles. *Acta Derm Venereol.* 2015;95(2):177–180.
10. Tan E, Martinka M, Ball N, Shapiro J. Primary cicatricial alopecias: clinicopathology of 112 cases. *J Am Acad Dermatol.* 2004;50(1):25–32.
11. Lyakhovitsky A, Amichai B, Sizopoulou C, Barzilai A. A case series of 46 patients with lichen planopilaris: demographics, clinical evaluation, and treatment experience. *J Dermatolog Treat.* 2015;26(3):275–279.
12. Abbasi NR, Orlow SJ. Lichen planopilaris noted during etanercept therapy in a child with severe psoriasis. *Pediatr Dermatol.* 2009;26(1):118.
13. Almaani N, Liu L, Perez A, Robson A, Mellerio JE, McGrath JA. Epidermolysis bullosa pruriginosa in association with lichen planopilaris. *Clin Exp Dermatol.* 2009;34(8):e825–e828.
14. Moravedge H, Salamat A. Dermatitis herpetiformis in association with lichen planopilaris. *J Am Acad Dermatol.* 2002;46(3):467–468.
15. Muñoz-Pérez MA, Camacho F. Lichen planopilaris and scleroderma en coup de sabre. *J Eur Acad Dermatol Venereol.* 2002;16(5):542–544.
16. Metin A, Calka O, Ugras S. Lichen planopilaris coexisting with erythema dyschromicum perstans. *Br J Dermatol.* 2001;145(3):522–523.
17. Atanaskova Mesinkovska N, Brankov N, Piliang M, Kyei A, Bergfeld WF. Association of lichen planopilaris with thyroid disease: a retrospective case-control study. *J Am Acad Dermatol.* 2014;70(5):889–892.
18. Ranasinghe GC, Piliang MP, Bergfeld WF. Prevalence of hormonal and endocrine dysfunction in patients with lichen planopilaris (LPP): a retrospective data analysis of 168 patients. *J Am Acad Dermatol.* 2017;76(2):314–320.
19. Garcovich S, Manco S, Zampetti A, Amerio P, Garcovich A. Onset of lichen planopilaris during treatment with etanercept. *Br J Dermatol.* 2008;158(5):1161–1163.
20. Fernández-Torres R, Paradela S, Valbuena L, Fonseca E. Infliximab-induced lichen planopilaris. *Ann Pharmacother.* 2010;44(9):1501–1503.

21. Drummond A, Pichler J, Argenziano G, et al. Lichen planopilaris after imiquimod 5% cream for multiple BCC in basal cell naevus syndrome. *Australas J Dermatol.* 2015;56(4):e105–e107.

22. Donovan J. Lichen planopilaris after hair transplantation: report of 17 cases. *Dermatol Surg.* 2012;38(12):1998–2004.

23. Stenn KS, Sundberg JP, Sperling LC. Hair follicle biology, the sebaceous gland, and scarring alopecias. *Arch Dermatol.* 1999;135(8):973–974.

24. Stenn KS. Insights from the asebia mouse: a molecular sebaceous gland defect leading to cicatricial alopecia. *J Cutan Pathol.* 2001;28(9):445–447.

25. Zheng Y, Eilertsen KJ, Ge L, et al. Scd1 is expressed in sebaceous glands and is disrupted in the asebia mouse. *Nat Genet.* 1999;23(3):268–270.

26. Sundberg JP, Boggess D, Sundberg BA, et al. Asebia-2J (Scd1(ab2J)): a new allele and a model for scarring alopecia. *Am J Pathol.* 2000;156(6):2067–2075.

27. Lu Y, Bu L, Zhou S, et al. Scd1ab-Xyk: a new asebia allele characterized by a CCC trinucleotide insertion in exon 5 of the stearoyl-CoA desaturase 1 gene in mouse. *Mol Genet Genomics.* 2004;272(2):129–137.

28. Stenn KS, Cotsarelis G, Price VH. Report from the cicatricial alopecia colloquium. *J Invest Dermatol.* 2006;126(3):539–541.

29. Al-Zaid T, Vanderweil S, Zembowicz A, Lyle S. Sebaceous gland loss and inflammation in scarring alopecia: a potential role in pathogenesis. *J Am Acad Dermatol.* 2011;65(3):597–603.

30. Mirmirani P, Willey A, Headington JT, Stenn K, McCalmont TH, Price VH. Primary cicatricial alopecia: histopathologic findings do not distinguish clinical variants. *J Am Acad Dermatol.* 2005;52(4):637–643.

31. Karnik P, Tekeste Z, McCormick TS, et al. Hair follicle stem cell-specific PPARgamma deletion causes scarring alopecia. *J Invest Dermatol.* 2009;129(5):1243–1257.

32. Zinkernagel MS, Trüeb RM. Fibrosing alopecia in a pattern distribution: patterned lichen planopilaris or androgenetic alopecia with a lichenoid tissue reaction pattern? *Arch Dermatol.* 2000;136(2):205–211.

33. Abbasi A, Kamyab-Hesari K, Rabbani R, Mollaee F, Abbasi S. A new subtype of lichen planopilaris affecting vellus hairs and clinically mimicking androgenetic alopecia. *Dermatol Surg.* 2016;42(10):1174–1180.

34. Fergie B, Khaira G, Howard V, de Zwaan S. Diffuse scarring alopecia in a female pattern hair loss distribution. *Australas J Dermatol.* 2017.

35. Kaliyadan F, Ameer AA. Localized and linear lichen planopilaris over the face and scalp with associated alopecia - clinical and dermoscopy pattern. *Dermatol Online J.* 2015;21(9).

36. Asz-Sigall D, González-de-Cossio-Hernández AC, Rodríguez-Lobato E, Ortega-Springall MF, Vega-Memije ME, Arenas Guzmán R. Linear lichen planopilaris of the face: case report and review. *Skin Appendage Disord.* 2016;2(1–2):72–75.

37. Gerritsen MJ, de Jong EM, van de Kerkhof PC. Linear lichen planopilaris of the face. *J Am Acad Dermatol.* 1998;38(4):633–635.

38. Küster W, Kind P, Hölzle E, Plewig G. Linear lichen planopilaris of the face. *J Am Acad Dermatol.* 1989;21(1):131–132.

39. Zhao N, Qu T. Linear lichen planopilaris of the face. *Eur J Dermatol.* 2012;22(5):691–692.

40. Baker K, Pehr K. Linear lichen planopilaris of the trunk: first report of a case. *J Cutan Med Surg.* 2006;10(3):136–138.

41. Vendramini DL, Silveira BR, Duque-Estrada B, Boff AL, Sodré CT, Pirmez R. Isolated body hair loss: an unusual presentation of lichen planopilaris. *Skin Appendage Disord.* 2017;2(3–4):97–99.

42. Grunwald MH, Zvulunov A, Halevy S. Lichen planopilaris of the vulva. *Br J Dermatol.* 1997;136(3):477–478.

43. Bolduc C, Sperling LC, Shapiro J. Primary cicatricial alopecia: lymphocytic primary cicatricial alopecias, including chronic cutaneous lupus erythematosus, lichen planopilaris, frontal fibrosing alopecia, and Graham-Little syndrome. *J Am Acad Dermatol.* 2016;75(6):1081–1099.

44. Miteva M, Tosti A. Dermoscopy guided scalp biopsy in cicatricial alopecia. *J Eur Acad Dermatol Venereol.* 2013;27(10):1299–1303.

45. Price VH. The medical treatment of cicatricial alopecia. *Semin Cutan Med Surg.* 2006;25(1):56–59.

46. Nguyen JV, Hudacek K, Whitten JA, Rubin AI, Seykora JT. The HoVert technique: a novel method for the sectioning of alopecia biopsies. *J Cutan Pathol.* 2011;38(5):401–406.

47. Headington JT. Cicatricial alopecia. *Dermatol Clin.* 1996;14(4):773–782.

48. Whiting D. The value of horizontal sections of scalp biopsies. *J Cutan Aging Cosmet Dermatol.* 1990;1:165–173.

49. Templeton SF, Santa Cruz DJ, Solomon AR. Alopecia: histologic diagnosis by transverse sections. *Semin Diagn Pathol.* 1996;13(1):2–18.

50. Miteva M, Torres F, Tosti A. The 'eyes' or 'goggles' as a clue to the histopathological diagnosis of primary lymphocytic cicatricial alopecia. *Br J Dermatol.* 2012;166(2):454–455.

51. Chiang C, Sah D, Cho BK, Ochoa BE, Price VH. Hydroxychloroquine and lichen planopilaris: efficacy and introduction of Lichen Planopilaris Activity Index scoring system. *J Am Acad Dermatol.* 2010;62(3):387–392.

52. Fisher DA. Adverse effects of topical corticosteroid use. *West J Med.* 1995;162(2):123–126.

53. Racz E, Gho C, Moorman PW, Noordhoek Hegt V, Neumann HA. Treatment of frontal fibrosing alopecia and lichen planopilaris: a systematic review. *J Eur Acad Dermatol Venereol.* 2013;27(12):1461–1470.

54. Nic Dhonncha E, Foley CC, Markham T. The role of hydroxychloroquine in the treatment of lichen planopilaris: a retrospective case series and review. *Dermatol Ther.* 2017;30.

55. Marmor MF, Kellner U, Lai TY, Melles RB, Mieler WF. American academy of O. Recommendations on screening for chloroquine and hydroxychloroquine retinopathy (2016 revision). *Ophthalmology.* 2016;123(6):1386–1394.

56. Lewis JD, Ferrara A, Peng T, et al. Risk of bladder cancer among diabetic patients treated with pioglitazone: interim report of a longitudinal cohort study. *Diabetes Care.* 2011;34(4):916–922.
57. Lewis JD, Habel LA, Quesenberry CP, et al. Pioglitazone use and risk of bladder cancer and other Common cancers in persons with diabetes. *JAMA.* 2015;314(3):265–277.
58. Li Z, Sun M, Wang F, Shi J, Wang K. Association between pioglitazone use and the risk of bladder cancer among subjects with diabetes mellitus: a dose-response meta-analysis. *Int J Clin Pharmacol Ther.* 2017;55(3):210–219.
59. Baibergenova A, Walsh S. Use of pioglitazone in patients with lichen planopilaris. *J Cutan Med Surg.* 2012;16(2):97–100.
60. Mesinkovska NA, Tellez A, Dawes D, Piliang M, Bergfeld W. The use of oral pioglitazone in the treatment of lichen planopilaris. *J Am Acad Dermatol.* 2015;72(2):355–356.
61. Spring P, Spanou Z, de Viragh PA. Lichen planopilaris treated by the peroxisome proliferator activated receptor-γ agonist pioglitazone: lack of lasting improvement or cure in the majority of patients. *J Am Acad Dermatol.* 2013;69(5):830–832.
62. Cribier B, Frances C, Chosidow O. Treatment of lichen planus. An evidence-based medicine analysis of efficacy. *Arch Dermatol.* 1998;134(12):1521–1530.
63. Laurberg G, Geiger JM, Hjorth N, et al. Treatment of lichen planus with acitretin. A double-blind, placebo-controlled study in 65 patients. *J Am Acad Dermatol.* 1991;24(3):434–437.
64. Spano F, Donovan JC. Efficacy of oral retinoids in treatment-resistant lichen planopilaris. *J Am Acad Dermatol.* 2014;71(5):1016–1018.
65. Cho BK, Sah D, Chwalek J, et al. Efficacy and safety of mycophenolate mofetil for lichen planopilaris. *J Am Acad Dermatol.* 2010;62(3):393–397.
66. Buell C, Koo J. Long-term safety of mycophenolate mofetil and cyclosporine: a review. *J Drugs Dermatol.* 2008;7(8):741–748.
67. Gafter-Gvili A, Sredni B, Gal R, Gafter U, Kalechman Y. Cyclosporin A-induced hair growth in mice is associated with inhibition of calcineurin-dependent activation of NFAT in follicular keratinocytes. *Am J Physiol Cell Physiol.* 2003;284(6):C1593–C1603.
68. Mirmirani P, Willey A, Price VH. Short course of oral cyclosporine in lichen planopilaris. *J Am Acad Dermatol.* 2003;49(4):667–671.
69. Menter A, Korman NJ, Elmets CA, et al. Guidelines of care for the management of psoriasis and psoriatic arthritis. Section 3. Guidelines of care for the management and treatment of psoriasis with topical therapies. *J Am Acad Dermatol.* 2009;60(4):643–659.

CHAPTER 13

Discoid Lupus Erythematosus

JADE FETTIG, MD • DANIEL CALLAGHAN III, MD • LYNNE J. GOLDBERG, MD

INTRODUCTION

Chronic cutaneous lupus erythematosus (CCLE) includes discoid lupus erythematosus (DLE), lupus erythematosus profundus/panniculitis (LEP), and chilblain lupus erythematosus. This chapter will focus only on DLE and LEP, as chilblain lupus does not occur on the scalp. The epidemiology, pathogenesis, and treatment of CCLE are not well characterized, as this condition is rare and the majority of research involves cutaneous symptoms of systemic lupus erythematosus (SLE). However, DLE is an important cause of alopecia, and as many as 50% of patients with DLE present with scalp lesions. The diagnosis depends on knowledge of the characteristic clinical, trichoscopic, and histologic features, as scalp DLE can be easily confused with other causes of alopecia, particularly lichen planopilaris (LPP).

EPIDEMIOLOGY

There is limited data on the epidemiology of CCLE. One large, prospective study evaluated 1002 patients from 29 European countries with cutaneous lupus erythematosus (CLE), including acute CLE, subacute CLE, and chronic CLE.[1] These investigators found a 2.5:1 female to male predominance, which is consistent with other research, indicating female predominance in this condition. This study found that the mean age of onset for CCLE was 41.2 ± 14.5 years. Another study showed that Raynaud's phenomenon, arthralgias, and SLE were more common in women with CLE than men. Some preliminary studies have shown that Maori, Pacific Islander, and part-Hawaiian individuals have a higher incidence of SLE and CCLE than individuals of European descent.[2] Overall, the incidence of CCLE is much lower among children compared with adults, but it does occur.[3]

ETIOLOGY AND PATHOGENESIS

DLE is an autoimmune disease resulting from a complex interplay of several factors. Although the specific pathogenesis remains unclear, it is thought to be triggered by an environmental stressor in the presence of an underlying genetic predisposition. Factors that have been implicated include ultraviolet (UV) irradiation, hormones, stress, drugs, chemicals, and infection. In this setting, immune dysregulation, autoantibodies, and aberrant cell signaling pathways unleash the inflammatory cascade with involvement of dendritic cells, T cells, and B cells. The result of this inflammation is apoptosis and necrosis, ultimately leading to the clinical picture of DLE.[4-6] Although DLE and SLE are clinically different diseases, the observation that up to 28% of patients with DLE are susceptible to transitioning to SLE suggests they share pathways and genetic backgrounds.[7]

The role genetics plays in the pathogenesis of lupus is highlighted by the fact that it has a 25% concordance rate among monozygotic twins compared with a 2% concordance rate for dizygotic twins.[8] Using genome-wide expression data from lesional and nonlesional skin of DLE patients, Dey-Rao et al. identified a subset of differentially expressed genes (DEGs) in DLE responsible for dysregulation of the complement cascade, apoptosis, and type 1 interferon (IFN) activation. Of these DEGs, 13% overlapped with genes previously associated with SLE; however, the other 87% did not overlap, suggesting that there are genetic abnormalities unique to DLE.[9] Specific genetic defects associated with an increased risk of DLE include TYK2, IRF5, and CLTA4.[10]

UV light is one of the most common triggers of DLE and is an important factor in the pathogenesis of the disease. It is thought to lead to aberrant apoptosis of keratinocytes and the release of proinflammatory compounds, including cytokines, chemokines, and autoantigens.[11]

Smoking has also been implicated in DLE and has been found to be associated with higher disease severity, lower quality of life, and worse response to treatment, particularly to antimalarials.[12-14] Although smoking is also linked to SLE, it is thought to be more strongly associated with DLE. Its role in the pathogenesis of DLE is likely because of its ability to generate free radicals, inflammatory cytokines, and apoptosis.[14]

Given the observation that DLE has a female predominance, sex hormones are thought to play a key role in its pathogenesis as well. Other etiologic factors that have been implicated in the pathogenesis of DLE include medications, chemicals, stress, and infections; however, more studies need to be performed to substantiate these claims.[5]

The IFN system is thought to play a critical role in the pathogenesis of DLE. Braunstein et al. demonstrated that the level of IFN gene expression correlates with cutaneous disease activity in DLE patients.[15] IFN-α acts to increase production of chemokines and chemokine receptors, which in turn act to stimulate migration of immune cells to DLE lesions. IFN-α has also been implicated in local keratinocyte cytotoxicity, further propagating the development of DLE lesions.[4]

DLE patients have been shown to have increased TNF-α production by peripheral blood monocytes, which may explain why a greater number of inflammatory cells are seen in DLE lesions as compared with other forms of CLE.[16] That said, the ineffectiveness TNF-α inhibitors have in the management of DLE lesions has called into question the role this cytokine plays in its pathogenesis. Other chemokines and cytokines that have been implicated in the pathogenesis of DLE include B-lymphocyte stimulator (BLyS/BAFF), IL-6, IL-10, IL-17, CXCl9, CXCL10, and CSCL11.[4]

Inflammatory cells involved in the pathogenesis of DLE include those of the innate immune system, particularly dendritic cells, and those of the adaptive immune system, including T cells and B cells. Although DLE is considered an autoimmune disease, antibodies commonly associated with SLE do not have as clear of an association in DLE, including antinuclear antibodies (ANAs), anti-dsDNA, anti-SSA/Ro, anti-SSB/La, and anti-Smith. A study of 115 patients with DLE found an observed prevalence of ANA (47.3%), anti-Ro (25.6%), and anti-ds-DNA (16.3%).[17] Kretz et al. found a significantly higher level of anti-annexin-1 antibodies in patients with DLE, suggesting it may be a promising candidate to be used as a diagnostic tool for DLE. Annexin-1 is externalized during apoptosis and has been shown to have antiinflammatory properties.[18] Kim et al. demonstrated that anti-RNP immunoglobulin G (IgG) correlated with disease activity in DLE patients; however, it was unclear if these antibodies contributed to skin disease or were byproducts of inflammation.[19]

Recently, O'Brien et al. demonstrated that the inflammatory infiltrate found in DLE lesions changes as they progress. CD8+ T cells were found to be more prominent in early lesions, whereas CD20+ B cells were

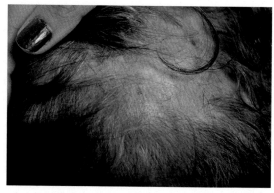

FIG. 13.1 Early lesion of discoid lupus erythematosus on the scalp. Note follicular plugging (centrally), faint erythema, and hair loss.

a greater component of end-stage lesions that lacked clinically apparent inflammation and demonstrated scarring alopecia. This is consistent with the understanding that B cells produce cytokines and autoantibodies, leading to increased collagen production, fibroblast proliferation, and ultimately fibrosis of the skin.[20]

In conclusion, the pathogenesis of DLE involves a complex picture of provocation, upregulation of the immune system, inflammation, and cell death. A better understanding of the specific etiologic factors involved in DLE will lead to more targeted and improved management options.

CLINICAL FINDINGS

DLE is characterized by erythematous plaques with scale. The typical skin finding of DLE is a well-defined erythematous patch with adherent follicular hyperkeratosis (Fig. 13.1), which, if removed, shows hyperkeratotic spikes known as the "carpet tack" sign.[21] The lesions then expand and result in hypopigmented, atrophic scars (Fig. 13.2). The lesions most commonly occur on UV exposed skin, including the scalp. In fact, more than half of the patients with DLE first present with scalp involvement, so this should be on the differential diagnosis for patients who present with scarring alopecia.[22] Advanced lesions can present as smooth, centrally hypopigmented or depigmented atrophic scars with complete or partial loss of follicular ostia (Fig. 13.3). The lesions of DLE on the scalp may resemble LPP or pseudopelade of Brocq (Fig. 13.4). Differentiating between LPP and DLE clinically can be difficult; lack of follicular plugging combined with perifollicular erythema and scale favors LPP over DLE.

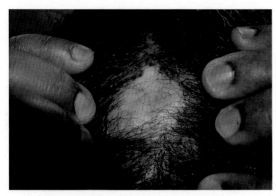

FIG. 13.2 Late lesion of discoid lupus erythematosus on the scalp showing erythema and scarring alopecia.

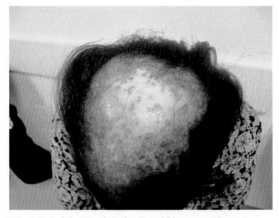

FIG. 13.3 Advanced scalp discoid lupus erythematosus resulting in scarring alopecia and central depigmentation.

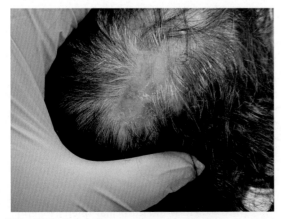

FIG. 13.4 Discoid lupus erythematosus lesions on scalp resembling lichen planopilaris or pseudopelade of Brocq.

Central depigmentation can be present in both LPP and DLE.[23] Rarely, untreated lesions of DLE may progress to squamous cell carcinoma or, less commonly, keratoacanthoma, basal cell carcinoma, malignant fibrous histiocytoma, or atypical fibroxanthoma.[24] There is an uncommon, disseminated form of discoid lupus that involves nonphotoexposed areas, such as the trunk, that has a higher likelihood than local DLE of progressing to SLE.

Lupus panniculitis can be associated with SLE or with discoid lesions and presents with indurated, painful nodules and plaques that eventually progress to lipoatrophy. These lesions are usually located on the proximal extremities and trunk.[25] When lupus panniculitis occurs on the scalp, patients can present with plaques of alopecia that may be erythematous, indurated, and painful. The overlying skin may be normal, erythematous, or clinically similar to discoid lupus, and lesions can be misdiagnosed as alopecia areata.[26] Uncommonly, lupus profundus can present with ulcerations that may be clinically consistent with squamous cell carcinoma of the scalp.[25] The diagnosis of lupus profundus of the scalp requires high clinical suspicion to correlate clinical, histopathologic, and serologic findings. The differential diagnosis includes traumatic and factitial panniculitis along with subcutaneous panniculitis-like T cell lymphoma.[25]

DERMATOSCOPIC FINDINGS

Characteristic trichoscopy findings of DLE include loss of follicular orifices, follicular keratotic plugs, variable scaling, scattered dark-brown discoloration, bluish-gray bluntly demarcated areas, large yellow dots, and thick arborizing vessels (Fig. 13.5).[27,28]

Active DLE lesions are more likely to have dark-brown discoloration (46.6% of cases) and large yellow dots (93.3% of cases). The dark-brown discoloration likely corresponds to the histopathologic feature of pigment incontinence and epidermal atrophy. The large yellow dots in DLE differ from the yellow dots seen in alopecia areata and androgenetic alopecia because they have a greater diameter (roughly three times as large) and are often darker in color.[28] Follicular orifices are preserved in active DLE lesions as they have not yet led to scarring. Conversely, inactive, burnt out DLE lesions are more likely to have loss of follicular orifices, porcelain-white to milky-red areas and yellow dots with radial, thin arborizing vessels.[28]

A hallmark sign of almost all patients with active or inactive DLE is thick arborizing vessels, similar to those seen in basal cell carcinoma. This can be a

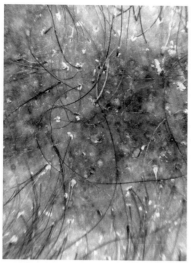

FIG. 13.5 Scalp trichoscopy of active discoid lupus erythematosus revealing follicular plugging and *brown* and *blue-gray* hyperpigmentation.

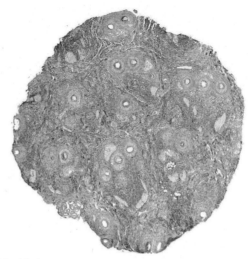

FIG. 13.6 Histopathology of discoid lupus erythematosus. Scanning magnification showing marked perifollicular and interfollicular inflammation (hematoxylin and eosin, 4×).

distinguishing trichoscopic feature when compared with other causes of alopecia, as they are very rarely seen in any other cause of cicatricial or noncicatricial alopecia other than a small proportion of patients with LPP.[28]

The presence of follicular red dots has been reported to be a feature of active DLE by Tosti et al., who observed it in 5 of 13 patients.[27] However, Rakowska et al. reported this finding in only 1 of 20 patients.[28] When present, it is thought that this may be a good prognostic feature, indicating a high probability of hair regrowth.

HISTOPATHOLOGIC FINDINGS

The changes on the biopsy of a lesion of DLE depend on the duration of the lesion and where the lesion specimen was taken from. The active border will have more inflammation (Fig. 13.6), and the atrophic center more fibrosis and scarring. In general, biopsies reveal interface dermatitis, with vacuolar alteration of the basal cell layer and follicular epithelium (Fig. 13.7). There is epidermal atrophy, variable hyperkeratosis with follicular plugging, and a dense superficial and deep perivascular and periadnexal lymphocytic infiltrate with admixed plasma cells.[29] Interstitial mucin is common (Fig. 13.8). Sebaceous glands are decreased. Over time the basement membrane zone thickens, which can be readily visualized by periodic acid–Schiff staining (Fig. 13.9), and eventually hair follicles are destroyed.

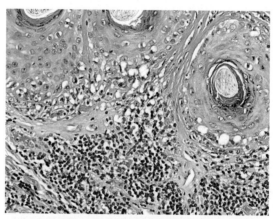

FIG. 13.7 Histopathology of discoid lupus erythematosus. Vacuolar alteration of follicular epithelium and a dense lymphocytic infiltrate are present (hematoxylin and eosin, 20×).

When DLE affects the scalp, a biopsy is often done to distinguish the resultant hair loss from other types of inflammatory alopecia. Histopathologic changes of DLE of the scalp are similar to those of DLE elsewhere, although, in addition, the typical epidermal changes of interface dermatitis and thickening of the basement membrane zone can also be seen along the follicular infundibulum. Sometimes LPP can resemble CCLE both clinically and histologically; in cases of LPP where there is interfollicular interface dermatitis, the presence of deep perivascular lymphocytic inflammation (Fig. 13.10) in addition to perifollicular

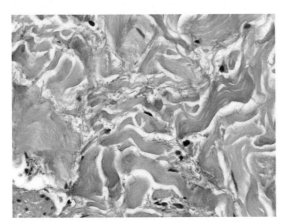

FIG. 13.8 Histopathology of discoid lupus erythematosus. Increased interstitial mucin is readily appreciated (hematoxylin and eosin, 40×).

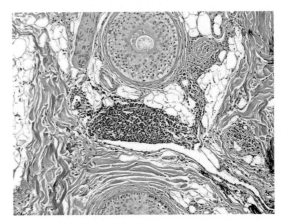

FIG. 13.10 Histopathology of discoid lupus erythematosus. Dense perivascular inflammation at the junction of the dermis and subcutis (hematoxylin and eosin, 20×).

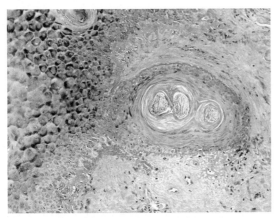

FIG. 13.9 Histopathology of discoid lupus erythematosus. Periodic acid–Schiff stain reveals a thickened basement membrane in both the epidermis and follicular infundibulum (hematoxylin and eosin, 20×).

inflammation and interstitial, rather than perifollicular, deposition of mucin can be helpful to distinguish CCLE.[23]

Cutaneous lupus can primarily affect the panniculus, where it causes a lobular lymphocytic panniculitis, often with increased mucin deposition. The overlying epidermis and dermis can be spared, although in up to half of cases there are overlying changes of DLE.[30] The inflammation can spill into the septae, and sometimes plasma cells, lymphoid follicles, and lymphocytic vasculitis can be seen. Hyalinization around blood vessels and in the fat is a helpful finding when present. The main differential diagnosis is subcutaneous panniculitis-like T-cell lymphoma.

Direct immunofluorescence (DIF) can be used as an adjunctive measure to routine microscopy in the diagnosis of DLE. In a recent review of 75 patients with DLE, DIF was positive in 68% of cases, with IgG at the dermoepidermal junction being the most common immunoreactant, followed by IgM and IgA. Combinations of two or more reactants were common. When added to the light microscopic findings, a conclusive diagnosis could be made in 85% of cases versus 60% with histopathology alone.[31]

A small percentage (2%) of DLE lesions will exhibit hyperplasia rather than atrophy.[32] Lesions of hypertrophic DLE can exhibit papillomatosis or a crateriform architecture mimicking squamous cell carcinoma and keratoacanthoma and can have a lichenoid infiltrate simulating lichen planus. Several studies have demonstrated the utility of immunoperoxidase staining for CD123, the interleukin-3 receptor α chain expressed on plasmacytoid dendritic cells, in the diagnosis of hypertrophic LE.[33,34] A heavy band of CD123 positive cells was found at the dermoepidermal junction in cases of hypertrophic DLE, as opposed to individual or small clusters of positive cells in squamous cell carcinoma and actinic keratosis.[33] The presence of CD123 positive cells was found to increase the accuracy of the diagnosis of hypertrophic DLE[34] and has been used to distinguish DLE from other lymphocytic scarring alopecias.[35]

PATIENT MANAGEMENT

There have been many formal studies evaluating various agents in the treatment of SLE; however, there have only been two randomized, placebo-controlled trials evaluating outcomes in CLE specifically.[36] As a result, the majority of topical and systemic treatments are off-label.

Research has shown that the skin lesions of CLE can be induced by exposure to UVA and UVB radiation.[37] As a result, photoprotection is the most important component of preventive management for patients with CLE. Patients should be advised to avoid tanning salons and sunbathing to avoid exacerbating existing lesions and inducing the formation of new lesions. In addition, patients should be advised to avoid traveling to sunny regions and may want to avoid careers that involve extensive time outdoors. Because glass windows are permeable to UVA, and some indoor lights and copying machines also emit UVA radiation, very photosensitive patients should adjust their lifestyles accordingly. Patients should be advised to apply sunscreen with at least a sun protection factor of 50 at least half an hour prior to sun exposure and to reapply frequently. The sunscreens that have been found to be the most effective in patients with CLE contain titanium oxide, a physical blocker, or are formulated with octocrylene as the UVB protectant and mexoryl SX, mexoryl XL, and parsol 1789 as the UVA protectants.[36] Patients should be advised to take a dietary supplement of 400 IU of vitamin D3 (cholecalciferol) daily while avoiding the sun and wearing sunscreens.

First-Line Therapy
Topical/intralesional steroids and calcineurin inhibitors

Although topical corticosteroids are usually the first-line agent for treatment of CLE, there has been only one randomized controlled trial studying topical steroids in CLE. This study compared application of fluocinonide 0.05% cream with 1% hydrocortisone cream and found that application of high-potency corticosteroids was more effective than low-potency corticosteroids.[38] Most clinicians recommend intermittent treatment with corticosteroids to avoid side effects, such as atrophy and telangiectasia. Application of topical steroids under occlusion can increase efficacy. Intralesional injection of corticosteroids into the dermis every 4–6 weeks has also been shown to be effective in the treatment of CLE.[36]

The topical calcineurin inhibitors tacrolimus and pimecrolimus have also been shown to be effective in the treatment of cutaneous lupus lesions. Application of calcineurin inhibitors once daily for

4–8 weeks resulted in improvement of erythematous plaques of CLE without atrophic side effects.[39] However, these agents are only approved for the treatment of atopic dermatitis in children and adults. Using topical retinoids and topical imiquimod to treat CLE has been described in case reports but has not been shown to be effective.[36] Similarly, there have been case reports of treatment of DLE lesions with laser and cryotherapy, but this approach should be used with extreme caution as DLE lesions are known to koebnerize, and physical treatments may actually worsen DLE plaques.[36]

Antimalarials

Systemic therapy is warranted when DLE lesions are not responsive to topical therapy. Although antimalarials are the first-line systemic agents, there was only one randomized controlled trial comparing hydroxychloroquine (400 mg/day) with acitretin (50 mg/day). This study found that about 50% of patients in both treatment arms experienced improvement; however, the incidence of side effects was higher among the patients taking acitretin.[40] High-quality evidence regarding the efficacy of antimalarials in the treatment of DLE lesions on the scalp is lacking. In general, 50%–90% of individuals with DLE who are treated with a systemic antimalarial agent (usually either chloroquine or hydroxychloroquine) exhibit some clinical improvement. The risk of ophthalmologic toxicity can be reduced by limiting dosing to maximum daily dosing based on ideal body weight (adults: hydroxychloroquine: 6.0–6.5 mg/kg ideal body weight per day; chloroquine: 3.5–4.0 mg/kg ideal body weight per day).[36] As mentioned earlier, smoking is associated with the pathogenesis of DLE, and patients should be strongly encouraged to quit smoking. In addition, they should be counseled that nicotine is known to interfere with the mechanism of action of antimalarial medications and has been shown to reduce the likelihood that their symptoms will improve while taking antimalarial treatments.[41]

Second-Line Therapy

No therapies have been specifically indicated for the treatment of CCLE, and second-line therapies are generally agents that are used in other rheumatologic conditions. Small studies have shown that 7.5–25 mg of methotrexate weekly in either oral or subcutaneous formulations can improve CCLE.[42,43] As mentioned earlier, the oral retinoids acitretin and isotretinoin dosed from 0.2 to 1.0 mg/kg body weight have been shown to be effective in treating CCLE in 50%–86% of patients, although these studies also had limited numbers of participants.[40,44] Dapsone, mycophenolate, thalidomide, clofazimine, azathioprine, cyclophosphamide, and cyclosporine have been described in small studies or case reports to be effective for the treatment of CCLE in refractory cases.[45] Kuhn et al. have developed a helpful treatment algorithm for CCLE.[45]

Biologic agents

A tool called the Cutaneous Lupus Area and Severity Index (CLASI) is used to assess clinical response to treatment in clinical studies of CLE and is also used to measure cutaneous response to treatment in studies of biologic agents for SLE.[46] Two anti-IFN-α monoclonal antibodies, sifalimumab and anifrolumab, have resulted in significant reduction in CLE activity using the CLASI tool.[46] The anti-IL-12/IL-23 monoclonal antibody ustekinumab is currently only approved for the treatment of psoriatic arthritis and moderate-to-severe plaque psoriasis, but case reports have shown efficacy in treating CLE.[46] There are mixed results regarding the efficacy of intravenous IG (IVIG) in the treatment of CLE, with some reports showing worsening of disease and others showing improvement. There have not been any randomized controlled trials evaluating the efficacy of IVIG for CLE. Overall, for patients with treatment-resistant CLE, no biologic agents have been approved.

CONCLUSION

Although CCLE is an uncommon cause of scarring alopecia, it is important to understand the clinical, trichoscopic and histopathologic features that differentiate it from other causes of scarring alopecia because effective treatments are available and untreated lesions can rarely progress to malignancy.

REFERENCES

1. Biazar C, Sigges J, Patsinakidis N, et al. Cutaneous lupus erythematosus: first multicenter database analysis of 1002 patients from the European Society of Cutaneous Lupus Erythematosus (EUSCLE). *Autoimmun Rev.* 2013;12(3): 444–454. https://doi.org/10.1016/j.autrev.2012.08.019.
2. Jarrett P, Thornley S, Scragg R. Ethnic differences in the epidemiology of cutaneous lupus erythematosus in New Zealand. *Lupus.* 2016;25(13):1497–1502. https://doi.org/10.1177/0961203316651745.
3. AlKharafi NNAH, Alsaeid K, AlSumait A, et al. Cutaneous lupus erythematosus in children: experience from a tertiary care pediatric Dermatology clinic. *Pediatr Dermatol.* 2016;33(2):200–208. https://doi.org/10.1111/pde.12788.
4. Kirchhof MG, Dutz JP. The immunopathology of cutaneous lupus erythematosus. *Rheum Dis Clin N Am.* 2014;40(3):455–474. https://doi.org/10.1016/j.rdc.2014.04.006.
5. Grönhagen CM, Nyberg F. Cutaneous lupus erythematosus: an update. *Indian Dermatol Online J.* 2014;5(1):7–13. https://doi.org/10.4103/2229-5178.126020.
6. Privette ED, Werth VP. Update on pathogenesis and treatment of CLE. *Curr Opin Rheumatol.* 2013;25(5):584–590. https://doi.org/10.1097/BOR.0b013e32836437ba.
7. Chong BF, Song J, Olsen NJ. Determining risk factors for developing systemic lupus erythematosus in patients with discoid lupus erythematosus. *Br J Dermatol.* 2012;166:29–35. https://doi.org/10.1111/j.1365-2133.2011.10610.x.
8. Sullivan KE. Genetics of systemic lupus erythematosus. Clinical implications. *Rheum Clin North Am.* 2000; 26(2):229–256, v–vi.
9. Dey-Rao R, Smith JR, Chow S, Sinha AA. Differential gene expression analysis in CCLE lesions provides new insights regarding the genetics basis of skin vs. Systemic disease. *Genomics.* 2014;104(2):144–155. https://doi.org/10.1016/j.ygeno.2014.06.003.
10. Järvinen TM, Hellquist A, Koskenmies S, et al. Tyrosine kinase 2 and interferon regulatory factor 5 polymorphisms are associated with discoid and subacute cutaneous lupus erythematosus. *Exp Dermatol.* 2010;19(2):123–131. https://doi.org/10.1111/j.1600-0625.2009.00982.x.
11. Kuhn A, Wenzel J, Weyd H. Photosensitivity, apoptosis, and cytokines in the pathogenesis of lupus erythematosus: a critical review. *Clin Rev Allergy Immunol.* 2014;47(2):148–162. https://doi.org/10.1007/s12016-013-8403-x.
12. Miot HA, Bartoli Miot LD, Haddad GR. Association between discoid lupus erythematosus and cigarette smoking. *Dermatol Basel Switz.* 2005;211(2):118–122. https://doi.org/10.1159/000086440.
13. Boeckler P, Cosnes A, Francès C, Hedelin G, Lipsker D. Association of cigarette smoking but not alcohol consumption with cutaneous lupus erythematosus. *Arch Dermatol.* 2009; 145(9):1012–1016. https://doi.org/10.1001/archdermatol.2009.199.
14. Piette EW, Foering KP, Chang AY, et al. Impact of smoking in cutaneous lupus erythematosus. *Arch Dermatol.* 2012;1 48(3):317–322. https://doi.org/10.1001/archdermatol.2011.342.
15. Braunstein I, Klein R, Okawa J, Werth VP. The interferon-regulated gene signature is elevated in subacute cutaneous lupus erythematosus and discoid lupus erythematosus and correlates with the cutaneous lupus area and severity index score. *Br J Dermatol.* 2012;166(5):971–975. https://doi.org/10.1111/j.1365-2133.2012.10825.x.

16. Nabatian AS, Bashir MM, Wysocka M, Sharma M, Werth VP. Tumor necrosis factor α release in peripheral blood mononuclear cells of cutaneous lupus and dermatomyositis patients. *Arthritis Res Ther.* 2012;14(1):R1. https://doi.org/10.1186/ar3549.

17. Patsinakidis N, Gambichler T, Lahner N, Moellenhoff K, Kreuter A. Cutaneous characteristics and association with antinuclear antibodies in 402 patients with different subtypes of lupus erythematosus. *J Eur Acad Dermatol Venereol.* 2016;30(12):2097-2104. https://doi.org/10.1111/jdv.13769.

18. Kretz CC, Norpo M, Abeler-Dörner L, et al. Anti-annexin 1 antibodies: a new diagnostic marker in the serum of patients with discoid lupus erythematosus. *Exp Dermatol.* 2010;19(10):919-921. https://doi.org/10.1111/j.1600-0625.2010.01145.x.

19. Kim A, O'Brien J, Tseng L, Zhang S, Chong B. Autoantibodies and disease activity in patients with discoid lupus erythematosus. *JAMA Dermatol.* 2014;150(6):651-654.

20. O'Brien JC, Hosler GA, Chong BF. Changes in T cell and B cell composition in discoid lupus erythematosus skin at different stages. *J Dermatol Sci.* 2017;85(3):247-249. https://doi.org/10.1016/j.jdermsci.2016.12.004.

21. Kuhn A, Landmann A. The classification and diagnosis of cutaneous lupus erythematosus. *J Autoimmun.* 2014;48-49:14-19. https://doi.org/10.1016/j.jaut.2014.01.021.

22. Milam EC, Ramachandran S, Franks AG. Treatment of scarring alopecia in discoid variant of chronic cutaneous lupus erythematosus with tacrolimus lotion, 0.3. *JAMA Dermatol.* 2015;151(10):1113-1116. https://doi.org/10.1001/jamadermatol.2015.1349.

23. Nambudiri VE, Vleugels RA, Laga AC, Goldberg LJ. Clinicopathologic lessons in distinguishing cicatricial alopecia: 7 cases of lichen planopilaris misdiagnosed as discoid lupus. *J Am Acad Dermatol.* 2014;71(4):e135-e138. https://doi.org/10.1016/j.jaad.2014.04.052.

24. Sherman RN, Lee CW, Flynn KJ. Cutaneous squamous cell carcinoma in black patients with chronic discoid lupus erythematosus. *Int J Dermatol.* 1993;32(9):677-679.

25. Mesinkovska NA, Galiczynski EM, Billings SD, Khera P. Nonhealing ulcers on the scalp. Diagnosis: lupus erythematosus panniculitis (LEP). *Arch Dermatol.* 2011;147(12):1443, 1448. https://doi.org/10.1001/archderm.147.12.1443-d.

26. Mitxelena J, Martínez-Peñuela A, Cordoba A, Yanguas I. Linear and annular lupus panniculitis of the scalp. *Actas Dermosifiliogr.* 2013;104(10):936-939. https://doi.org/10.1016/j.ad.2012.12.014.

27. Tosti A, Torres F, Misciali C, et al. Follicular red dots. *Arch Dermatol.* 2009;145(12):1406-1409. https://doi.org/10.1001/archdermatol.2009.277.

28. Rakowska A, Slowinska M, Kowalska-Oledzka E, et al. Trichoscopy of cicatricial alopecia. *J Drugs Dermatol.* 2012;11(6):753-758.

29. Bolduc C, Sperling LC, Shapiro J. Primary cicatricial alopecia: lymphocytic primary cicatricial alopecias, including chronic cutaneous lupus erythematosus, lichen planopilaris, frontal fibrosing alopecia, and Graham-Little syndrome. *J Am Acad Dermatol.* 2016;75(6):1081-1099. https://doi.org/10.1016/j.jaad.2014.09.058.

30. Patterson J. *Weedon's Skin Pathology.* 4th ed. Elsevier; 2015.

31. Bharti S, Dogra S, Saikia B, Walker RM, Chhabra S, Saikia UN. Immunofluorescence profile of discoid lupus erythematosus. *Indian J Pathol Microbiol.* 2015;58(4):479-482. https://doi.org/10.4103/0377-4929.168850.

32. Arps DP, Patel RM. Cutaneous hypertrophic lupus erythematosus: a challenging histopathologic diagnosis in the absence of clinical information. *Arch Pathol Lab Med.* 2013;137(9):1205-1210. https://doi.org/10.5858/arpa.2013-0241-CR.

33. Ko CJ, Srivastava B, Braverman I, Antaya RJ, McNiff JM. Hypertrophic lupus erythematosus: the diagnostic utility of CD123 staining. *J Cutan Pathol.* 2011;38(11):889-892. https://doi.org/10.1111/j.1600-0560.2011.01779.x.

34. Walsh NM, Lai J, Hanly JG, et al. Plasmacytoid dendritic cells in hypertrophic discoid lupus erythematosus: an objective evaluation of their diagnostic value. *J Cutan Pathol.* 2015;42(1):32-38. https://doi.org/10.1111/cup.12416.

35. Fening K, Parekh V, McKay K. CD123 immunohistochemistry for plasmacytoid dendritic cells is useful in the diagnosis of scarring alopecia. *J Cutan Pathol.* 2016;43(8):643-648. https://doi.org/10.1111/cup.12725.

36. Kuhn A, Ruland V, Bonsmann G. Cutaneous lupus erythematosus: update of therapeutic options part I. *J Am Acad Dermatol.* 2011;65(6):e179-e193. https://doi.org/10.1016/j.jaad.2010.06.018.

37. Kuhn A, Sonntag M, Richter-Hintz D, et al. Phototesting in lupus erythematosus: a 15-year experience. *J Am Acad Dermatol.* 2001;45(1):86-95. https://doi.org/10.1067/mjd.2001.114589.

38. Roenigk HH, Martin JS, Eichorn P, Gilliam JN. Discoid lupus erythematosus. Diagnostic features and evaluation of topical corticosteroid therapy. *Cutis.* 1980;25(3):281-285.

39. Sugano M, Shintani Y, Kobayashi K, Sakakibara N, Isomura I, Morita A. Successful treatment with topical tacrolimus in four cases of discoid lupus erythematosus. *J Dermatol.* 2006;33(12):887-891. https://doi.org/10.1111/j.1346-8138.2006.00203.x.

40. Ruzicka T, Sommerburg C, Goerz G, Kind P, Mensing H. Treatment of cutaneous lupus erythematosus with acitretin and hydroxychloroquine. *Br J Dermatol.* 1992;127(5):513-518.

41. Jewell ML, McCauliffe DP. Patients with cutaneous lupus erythematosus who smoke are less responsive to antimalarial treatment. *J Am Acad Dermatol.* 2000;42(6):983-987.

42. Huber A, Tüting T, Bauer R, Bieber T, Wenzel J. Methotrexate treatment in cutaneous lupus erythematosus: subcutaneous application is as effective as intravenous administration. *Br J Dermatol.* 2006;155(4):861-862. https://doi.org/10.1111/j.1365-2133.2006.07431.x.

43. Bottomley WW, Goodfield MJ. Methotrexate for the treatment of discoid lupus erythematosus. *Br J Dermatol.* 1995;133(4):655–656.

44. Shornick JK, Formica N, Parke AL. Isotretinoin for refractory lupus erythematosus. *J Am Acad Dermatol.* 1991;24(1):49–52.

45. Kuhn A, Ruland V, Bonsmann G. Cutaneous lupus erythematosus: update of therapeutic options part II. *J Am Acad Dermatol.* 2011;65(6):e195–e213. https://doi.org/10.1016/j.jaad.2010.06.017.

46. Presto JK, Hejazi EZ, Werth VP. Biological therapies in the treatment of cutaneous lupus erythematosus. *Lupus.* 2016. https://doi.org/10.1177/0961203316670731.

CHAPTER 14

Folliculitis Decalvans

LAURA MIGUEL-GÓMEZ, MD, PHD • DAVID SACEDA-CORRALO, MD, PHD •
RITA RODRIGUES-BARATA, MD • SERGIO VAÑÓ-GALVÁN, MD, PHD

HISTORY AND DEFINITION

History

Folliculitis decalvans (FD) was first described by Quinquaid in 1888; he named this disease as "folliculite épilante,"[1] but Brocq and colleagues, 13 years later, described this disease as "folliculitis decalvans" and determined its cicatricial character, derived from a chronic inflammatory process that causes definitive destruction of hair follicles, distinguishing it from other types of alopecia.[2] In 1971, Smith and Sanderson[3] used the name "tufted folliculitis" to refer to a clinical peculiarity that is not specific, because it can appear in other types of alopecia, but it is very characteristic of this disease, which occurs when several follicles emerge from the same orifice or follicular ostium.

Definition

FD is a rare variant of primary cicatricial alopecia that causes a painful inflammation around the hair follicles with an irreversible follicular destruction. Predominantly, it affects young and middle-aged adults.[4] Clinically, inflammatory cutaneous lesions and alopecic patches occur over the vertex and occipital area of the scalp.[5] Etiopathogenesis of this disease is not yet well known; however, the presence of *Staphylococcus aureus* in most cases and the abnormal alteration of the patient's local immune response have been suggested as possible triggers.[6] Histopathology is considered the gold standard for diagnosis of FD, and the objective of treatment is to avoid the progression of this disease.

EPIDEMIOLOGY

There are no adequate epidemiologic studies for this disease. FD represents approximately 9%–11% of all cases of primary cicatricial alopecia.[7] It appears in middle-aged adults around the age of 35 years and affects both sexes equally. In several studies, certain predominance has been found in males.[4,5,7] A curious fact is the predominance of females in patients over 50 years of age who suffer from this disease.[5,8] There is no clear association established with a particular race.

ETIOPATHOGENESIS

Etiopathogenesis of FD is unclear; the most supported hypothesis is that in genetically predisposed individuals,[5,9–12] *S. aureus* infection and liberation of cytotoxic substances (superantigens) in the hair follicles induce an intense migration of neutrophils toward epidermis and perifollicular dermis, recruited by mechanisms of innate immunity. Neutrophils damage the follicular epithelium and penetrate the follicle where phagocytosis of *S. aureus* triggers a process of chronic inflammation, which evolves into a fibrous and atrophic stage and eventually cicatricial, with a complete destruction of the pilosebaceous unit.[13] Nasal carriage of *S. aureus* can also have an important role in the chronicity of FD.[4]

CLINICAL PRESENTATION: SIGNS AND SYMPTOMS

The vertex and the occipital area of the scalp are most commonalty affected, but other involved locations have been described, such as the facial area, including beard and eyebrows, and nape. This affectation outside the scalp is exceptional.[5,14] In early stages (Fig. 14.1), several clinical and trichoscopic signs can be observed:

- follicular pustules and papules
- erythema
- perifollicular hyperkeratosis
- "tufted hairs": several follicles (6–20) emerge from the same orifice or follicular ostium. They are very characteristic of this disease
- yellowish scales and crusts

In the late stages of FD, irreversible destruction of hair follicles occurs and irregular, atrophic, flesh-colored patches of scarring alopecia appear where the inflammatory process was originated. Most cases are usually limited to a specific area; however, sometimes the coalescence of the lesions can cause extensive scarring areas leading to a great aesthetic problem (Fig. 14.2).

Localized pruritus, trichodynia, and burning sensation are the most common symptoms, and they are often associated with the degree of local inflammation

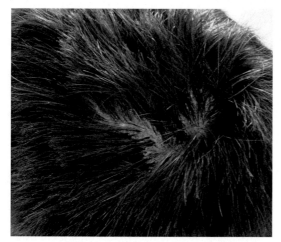

FIG. 14.1 A 33-year-old male diagnosed with folliculitis decalvans 5 years ago. Alopecic patch with perifollicular hyperkeratosis, tufted hairs, yellowish crusts, and scales.

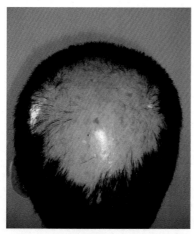

FIG. 14.2 A 40-year-old man diagnosed with folliculitis decalvans 16 years ago presents an extensive cicatricial alopecic patch. This case is an example of a late and severe stage of disease.

intensity. However, there is not always a direct relationship between inflammatory intensity and clinical manifestations; thus, some patients may remain asymptomatic, whereas others, with the same form of the disease, have very evident symptoms.

TRICHOSCOPY

A noninvasive tool that can be used in the differential diagnosis of cicatricial alopecia is trichoscopy (Fig. 14.3).

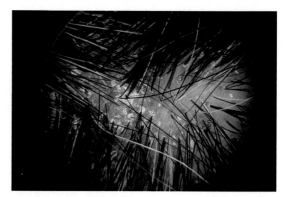

FIG. 14.3 Trichoscopy shows tufted hairs, crusts, and perifollicular hyperkeratosis over a scarring alopecic patch during an outbreak of disease.

The characteristic sign of this disease that can be observed through the trichoscopy is the polytrichia or "tufted hairs." Other additional trichoscopic findings include diffuse erythema, hyperkeratosis and perifollicular fibrotic linear bands, yellowish scales, crusts, and follicular pustules. In late stages, red-milky and ivory-colored areas appear, with absence of follicular orifices. White or yellow dots are rare, present in less than 20% of patients, and there is no characteristic vascular pattern.[15]

HISTOPATHOLOGY

In early stage, several histopathologic findings, such as an infundibular acneiform dilation accompanied by an intra- and perifollicular infiltrate, composed of neutrophilic granulocytes, are observed (Figs. 14.4 and 14.5). As it progresses, the infiltrate is mixed, composed of neutrophils, lymphocytes, plasma cells, and foreign body–type multinucleated giant cells, extending to the adventitial dermis. In later stage, periadnexal dermal fibrosis predominates.[16]

DIAGNOSIS

Clinical History

A complete clinical history should be made, including age, race, gender, drugs taken by the patient,[17] history of dermatologic or autoimmune diseases, history of recurrent infections or signs of immunodeficiency,[9,18] family history of FD,[12] the time-to-onset, the progression of the initial clinical presentation, and associated symptoms.

Dermatologic Examination

In addition to the clinical and trichoscopical signs that can be seen in FD, we must make a complete physical

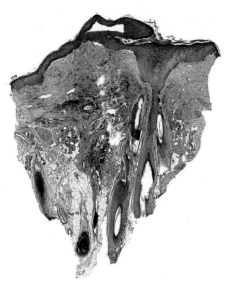

FIG. 14.4 Histology: several follicles emerging from a single follicular orifice (hematoxylin-eosin, original magnification ×20). (Courtesy of Dr. Rosario Carrillo.)

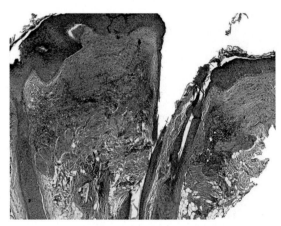

FIG. 14.5 Histology: Chronic inflammatory infiltrate and perifollicular scar reaction (hematoxylin-eosin, original magnification ×40). (Courtesy of Dr. Rosario Carrillo.)

examination and look for signs that might point to other diseases, such as lichen planopilaris (e.g., trachyonychia, involvement of oral mucosae, purple and pruritic papules on wrists of the hands), fungal infection (e.g., onychomycosis, erythematous plaques with pustules on the trunk or extremities), or discoid lupus erythematosus (atrophic plaques in ear lobes and face).

Photography
Digital photographs (photo dermoscopy and global photography) as well as measures of the alopecic patch are very useful to monitor progression of the disease.

Bacterial Cultures
A culture and antibiogram (antibiotic sensitivity test) of one of the pustules should be taken. *S. aureus* is isolated in many patients; this fact supports the hypothesis of its implication in the etiopathogenesis of FD.[19] In addition, a nasal culture is recommended to study the existence of nasal carrier of this microorganism.[20]

Skin Biopsy
Skin biopsy is the gold-standard test that confirms the clinical suspicion. It is very important to choose the right place to perform the biopsy; it must be taken of the edge of the patch where there is inflammatory activity.[20]

DIFFERENTIAL DIAGNOSIS
A clinical pattern similar to FD can be observed in other hair diseases, so knowing their differences to avoid a misdiagnosis or delayed diagnosis is very important.

- **Bacterial folliculitis:** scattered pustules are observed over the scalp and they do not cause any alopecic patches.
- **Tinea capitis:** follicular pustules can be present but "comma," "corkscrew," and dystrophic broken hairs are characteristic trichoscopic features of this disease, and KOH examination and fungal culture are helpful for the diagnosis.
- **Discoid lupus erythematosus, lichen planopilaris, central centrifugal cicatricial alopecia, and classic pseudopelade of Brocq:** all of them present scarring alopecic patches such as FD but lymphocytic infiltration is observed in histopathology. Inflammatory lesions such as pustules are rare.
- **Acne keloidalis nuchae:** typically it affects young black male patients. Firm papules with pustules over the occipital area and neck coalesce giving rise to hairless, keloid-like painful nodules and plaques, which can be very disfiguring.
- **Acne necrotica varioliformis:** it presents with follicular pustules and papules on the scalp (frontal hairline), face, and rarely upper trunk, with a tendency to central necrosis, hemorrhagic crusting, and formation of depressed scars.
- **Erosive pustular dermatosis of the scalp:** typically it affects elderly patients with a history of extensive sun exposure. Pustules, crusts, erosions, and residual cicatricial areas over the vertex or occipital

area are observed. Histology shows mixed inflammatory infiltrate.

- **Dissecting cellulitis of the scalp:** multiple and fluctuating painful nodules appear over the scalp that interconnect through sinus tracts and finally discharge purulent material. The inflammation is deep at the level of dermis and subcutaneous fat.

TREATMENTS

Patient's education is necessary to achieve a good therapeutic compliance. Explaining that therapy is not curative but is important to stop the progression of alopecia is a priority.

Local Treatment (in Mild Forms and in Combination With Oral Treatment in Moderate/Severe Forms)

- **Antistaphylococcal topical antibiotics** (mupirocin, fusidic acid) with or without topical corticosteroids (betamethasone dipropionate, fluticasone): 3 days a week.
- **Intralesional corticosteroids** (triamcinolone): every 3 months if there is no control with topical treatment.

Oral Treatment (Table 14.1)

- **Oral antibiotic** (with or without oral corticosteroids if there is a severe inflammation).
  1. **Tetracyclines** (minocycline, doxycycline): for 8 to 12 weeks. Generally, in combination with topical treatment.[21]
  2. **Rifampicin and clindamycin:** a 10-week course of rifampicin and clindamycin (both 300 mg twice daily) has been shown to induce remission.[5]
  3. **Others:** azithromycin, dapsone,[22] sulfamethoxazole-trimethoprim, oral fusidic acid.
- **Other oral treatments:** isotretinoin, biologic drugs,[23,24] human immunoglobulin.[25]
- **Other therapies:**
  1. **Photodynamic therapy:** improvement and stability of the disease have been obtained in certain cases, some of them in association with topical and/or oral treatment.[26]
  2. **Laser[27] and radiotherapy[28]:** in highly selected cases.
  3. **Restoration surgery:** in highly selected cases with no signs of disease activity for several years without any treatment.

TABLE 14.1
Summary of Oral Treatments Regimen Most Used in Folliculitis Decalvans

	Posology	Contraindications	Pregnancy and Breast Feeding	Patient Information
Doxycycline, Minocycline	100 mg/day for 2–3 months	Allergy to tetracyclines Porphyria	Contraindicated (dental discoloration, alterations in growth)	Two hours before and after taking the tetracyclines, no dairy products should be consumed.
Rifampicin + clindamycin	300 mg/12 h for 10 weeks	Rifampicin: Allergy to rifamycins Acute hepatitis Porphyria Clindamycin: meningitis	Contraindicated (neonatal hemorrhage, malformations)	Urine and other secretions orange-colored (tears)
Azithromycin	500 mg/3 times a week for 3 months	Allergy to macrolides	FDA category B	–
Isotretinoin	20 mg/day for 3–6 months	Severe dyslipidemia Liver failure Simultaneous treatment with tetracyclines	Contraindicated (severe malformations)	Avoid drinking alcohol Skin hydration Use contraceptive methods
Dapsone	50–100 mg/day for 3–6 months	G6PD deficiency Allergic to sulfones	Contraindicated	–
Corticosteroids	0.5–1 mg/kg/day during the first weeks of the outbreak	Severe systemic infections	Contraindicated, if necessary, use the lowest possible dose	Stretch marks Weight gain Hyperexcitability Osteoporosis

PROGNOSIS

FD is a chronic disease with continuous outbreaks that decrease as the evolution time advances; nonetheless, treatment should be started immediately to prevent the progression of the irreversible alopecic patch. Fortunately, there is no increase in mortality because of this disease, but there are aesthetic problems and local discomfort that may affect psychologic health of patient, sometimes being an important limitation in his social and work environment. There are new therapies available that can have good results if used in combination with existing therapies.[25]

REFERENCES

1. Quinquaud E. Folliculite épilante et destructive des régions velues. *Bull Mem Soc Med Paris.* 1888;5:395–398.
2. Brocq L, Leglet J, Ayrignaq J. Recherches sur l'alopécie atrophicante. *Ann Dermatol Syphil.* 1905;6:1–32.
3. Smith NP, Sanderson KV. Tufted folliculitis of the scalp. *J R Soc Med.* 1971;71:606–608.
4. Otberg N, Kang H, Alzolibani AA, Shapiro J. Folliculitis decalvans. *Dermatol Ther.* 2008;21:238–244.
5. Vano Galvan S, Molina Ruiz AM, Fernandez Crehuet P, et al. Folliculitis decalvans: a multicentre review of 82 patients. *J Eur Acad Dermatol Venereol.* 2015;29:1750–1757.
6. Ekmekci TR, Koslu A. Tufted hair folliculitis causing skullcap-pattern cicatricial alopecia. *J Eur Acad Dermatol Venereol.* 2006;20:227–229.
7. Tan E, Martinka M, Ball N, Shapiro J. Primary cicatricial alopecias: clinicopathology of 112 cases. *J Am Acad Dermatol.* 2004;50:25–32.
8. Bunagan MJ, Banka N, Shapiro J. Retrospective review of folliculitis decalvans in 23 patients with course and treatment analysis of long-standing cases. *J Cutan Med Surg.* 2014;18:1–5.
9. Shitara A, Igareshi R, Morohashi M. Folliculitis decalvans and cellular immunity-two brothers with oral candidosis. *Jpn J Dermatol.* 1974;28:133–140.
10. Vaughan Jones S, Black M. Cicatricial alopecia occurring in two sisters from Ghana. *Clin Exp Dermatol.* 1994;19:500–502.
11. Douwes KE, Landthaler M, Szeimies RM. Simultaneous occurrence of folliculitis decalvans capillitii in identical twins. *Br J Dermatol.* 2000;143:195–197.
12. Jaiswal AK, Vaishampayan S, Walia NS, Verma R. Folliculitis decalvans in a family. *Indian J Dermatol Venereol Leprol.* 2000;66:216–217.
13. Chiarini C, Torchia D, Bianchi B, Volpi W, Caproni M, Fabbri P. Immunopathogenesis of folliculitis decalvans: clues in early lesions. *Am J Clin Pathol.* 2008;130:526–534.
14. Karakuzu A, Erdem T, Aktas A, Atasoy M, Gulec AI. A case of folliculitis decalvans involving the beard, face and nape. *J Dermatol.* 2001;28:329–331.
15. Fernández-Crehuet P, Vañó-Galván S, Molina-Ruiz AM, et al. Trichoscopic features of folliculitis decalvans: results in 58 patients. *Int J Trichology.* 2017;9:140–141.
16. Ross EK, Tan E, Shapiro J. Update on primary cicatricial alopecias. *J Am Acad Dermatol.* 2005;53:1–37.
17. Hoekzema R, Drillenburg P. Folliculitis decalvans associated with erlotinib. *Clin Exp Dermatol.* 2010;35:916–918.
18. Frazer N, Grant P. Folliculitis decalvans with hypocomplementemia. *Br J Dermatol.* 1982;107:88.
19. Chandrawansa PH, Giam YC. Folliculitis decalvans–a retrospective study in a tertiary referred centre, over five years. *Singapore Med J.* 2003;44:84–87.
20. Olsen EA, Bergfeld WF, Cotsarelis G, et al. Summary of North American Hair Research Society (NAHRS)-sponsored workshop on cicatricial alopecia, Duke University Medical Center, February 10 and 11, 2001. *J Am Acad Dermatol.* 2003;48:103–110.
21. Sillani C, Bin Z, Ying Z, Zeming C, Jian Y, Xingqi Z. Effective treatment of folliculitis decalvans using selected antimicrobial agents. *Int J Trichol.* 2010;2:20–23.
22. Paquet P, Pierard GE. Dapsone treatment of folliculitis decalvans. *Ann Dermatol Venereol.* 2004;131:195–197.
23. Mihaljevic N, von den Driesch P. Successful use of infliximab in a patient with recalcitrant folliculitis decalvans. *J Dtsch Dermatol Ges.* 2012;10:589–590.
24. Kreutzer K, Effendy I. Therapy-resistant folliculitis decalvans and lichen planopilaris successfully treated with adalimumab. *J Dtsch Dermatol Ges.* 2014;12:74–76.
25. Ismail N, Ralph N, Murphy G. Intravenous human immunoglobulin for treatment of folliculitis decalvans. *J Dermatol Treat.* 2015;26:471–472.
26. Miguel-Gomez L, Vano-Galvan S, Perez-Garcia B, Carrillo-Gijon R, Jaen-Olasolo P. Treatment of folliculitis decalvans with photodynamic therapy: results in 10 patients. *J Am Acad Dermatol.* 2015;72:1085–1087.
27. Parlette EC, Kroeger N, Ross EV. Nd:YAG laser treatment of recalcitrant folliculitis decalvans. *Dermatol Surg.* 2004;30:1152–1154.
28. Elsayad K, Kriz J, Haverkamp U, et al. Treatment of folliculitis decalvans using intensity-modulated radiation via tomotherapy. *Strahlenther Onkol.* 2015.

CHAPTER 15

Dissecting Cellulitis of the Scalp

DAVID SACEDA-CORRALO, MD, PHD • LAURA MIGUEL-GÓMEZ, MD, PHD •
RITA RODRIGUES-BARATA, MD • SERGIO VAÑÓ-GALVÁN, MD, PHD

DEFINITION

Dissecting cellulitis of the scalp (DC) is a rare neutrophilic alopecia in which inflammatory nodules, abscesses, and painful plaques on the scalp progress chronically to permanent hair loss.[1] It predominantly occurs in African-American men. Involved areas are principally located on the vertex and the occiput.

EPIDEMIOLOGY

DC is an unfrequent scarring alopecia; it represents only 1.4%–4.5% of the cases.[2,3] It mostly occurs in 20- to 40-year-old African-American males,[4] but it also affects Caucasians and women rarely.[5,6] The onset of DC usually occurs after puberty, although it has been reported in children.[7]

ETIOLOGY

The etiology of DC remains unclear. Along with hidradenitis suppurativa (HS), pilonidal cyst, and acne conglobata, DC forms the follicular occlusion tetrad.[8] These diseases have a common etiopathogenic mechanism, in relation to follicular hyperkeratosis, follicular occlusion, secondary bacterial infection, and subsequent neutrophilic and granulomatous inflammatory response with follicular destruction.[9,10] New insights into the molecular basis of inflammation in DC, especially via interleukin 1, have been discovered.[11]

DC has been related to working with oily substances (mechanics, sweet-fried "churros" makers) that could act as a trigger of the disease in individuals who are predisposed to this condition and working in contact with exhaust fumes (bus drivers, gas-station sellers, mechanics) that may induce the activation of the DC as smoking in HS.[5]

Hormonal influence may also play a role in DC. The disorder is mainly localized on the vertex, and response to finasteride has been observed in some cases.[5,6] Furthermore, three cases of DC associated with the use of anabolic-androgenic steroids in gyms have been described.[5]

Despite the fact that the fluid of the abscesses in DC is usually sterile, some reports point to the role of the bacteria in the pathogenesis of the disease. The most common bacteria revealed in discharged pus are coagulase-negative staphylococci (*Staphylococcus epidermidis*, mainly, and *Propionibacterium acnes*), followed by *Staphylococcus aureus*.[5,12–14] Response to oral antibiotics supports this theory as well.[12]

The genetic base for DC has not been elucidated. Probably the disease does not depend on a specific gene defect; however, the male dominance, the young age of onset, and the occurrence in afro-Caribbean patients predominantly suggest a genetic risk factor.[11] There are some cases of familiar DC in the literature.[5,7]

CLINICAL FEATURES

DC shows clinically few to several firm or fluctuant subcutaneous nodules with a patch of alopecia on the skin surface. Often these nodules evolve to abscesses and sinus tracts. Abscesses contain hemorrhagic or purulent aseptic material, which may drain spontaneously or after puncture.[15]

The most common location is the vertex (49%–71%) and the occiput (47%) (Fig. 15.1),[5,6] but isolated temporal and parietal location has also been described.[5] Long-term cases have diffuse skin lesions over the entire scalp and may have cerebriform configuration.[6,15] Associated cervical lymphadenopathy is frequent when the condition is active.[15,16]

The symptoms commonly related to DC are pruritus and pain, although their prevalence is not well defined.[5,6]

TRICHOSCOPY

Trichoscopy may help make a correct diagnosis of DC and treat it properly in early stages of the disease.[17,18] Patches of alopecia show loss of follicular openings confirming the diagnosis of scarring alopecia. Sometimes the skin surface may contain large, yellow amorphous areas.[17] A study carried out by Rudnicka et al. in 1884 patients presenting with hair loss described the presence of "3D" yellow dots

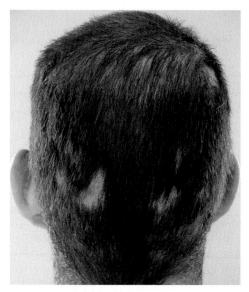

FIG. 15.1 Early stages of dissecting cellulitis of the scalp. Patches of alopecia may mimic other causes of focal alopecia, such as alopecia areata or trichotillomania.

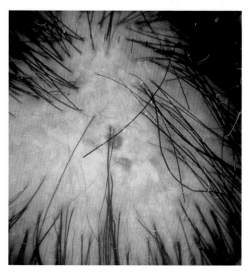

FIG. 15.3 Trichoscopic findings in late stages of dissecting cellulitis of the scalp. Patch of alopecia with loss of follicular openings, isolated vellus hairs, and keratotic plugs. We can observe telangiectasias because of previous corticosteroid injections.

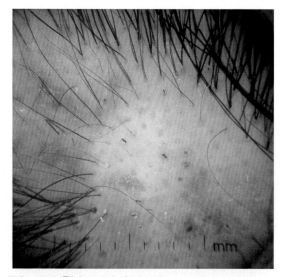

FIG. 15.2 Trichoscopic findings in early stages of dissecting cellulitis of the scalp. Multiple "3D" *yellow dots*, *black dots*, and broken hair. There is no evidence of loss of follicular openings.

in eight patients with DC.[3] This finding corresponds to common yellow dots imposed over dystrophic hairs. It is considered one of the most characteristic trichoscopic features of DC (Fig. 15.2).[3] Common black dots and isolated yellow dots can also be found in DC.[19–21] Red dots

were described in DC, although they are not a characteristic finding of the disease.[21] Broken hairs and exclamation mark hairs can be detected in patients with recent-onset DC (mean time of 0.75 years).[19,21]

White dots are present in long-standing disease, when patches of scarring alopecia are established, and correspond to follicular fibrosis (Fig. 15.3).[3,21] As most of the patients are of African descent, they must not be misdiagnosed with pinpoint white dots. A whitish halo surrounding these dots has also been described in DC.[17]

PATHOLOGY

Histopathology of DC is similar to HS and other disorders of the follicular occlusion tetrad.[22–25] Biopsies obtained from early lesions of DC feature distension of the follicles with keratotic plugs and neutrophilic infiltrate.[22] At this stage, a deep peribulbar and subfollicular lymphocytic, histiocytic, and plasma cellular infiltrate can also be observed.[26] When inflammation breaks the follicular epithelium, abscesses in the dermis and subcutaneous tissue appear, which are connected by sinus tracts.[13,24,27]

Hairs in catagen and telogen stages are increased in number, as the inflammation results in acute catagen transition.[15,28] As in acute or subacute alopecia areata, pigmented casts in the fibrous streamers are a common

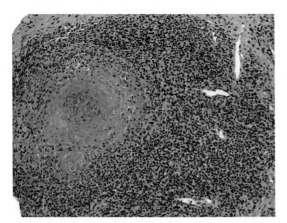

FIG. 15.4 Biopsy from late-stage lesions of dissecting cellulitis of the scalp. Chronic granulomas consisting in lymphocytes, plasma cells, and foreign-body giant cells can be observed. (Courtesy of Dr. Jesús Cuevas.)

TABLE 15.1
Comorbidities in Dissecting Cellulitis
CUTANEOUS DISORDERS
Hidradenitis[6,29]
Acne conglobata[6,29]
Pilonidal cysts[4]
Pyoderma[29,34]
Psoriasis[4]
Pityriasis rubra pilaris[34]
Squamous cell carcinoma (in longstanding DC)[4]
Malignant proliferating pilar cysts[51]
OSTEOARTICULAR DISORDERS
Spondyloarthritis[51]
Osteomyelitis[52]
Sternocostoclavicular hyperostosis[52]
Arthropathy[52]
Arthritis[52]
GASTROINTESTINAL DISORDERS
Crohn's disease[34]
Nonalcoholic steatohepatitis[40]
OTHER DISORDERS
Keratitis-ichthyosis-deafness syndrome[44,51,53]
Marginal keratitis[34,54]

finding in DC.[28] Sebaceous glands are not involved in the early course of the disease, but eventually they will be destroyed.[15]

In later stages, chronic granulomas consisting of lymphocytes, plasma cells, and foreign-body giant cells can be observed (Fig. 15.4).[15,24] These granulomas occur in all the disorders of the follicular occlusion tetrad but seem more common in DC.[24] True sinus tracts are lined by a multilayered squamous epithelium. This epithelium belongs to the outer follicular sheath, and it is the most characteristic histopathologic feature in DC.[15,22] The destruction of hair follicles results in scarring alopecia.[27]

ASSOCIATED CONDITIONS

DC is frequently associated with other disorders included in the follicular occlusion tetrad. Large case series detected the presence of HS in 12%–24% and acne conglobata in 14%–16% of patients.[5,6] Associated pilonidal cyst has also been described.[29] Another related disorder described in patients with DC is arthritis similar to that described in spondyloarthropathies (axial and peripheral arthritis). Combinations of different diseases have been reported frequently.[29] All associated conditions, including uncommon disorders, are summarized in Table 15.1.

DIFFERENTIAL DIAGNOSIS

The condition has a distinctive clinical appearance in advanced cases. However, early stages of DC may resemble other diseases.

The differential diagnosis includes inflammatory tinea capitis (kerion celsi), folliculitis decalvans (FD), and cutis verticis gyrata. Special stains for fungal organisms and cultures will rule out tinea. FD is characterized by superficial inflammation (perifollicular pustules), and DC is a deeper process (superficial fat tissue).

Alopecic and aseptic nodules of the scalp (AANS) has been proposed as a distinct clinical entity. AANS is infrequent, affects predominantly young white or Asian males, and most patients have one or two firm, dome-shaped nodules on the occiput or vertex of the scalp without scarring alopecia.[30]

Early DC simulates alopecia areata on trichoscopy, but loss of follicular openings and absence of exclamation mark hairs rule it out.[31] Also trichotillomania may resemble early DC, but classic trichoscopic findings help distinguish both.[32]

TREATMENT

Treatment includes improved scalp hygiene, topical antiseptics, and topical antibiotics. There are no clinical trials proving the efficacy of any therapy in DC; most of the therapeutic options are based on case series and personal experiences. The combination of different treatment options is a common practice.

Corticosteroids

Corticosteroids have been used in DC looking for their antiinflammatory effects. Oral steroids have not been proved to be useful in clinical management of DC, and they are associated with short- and long-term adverse effects. Corticosteroids injections are commonly used to treat inflammatory subcutaneous nodules and for speed healing.[33]

Oral Antibiotics

Different treatment regimens have shown to reduce the inflammatory activity and improve acute symptoms. Possible options include tetracyclines (oxytetracycline, 1g daily or doxycycline 100 mg daily), macrolides (azythromycin, 500 mg daily three times a week), quinolones (ciprofloxacin, 500 mg twice daily), and combination of several antibiotics (e.g., rifampicin and clindamycin, 300 mg twice daily for 10 weeks).[5,6,34] The length of the antibiotic treatment is controversial because there is no evidence that longer regimens delay new flares of the disease.

Oral Retinoids

Some authors consider that oral retinoids must be the initial treatment of choice.

Oral isotretinoin (0.5–0.8 mg/kg daily) has been proved to be effective, with complete remission after 3 months of treatment, but frequent relapse after discontinuation.[6] There are also reported cases treated with acitretin (30 mg daily, outcome unknown) and alitretinoin in patients with keratitis-ichthyosis-deafness syndrome and DC.[6,35,36]

Other Treatments

- *Infliximab*: this intravenous tumor necrosis factor α inhibitor has been effective in treating DC according to isolated case reports. Authors described a decrease of inflammatory activity and 1-year remission after infusion of 5 mg/kg at 8-week interval for a year. Other studies did not show significant improvement.[6,37–39]
- *Adalimumab*: considering DC as an entity grouped in the follicular occlusion tetrad, adalimumab would work as it does in HS. This tumor necrosis factor α inhibitor has been used in DC at psoriasis dosage (80 mg, followed by 40 mg 1 week later and 40 mg every other week) with successful clinical remission, but with early relapses. As in HS, higher doses might be required to reduce

the inflammation and stop progression of the disease.[39–43]
- *Finasteride*: 1 mg daily of finasteride was administrated in three DC patients with significant improvement in two.[5]
- *Photodynamic therapy (PDT)*: good experiences with PDT in DC have been reported.[44] However, therapeutic failures have also been described.[5]
- *Surgery*: scalp resection may be performed to galeal or just subgaleal level. The periosteum must be preserved to have a base of granulation tissue upon which a skin graft can be performed.[33,45–47]
- *Brachytherapy*: an isolated case report showed that brachytherapy may be a useful therapeutic for some patient with DC. Further investigations are needed to determine the target patient population.[48]

PROGNOSIS

As it is an uncommon disease, DC patients do not usually receive an early diagnosis, and treatment is not started soon enough to stop disease progression at early stages. Patients under medical treatment could control the DC in many cases, and medical complications are not frequent. However, advanced DC may result in severe complications, such as osteomyelitis of the underlying cranium and squamous cell carcinoma established in chronic ulcers.[33,49] A very important issue to keep in mind is the significant psychologic distress and loss of quality of life associated to DC.[50]

REFERENCES

1. Spitzer L. Dermatitis follicularis et perifollicularis conglobate. *Dermatol Z*. 1903;10:109–120.
2. Tan E, Martinka M, Ball N, Shapiro J. Primary cicatricial alopecias: clinicopathology of 112 cases. *J Am Acad Dermatol*. 2004;50(1):25–32. https://doi.org/10.1016/j.jaad.2003.04.001.
3. Rudnicka L, Olszewska M, Rakowska A, Slowinska M. Trichoscopy update 2011. *J Dermatol Case Rep*. 2011;5(4):82–88. https://doi.org/10.3315/jdcr.2011.1083.
4. Scheinfeld N. Dissecting cellulitis (Perifolliculitis Capitis Abscedens et Suffodiens): a comprehensive review focusing on new treatments and findings of the last decade with commentary comparing the therapies and causes of dissecting cellulitis to hidradenitis suppura. *Dermatol Online J*. 2014;20(5):2.
5. Segurado-Miravalles G, Camacho-Martínez FM, Arias-Santiago S, et al. Epidemiology, clinical presentation and therapeutic approach in a multicentre series of dissecting cellulitis of the scalp. *J Eur Acad Dermatol Venereol*. 2016:0–1. https://doi.org/10.1111/jdv.13948.

6. Badaoui A, Reygagne P, Cavelier-Balloy B, et al. Dissecting cellulitis of the scalp: a retrospective study of 51 patients and review of literature. *Br J Dermatol.* 2016;174(2):421–423. https://doi.org/10.1111/bjd.13999.

7. Ramesh V. Dissecting cellulitis of the scalp in 2 girls. *Dermatologica.* 1990;180(1):48–50. http://www.ncbi.nlm.nih.gov/pubmed/2106459.

8. Chicarilli ZN. Follicular occlusion triad: hidradenitis suppurativa, acne conglobata, and dissecting cellulitis of the scalp. *Ann Plast Surg.* 1987;18(3):230–237. http://www.ncbi.nlm.nih.gov/pubmed/2954503.

9. Van der Zee HH, Laman JD, Boer J, Prens EP. Hidradenitis suppurativa: viewpoint on clinical phenotyping, pathogenesis and novel treatments. *Exp Dermatol.* 2012;21(10):735–739. https://doi.org/10.1111/j.1600-0625.2012.01552.x.

10. Hoffman E. Perifolliculitis capitis abscedens et suffodiens. *Dermatol Z.* 1908;15:122–123.

11. Kong HH, Segre JA. Skin microbiome: looking back to move forward. *J Invest Dermatol.* 2012;132(3 Pt 2):933–939. https://doi.org/10.1038/jid.2011.417.

12. Bjellerup M, Wallengren J. Familial perifolliculitis capitis abscedens et suffodiens in two brothers successfully treated with isotretinoin. *J Am Acad Dermatol.* 1990;23(4 Pt 1):752–753. http://www.ncbi.nlm.nih.gov/pubmed/2229506.

13. Navarini AA, Trüeb RM. 3 cases of dissecting cellulitis of the scalp treated with adalimumab: control of inflammation within residual structural disease. *Arch Dermatol.* 2010;146(5):517–520. https://doi.org/10.1001/archdermatol.2010.16.

14. Mihić LL, Tomas D, Situm M, et al. Perifolliculitis capitis abscedens et suffodiens in a caucasian: diagnostic and therapeutic challenge. *Acta Dermatovenerol Croat.* 2011;19(2):98–102. http://www.ncbi.nlm.nih.gov/pubmed/21703156.

15. Bolduc C, Sperling LC, Shapiro J. Primary cicatricial alopecia: other lymphocytic primary cicatricial alopecias and neutrophilic and mixed primary cicatricial alopecias. *J Am Acad Dermatol.* 2016;75(6):1101–1117. https://doi.org/10.1016/j.jaad.2015.01.056.

16. Torok RD, Bellet JS. Tinea capitis mimicking dissecting cellulitis. *Pediatr Dermatol.* 2013;30(6):753–754. https://doi.org/10.1111/pde.12235.

17. Rakowska A, Slowinska M, Kowalska-Oledzka E, et al. Trichoscopy of cicatricial alopecia. *J Drugs Dermatol.* 2012;11(6):753–758. http://www.ncbi.nlm.nih.gov/pubmed/22648224.

18. Olszewska M, Rudnicka L, Rakowska A, Kowalska-Oledzka E, Slowinska M. Trichoscopy. *Arch Dermatol.* 2008;144(8):1007. https://doi.org/10.1001/archderm.144.8.1007.

19. Tosti A, Torres F, Miteva M. Dermoscopy of early dissecting cellulitis of the scalp simulates alopecia areata. *Actas Dermosifiliogr.* 2013;104(1):92–93. https://doi.org/10.1016/j.ad.2012.05.008.

20. Kowalska-Oledzka E, Slowinska M, Rakowska A, et al. "Black dots" seen under trichoscopy are not specific for alopecia areata. *Clin Exp Dermatol.* 2012;37(6):615–619. https://doi.org/10.1111/j.1365-2230.2012.04401.x.

21. Segurado-Miravalles G, Camacho-Martinez F, Arias-Santiago S, et al. Trichoscopy of dissecting cellulitis of the scalp: exclamation mark hairs and white dots as markers of disease chronicity. *J Am Acad Dermatol.* 2016;75(6):1267–1268. https://doi.org/10.1016/j.jaad.2016.08.035.

22. Bernárdez C, Molina-Ruiz AM, Requena L. Histopatología de las alopecias. Parte II: alopecias cicatriciales. *Actas Dermosifiliogr.* 2015;106(4):260–270. https://doi.org/10.1016/j.ad.2014.06.016.

23. Stenn KS, Sundberg JP, Sperling LC. Hair follicle biology, the sebaceous gland, and scarring alopecias. *Arch Dermatol.* 1999;135(8):9–12. https://doi.org/10.1001/archderm.135.8.973.

24. Childs JM, Sperling LC. Histopathology of scarring and nonscarring hair loss. *Dermatol Clin.* 2013;31(1). https://doi.org/10.1016/j.det.2012.08.001.

25. Thakur BK, Verma S, Raphael V. Clinical, trichoscopic, and histopathological features of primary cicatricial alopecias: a retrospective observational study at a tertiary care centre of North East India. *Int J Trichol.* 2015;7(3):107–112. https://doi.org/10.4103/0974-7753.167459.

26. Sperling LC, Cowper SE, Knopp EA. Dissecting cellulitis of the scalp (perifolliculitis capitis abscedens et suffodiens). In: *An Atlas of Hair Pathology with Clinical Correlations.* 2nd ed. London: Informa Healthcare; 2012:166–170.

27. Sperling LC. Scarring alopecia and the dermatopathologist. *J Cutan Pathol.* 2001;28(7):333–342.

28. Miteva M, Romanelli P, Tosti A. Pigmented casts. *Am J Dermatopathol.* 2014;36(1):58–63. https://doi.org/10.1097/DAD.0b013e3182919ac7.

29. Koshelev MV, Garrison PA, Wright TS. Concurrent hidradenitis suppurativa, inflammatory acne, dissecting cellulitis of the scalp, and pyoderma gangrenosum in a 16-year-old boy. *Pediatr Dermatol.* 2014;31(1). https://doi.org/10.1111/pde.12196.

30. Abdennader S, Reygagne P. Alopecic and aseptic nodules of the scalp. *Dermatology.* 2008;218(1):86. https://doi.org/10.1159/000165608.

31. Miteva M, Tosti A. Hair and scalp dermatoscopy. *J Am Acad Dermatol.* 2012;67(5):1040–1048. https://doi.org/10.1016/j.jaad.2012.02.013.

32. Miteva M, Tosti A. Flame hair. *Ski Appendage Disord.* 2015;1(2):105–109. https://doi.org/10.1159/000438995.

33. Jerome MA, Laub DR. Dissecting cellulitis of the scalp: case discussion, unique considerations, and treatment options. *Eplasty.* 2014;14:ic17. http://www.ncbi.nlm.nih.gov/pubmed/24966998.

34. Scheinfeld NS. A case of dissecting cellulitis and a review of the literature. *Dermatol Online J.* 2003;9(1):87–93. https://doi.org/10.1007/s11845-008-0177-4.

35. Werchau S, Toberer F, Enk A, Helmbold P. Keratitis-ichthyosis-deafness syndrome: response to alitretinoin and review of literature. *Arch Dermatol.* 2011;147(8):993. https://doi.org/10.1001/archdermatol.2011.216.

36. Prasad S, Bygum A. Successful treatment with alitretinoin of dissecting cellulitis of the scalp in keratitis-ichthyosis-deafness syndrome. *Acta Derm Venereol.* 2013;93(4):473–474. https://doi.org/10.2340/00015555-1499.

37. Brandt HRC, Malheiros APR, Teixeira MG, Machado MCR. Perifolliculitis capitis abscedens et suffodiens successfully controlled with infliximab. *Br J Dermatol*. 2008;159(2):506–507. https://doi.org/10.1111/j.1365-2133.2008.08674.x.

38. Wollina U, Gemmeke A, Koch A. Dissecting cellulitis of the scalp responding to intravenous tumor necrosis factor-alpha antagonist. *J Clin Aesthet Dermatol*. 2012;5(4):36–39. http://www.ncbi.nlm.nih.gov/pubmed/22708007.

39. Sand FL, Thomsen SF. Off-label use of TNF-alpha inhibitors in a dermatological university department: retrospective evaluation of 118 patients. *Dermatol Ther*. 2015;28(3):158–165. https://doi.org/10.1111/dth.12222.

40. Mansouri Y, Martin-Clavijo A, Newsome P, Kaur MR. Dissecting cellulitis of the scalp treated with tumour necrosis factor-alpha inhibitors: experience with two agents. *Br J Dermatol*. 2016;174(4):916–918. https://doi.org/10.1111/bjd.14269.

41. Navarini AA, Trüeb RM. 3 cases of dissecting cellulitis of the scalp treated with adalimumab. *Arch Dermatol*. 2010;146(5). https://doi.org/10.1001/archdermatol.2010.16.

42. Sukhatme SV, Lenzy YM, Gottlieb AB. Refractory dissecting cellulitis of the scalp treated with adalimumab. *J Drugs Dermatol*. 2008;7(10):981–983. http://www.ncbi.nlm.nih.gov/pubmed/19112766.

43. Martin-García RF, Rullán JM. Refractory dissecting cellulitis of the scalp successfully controlled with adalimumab. *P R Health Sci J*. 2015;34(2):102–104. http://www.ncbi.nlm.nih.gov/pubmed/26061062.

44. Liu Y, Ma Y, Xiang LH. Successful treatment of recalcitrant dissecting cellulitis of the scalp with ALA-PDT: case report and literature review. *Photodiagnosis Photodyn Ther*. 2013;10(4):410–413. https://doi.org/10.1016/j.pdpdt.2013.03.008.

45. Housewright CD, Rensvold E, Tidwell J, Lynch D, Butler DF. Excisional surgery (scalpectomy) for dissecting cellulitis of the scalp. *Dermatol Surg*. 2011;37(8):1189–1191. https://doi.org/10.1111/j.1524-4725.2011.02049.x.

46. Bellew SG, Nemerofsky R, Schwartz RA, Granick MS. Successful treatment of recalcitrant dissecting cellulitis of the scalp with complete scalp excision and split-thickness skin graft. *Dermatol Surg*. 2003;29(10):1068–1070. http://www.ncbi.nlm.nih.gov/pubmed/12974708.

47. Arneja JS, Vashi CN, Gursel E, Lelli JL. Management of fulminant dissecting cellulitis of the scalp in the pediatric population: case report and literature review. *Can J Plast Surg*. 2007;15(4):211–214. http://www.ncbi.nlm.nih.gov/pubmed/19554179.

48. Paul S, Bach D, Leboeuf NR, Devlin PM, Lipworth AD. Successful use of brachytherapy for a severe hidradenitis suppurativa variant. *Dermatol Ther*. 2016;29:455–458.

49. Curry SS, Gaither DH, King LEJ. Squamous cell carcinoma arising in dissecting perifolliculitis of the scalp. A case report and review of secondary squamous cell carcinomas. *J Am Acad Dermatol*. 1981;4(6):673–678. https://doi.org/10.1016/S0190-9622(81)70068-9.

50. Chiang YZ, Bundy C, Griffiths CEM, Paus R, Harries MJ. The role of beliefs: lessons from a pilot study on illness perception, psychological distress and quality of life in patients with primary cicatricial alopecia. *Br J Dermatol*. 2015;172(1):130–137. https://doi.org/10.1111/bjd.13259.

51. Nyquist G, Mumm C, Grau R, et al. Malignant proliferating pilar tumors arising in KID syndrome: a report of two patients. *Am J Med Genet A*. 2007;143(7):734–741.

52. Wasserman E. Perifolliculitis capitis abscedens et suffodiens with rheumatoid arthritis; report of a case. *AMA Arch Derm Syphilol*. 1951;64(6):787–789.

53. Coggshall K, Farsani T, Ruben B, et al. Keratitis, ichthyosis, and deafness (KID) syndrome: a review of infectious and neoplastic complications. *J Am Acad Dermatol*. 2013;69(1):127–134. https://doi.org/10.1016/j.jaad.2012.12.965.

54. Enrenreich E. Perifolliculitis capitis abscedens et suffodiens. Interstitial keratitis. *AMA Arch Derm Syphilol*. 1953;68(6):744–746.

CHAPTER 16

Acne Keloidalis Nuchae

RITA RODRIGUES-BARATA, MD • LAURA MIGUEL-GÓMEZ, MD, PHD •
DAVID SACEDA-CORRALO, MD, PHD • SERGIO VAÑÓ-GALVÁN, MD, PHD

INTRODUCTION

Acne keloidalis, or folliculitis keloidalis nuchae, is a form of chronic cicatricial alopecia, most commonly observed in men of African origin.[1] It was originally recognized by Hebra in 1860, although later in 1896, Kaposi described it as a differentiated entity—dermatitis papillaris capillittii.[2] Lastly, Bazin in 1872 called it acne keloidalis nuchae (AKN).[3] Clinically it is characterized by the appearance of papules, pustules, and even occasionally of keloid-like masses in the occipital and nuchal region.[4] There are known factors that favor the onset of the disease in predisposed individuals, such as androgens, infections, inflammatory processes, trauma, and ingrown hairs.[5,6] It was classified as a mixed cicatricial alopecia, as it holds similar characteristics of other forms of scarring alopecias, as well as because it can coexist simultaneously with them.[7] Therapeutic intervention is mandatory to prevent disease progression and the development of subsequent cicatricial alopecia.

EPIDEMIOLOGY

It occurs mainly in young male patients of African origin.[4] Is has been reported also in Caucasians and in other racial groups.[8,9] It occurs 20 times more frequently in men than in women.[9–11] The exact disease prevalence rate is unknown, but reports in literature range from 0.45% in Afro-Caribbean population to 13.6% in American football players.[4,12–18]

PATHOGENESIS

The distinguished texture and curvature of the African patient's hair is believed to be a necessary, but not unique, factor in the development of the disease.[19] Association of other factors occurring at the puberty age would act in promoting the symptoms, such as increase of androgens levels, sebaceous gland activity, and activity of androgen receptors in the follicles.[6,20] It is also considered that a genetic component exists because the majority of affected patients are of African origin.

Moreover, it has been proposed that the shaving practices along with the kinky nature of this patient's hair induces follicular irritation and transepithelial elimination of hair follicles, facilitating the phenomena of ingrown hairs, in a similar mechanism as it occurs in the pseudofolliculitis of the beard.[21] Nevertheless, dermoscopy and histopathologic findings do not corroborate this theory.[22–24] Also AKN associated with pseudofolliculitis barbae has not yet been described.

Local trauma to the site from scratching, picking, occlusion and friction from tight headwear in the area, and obesity contributes to inducing chronic inflammation, but the underlying mechanism is not yet known.[1,25,26] A few theories have been proposed. Some relate it to a papular lichen simplex chronicus–like reaction, which these patients are especially predisposed to.[27] Others have hypothesized that it would be a mechanical irritation in an existing incipient folliculitis or that local trauma could induce abnormal keratin expression.[28,29] Nevertheless it is considered a primary cicatricial alopecia.[23]

Herzberg et al. have proposed the theory of an autoimmune reaction toward the follicle by unknown antigens present in the same follicle or in the surrounding epithelium, which will set up the inflammatory process and subsequent destruction of the pilosebaceous units and the development of fibrosis.[19] *Demodex*, skin flora, desquamated keratinocyte, and sebum could act as potential antigens, as well as hair cosmetics. On the other hand, the role of bacteria, especially *Staphylococcus aureus* and fungal elements such as *Malassezia* in the pathogenesis of AKN is thought to have a secondary relevance. Reports of drug-induced AKN have implicated certain medications such as cyclosporine, diphenylhydantoin and carbamazepine in some patients.[8,30,31]

CLINICAL FINDINGS

It manifests in the nuchal and/or occiput region after puberty, with a mean age of onset of 29 years.[4] Affected individuals do not have the tendency to develop keloids in other areas of the body, neither the lesions show keloid histologic criteria. Initially different-sized

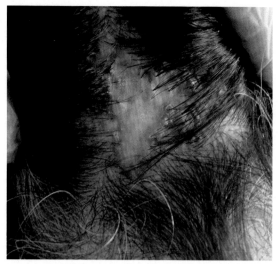

FIG. 16.1 Alopecia patch with loss of follicular ostia, tufted hairs, and small papules on the borders of the patch.

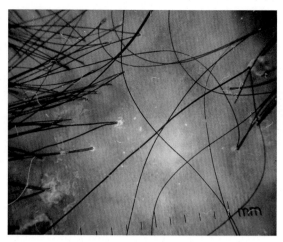

FIG. 16.2 Late stage of acne keloidalis nuchae with *white dots*, follicular hyperkeratosis, and loss of follicular openings.

flesh-colored or pink papules develop progressively in the neck or occipital region with lateral progression or onto the vertex. The high concentration of mast cells and the characteristic widening of the papillary dermis in this region can explain the characteristic localization of AKN in occipital or nape area.[20]

The clinical presentations of AKN lesions are variable. Patients often complain of itching or pain, starting hours before the appearance of the lesions. Pruritus leads to scratching, irritation, and consequent inflammation. Secondary bacterial infection complicates the disease, predisposing to the development of pustules, sinus, and abscesses with purulent discharge. Some lesions can turn up to develop rapidly nodules and tumorous or keloid masses. In a few patients, it manifests initially as a generalized folliculitis. Androgenetic alopecia, central centrifugal cicatricial alopecia and folliculitis decalvans have been described in association with AKN.[7,32,33] Verma also have pointed the coexistence of metabolic syndrome in some patients and postulate that acne keloidalis could constitute an additional symptom of the syndrome.[34] One report has described the appearance of keloids in another part of the body, but it is a rare association.[14] In latter stages, destruction of hair follicles leads to cicatricial alopecia with loss of follicular openings (Fig. 16.1).

TRICHOSCOPY

At dermatoscopy, in early stages tufted hair folliculitis and follicular hyperkeratosis can be observed, and in latter stages white dots and loss of follicular openings. No ingrowth hairs have been described (Fig. 16.2).

PATHOLOGY

Pathologic findings in AKN are variable and depend on the stage of the disease.[35,36] They are not specific as they can be observed in other forms of cicatricial alopecias. Sperling described chronic perifollicular inflammation with plasma cells and lymphocytic cells, more pronounced at the isthmus and deep infundibulum.[23] Also at the level of the isthmus, lamellar fibroplasia and thinning of the follicular epithelium can be observed. Sebaceous glands are absent or destroyed.[37] And it is not clear yet whether the sebaceous gland constitutes the main target of the inflammatory process or it is damaged as a secondary mechanism.

Granulomatous reaction, desquamation of the inner root sheath, and polytrichia are also described. Later on, hair follicles disappearance and replacement by connective tissue is remarkable. Signs of secondary bacterial infection, microabscesses, and sinus tract formation can also conduce to the pathologic findings.

DIFFERENTIAL DIAGNOSIS

- **Folliculitis decalvans**: although many features are shared, there is typically significantly less fibrosis in this condition. Clinical discrimination is reliable.

- **Deep infectious folliculitis**: the inflammatory infiltrate tends to form tightly around the involved follicle with less extensive follicular disruption or dermal scarring. Special stains are also of assistance here. In cases of doubt, culture studies should be recommended.
- **Hidradenitis suppurativa**: although location and clinical details are discriminatory, this condition also shows sinus tracts and large areas of abscess formation.

TREATMENT

Early therapeutic intervention is mandatory to prevent disease progression and the appearance of ultimate cicatricial alopecia. Patients should avoid precipitating factors, such as frequent haircuts, tight headwear, and scratching.[38,39]

Early disease can be treated with **potent topical corticosteroids**. Callender et al. found Clobetasol propionate 0.05% foam, twice daily in a pulse-dose regimen during 8–12 weeks, to be effective in improving AKN in African-descendent patients.[40] If pustular lesions are present, **topical antibiotics** can be used in combination with corticosteroids; 1% Clindamycin lotion was used twice daily in 10 patients with AKN, with improvement in all patients.[41] In extensive disease, **oral antibiotics** are usually necessary. The most used oral antibiotics include doxycycline, minocycline, and tetracycline at acne dosages.[1,32,42] Cephalosporins and penicillins can also be useful.[33] The use of **antiseptic solutions** should be given to prevent secondary bacterial infections.[38]

In mild to moderate diseases, with the presence of large papular to nodular lesions, **intralesional triamcinolone** (5–40 mg/mL at 4 weeks intervals) is also recommended.[39] Triamcinolone doses should be limited to prevent side effects such as hypopigmentation and skin atrophy. In patients with associated folliculitis decalvans, adding a long-term regimen of oral retinoids can help controlling both disorders.[32,33]

Additional treatments have been used in AKN with variable results. Cryotherapy has proved its effectiveness in both early and fibrotic lesions (two freeze-thaw cycles of 20 s in each cycle); care should be taken to avoid possible permanent depigmentation if done too strongly.[43] Tretinoin combinations and imiquimod have been used with variable outcomes.[44,45] Imiquimod, once daily for 5 days/week for 8 weeks, has shown an average of 28% reduction on the number of lesions, compared with 17% reduction with pimecrolimus twice daily, during 8 weeks.[46]

Surgical treatment is reserved to diseases unresponsive to medical treatment or to those patients with presence of cosmetically disfiguring extensive fibrosis.[47] Small punches passing deeply the follicular bulb are useful in removing fibrotic lesions. Electrosurgery and cryosurgery have been used as well, and fusiform excision is necessary in extensive refractory and disfiguring cases, leaving to heal by primary or secondary intention (the latter favored by most authors).[43,48–51] A semilunar tissue expander was used in a 40-year-old male patient with a successful outcome.[52]

More recently, postoperative radiation therapy has been used to treat a refractory AKN case, which managed to prevent recurrences.[52,53] Treatment with 1064 nm Nd:YAG laser, 595 nm PDL, and 810 nm Diode laser has been shown to reduce significantly the number and size of lesions in patients with AKN.[54,55] Diode laser has been used in two East Indian males, with an overall improvement of 90% after four sessions each 4 to 6 week, in combination with tretinoin 0.025% cream and betamethasone dipropionate 0.05% cream.[56] CO_2 Laser and UVB-BE have also proved its effectiveness and can be considered as an alternative treatment in selected and refractory cases[8,57–59] (Table 16.1).

TABLE 16.1
Treatment Modalities in AKN

	Treatment Regimen	Indication
Potent corticosteroids	Clobetasol propionate 0.05% foam, twice daily, 8–12 weeks[40]	Early disease
Topical antibiotics	1% Clindamycin lotion twice daily[41]	If pustular lesions are present, in combination with corticosteroids
Oral antibiotics	Doxycycline, minocycline and tetracycline at acne dosages[1,32,42]	Extensive disease
	Cephalosporins and penicillins[33]	

continued

TABLE 16.1
Treatment Modalities in AKN—cont'd

	Treatment Regimen	Indication
Intralesional corticosteroids	Triamcinolone acetonide 5–40 mg/mL at 4 weeks intervals[39]	In mild to moderate disease, with the presence of large papular to nodular lesions
Oral retinoids	Isotretinoin[32,33]	In patients with associated folliculitis decalvans
Other topical agents	Retinoid combinations[44]	In mild to moderate disease
	Imiquimod once a day or 5 days/week for 8 weeks[45]	
	Pimecrolimus twice a day, during 8 weeks[46]	
Cryotherapy[43]	2 freeze-thaw cycles of 20 s each cycle	Early disease and fibrotic lesions
Surgical treatment[43,48–51]	Punch excision	Extensive refractory and disfiguring disease
	Electrosurgery	
	Cryosurgery	
	Fusiform excisions	
	Tissue expanders	
Postoperative radiotherapy[52,53]		Refractory AKN
Light therapies[54–59]	1064 nm Nd:YAG laser	Alternative treatment in selected and refractory cases
	595 nm PDL	
	810 nm Diode laser	
	CO_2 Laser	
	UVB-BE	

AKN, acne keloidalis nuchae.

PROGNOSIS

Therapeutic intervention is mandatory to prevent disease progression and the development of subsequent cicatricial alopecia. Haircuts, other forms of local irritation, or the use of caps or helmets usually precede the appearance of the lesions. Avoiding these actions can help preventing its appearance or reappearance.

REFERENCES

1. Dinehart SM, Herzberg AJ, Kerns BJ, Pollack SV. Acne keloidalis: a review. *J Dermatol Surg Oncol.* 1989;15(6):642–647.
2. Adamson H. Dermatitis papillaris capillitii (Kaposi): acne keloid. *Br Dermatol.* 1914;26:69–83.
3. Fox H. Folliculits keloidalis a better term than dermatitis papillaris capillitii. *Arch Dermatol Syphilol.* 1947;55:112–113.
4. Adegbidi H, Atadokpede F, do Ango-Padonou F, Yedomon H. Keloid acne of the neck: epidemiological studies over 10 years. *Int J Dermatol.* 2005;44(suppl 1):49–50.
5. Ogunbiyi AO, Adedokun B. Perceived etiological factors of folliculitis keloidalis nuchae and treatment options amongst Nigerian men. *Br J Dermatol.* 2015;173(suppl 2):22–25.
6. Ogunbiyi AO. Acne keloidalis nuchae: prevalence, impact, and management challenges. *Clin Cosmet Investig Dermatol.* 2016;14(9):483–489.
7. Olsen EA, Bergfeld WF, Cotsarelis G, et al. Summary of North American Hair Research Society (NAHRS)-sponsored workshop on cicatricial alopecia, Duke Medical Centre, February 10 and 11, 2001. *J Am Acad Dermatol.* 2003;48(1):103–110.
8. Azurdia RM, Graham RM, Wesmann K, Guerin DM. Acne keloidalis in Caucasian patients on cyclosporine following organ transplantation. *Br J Dermatol.* 2000;143(2):465–467.

9. Loayza E, Cazar T, Uraga V, Lubkov A, Garces JC. Acne keloidalis nuchae in Latin American women. *Int J Dermatol.* 2015;54(5):e183–e185.

10. Dinehart SM, Tanner L, Mallory SB, Herzberg AJ. Acne keloidalis in women. *Cutis.* 1989;44(3):250–252.

11. Ogunbiyi AO, George AO. Acne keloidalis in females; case report and review of literature. *JNMA.* 2005;97:736–738.

12. Dunwell P, Rose A. Study of the skin disease spectrum occurring in an Afro-Caribbean population. *Int J Dermatol.* 2003;42(4):287–289.

13. Ogunbiyi AO, Daramola OO, Alese OO. Prevalence of skin diseases in Ibadan, Nigeria. *Int J Dermatol.* 2004;43(1):32–36.

14. Salami T, Omeife H, Samuel S. Prevalence of acne keloidalis nuchae in Nigerians. *Int J Dermatol.* 2007;46:482–484.

15. Ogunbiyi AO, Owoaje E, Ndahi A. Prevalence of skin diseases in school children. *Pediatr Dermatol.* 2005;22:6–10.

16. Child FJ, Fuller LC, Higgind EM, Du Vivier AW. A study of the spectrum of skin disease occurring in the black population in South East London. *Br J Dermatol.* 1991;141:512–517.

17. Khumalo NP, Jessop S, Gumedze F, Ehrlich R. Hair dressing is associated with scalp disease in African school children. *Br J Dermatol.* 2007;157:106–110.

18. Knable Jr AL, Hanke CW, Gonin R. Prevalence of acne keloidalis nuchae in football players. *J Am Acad Dermatol.* 1997;37(4):570–574.

19. Herzberg AJ, Dinehart SM, Kerns BJ, Pollack SV. Acne keloidalis. Transverse microscopy, immmunohistochemistry, and electron microscopy. *Am J Dermatopathol.* 1990;12(2):109–121.

20. George AO, Akanji AO, Nduka EU, Olasode O. Clinical biochemistry and morphological features of acne keloidalis in a black population of acne keloidalis in a black population. *Int J Dermatol.* 1993;32(10):714–716.

21. Kelly AP. Psuedofolliculitis barbae and acne keloidalis nuchae. *Dermatol Clin.* 2003;21(4):645–653.

22. Sperling LC, Skelton 3rd HG, Smith KJ, Sau P, Friedman K. Follicular degeneration syndrome in men. *Arch Dermatol.* 1994;130(6):763–769.

23. Sperling LC, Homoky C, Prat L, Sau P. Acne keloidalis is a form of primary scarring alopecia. *Arch Dermatol.* 2000;136:479–484.

24. Tosti A. Acne keloidalis nuchae. In: Tosti A, ed. *Dermoscopy of the Hair and Nails.* 2nd ed. Boca Raton, Florida: Taylor & Francis group; 2016:65.

25. Smith JD, Odom RB. Pseudofolliculitis of the beard. *Arch Dermatol.* 1977;113:328–329.

26. Halder RM. Hair and scalp disorders in blacks. *Cutis.* 1983;32(4):378–380.

27. Burkhart CG, Burkhart CN. Acne keloidalis is lichen simplex chronicus with fibrotic keloidal scarring. *J Am Acad Dermatol.* 1998;39(4 Pt 1):661.

28. Winter H, Schissel D, Parry D, et al. Unusual Ala12Thr polymorphism in the 1A-helical segment of the companion layer-specific keratin K6hf: evidence for a risk factor in etiology of the common hair disorder pseudofolliculitis barbae. *J Invest Dermatol.* 2004;122:652–657.

29. Kurokawa I, Konishi T, Kakuno A, Tsubura A. Keratin and filaggrin expression in dermatitis papillaris capilliti. *Int J Dermatol.* 2014;53(9):e392–e395.

30. Grunwals MH, Ben-Dor D, Livini E, Halevy S. Acne keloidalis-like lesions n the scalp associated with antiepileptic drugs. *Int J Dermatol.* 1990;29(8):559–561.

31. Wu WY, Otberg N, McElwee KJ, Shapiro J. Diagnosis and management of primary cicatricial alopecia: part II. *Skinmed.* 2008;7(2):78–83.

32. Goh MSY, Magee J, Chong AH. Keratosis follicularis spinulosa decalvans and acne keloidalis nuchae. *Australas J Dermatol.* 2005;46(4):257–260.

33. Janjua SA, Iftikhar N, Pastar Z, Hosler GA. Keratosis follicularis spinulosa decalvans associated with acne keloidalis nuchae and tufted hair folliculitis. *Am J Clin Dermatol.* 2008;9(2):137–140.

34. Verma SB, Wollina U. Acne keloidalis nuchae; another cutaneous symptom of metabolic syndrome, truncal obesity and impending overt diabetes mellitus. *Am J Clin Dermatol.* 2010;11(6):433–436.

35. Tan E, Martinka M, Ball N, Shapiro J. Primary cicatricial alopecias – a clinicopathologic review of 112 cases. *J Am Acad Dermatol.* 2004;50(1):25–32.

36. Bernárdez C, Molina-Ruiz AM, Requena L. Histologic features of alopecias: part II: scarring alopecias. *Actas Dermosifiliogr.* 2015;106(4):260–270.

37. Al-Zaid T, Vanderwell S, Genbowic A, Lyle S. Sebaceous gland loss and inflammation in scarring alopecia: a potential role in pathogenesis. *J Am Acad Dermatol.* 2011;65:597–603.

38. Alexis A, Heath CR, Halder RM. Folliculitis keloidalis nuchae and pseudofolliculitis barbae: are prevention and effective treatment within reach? *Dermatol Clin.* 2014;32(2):183–191.

39. Maranda EL, Simmons BJ, Nguyen AH, Lim VM, Keri JE. Treatment of acne keloidalis nuchae: a systematic review of the literature. *Dermatol Ther (Heidelb).* 2016;6(3):363–378.

40. Callender VD, Young CM, Haverstock CL, et al. An open label study of clobetasol propionate 0.05% and betamethasone valerate 0.12% foams in treatment of mild to moderate acne keloidalis. *Cutis.* 2005;75(6):317–321.

41. Chu T. Pseudofolliculitis barbae. *Practitioner.* 1989;233 (1464):307–309.

42. Bajaj V, Langtry JAA. Surgical excision of acne keloidalis nuchae with secondary intention healing. *Clin Exp Dermatol.* 2008;9(2):137–140.

43. Layton AM, Yip J, Cunliffe WJ. A comparison of intralesional triamcinolone and cryosurgery in the treatment of acne keloids. *Br J Dermatol.* 1994;130(4):498–501.

44. Karpouzis A, Giatromanolaki A, Sivridis E, Kouskoukis C. Perifolliculitis capitis abscedens et suffodiens successfully controlled with topical isotretinoin. *Eur J Dermatol.* 2003;13(2):192–195.

45. Shaffer N, Billick RC, Srolovitz H. Perifolliculitis capitis abscedens et suffodiens. Resolution with combination therapy. *Arch Dermatol.* 1992;128(10):1329–1331.

46. Barr J, Friedman A, Baldwin H. Use of imiquimod and pimecrolimus in the treatment of acne keloidalis nuchae (Poster abstract). *J Am Acad Dermatol.* 2005; 3(suppl):P64.

47. Gloster HMJ. The surgical management of extensive cases of acne keloidalis nuchae. *Arch Dermatol.* 2000;136(11):1376–1379.

48. Glenn MJ, Bennett RG, Kelly AP. Acne keloidalis nuchae treatment with excision and secondary intention healing. *J Am Acad Dermatol.* 1995;33(1):243–246.

49. Beckett N, Lawson C, Cohen G. Electrosurgical excision acne keloidalis with secondary intention healing. *J Clin Aesthet Dermatol.* 2011;4(1):36–39.

50. Califano J, Miller S, Frodel L. Treatment of occipital acne keloidalis by excision followed by secondary intention healing. *Arch Facial Plast Surg.* 1999;1(4):308–311.

51. Etzkorn JR, Chitwood K, Cohen G. Tumor stage acne keloidalis nuchae treated with surgical excision and secondary intention healing. *J Drugs Dermatol.* 2012;11(4):540–541.

52. Pestalardo CM, Cordero AJ, Ansorena JM, Bestue M, Martinho A. Acne keloidalis nuchae. Tissue expansion treatment. *Dermatol Surg.* 1995;21(8):723–724.

53. Millan-Cayetano JF, Repiso-Jimenez JB, Del Boz J, de Troya-Martin M. Refractory acne keloidalis nuchae treated with radiotherapy. *Australas J Dermatol.* 2017;58(1):e11–e13.

54. Esmat SM, Abdel Hay RM, Abu Zeid OM, et al. The efficacy of laserassisted hair removal in the treatment of acne keloidalis nuchae: a pilot study. *Eur J Dermatol.* 2012;22(5):645–650.

55. Dragoni F, Bassi A, Cannarozzo G, Bonan P, Moretti S, Campolmi P. Successful treatment of acne keloidalis nuchae resistant to conventional therapy with 1064-nm ND:YAG laser. *G Ital Dermatol Venereol.* 2013:231–232.

56. Shah GK. Efficacy of diode laser for treating acne keloidalis nuchae. *Indian J Dermatol Vnereol Leprol.* 2005;71(1):31–34.

57. Kantor GR, Ratz JL, Wheeland RG. Treatment of acne keloidalis nuchae with carbon dioxide laser. *J Am Acad Dermatol.* 1986;14:263–267.

58. Sattler ME. Folliculitis keloidais nuchae. *WMJ.* 2001;100(1):37–38.

59. Okoye GA, Rainer BM, Leung SG, et al. Improving acne keloidalis nuchae with targeted ultraviolet B treatment: a prospective, randomized split-scalp study. *Br J Dermatol.* 2014;171(5):1156–1163.

CHAPTER 17

Erosive Pustular Dermatosis of the Scalp

RITA RODRIGUES-BARATA, MD • DAVID SACEDA-CORRALO, MD, PHD • LAURA MIGUEL-GÓMEZ, MD, PHD • SERGIO VAÑÓ-GALVÁN, MD, PHD

INTRODUCTION

Erosive pustular dermatosis of the scalp (EPDS) is a rare, but probably underdiagnosed, form of scarring alopecia initially described by Burton in 1977,[1] occurring manly in elderly patients, and it is characterized by the appearance of a progressive eruption of sterile pustules and erosions on the scalp, with subsequent crusting, and lastly, cicatricial alopecia and skin atrophy.[2] It is of unknown etiology, but a prior history of trauma to the scalp, surgery, or actinic damage is usually present.[3] A similar eruption can occur on the legs. Microbiologic cultures are commonly negative and histopathologic findings typically nonspecific. Its course tends to be chronic and scarcely responsive to medical treatments.

EPIDEMIOLOGY

EPDS is a very uncommon condition, with unknown prevalence, probably higher than that reported in literature. It majorly affects elderly patients, with a female predominance estimated of 2:1.[4,5] The largest case series reported in the literature included 20 patients, with a mean age of 59.4 years, concordant with other case reports.[2] Nevertheless, it can manifest in younger patients. Patton et al.[4] described an EPDS in a 15-year-old patient and Shimada et al.[6] in a 6-month-old girl with Klippel-Feil syndrome. Apparently, there is no racial predominance, although it has not been reported in the black race.

PATHOGENESIS

The exact pathophysiology of EPDS is not well known. It is frequent to find the existence of a prior induced chemical or mechanical trauma on the scalp that precedes in weeks to months the appearance of the condition.[7,8] Some authors have established the hypothesis that the pathogenesis of the entity is an autoimmune response toward the hair follicle induced by trauma with consequent chronic inflammation and scarring.[9,10]

The frequent association of the entity with other autoimmune disorders, such as rheumatoid arthritis, Takayasu arteritis, or Hashimoto thyroiditis, and its good response to corticosteroids and antiinflammatory medication corroborate this hypothesis that it is an autoimmune-based disease.[11,12] In the largest case series of Starace et al.,[2] 25% of their patients had an associated autoimmune disease. On the other hand, other authors have hypothesized the existence of an impaired mechanism of neutrophil chemotaxis and/or a dysfunction of cytokine production.[13,14] Impaired cellular immunity pathways in EPDS have not been demonstrated.

Traumas that have been associated with the development of EPDS include sun damage, skin grafting, laser, cryotherapy, radiotherapy, carbon dioxide laser therapy, hair transplant, as well as photodynamic therapy.[7,15-18] In addition, erosive lesions can appear in sites of previous herpes zoster or after implantation of a cochlear prosthesis.[19,20] There are also reports of association of EPDS with medications, such as minoxidil, and other topical treatments, such as tretinoin, topical latanoprost, imiquimod, and mebutate ingenol.[21-25] Toda et al. described an erosive pustular dermatosis–like eruption on the scalp in a patient who received Gefitinib therapy.[26] A total of 11 similar cases were described when taking antiepidermal growth factor receptor therapies. Another report describes the case of a female patient who developed EPDS in an area of a scalp wound after child delivery.[4] In this case, the imbalance of the hormonal status may have triggered the inflammatory response. Similarly, the role of androgenetic alopecia and chronic actinic damage are considered as predisposing factors in the development of EPDS.[2,9] This is explained by the fact that the atrophic skin is associated with impaired healing mechanisms, predisposing the development of an autoimmune response to skin antigens that is still not identified.[11,12] Recently Herbst et al. described an EPDS after contact dermatitis from a prosthetic hair piece[27] (Table 17.1).

TABLE 17.1
Precipitating Factors in Relation With Erosive Pustular Dermatosis of the Scalp

Local trauma[7,15–18,20]
Sun damage, skin grafting, cryotherapy, radiotherapy, laser therapy
Photodynamic therapy
Hair transplant
Implantation of a cochlear prosthesis

Infections[19]
Herpes zoster

Medications[21–26]
Minoxidil, Tretinoin, Latanoprost, Imiquimod
Mebutate ingenol
Antiepidermal growth factor therapies

Contact dermatitis from a prosthetic hair piece[27]

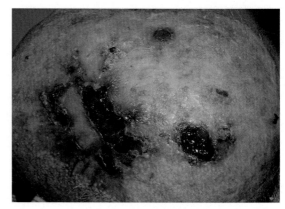

FIG. 17.1 An 80-year-old man with extensive erosions and crusts along the scalp, with pinpoint pustules on the sides.

CLINICAL FINDINGS

This condition most often affects older individuals with actinic damage in a bald scalp. The existence of a traumatic or previous viral infection in the area is highly suggestive of EPDS. In the recent series of Starace et al., mechanical trauma was the most frequent precipitating factor.[2] Lesions consist of eroded and exudative plaques that progressively increase in size and develop scarring phenomena. The presence of pustules indicates the condition but can be absent as well (Fig. 17.1).

TRICHOSCOPY

Trichoscopy is quite useful in the diagnosis of the disease and in differentiating it from other forms of cicatricial alopecias. Specific signs include severe cutaneous atrophy, absence of follicular openings, presence of erosions and scabs, consistent yellowish exudate, and hair bulbs visible through the epidermis.[2,28] The latter sign has only been described in aplasia cutis congenita.[29] A pattern of hyperpigmentation consistent of brownish-grey plaques has also been described, as well as tortuous and curved hair shafts, broken at few millimeters from the follicular opening. Tufted hairs with no more than four shafts emerging from the same follicular ostium were observed in two patients.[2]

Usually microbiologic culture results are negative for bacteria and fungi. If they are positive, it usually indicates secondary colonization.

PATHOLOGY

Reports lack to confirm primary participation of the hair follicle, although EPDS is classified as a primary cicatricial alopecia. Pathology findings are generally nonspecific and need to be interpreted in a suggestive clinical context.[27,30] Epidermis can appear atrophic, normal, parakeratotic, or eroded, depending where the biopsy is performed. A mixed chronic inflammatory infiltrate, which is nonfolliculocentric and consists of lymphocytes, plasma cells, and occasionally neutrophils, is observed in the dermis. Consequently, this induces an acute alopecia evidenced by an increase in catagen follicles. Inflammation then persists because of poor healing mechanisms, and foreign body granulomas against naked hair shafts have also been described. In latter stages, follicular units and sebaceous glands are reduced or absent. The results of immunofluorescence examinations are negative.

DIFFERENTIAL DIAGNOSIS

The differential diagnosis is based on clinical, dermatoscopic, and histologic findings and microbial cultures.[7,10,31] It includes infections (pyoderma, kerion, and atrophic candidiasis) and noninfectious entities, such as folliculitis decalvans, pemphigus vulgaris, pemphigus foliaceus, cicatricial pemphigoid, ulcerative lichen planus, squamous cell carcinoma, or dermatitis artefacta. Amicrobial pustulosis of the folds, a rare form of neutrophilic dermatosis, must also be taken into consideration, although the latter normally affects young female patients presenting with pustulosis in cutaneous folds and associated autoimmune disorders.[32]

TREATMENT

EPDS is a chronic disease that requires long-term treatment. Multiple therapeutic modalities have been tested, but potent topical corticosteroids and tacrolimus are the top-line treatments.[2,33] Oral and topical antibiotics have shown poor response. Other reported treatments in the literature are considered as second- or third-line therapies.[34]

Topical potent corticosteroids have been used in most reported cases, with considerable efficacy and relative safety. However, the main disadvantage is that prolonged use may worsen skin atrophy. In addition, EPDS usually relapses when treatment is discontinued in patients who experienced initial improvement with topical corticosteroids. Starace et al., in their case series, have observed that 16 of 18 patients responded to clobetasol propionate 0.5% cream and that only two patients required different treatment modalities.[2] Guarneri and Vaccaro have used oral corticosteroids in tapering dosage schedule for 12 weeks with complete clearance of lesions, with residual cicatricial alopecia in a patient with EPDS induced by photodynamic therapy.[16]

Topical tacrolimus 0.1% ointment is considered an alternative treatment to avoid corticosteroid side effects, with reported similar efficacy.[19,20,34,35] It can be used once or twice daily, with proven efficacy not only in scalp EPDS but also in EPD on the legs. According to the literature, improvement is seen after 1–2 weeks of treatment, but complete resolution may take up to 16 weeks to achieve. Topical tacrolimus may be used either as monotherapy, in combination with topical corticosteroids, or as a maintenance regimen after initial improvement with corticosteroids. In a patient with EPD of the legs, tacrolimus two times a week for 1 year as a maintenance treatment was capable to avoid recurrences.[36] Tacrolimus has the advantage over topical corticosteroids to prevent skin atrophy and has also shown to reverse partially skin atrophy associated with EPDS.

Boffa used **0.005% calcipotriol cream** in a patient with EPDS, with striking improvement at the eighth week of treatment and partial hair regrowth after 12 weeks of therapy.[37] **Oral Dapsone** has been tried in EPDS with disappointing results. Some have hypothesized that the lack of response could be because of the fact that local concentration following systemic administration only reaches subtherapeutic levels.[13] Then again, **5% Dapsone gel** has been used in four patients, with complete disappearance of skin lesions and a considerable long period of time free of recurrences without treatment. The improvement was observed between 2 weeks and 2 months after starting the treatment, and the complete clearance was observed between 1 and 4 months. No side effects were mentioned.[13]

Other treatments have also shown utility, such as oral isotretinoin, nimesulide, and zinc sulphate.[9,38] Acitretin may be useful in some patients, although there is the need for laboratory and contraceptive controls.[39] Oral treatments in the EPDS have shown varied responses, but always requiring prolonged periods of time, with risk of relapses. Therefore, maintenance treatment with calcineurin inhibitors is recommended.

Significant improvement has been observed in a patient treated with photodynamic therapy, although it has been reported that the same treatment could be related with the development of EPDS.[40,16] Meyer et al. used methyl 5 aminolevulinic acid in cream with 603 nm irradiation with two sessions of photodynamic therapy, with 1 week interval between sessions, with very good results at the week 12.[40] It can be considered as a third-line treatment, although it should be assessed with caution for the possibility that it could trigger the onset of EPDS. Surgery has been used on occasions to rule out squamous cell carcinoma, with goods results.

PROGNOSIS

Its course tends to be chronic and dependent of medical treatments for long periods of time. Preventive measures such as the use of hats to prevent sun exposure on the scalp and avoidance of physical and/or chemical trauma are recommended.

REFERENCES

1. Burton JL. Case for diagnosis. Pustular dermatosis of the scalp. *Br J Dermatol*. 1977;97(suppl 15):67–69.
2. Starace M, Loi C, Bruni F, et al. Erosive pustular dermatosis of the scalp: clinical, trichoscopic, and histopathologic features of 20 cases. *J Am Acad Dermatol*. 2017;76(6). 1109–1114.e2.
3. Vano-Galvan S, Martorell-Catayud A, Jaen P. Erosive pustular dermatosis of the scalp. *J Pak Med Assoc*. 2012;62: 501–502.
4. Patton D, Lynch PJ, Fung MA, et al. Chronic atrophic erosive dermatosis of the scalp and extremities: a recharacterization of erosive pustular dermatosis. *J Am Acad Dermatol*. 2007;57(3):421–427.
5. Pye RJ, Peachey RD, Burton JL. Erosive pustular dermatosis of the scalp. *Br J Dermatol*. 1979;100(5):559–566.
6. Shimada R, Masu T, Hanamizu H, Aiba S, Okuyama R. Infantile erosive pustular dermatosis of the scalp associated with Klippel-Feil syndrome. *Acta Derm Venereol*. 2010;90(2):73–77.
7. Grattan CE, Peachey RD, Boon A. Evidence for a role of local trauma in the pathogenesis of erosive pustular dermatosis of the scalp. *Clin Exp Dermatol*. 1988;13:7–10.

8. Layton AM, Cunliffe WJ. Acase of erosive pustular dermatosis of the scalp following surgery and a literature review. *Br J Dermatol.* 1995;132:472–473.

9. Mastroianni A, Cota C, Minutilli E, et al. Erosive pustular dermatosis of the scalp: a case report and review of the literature. *Dermatology.* 2005;211:273–276.

10. Van Exel CE, English III JC. Erosive pustular dermatosis of the scalp and nonscalp. *J Am Acad Dermatol.* 2007;57(2 suppl):S11–S14.

11. Hashimoto N, Ishibashi Y. Pustular dermatosis of the scalp associated with autoimmune diseases. *J Dermatol.* 1989;16:383–387.

12. Yamamoto T, Furuse Y. Erosive pustular dermatosis of the scalp in association with rheumatoid arthritis. *Int J Dermatol.* 1995;34:148.

13. Broussard KC, Berger TG, Rosenblum M, et al. Erosive pustular dermatosis of the scalp: a review with a focus on dapsone therapy. *J Am Acad Dermatol.* 2012;66(4):680–686.

14. Yang CS, Kuhn H, Cohen LM, et al. Aminolevulinic acid photodynamic therapy in the treatment of erosive pustular dermatosis of the scalp: a case series. *JAMA Dermatol.* 2016;152(6):694–697.

15. Mehmi M, Abdullah A. Erosive pustular dermatosis of the scalp occurring after partial thickness skin graft for squamous cell carcinoma. *Br J Plast Surg.* 2004;57(8):806–807.

16. Guarneri C, Vaccaro M. Erosive pustular dermatosis of the scalp following topical methylaminolaevulinate photodynamic therapy. *J Am Acad Dermatol.* 2009;60:521–522.

17. Tavares-Bello R. Erosive pustular dermatosis of the scalp. A chronic recalcitrant dermatosis developed upon CO_2 laser treatment. *Dermatology.* 2009;219(1):71–72.

18. Shahmoradi Z, Abtahi-Naeini B, Pourazizi M. Erosive pustular dermatosis of the scalp following hair transplantation. *Adv Biomed Res.* 2014;3:176.

19. Kim KR, Lee JY, Kim MK, Yoon TY. Erosive pustular dermatosis of the scalp following herpes zoster: successful treatment with topical tacrolimus. *Ann Dermatol.* 2010;22(2):232–234.

20. Marzano AV, Ghislanzoni M, Zaghis A, Spinelli D, Crosti C. Localized erosive pustular dermatosis of the scalp at the site of a cochlear implant: successful treatment with topical tacrolimus. *Clin Exp Dermatol.* 2009;34(5):157–159.

21. Guarneri C, Cannavo SP. Erosive pustular dermatosis of the scalp from topical minoxidil 5% solution. *Int J Dermatol.* 2013;52(4):507–509.

22. Rongioletti F, Delmonte S, Rossi ME, et al. Erosive pustular dermatosis of the scalp following cryotherapy and topical tretinoin for actinic keratoses. *Clin Exp Dermatol.* 1999;24(6):499–500.

23. Vaccaro M, Barbuzza O, Borgia F, et al. Erosive pustular dermatosis of the scalp following topical latanoprost for androgenetic alopecia. *Dermatol Ther.* 2015;28(2):65–67.

24. Vaccaro M, Barbuzza O, Guarneri B. Erosive pustular dermatosis of the scalp following treatment with topical imiquimod for actinic keratosis. *Arch Dermatol.* 2009;145(11):1340–1341.

25. Rongioletti F, Chinazzo C, Javor S. Erosive pustular dermatosis of the scalp induced by ingenol mebutate. *J Eur Acad Dermatol Venereol.* 2016;30:e110–e111.

26. Toda N, Fujimoto N, Kato T, et al. Erosive pustular erosive dermatosis of the scalp-like eruption due to gefitinib: case report and review of the literature of alopecia associated with EGFR inhibitors. *Dermatology.* 2012;225(1):18–21.

27. Herbst JS, Herbst AT. Erosive pustular dermatosis of the scalp after contact dermatitis from a prosthetic hair piece. *JAAD Case Rep.* 2017;3:121–123.

28. Starace M, Patrizi A, Piraccini BM. Visualization of hair bulbs through the scalp: a trichoscopic feature of erosive pustular dermatitis of the scalp. *Int J Trichology.* 2016;8(2):91–93.

29. Kowalska-Oledzka E, Slowinska M, Rakowska A, et al. 'Black dots' seen under trichoscopy are not specific for alopecia areata. *Clin Exp Dermatol.* 2012;37(6):615–619.

30. Bernárdez C, Molina-Ruiz AM, Requena L. Histologic features of alopecias: part II: scarring alopecias. *Actas Dermosifiliogr.* 2015;106(4):260–270.

31. Lugovic-Mihie L, Barisie F, Bulat V, et al. Differential diagnosis of the scalp hair folliculitis. *Acta Clin Croat.* 2011;50(3):395–402.

32. Marzano AV, Ramoni S, Caputo R. Amicrobial pustulosis of the folds. Report of 6 cases and a literature review. *Dermatology.* 2008;216(4):305–311.

33. Cenkowski MJ, Silver S. Topical tacrolimus in the treatment of erosive pustular dermatosis of the scalp. *J Cutan Med Surg.* 2007;11:222–225.

34. Semkova K, Tchernev G, Wollina U. Erosive pustular dermatosis (chronic atrophic dermatosis of the scalp and extremities). *Clin Cosmet Investig Dermatol.* 2013:177–182.

35. Tardio NB, Daly TJ. Erosive pustular dermatosis of the scalp and associated alopecia successfully treated with topical tacrolimus. *J Am Acad Dermatol.* 2011;65(3):93–94.

36. Dal'Olio E, Rosina P, Girolomoni G. Erosive pustular dermatosis of the leg: long-term control with topical tacrolimus. *Australas J Dermatol.* 2011;52(1):e15–e17.

37. Boffa MJ. Erosive pustular dermatosis of the scalp successfully treated with calcipotril cream. *Br J Dermatol.* 2003;148(3):593–595.

38. Caputo R, Veraldi S. Erosive pustular dermatosis of the scalp. *J Am Acad Dermatol.* 1993;28:96–98.

39. Darwich E, Muñoz-Santos C, Mascaró Jr JM. Erosive pustular dermatosis of the scalp responding to acitetin. *Arch Dermatol.* 2011;147:252–253.

40. Meyer T, Lopez-Navarro N, Herrera-Costa E, Jose A, Herrera E. Erosive pustular dermatosis of the scalp: a successful treatment with photodynamic therapy. *Photodermatol Photoimmunol Photomed.* 2010;26(1):44–45.

CHAPTER 18

Hair and Scalp Disorders Associated With Systemic Disease (Secondary Alopecia)

SEBASTIAN VERNE, MD • MARIYA MITEVA, MD

Alopecia is classically divided into scarring and nonscarring, with scarring alopecia being further divided into primary and secondary.[1] Primary alopecia arises from a process that originates from the hair follicles, whereas secondary alopecia, classically referring to secondary scarring alopecia, is due to all other causes. This chapter covers diseases that may lead to secondary alopecia with a focus on scalp involvement (Table 18.1). Secondary alopecia associated with lupus erythematosus (LE), dermatomyositis (DM), and psoriasis will be discussed in detail in separate chapters. The treatment of secondary alopecia involves the treatment of the underlying disease.

AMYLOIDOSIS

Amyloidosis encompasses a group of diseases that are characterized by the extracellular deposition of amyloid. It can be divided into three entities: deposition of an abnormal protein (monoclonal light-chain immunoglobulins) as in acquired systemic (AL) amyloidosis, deposition of nonimmunoglobulinemic acute phase proteins as in reactive systemic (AA) amyloidosis, and for unknown reasons as in wild-type transthyretin amyloidosis.[2] Mucocutaneous manifestations of systemic amyloidosis include macroglossia, periorbital purpura, waxy infiltrate of the palm and volar fingertips, nontender papular or nodular lesions on the face, neck, scalp, and anogenital area, and nail dystrophy.[2,3] The presence of alopecia has been reported in systemic amyloidosis and can involve any hair-bearing area ranging from isolated nonscarring alopecia to alopecia universalis, with all patients displaying some degree of plasma cell dyscrasia including multiple myeloma.[4-9] Physical examination reveals patchy or diffuse nonscarring alopecia (Fig. 18.1A), and on dermoscopy, there are peripilar salmon-colored halos that are seen around empty follicles as well as around

follicles containing terminal and vellus hairs, black dots, and/or broken hairs (Fig. 18.1B).[4,6] On horizontal sections of scalp biopsies, there is preserved follicular architecture with intact sebaceous glands and persistent telogen germinal units with only a few anagen follicles demonstrating hair cycle arrest.[4,6] The most prominent finding is the presence of homogenous, eosinophilic deposits of amyloid surrounding follicular structures (Fig. 18.1C). These compressed follicular structures correspond to the dystrophic hairs surrounded by the salmon-colored halo on

TABLE 18.1 Most Common Conditions Associated With Secondary Alopecia	
Nonscarring pattern	Amyloidosis
	Pemphigus foliaceus
	Dermatomyositis
	Systemic lupus erythematosus
	Leprosy
Scarring pattern	Cicatricial pemphigoid
	Epidermolysis bullosa
	Morphea
	Discoid lupus erythematosus
	Sarcoidosis
	Cutaneous T-cell lymphoma
	Alopecia neoplastica
	Mastocytosis
Mixed pattern	Pemphigus vulgaris
	Postoperative alopecia
	Graft-versus-host disease

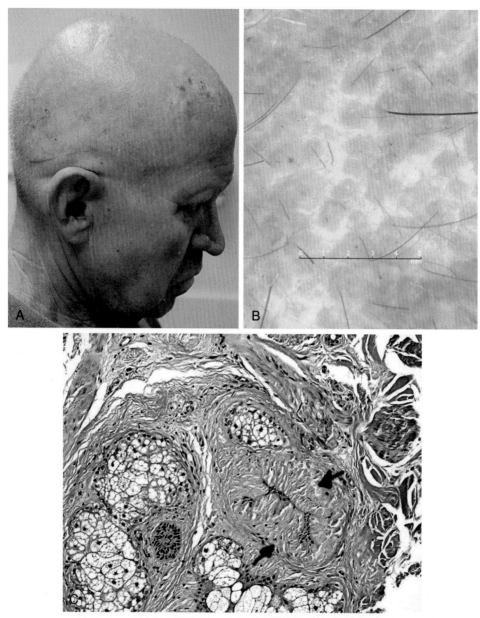

FIG. 18.1 **(A)** Amyloidosis of the scalp in a patient with multiple myeloma. Note the diffuse hair loss with only short sparse hair. The skin is thickened, and there are focal petechiae. **(B)** On dermoscopy, there are prominent salmon-colored peripilar halos surrounding the emergences of vellus hairs, broken hairs, and *black dots* (handyscope FotoFinder Systems, ×20). **(C)** On horizontal section at the level of the isthmus, there are intact sebaceous glands. There are two telogen follicles, one of which shows only focal epithelial remnants as it is almost completely obliterated by thick pink homogenous material (amyloid, *arrows*) (hematoxylin and eosin, ×40).

dermoscopy. Previous reports based on vertical sections of scalp biopsies have shown loss of follicular units and atrophic sebaceous glands, suggesting a scarring component.[7,9]

BULLOUS DISEASE

Autoimmune bullous disorders develop as autoantibodies target epidermal or subepidermal antigens. The type and location of antigens targeted define the disease and correspond to the clinical presentation. The presence of targeted antigens in the scalp of patients who develop antibodies may result in involvement, and possibly alopecia.[10] Many basement membrane zone and intraepithelial components found in the interfollicular epidermis have been found in hair follicles, including bullous pemphigoid antigens 180 and 230, a6b4 integrin, laminins 311 and 332, collagen types IV and VII, and desmogleins 1 and 3, albeit not uniformly distributed throughout.[11–14] Basement membrane zone components BP180, BP230, a6b4 integrin, laminin 332, and collagen type IV stain similar to the interfollicular epidermis at the upper follicle, gradually decrease at the lower portion, and become discontinuous around the hair bulb.[12] Desmoglein 1 is expressed by the more differentiated cells including the suprabasal cells of the outer root sheath (ORS) and the inner root sheath (IRS) in the lower follicle. Desmoglein 3 is expressed throughout the suprabasal cells of the ORS, gradually lost through the isthmus leading to the infundibulum where staining is present in the basal layer, and not expressed in the IRS.[14]

Pemphigus

Pemphigus vulgaris (PV) commonly affects the scalp; however, associated hair loss is much less commonly reported. One study that performed direct immunofluorescence on 50 plucked hairs of 15 patients with pemphigus found a distinct to strong pattern of immunofluorescence of the ORS, even in subsets of patients with stable disease or clinically uninvolved scalp.[15] PV has been associated with anagen shedding with or without alopecia, and some reports exist of scarring alopecia following tufted folliculitis and secondary bacterial infection.[10,16,17]

PV is mostly associated with anagen shedding (anagen effluvium) without alopecia that presents within lesional and perilesional areas (Fig. 18.2A and B). The hairs can be easily plucked with intact root sheaths, and direct immunofluorescence reveals IgG and C3 deposits with clefting of the ORS. Following disease control, patients regrow their hair.[16]

Pemphigus vegetans, a variation of PV, rarely involves the scalp and has not been described with any particular hair loss pattern.[18] Pemphigus foliaceus (PF)–associated alopecia has been described as a nonscarring patchy alopecia that develops over severely involved erythematous scaling and crusting. This entity is thought to present as a nonscarring alopecia because desmoglein 1, the target antigen of PF, is present throughout the hair follicle but spares the follicular bulge allowing for hair regrowth.[10] Lesional scalp biopsies demonstrate subcorneal acantholysis to the infundibular epithelium, with perilesional direct immunofluorescence displaying intercellular IgG and ELISA demonstrating Dsg1 antibodies.[19]

Pemphigoid

Bullous pemphigoid has not been described as a cause of alopecia. Cicatricial pemphigoid (CP), an entity similar to bullous pemphigoid, leading to scarring alopecia in several patients was first described by Brunsting and Perry in 1957.[20] The target antigens in CP are BP180, BP230, and laminin 5, which have been found within hair follicles. Although there is consistent presence of the antigens, CP causes alopecia in only a small subset of patients. The theories behind this selectiveness include lack of antibody-antigen target binding or ubiquitous binding with varying scarring responses between patients. Histology shows dermal-epidermal separation at the basal lamina with occasional monocytes in the dermis, and salt-split skin demonstrates IgG on the epidermal side.[21]

Epidermolysis Bullosa

Alopecia universalis and occasional congenital alopecia have been described in patients with lethal acantholytic epidermolysis bullosa (EB) and EB simplex with muscular dystrophy, respectively.[22,23] In junctional and dystrophic EB, blistering of the lamina lucida and below causes inflammation leading to a cicatricial alopecia. The relationship between blister formation and trauma results in hair loss in the occipital area most commonly.[24] Of the junctional EB types, Herlitz junctional EB, non-Herlitz junctional EB, and junctional EB with pyloric atresia can lead to patchy or diffuse cicatricial alopecia.[25–27] Dystrophic EB may also result in sparse hair followed by cicatricial alopecia or folliculitis-like lesions.[28,29]

Other bullous diseases including dermatitis herpetiformis and linear IgA bullous dermatosis have not been reported to cause alopecia although they have been reported in patients with alopecia areata (AA) and Vogt-Koyanagi-Harada disease, respectively.[30,31]

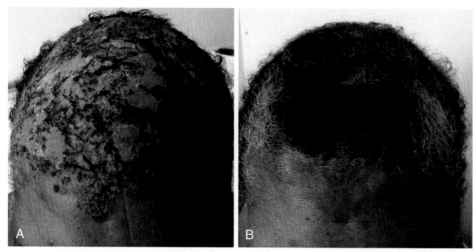

FIG. 18.2 **(A** and **B)** Pemphigus vulgaris involving the scalp. Note the extensive erosions and hemorrhagic crusts healing after treatment with complete hair regrowth. (Image courtesy of Rodrigo Pirmez MD.)

CONNECTIVE TISSUE DISEASE

Scleroderma

Scleroderma is an autoimmune disease with excessive deposition of collagen that can be divided into generalized and localized forms. Of these two forms, only localized scleroderma (morphea) is known to cause alopecia. Localized scleroderma on the scalp usually has a linear presentation and is thus termed *en coup de sabre* (ECDS) because of the resemblance to the cut from a sword. Although there is debate as to whether linear scleroderma follows Blaschko's lines, it is clear that the most common pattern for ECDS is a single vertical line adjacent to the midline of the frontal scalp and forehead.[32] However, variations of this have been described including two lines either on the same side or bilaterally, three lines on the same side, involvement of the vertex, and occiput.[32-35] Although classically a linear lesion on the scalp, ECDS has also been reported as a round atrophic patch on the occipital scalp.[36] The cicatricial alopecia and the skin involvement usually do not extend beyond the eyebrow. It is important to make the distinction between ECDS and progressive hemifacial atrophy, which is associated with more extensive atrophy and ophthalmologic and neurologic sequelae.[37] The differential diagnosis for ECDS should also include linear lesions of discoid lupus erythematosus (DLE), lichen planopilaris, and erosive pustular dermatosis of the scalp.[38]

Histologically, there are dermal sclerosis, atrophy of the eccrine glands, collagenous replacement of adipose tissue, absence of sebaceous glands but preservation of the arrector pili muscles. Transverse sections

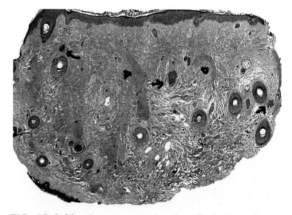

FIG. 18.3 Morphea *en coup de sabre*. On horizontal sections, there are altered follicular architecture with thickened collagen in the dermis, loss of sebaceous glands, but preserved arrector pili muscles (*triangles*). Note the atrophic follicular epithelial structures resembling telogen germinal units (*arrows*) (hematoxylin and eosin, ×10).

reveal columnar and slender follicular epithelial structures that resemble telogen germinal units (Fig. 18.3).[39] Perineural lymphocytic and plasmocytic infiltrate extending into the subcutis and fascia may also be present.[40]

Dermatomyositis

DM is an idiopathic inflammatory myopathy with classic cutaneous findings. The pathognomonic dermatologic features include Gottron's papules of the hands and a heliotrope rash around the eyes, whereas

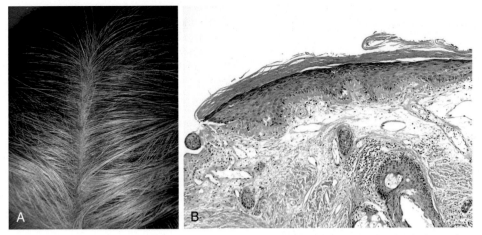

FIG. 18.4 **(A)** Dermatomyositis (DM) of the scalp: There are diffuse erythema and scaling in the scalp simulating seborrheic dermatitis. (**(A)** Image courtesy of Julio Jasso-Olivares MD.) **(B)** DM of the scalp. Note the interface dermatitis, the thick basement membrane, telangiectasia, and mucin deposition in the dermis (hematoxylin and eosin, ×10).

other characteristic features are malar rash, poikiloderma in a photosensitive distribution described as the shawl sign on the upper back and v-sign on the neck and chest, and periungual changes including telangiectasia.[41] Scalp involvement is commonly seen in DM and presents as a diffuse, erythematous, scaly, atrophic dermatosis with significant symptoms of burning and pruritus unlike lupus (Fig. 18.4A). There is a nonscarring alopecia in 33%–43% of cases.[42,43] The scalp involvement can be confused for seborrheic dermatitis or psoriasis.[42,44] Histologically, scalp-involved skin is similar to other sites showing hyperkeratosis, follicular plugging, variable epidermal atrophy, basal layer vacuolar degeneration, thickened basement membrane zone, and perivascular lymphocytic infiltrate (Fig. 18.4B).[42]

Lupus Erythematosus
LE is a chronic autoimmune inflammatory disease encompassing many disease subsets. Cutaneous manifestations can be seen in systemic lupus erythematosus (SLE) or cutaneous LE, which is further divided into acute cutaneous LE, subacute cutaneous LE, and chronic cutaneous LE. Scalp involvement with hair loss is classically described in SLE and DLE, a subtype of chronic cutaneous LE (see Chapter 3). In short, characteristic scalp lesions in DLE present as erythematous or violaceous scaling papules expanding to plaques with atrophy, follicular plugging, telangiectasia, and dyspigmentation with the end result of scarring.[45] Dermoscopy features of DLE scalp lesions include loss of follicular ostia, white patches,

branching capillaries, keratin plugs, blue-gray dots, follicular red dots, and blue-white veil.[46–49] Histologic features of DLE lesions include vacuolar interface changes, superficial and deep perivascular and periadnexal lymphocytic infiltration, keratin filling follicular ostia, pigmentary incontinence with melanophages in the papillary dermis, basement membrane thickening, and superficial and deep dermal mucin (see Chapter 3). Direct immunofluorescence shows granular deposition of immunoglobulin, primarily IgG, and C3 at the dermal-epidermal junction.[50] In contrast to DLE, SLE typically presents with a nonscarring alopecia akin to AA. The histology shows the classic histologic features of LE but with normal terminal and vellus follicular counts and deeper inflammatory infiltrates.[50,51]

GRANULOMATOUS DERMATITIS
Sarcoidosis
Sarcoidosis is a systemic granulomatous disease that can affect the skin and rarely the scalp. Scalp involvement seldom exists without other cutaneous lesions or systemic involvement.[52] Clinically, alopecia associated with sarcoidosis presents as localized areas of cicatricial alopecia with diverse morphology: erythema and scaling, an infiltrative lesion and border, indurated plaques and nodules (Fig. 18.5), superficial ulcerations, and may resemble DLE.[52,53] Two cases of nonscarring alopecia have been described, but there were no clinically apparent scalp lesions suggesting perhaps early cutaneous involvement.[54,55] Dermoscopy shows decreased

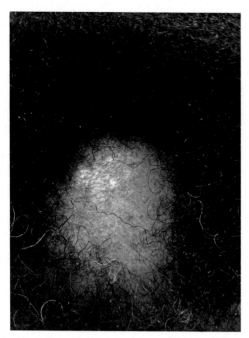

FIG. 18.5 Sarcoidosis of the scalp. There is a plaque of scarring alopecia simulating central centrifugal cicatricial alopecia. The patient had concomitant plaques on the lower legs and pulmonary involvement. (Image courtesy of Rodrigo Pirmez MD.)

hair density, absence of follicular ostia, perifollicular and follicular or diffuse orange discoloration. Perifollicular scaling, dystrophic hairs and telangiectasia can also be detected.[56] Histologically, vertical sections show sarcoidal granulomas consisting of epithelioid histiocytes surrounded by lymphocytes throughout the papillary and middermis. Horizontal sections have been reported and reveal at the level of the isthmus, destruction of follicular units by granulomas and scattered miniaturized anagen follicles surrounded by epithelioid giant cells.[56,57]

Leprosy

Leprosy is an infectious disease caused by *Mycobacterium leprae*. Scalp involvement of leprosy is rare because of the scalp's relatively higher temperature compared with other areas of the body. Although rare, alopecia has been described in patients along the whole spectrum of disease from tuberculoid leprosy to lepromatous leprosy.[58] Clinically, there are infiltrated nontender erythematous to hypopigmented plaques with nonscarring alopecia displaying classic hypoesthesia of lepromatous lesions.[59] Histology shows a dense infiltrate of lymphocytes with multinucleate giant cells forming granulomas throughout the dermis and spreading around skin adnexa, blood vessels, and nerve fibers.[58,59] Multidrug therapy can lead to partial or complete lesion resolution and hair regrowth.

MALIGNANCY

Lymphoproliferative Disorders

Mycosis fungoides (MF) and Sezary syndrome (SS), both subtypes of cutaneous T-cell lymphoma (CTCL), have been described to cause alopecia. One large retrospective analysis study reviewed 1550 cases of biopsy-proven MF or SS and queried the National Alopecia Areata Registry of 5000 patients.[60] In this study 2.5% of their population with MF/SS also had alopecia, whereas no members of the registry self-reported having MF/SS. Of these patients, 34% had patchy hair loss clinically identical to AA and 66% had alopecia within overt MF lesions. Total-body hair loss was present only in patients with SS and generalized erythroderma. Folliculotropic MF (F-MF), an uncommon variant of MF characterized by the presence of atypical T lymphocytes preferentially within the follicular epithelium, was present in some but not all patients with patchy alopecia.

Another report describes F-MF presenting on the pubis as AA both clinically and on initial biopsy but diagnosed as F-MF after continued nonresolving alopecia with new lesions and repeated biopsies.[61] Although AA universalis and CTCL-related alopecia universalis can be clinically indistinguishable with hairless smooth skin when the CTCL variant does not present with erythematous plaques, there are dermoscopic and histologic distinctions. On dermoscopy, CTCL reveals follicular or diffuse scaling with reduced follicular openings containing broken hairs, short hairs, or keratotic filiform spicules, whereas AA demonstrates yellow dots and dystrophic hairs represented by black dots, broken hairs, and exclamation mark hairs. On histology, CTCL may have loss of sebaceous glands, which are preserved in AA, and follicular mucinosis. In scalp biopsies from patients with CTCL alopecia, the epidermotropic CD4 T-cell infiltrate is noted at all follicular levels, whereas in AA it is restricted to peri- or intrabulbar CD4 T-cell infiltrate (Fig. 18.6).[62]

Alopecia Neoplastica

Alopecia neoplastica (AN) in this discussion refers to hair loss secondary to scalp metastasis of a visceral malignancy, which has been called secondary

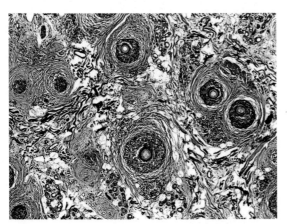

FIG. 18.6 Cutaneous T-cell lymphoma associated with alopecia areata–like hair loss. At the level of the lower follicle, most follicles are miniaturized or in telogen phase and reveal epidermotropism of the follicular epithelium with atypical lymphocytes accompanied by mucin. There are lichenoid infiltrate and wiry thin perifollicular fibrosis (hematoxylin and eosin, ×4).

AN to differentiate it from primary AN that can be used to describe cancer originating in the cutaneous scalp.[63] Since first being described in 1949,[64] AN has been reported in patients with breast cancer (ductal, intraductal, infiltrating ductal, adenocarcinoma, and scirrhous types),[65] gastrointestinal cancer (gastric and colon adenocarcinomas and singlet ring cell types),[66] pulmonary adenocarcinoma,[67] cervical squamous cell cancer,[68] and placental trophoblastic tumor.[69] Although uncommon, the presence of AN can precede and lead to the diagnosis of a primary malignancy,[67,69–71] or more commonly it is diagnosed in patients with an established history of malignancy, even after more than a decade.[72] Early lesions can present as solitary or multiple, plaques or patches, small or large, that can be easily confused for AA. Lesions may present also as cicatricial alopecia. Histology of lesional skin reveals the infiltration of tumor cells consistent with the primary malignancy throughout the dermis and atrophic or absent pilosebaceous units.[73]

MISCELLANEOUS

Mastocytosis

Cutaneous mastocytosis (CM) is a group of disorders defined by the accumulation of mast cells in the skin. CM has rarely been described to affect the scalp and cause alopecia. One case describes an irregularly shaped area of scarring alopecia on the vertex and superior scalp of a patient with no other cutaneous lesions. Histology revealed dense fibrosis in the upper dermis, decreased number of hair follicles, follicles with perifollicular fibrosis, fibrous tracts at sites of previous follicular structures, and perifollicular mixed cell infiltrate with mast cells. Staining revealed diffuse mast cells in the dermis and focally perifollicular.[74] Another case reported a patient with congenital alopecia with yellowish to brown nodules with erythematous patches in areas of scalp alopecia. Histology revealed significant hyperplasia of mast cells in the papillary dermis and around blood vessels. Patchy hair regrowth occurred during early years and further after treatment indicating a nonscarring alopecia.[75]

Postoperative

Postoperative alopecia (PA), also known as pressure alopecia, refers to hair loss primarily of the vertex and occiput due to pressure-induced hypoxia. PA was first reported in eight patients undergoing prolonged gynecologic procedures and has since been described in multiple surgical fields, most commonly after lengthy surgical procedures and immobilization.[76,77] The onset of alopecia has been described from 3 to 28 days postoperatively with hair regrowth ranging from 28 to 120 days. In the days following surgery, patients typically are symptomatic with occipital discomfort followed by edematous and crusted erosions, or may be completely asymptomatic.[78] This is followed by a patch of hair loss clinically similar to that in AA (Fig. 18.7). Although more commonly a nonscarring alopecia, studies have found PA to include a spectrum from nonscarring to scarring alopecia dependent on the duration of immobilization during surgery, correlating with duration of local scalp hypoxia.[79] Dermoscopy shows broken hairs at different length, cadaverized hairs, black dots, and yellow dots. Histology of a nonscarring PA shows all follicles in the catagen phase with no follicular disruption or atrophy and no perivascular, periadnexal, or peribulbar infiltrates. Apoptotic bodies are seen in the follicular epithelium. Pigment casts are also seen in the follicular infundibulum.[78] The natural course of PA may result in complete resolution or permanent alopecia dependent on the severity of the initial insult. To help prevent PA, it is important that physicians are familiar with this entity and perform periodic patient repositioning during surgery or other times of prolonged immobilization.

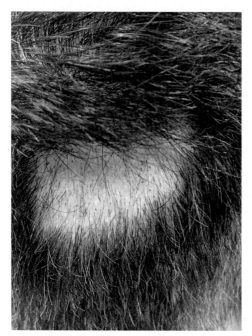

FIG. 18.7 Pressure-induced alopecia after prolonged orthopedic surgery. The patch resembles the patches of alopecia areata or trichotillomania. The broken hairs are visible on clinical examination.

Graft-Versus-Host Disease

The development of alopecia after bone marrow transplant is most commonly associated with use of the chemotherapeutic agents (discussed in Chapter 5) used to prepare for transplant, but graft-versus-host disease (GVHD) in itself has also been shown to be associated with alopecia.[80] The development of AA in GVHD is well established and is in accordance with the dysregulation of immune mechanisms and may present in acute and chronic GVHD.[80-82] According to the NIH criteria for clinical trials in GVHD, new onset of scarring or nonscarring scalp alopecia, after recovery from chemotherapy, is considered a distinctive feature that may be seen in chronic GVHD.[83] Nevertheless, there are few reports in the literature detailing the clinical and histologic presentation.[84]

The presence of alopecia after bone marrow transplant can cause a significant impact on quality of life for an individual, and reaching an accurate diagnosis, whether reversible or irreversible hair loss, is important for the patient and can be reached with a combination of patient history, physical examination, and histologic examination.

REFERENCES

1. Sperling LC, Sinclair RD, Shabrawi-Caelen LE. Alopecias. In: Bolognia JL, Jorrizo JL, Schaffer JV, eds. *Dermatology.* 3rd ed. 2012.
2. Wechalekar AD, Gillmore JD, Hawkins PN. Systemic amyloidosis. *Lancet.* 2016;387(10038):2641–2654.
3. Wong CK. Mucocutaneous manifestations in systemic amyloidosis. *Clin Dermatol.* 1990;8(2):7–12.
4. Miteva M, Wei E, Milikowski C, Tosti A. Alopecia in systemic amyloidosis: trichoscopic-pathologic correlation. *Int J Trichol.* 2015;7(4):176–178.
5. Wheeler GE, Barrows GH. Alopecia universalis. A manifestation of occult amyloidosis and multiple myeloma. *Arch Dermatol.* 1981;117(12):815–816.
6. Hunt SJ, Caserio RJ, Abell E. Primary systemic amyloidosis causing diffuse alopecia by telogen arrest. *Arch Dermatol.* 1991;127(7):1067–1068.
7. Lutz ME, Pittelkow MR. Progressive generalized alopecia due to systemic amyloidosis. *J Am Acad Dermatol.* 2002; 46(3):434–436.
8. Renker T, Haneke E, Rocken C, Borradori L. Systemic light-chain amyloidosis revealed by progressive nail involvement, diffuse alopecia and sicca syndrome: report of an unusual case with a review of the literature. *Dermatology.* 2014;228(2):97–102.
9. Barja J, Pineyro F, Almagro M, et al. Systemic amyloidosis with an exceptional cutaneous presentation. *Dermatol Online J.* 2013;19(1):11.
10. Miteva M, Murrell DF, Tosti A. Hair loss in autoimmune cutaneous bullous disorders. *Dermatol Clin.* 2011;29(3):503–509. xi.
11. Chuang YH, Dean D, Allen J, Dawber R, Wojnarowska F. Comparison between the expression of basement membrane zone antigens of human interfollicular epidermis and anagen hair follicle using indirect immunofluorescence. *Br J Dermatol.* 2003;149(2):274–281.
12. Joubeh S, Mori O, Owaribe K, Hashimoto T. Immunofluorescence analysis of the basement membrane zone components in human anagen hair follicles. *Exp Dermatol.* 2003;12(4):365–370.
13. Kurzen H, Moll I, Moll R, et al. Compositionally different desmosomes in the various compartments of the human hair follicle. *Differentiation.* 1998;63(5):295–304.
14. Wu H, Stanley JR, Cotsarelis G. Desmoglein isotype expression in the hair follicle and its cysts correlates with type of keratinization and degree of differentiation. *J Invest Dermatol.* 2003;120(6):1052–1057.
15. Schaerer L, Trueb RM. Direct immunofluorescence of plucked hair in pemphigus. *Arch Dermatol.* 2003; 139(2):228–229.
16. Delmonte S, Semino MT, Parodi A, Rebora A. Normal anagen effluvium: a sign of pemphigus vulgaris. *Br J Dermatol.* 2000;142(6):1244–1245.
17. Petronic-Rosic V, Krunic A, Mijuskovic M, Vesic S. Tufted hair folliculitis: a pattern of scarring alopecia? *J Am Acad Dermatol.* 1999;41(1):112–114.

18. Danopoulou I, Stavropoulos P, Stratigos A, et al. Pemphigus vegetans confined to the scalp. *Int J Dermatol.* 2006; 45(8):1008–1009.

19. Mlynek A, Bar M, Bauer A, Meurer M. Juvenile pemphigus foliaceus associated with severe nonscarring alopecia. *Br J Dermatol.* 2009;161(2):472–474.

20. Brunsting LA, Perry HO. Benign pemphigold; a report of seven cases with chronic, scarring, herpetiform plaques about the head and neck. *AMA Arch Derm.* 1957;75(4):489–501.

21. Ball S, Walkden V, Wojnarowska F. Cicatricial pemphigoid rarely involves the scalp. *Australas J Dermatol.* 1998;39(4): 258–260.

22. Jonkman MF, Pasmooij AM, Pasmans SG, et al. Loss of desmoplakin tail causes lethal acantholytic epidermolysis bullosa. *Am J Hum Genet.* 2005;77(4):653–660.

23. Yin J, Ren Y, Lin Z, Wang H, Zhou Y, Yang Y. Compound heterozygous PLEC mutations in a patient of consanguineous parentage with epidermolysis bullosa simplex with muscular dystrophy and diffuse alopecia. *Int J Dermatol.* 2015;54(2):185–187.

24. Tosti A, Duque-Estrada B, Murrell DF. Alopecia in epidermolysis bullosa. *Dermatol Clin.* 2010;28(1):165–169.

25. Laimer M, Lanschuetzer CM, Diem A, Bauer JW. Herlitz junctional epidermolysis bullosa. *Dermatol Clin.* 2010; 28(1):55–60.

26. Hintner H, Wolff K. Generalized atrophic benign epidermolysis bullosa. *Arch Dermatol.* 1982;118(6):375–384.

27. Dang N, Klingberg S, Rubin AI, et al. Differential expression of pyloric atresia in junctional epidermolysis bullosa with ITGB4 mutations suggests that pyloric atresia is due to factors other than the mutations and not predictive of a poor outcome: three novel mutations and a review of the literature. *Acta Derm Venereol.* 2008;88(5): 438–448.

28. Horn HM, Tidman MJ. The clinical spectrum of dystrophic epidermolysis bullosa. *Br J Dermatol.* 2002;146(2): 267–274.

29. Fan YM, Yang YP, Li SF. Medical genetics: sporadic dystrophic epidermolysis bullosa with albopapuloid and prurigo- and folliculitis-like lesions. *Int J Dermatol.* 2009;48(8):855–857.

30. Reunala T, Collin P. Diseases associated with dermatitis herpetiformis. *Br J Dermatol.* 1997;136(3):315–318.

31. Yanagihara S, Mizuno N, Naruse A, Tateishi C, Tsuruta D, Ishii M. Linear immunoglobulin A/immunoglobulin G bullous dermatosis associated with Vogt-Koyanagi-Harada disease. *J Dermatol.* 2011;38(8):798–801.

32. Soma Y, Fujimoto M. Frontoparietal scleroderma (en coup de sabre) following Blaschko's lines. *J Am Acad Dermatol.* 1998;38(2 Pt 2):366–368.

33. Dilley JJ, Perry HO. Bilateral linear scleroderma en coup de sabre. *Arch Dermatol.* 1968;97(6):688–689.

34. McKenna DB, Benton EC. A tri-linear pattern of scleroderma 'en coup de sabre' following Blaschko's lines. *Clin Exp Dermatol.* 1999;24(6):467–468.

35. Asano Y, Ihn H, Tamaki K. An unusual manifestation of linear scleroderma 'en coup de sabre' on the vertex and frontoparietal regions. *Clin Exp Dermatol.* 2007;32(6):758–759.

36. Saceda-Corralo D, Nusbaum AG, Romanelli P, Miteva M. A case of circumscribed scalp morphea with perineural lymphocytes on pathology. *Skin Appendage Disord.* 2017;3:175–178.

37. Gambichler T, Kreuter A, Hoffmann K, Bechara FG, Altmeyer P, Jansen T. Bilateral linear scleroderma "en coup de sabre" associated with facial atrophy and neurological complications. *BMC Dermatol.* 2001;1:9.

38. Starace M, Loi C, Bruni F, et al. Erosive pustular dermatosis of the scalp: clinical, trichoscopic, and histopathologic features of 20 cases. *J Am Acad Dermatol.* 2017;76(6):1109–1114. e1102.

39. Pierre-Louis M, Sperling LC, Wilke MS, Hordinsky MK. Distinctive histopathologic findings in linear morphea (en coup de sabre) alopecia. *J Cutan Pathol.* 2013;40(6): 580–584.

40. Goh C, Biswas A, Goldberg LJ. Alopecia with perineural lymphocytes: a clue to linear scleroderma en coup de sabre. *J Cutan Pathol.* 2012;39(5):518–520.

41. Callen JP. Dermatomyositis. *Lancet.* 2000;355(9197): 53–57.

42. Kasteler JS, Callen JP. Scalp involvement in dermatomyositis. Often overlooked or misdiagnosed. *JAMA.* 1994;272(24):1939–1941.

43. Tilstra JS, Prevost N, Khera P, English 3rd JC. Scalp dermatomyositis revisited. *Arch Dermatol.* 2009;145(9): 1062–1063.

44. Moghadam-Kia S, Franks Jr AG. Autoimmune disease and hair loss. *Dermatol Clin.* 2013;31(1):75–91.

45. Trueb RM. Involvement of scalp and nails in lupus erythematosus. *Lupus.* 2010;19(9):1078–1086.

46. Cervantes J, Hafeez F, Miteva M. Blue-white veil as novel dermatoscopic feature in discoid lupus erythematosus in 2 African-American patients. *Skin Appendage Disord.* 2017;3:211–214.

47. Duque-Estrada B, Tamler C, Sodre CT, Barcaui CB, Pereira FB. Dermoscopy patterns of cicatricial alopecia resulting from discoid lupus erythematosus and lichen planopilaris. *An Bras Dermatol.* 2010;85(2):179–183.

48. Tosti A, Torres F, Misciali C, et al. Follicular red dots: a novel dermoscopic pattern observed in scalp discoid lupus erythematosus. *Arch Dermatol.* 2009;145(12): 1406–1409.

49. Lanuti E, Miteva M, Romanelli P, Tosti A. Trichoscopy and histopathology of follicular keratotic plugs in scalp discoid lupus erythematosus. *Int J Trichol.* 2012;4(1):36–38.

50. Trueb RM. Hair and nail involvement in lupus erythematosus. *Clin Dermatol.* 2004;22(2):139–147.

51. Ye Y, Zhao Y, Gong Y, et al. Non-scarring patchy alopecia in patients with systemic lupus erythematosus differs from that of alopecia areata. *Lupus.* 2013;22(14): 1439–1445.

52. Katta R, Nelson B, Chen D, Roenigk H. Sarcoidosis of the scalp: a case series and review of the literature. *J Am Acad Dermatol*. 2000;42(4):690–692.

53. Henderson CL, Lafleur L, Sontheimer RD. Sarcoidal alopecia as a mimic of discoid lupus erythematosus. *J Am Acad Dermatol*. 2008;59(1):143–145.

54. Greer KE, Harman Jr LE, Kayne AL. Unusual cutaneous manifestations of sarcoidosis. *South Med J*. 1977;70(6):666–668.

55. Smith SR, Kendall MJ, Kondratowicz GM. Sarcoidosis–a cause of steroid responsive total alopecia. *Postgrad Med J*. 1986;62(725):205–207.

56. Torres F, Tosti A, Misciali C, Lorenzi S. Trichoscopy as a clue to the diagnosis of scalp sarcoidosis. *Int J Dermatol*. 2011;50(3):358–361.

57. La Placa M, Vincenzi C, Misciali C, Tosti A. Scalp sarcoidosis with systemic involvement. *J Am Acad Dermatol*. 2008;59(5 suppl):S126–S127.

58. Macedo RB, Santos T, Ramos PB, Takano DM, Leal VS. Leprosy on the scalp. *An Bras Dermatol*. 2016;91(5 suppl 1):69–71.

59. Jadhav P, Zawar V. Interesting patchy alopecia. *Int J Trichol*. 2015;7(2):74–76.

60. Bi MY, Curry JL, Christiano AM, et al. The spectrum of hair loss in patients with mycosis fungoides and Sezary syndrome. *J Am Acad Dermatol*. 2011;64(1):53–63.

61. Iorizzo M, El Shabrawi Caelen L, Vincenzi C, Misciali C, Tosti A. Folliculotropic mycosis fungoides masquerading as alopecia areata. *J Am Acad Dermatol*. 2010;63(2):e50–e52.

62. Miteva M, El Shabrawi-Caelen L, Fink-Puches R, et al. Alopecia universalis associated with cutaneous T cell lymphoma. *Dermatology*. 2014;229(2):65–69.

63. Cohen PR. Primary alopecia neoplastica versus secondary alopecia neoplastica: a new classification for neoplasm-associated scalp hair loss. *J Cutan Pathol*. 2009;36(8):917–918.

64. Ronchese F. Alopecia due to metastases from adenocarcinoma of the breast; report of a case. *Arch Derm Syphilol*. 1949;59(3):329–332.

65. Conner KB, Cohen PR. Cutaneous metastasis of breast carcinoma presenting as alopecia neoplastica. *South Med J*. 2009;102(4):385–389.

66. Kim JH, Kim MJ, Sim WY, Lew BL. Alopecia neoplastica due to gastric adenocarcinoma metastasis to the scalp, presenting as alopecia: a case report and literature review. *Ann Dermatol*. 2014;26(5):624–627.

67. Cohen PR. Lung cancer-associated scalp hair loss: a rare cause of secondary alopecia neoplastica. *Cutis*. 2013;92(5):E7–E8.

68. Chung JJ, Namiki T, Johnson DW. Cervical cancer metastasis to the scalp presenting as alopecia neoplastica. *Int J Dermatol*. 2007;46(2):188–189.

69. Yuen YF, Lewis EJ, Larson JT, Wilke MS, Rest EB, Zachary CB. Scalp metastases mimicking alopecia areata. First case report of placental site trophoblastic tumor presenting as cutaneous metastasis. *Dermatol Surg*. 1998;24(5):587–591.

70. Carson HJ, Pellettiere EV, Lack E. Alopecia neoplastica simulating alopecia areata and antedating the detection of primary breast carcinoma. *J Cutan Pathol*. 1994;21(1):67–70.

71. Martin J, Ross JB. Alopecia totalis as a presentation of cutaneous metastasis (alopecia neoplastica). *Int J Dermatol*. 1983;22(8):487–489.

72. Haas N, Hauptmann S. Alopecia neoplastica due to metastatic breast carcinoma vs. extramammary Paget's disease: mimicry in epidermotropic carcinoma. *J Eur Acad Dermatol Venereol*. 2004;18(6):708–710.

73. Cohen I, Levy E. SCHREIBER H: Alopecia neoplastica due to breast carcinoma. *Arch Dermatol*. 1961;84:490–492.

74. Xu X, Solky B, Elenitsas R, Cotsarelis G. Scarring alopecia associated with mastocytosis. *J Cutan Pathol*. 2003;30(9):561–565.

75. Kim CR, Kim HJ, Jung MY, et al. Cutaneous mastocytosis associated with congenital alopecia. *Am J Dermatopathol*. 2012;34(5):529–532.

76. Abel RR, Lewis GM. Postoperative (pressure) alopecia. *Arch Dermatol*. 1960;81:34–42.

77. Davies KE, Yesudian P. Pressure alopecia. *Int J Trichol*. 2012;4(2):64–68.

78. Hanly AJ, Jorda M, Badiavas E, Valencia I, Elgart GW. Postoperative pressure-induced alopecia: report of a case and discussion of the role of apoptosis in non-scarring alopecia. *J Cutan Pathol*. 1999;26(7):357–361.

79. Lwason NW, Mills NL, Ochsner JL. Occipital alopecia following cardiopulmonary bypass. *J Thorac Cardiovasc Surg*. 1976;71(3):342–347.

80. Bresters D, Wanders DC, Louwerens M, Ball LM, Fiocco M, van Doorn R. Permanent diffuse alopecia after haematopoietic stem cell transplantation in childhood. *Bone Marrow Transpl*. 2017.

81. Sanli H, Kusak F, Arat M, Ekmekci P, Ilhan O. Simultaneous onset of chronic graft versus host disease and alopecia areata following allogeneic haematopoietic cell transplantation. *Acta Derm Venereol*. 2004;84(1):86–87.

82. Zuo RC, Naik HB, Steinberg SM, et al. Risk factors and characterization of vitiligo and alopecia areata in patients with chronic graft-vs-host disease. *JAMA Dermatol*. 2015;151(1):23–32.

83. Jagasia MH, Greinix HT, Arora M, et al. National institutes of health consensus development project on criteria for clinical trials in chronic graft-versus-host disease: I. The 2014 diagnosis and staging working group report. *Biol Blood Marrow Transpl*. 2015;21(3):389–401. e381.

84. Basilio FM, Brenner FM, Werner B, Rastelli GJ. Clinical and histological study of permanent alopecia after bone marrow transplantation. *An Bras Dermatol*. 2015;90(6):814–821.

CHAPTER 19

Hair Loss in Children

KATE E. OBERLIN, MD • LAWRENCE A. SCHACHNER, MD

INTRODUCTION

This chapter exhibits the most common causes and presentation of pediatric alopecia. The characteristic manifestations of disease, trichoscopy, and pathology are highlighted to enhance the diagnosis and management of hair loss in children. Pediatric alopecia can be categorized into hair disorders presenting with patchy or diffuse alopecia, and additionally, with and without increased hair shaft fragility to help delineate the presenting etiology. Hair shaft abnormalities can be caused by either genetic abnormalities or acquired through external physical injury. Etiology can be deduced by the history, by demographics of the patient, and, ultimately, by a thorough cutaneous and hair examination. A hair pull test and subsequent trichoscopy can be performed to look for characteristic findings. Trichoscopy is a noninvasive bedside tool that can be used for rapid hair loss diagnosis based on characteristic scalp and hair shaft findings. A punch biopsy may be necessary if the above information is inconclusive; however, it is rarely performed in children. Recently, a pediatric severity of alopecia score was implemented for the purpose of clinical monitoring and research.[1] The unique trichoscopic findings of pediatric alopecia are presented, as well as clinical clues and histologic findings to formulate the accurate diagnosis and optimize patient care.

PATCHY ALOPECIA IN CHILDHOOD

A vast array of diagnoses can present as patchy alopecia in childhood, which is the most typical presentation of alopecia in the pediatric population. The most common causes include alopecia areata, trichotillomania (TTM), temporal triangular alopecia (TTA), tinea capitis, aplasia cutis congenita (ACC), and traction alopecia. A recent study, based on 2800 children seen in the dermatology clinics in Jordan, reported tinea capitis as the most common cause of hair loss (40%), followed by alopecia areata (26.2%), and telogen effluvium (17.6%).[2] Conversely, primary cicatricial alopecia is rare in children. Clinical presentation, family history, association with abnormalities of the teeth and nails, and other signs of abnormal growth and development can point to the correct diagnosis. Trichoscopy is fundamental in this age group, as it is a noninvasive practical tool and can be used, alongside light microscopy, for the diagnosis of hair shaft disorders.

Alopecia Areata

Alopecia areata is an autoimmune condition resulting in nonscarring alopecic patches, which usually remain localized. However, the patches can wax and wane, remit, or result in progressive, complete alopecia of the scalp, known as alopecia areata totalis, or the entire body, known as alopecia areata universalis. The clinical findings and management of alopecia areata are discussed in detail in Chapter 4. Here we focus on the specifics in children.

Age

Children of any age may be affected. Furthermore, alopecia areata can even present in the neonatal period as congenital disease with either patchy or diffuse alopecia apparent at birth.[3]

Association with comorbidities

Alopecia areata is an autoimmune disease and can present with additional autoimmune manifestations. The most common autoimmune comorbidities include vitiligo, psoriasis, thyroid disease, juvenile idiopathic arthritis, and atopic dermatitis.[4,5] Children with alopecia areata may particularly be at risk for thyroid abnormalities if they have a medical history of Down syndrome, a personal history of atopy, a family history of thyroid disease, or clinical findings that are suggestive of thyroid dysfunction.[6]

Clinical presentation

The most common presentation of alopecia areata is a solitary alopecic patch (Fig. 19.1). The patch can occur on any hair-bearing surface such as the eyebrows; however, the scalp is the most common location. The ophiasis pattern of alopecia presents with balding of the posterior occipital scalp in a bandlike distribution and can be progressive in nature. A diffuse form of alopecia areata can also manifest with more generalized scalp

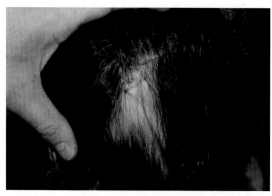

FIG. 19.1 A pediatric patient with alopecia areata demonstrating a well-demarcated alopecic patch on the vertex of the scalp.

TABLE 19.1
Treatment Options for Alopecia Areata

Topical	Corticosteroids
	Minoxidil
	Immunotherapy with contact sensitizers including diphenylcyclopropenone and squalene acid dibutyl ester
	Irritants including anthralin and retinoids
	Prostaglandin analogues
	Janus kinase inhibitors (ruxolitinib)
	Calcineurin inhibitors
	Excimer laser (308 nm)
Intralesional	Corticosteroids
Systemic	Corticosteroids (pulsed and daily regimens)
	Phototherapy
	Immunosuppressive agents (methotrexate, azathioprine, and cyclosporine)
	Janus kinase inhibitors (tofacitinib)

involvement, however, with a more subtle presentation, lacking the discrete alopecic patches. Nail changes may also be seen and commonly involve gridlike pitting of the nails, in addition to longitudinal ridging, and trachyonychia (rough, sandpaper nails).

Trichoscopy

To clinch the diagnosis, clinical history and trichoscopic findings are paramount. Trichoscopy demonstrates characteristic *"exclamation mark"* hairs with proximal tapering, broken hairs, short regrowing hairs, and black dots (which are a type of cadaverized hairs). Yellow dots, which correspond to empty follicles with dilated infundibulum filled with sebum and keratin, are less common in prepubertal children.[7]

Pathology

In the acute stage, histology reveals a characteristic peribulbar lymphocytic infiltrate, known as a *"swarm-of-bees"* appearance. The subacute stage is characterized by increased telogen count, and the chronic stage shows predominance of vellus follicles and nanogen follicles.

Management

Management of pediatric alopecia areata is particularly challenging given the early onset and chronic course. For instance, intralesional corticosteroid injections are the first-line therapy for patchy alopecia areata in adults; however, they are not suitable for young children because of fear of injections and needles and can be used only in some cases after application of topical anesthetic creams. A wait-and-see approach can be offered, particularly in very young children.

Table 19.1 summarizes the treatment approach in alopecia areata in children.[8,9]

Trichotillomania

TTM is a hair disorder caused by the compulsion to pull out one's own hair and is performed either consciously or subconsciously. The scalp is the most common site of involvement; however, the eyebrows, eyelashes, and body hair may also be affected by the patient plucking or rubbing the areas.

Age

TTM is seen in all age groups; however, females in the prepubertal age range predominate.

Association with comorbidities

Contributing psychosocial factors must be explored with the pediatrician. Additionally, both onychophagia and trichophagia are more common in individuals who have TTM; the chewing behavior of trichophagia can even lead to the formation of trichobezoars, a potentially life-threatening condition due to gastrointestinal dysfunction.[10]

Clinical presentation

TTM manifests as an irregular or rectangular alopecic patch and favors the frontal and vertex scalp, often more common favoring the side of the patient's dominant handedness.[10,11] On gross clinical examination,

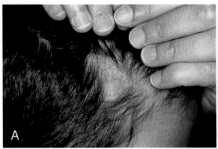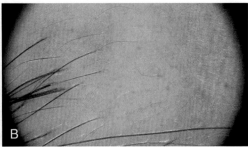

FIG. 19.2 **(A)** Temporal triangular alopecia manifesting with a well-defined, triangular alopecic patch in the frontotemporal scalp. **(B)** Trichoscopy of temporal triangular alopecia demonstrating upright regrowing hairs, vellus hairs, and pigtail hairs with peripheral terminal hairs. (Image courtesy of Giselle Martins, MD.)

alopecic patches with hairs of variable lengths and thickness may be observed, and most commonly seen is the tonsure pattern (Friar Tuck sign). The hair pull test is negative.

Trichoscopy

Broken hairs are a common feature, although this finding may also be seen in both alopecia areata and tinea capitis.[12] Coiled hairs may be seen in TTM and again are also seen in tinea capitis. Coiled hairs are the result of hair shaft fractures due to pulling; the residual distal part of the hair may then contract and coil back to the scalp.[12] Other trichoscopic findings include *flame hairs*, which are wavy and cone-shaped hair residues leftover after the pulling of anagen hairs; the *v-sign*, which refers to two hairs emerging from a single follicular opening that are broken at an equal level; and *tulip hairs*, which are short hairs with darker, flower-shaped ends, possibly due to diagonal fractures caused by pulling.[12] The *"hair powder" sign* may also be seen as hair shafts are damaged by mechanical forces and leave a sprinkled "hair powder" configuration.[12]

Pathology

Histologic examination reveals increased catagen/telogen count, trichomalacia, and pigmented casts.[13]

Management

Treatment is aimed at prevention and amelioration of stress-induced factors; therapy with systemic medications may be necessary in severe cases with input from psychiatry. In children, a referral to behavioral psychology is usually the first-line therapy. TTM is further discussed in Chapter 7.

Temporal Triangular Alopecia

TTA, or congenital triangular alopecia, is a nonscarring, localized alopecic process that presents in childhood.

Age

Most cases present in early childhood and are sporadic in inheritance. Yamakazi et al. reviewed 52 cases of TTA and found that the most common age of presentation was between 2 and 9 years, with equal gender predilection, and found that 3 cases occurred with a familial precedent.[14]

Association with comorbidities

Yamakazi et al. also found that four cases of TTA were associated with phakomatosis pigmentovascularis.[14] In 2000, Kim et al. additionally reported 3 cases of TTA in association with phakomatosis pigmentovascularis; an underlying pathogenesis or association remains to be deduced.[15]

Clinical presentation

TTA presents with a well-circumscribed, triangular alopecic patch in the frontotemporal scalp (Fig. 19.2A). The alopecia is nonscarring and usually located in a unilateral distribution. Vellus hairs may be observed in the patch. The most common clinical misdiagnosis includes alopecia areata, followed by TTM, traction alopecia, and congenital aplasia cutis.[16]

Trichoscopy

Trichoscopy is a simple tool to allow for the differentiation and conclusion of the diagnosis. Trichoscopy reveals follicular openings with upright regrowing hairs, vellus hairs, and pigtail hairs surrounded by a peripheral margin of terminal hairs (Fig. 19.2B).[17] No exclamation mark hairs or yellow or black dots should be present, which would favor the alternative diagnosis of alopecia areata.[16]

Pathology

TTA is clinically diagnosed; however, for a challenging case, histopathology can be pursued and will demonstrate miniaturized hair follicles and an absence of terminal hairs; the total number of follicles should be preserved.[14]

Management

Parents should be reassured about the nonprogressive nature of TTA; however, the condition will persist throughout life.

Aplasia Cutis Congenita

ACC is a localized, congenital absence of skin, readily identifiable at birth.

Clinical presentation

ACC can be diagnosed clinically as a well-defined circular atrophic lesion sometimes covered by a thin membrane.[10] Furthermore, ACC may occur in conjunction with the so-called *hair collar sign*. The *"hair collar sign"* was first described by Commens et al. in 1989 as a ring of dark, terminal hair surrounding an alopecic patch on the scalp; the two initial lesions were also associated with ectopic neural tissue.[18] It is imperative to perform imaging before obtaining a biopsy, as the lesions may be associated with neural tissue.

Association with comorbidities

After making the diagnosis, imaging should be performed to rule out any underlying connection. ACC with the *"hair collar sign"* has been associated with encephaloceles, meningoceles, and soft tissue and bony defects; thus, imaging is vital for optimal management.[19,20] Additionally, the presence of encephaloceles and meningoceles producing abnormal shearing forces is thought to drive the pathogenesis behind the hypertrophic peripheral tuft of hair by causing the developing follicles to point outward, away from the defect.[21]

Trichoscopy

Trichoscopy of the lesion also serves as a clue to the diagnosis and, alongside the clinical presentation, makes a biopsy unnecessary in most cases. In a retrospective analysis of five patients, Rakowska et al. demonstrated that the trichoscopic features of ACC included elongated hair bulbs visible through the semitranslucent epidermis, and were displayed in a radial configuration, which were observed at the periphery of the lesion.[17] The central parts of the lesion showed absence of follicular openings, but demonstrated prominent vasculature corresponding to the presence of skin atrophy; this finding was highly specific for ACC.[17] The differential diagnosis includes nevus sebaceus, which is distinguished on trichoscopy by the pattern of yellow dots not associated with hair follicles.[22]

Pathology

Histologic examination will show absence of the epidermis and dermal appendages and decreased elastic tissue.

Management

Lastly, the prognosis of ACC varies depending on the presence and type of neural tissue connection and associated intracranial abnormalities. Most cases, however, heal with only minor cosmetic complications.

Tinea Capitis

Tinea capitis is a cutaneous infection caused most commonly by dermatophyte fungi of the *Trichophyton* and *Microsporum* species.

Age

Tinea capitis affects mostly preadolescent children, with most cases occurring in children aged 4–7 years.

Clinical presentation

Tinea capitis manifests as scaly, localized alopecic patches, and occasionally, robust inflammation can result in the presence of a boggy subcutaneous abscess, known as a *kerion*.[10] The classic clinical triad consists of alopecia, scaling, and lymphadenopathy in the cervical, postauricular, or occipital nodes.

Trichoscopy

In a study by Amer et al., the trichoscopic findings of tinea capitis, in contrast to alopecia areata, were reviewed; patients with tinea capitis were found to have comma hairs, zigzag hairs, black dots, Morse code hairs, and corkscrew hairs, from most to least common, respectively.[23]

Comma hairs are considered specific for the diagnosis of tinea capitis and have been observed both in Caucasian and African children, whereas corkscrew hairs have been reported only in African children.[17,24] Both *zigzag* and *corkscrew hairs* are thought to be variations of the comma hair. The comma hair has a sharp slanting end, and homogenous pigmentation of the hair shaft is thought to be due to cracking and bending caused by the infiltration of hyphae.[24,25] *Morse code hairs* are seen as irregularly interrupted hairs with normally pigmented and paler narrowed intervals on trichoscopy and are thought to be caused by fungal penetration.[23] Similar to alopecia areata, broken hairs and coiled hairs may also be demonstrated as well.[12] Fig. 19.3 highlights the unique characteristics among the aforementioned hair types to help identify their presence on scalp examination.[23]

Management

A culture should be used to delineate the species for appropriate antifungal therapy. Potassium hydroxide examination of the hairs on microscopic examination may also be used for the visualization of hyphae

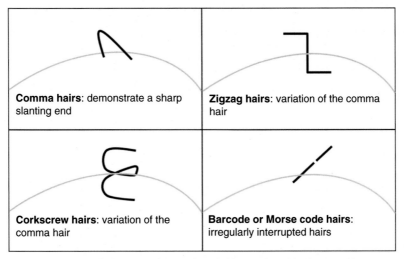

FIG. 19.3 Schematic of the various hair types found in tinea capitis.

and spores; however, it is not always reliable. Wood's lamp examination should be performed for findings of characteristic fluorescence (hair shafts infested with *Microsporum* spp. fluoresce in green). Empiric treatment should be initiated while awaiting culture results; griseofulvin at 20–25 mg/kg/daily for a period of at least 6–8 weeks is considered first-line therapy, particularly for *Microsporum* cases. Newer data suggest that terbinafine can be used with success for shorter durations in children "older than 4 years of age diagnosed with tinea capitis due to *Trichophyton* spp."[26] Tinea capitis is further reviewed in Chapter 20.

Traction Alopecia

Traction alopecia is hair loss due to excessive pulling or force due to tight hairstyles, most commonly demonstrated along the hairline of the scalp as marginal traction alopecia. However, a nonmarginal patchy variant also exists. This condition is more common in black females because of specific hairstyles used. In a survey conducted by Wright et al., more than 200 African-American girls, aged 1–15 years, were questioned regarding their hair care practices and then analyzed according to their specific hair condition; wearing cornrows in the last year and pulling chemically straightened hairstyles were both key risk factors significantly associated with the development of traction alopecia.[27] Hairstyle-related pulling forces cause mechanical damage to the hair follicles, resulting in inflammation that can present as follicular papules and pustules in areas of tension in acute traction alopecia.[28] If the pulling force is discontinued at this stage, the hair has a chance to regrow.

Clinical presentation

The periphery of the scalp is most commonly involved, particularly the frontal, temporal, and preauricular area. Gross examination will show lack of terminal hairs in the alopecic area and demonstrate, instead, preservation of the fine vellus hairs (the fringe sign).[29]

Trichoscopy

Trichoscopy may reveal perifollicular erythema, pustules, scaling, and broken hairs in the early phases.[30] Hair casts made of whitish yellow keratin cylinders may encircle the hair shaft and are freely movable; these casts can mimic the nits of pediculosis capitis and idiopathic hair casts in children.[30,31]

Management

After the clinical diagnosis is made, the majority of therapy rests on addressing specific grooming habits. Treatment of traction alopecia requires discontinuation of hairstyles that exert tension; loose and natural hairstyles should be used to prevent follicular destruction and scarring.

Pressure-Induced Alopecia

Pressure-induced alopecia, also known as postoperative alopecia when associated with surgery, may be demonstrated in children with prolonged bed rest, surgical intervention, and use of certain medical devices. The posterior scalp is most commonly involved; some patients have complete resolution with time, whereas others develop a scarring, permanent alopecia. There is a direct correlation between the length of surgery and the development of permanent alopecia; hypoxemia and hypotension may be exacerbating factors.[32]

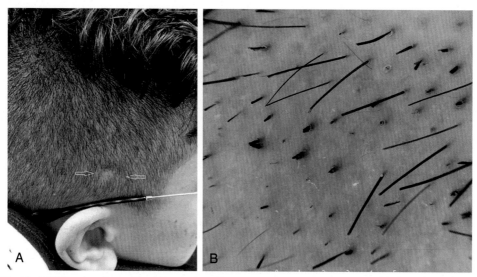

FIG. 19.4 **(A)** A young boy with a history of neck surgery developed small symmetric patches of hair loss on the bilateral parietal scalp at the site of the halo brace (*arrows*). **(B)** Trichoscopy shows dystrophic hairs at various lengths (handyscope, ×10). (Image courtesy of Mariya Miteva, MD.)

Postoperative alopecia can be prevented by frequent repositioning, both intraoperatively and on recovery. An example of pressure-induced alopecia is demonstrated with alopecia resulting from pressure due to a halo brace (Fig. 19.4A). Trichoscopy reveals dystrophic hairs at various lengths (Fig. 19.4B).

SCARRING ALOPECIAS

Although patchy scarring alopecias are rare in childhood, a variety of conditions has been reported in the literature.

Frontal Fibrosing Alopecia

Recently, scarring alopecia secondary to frontal fibrosing alopecia was reported in three children by Atarquine et al.[33] A set of twin sisters demonstrated frontotemporal symmetric and progressive alopecia beginning at age 5, and in association with follicular facial papules; additionally, a 7-year-old girl with a frontotemporal alopecic band and alopecia of the eyebrows had a biopsy-proven case of lichen planopilaris.[33] All three children were treated with monthly intralesional steroid injections with a favorable course.[33]

Discoid Lupus Erythematosus

Similarly, the diagnosis of discoid lupus erythematosus (DLE) is uncommon in the pediatric population with less than 3% of patients developing the disease before age 10. DLE in children manifests with characteristic alopecia of the scalp with keratotic scaling, loss of follicular openings, and enlarged branching vessels on dermoscopy.[34,35]

Lichen Planopilaris

Lichen planopilaris is a type of cicatricial alopecia that rarely presents in children. A retrospective study by Christensen et al. reviewed four cases of biopsy-proven lichen planopilaris in children, with ages ranging from 13 to 16 years.[36] Perifollicular scaling and scarring were the most common manifestations in the scalp (Fig. 19.5A). Trichoscopy reveals loss of follicular openings, perifollicular erythema, and peripilar casts (Fig. 19.5B). The authors further advised that lichen planopilaris can mimic alopecia areata in this population given the relatively asymptomatic presentation and subtle cutaneous findings; first-line therapy includes potent topical corticosteroids or intralesional steroids.[36]

Central Centrifugal Cicatricial Alopecia

In 2017, Eginli et al. reported six adolescents with biopsy-proven central centrifugal cicatricial alopecia (CCCA) between the ages of 14 and 19 years.[37] Interestingly, five of the six patients had scalp symptoms including tender papules and pruritus; additionally, five of the six patients also had a family history of CCCA.[37] These authors highlighted that although rare in the

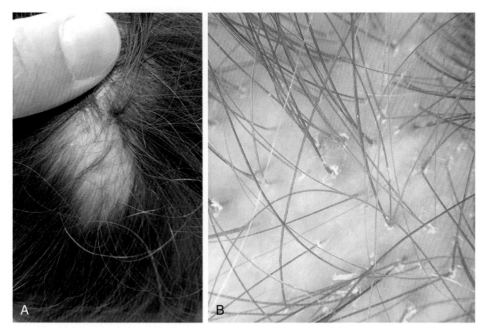

FIG. 19.5 **(A)** 10-year-old boy with a biopsy-proven diagnosis of lichen planopilaris. **(B)** Trichoscopy of the patch reveals loss of follicular openings, peripilar casts (some of which encircle the proximal portion of the hair shaft), and erythema (handyscope, ×10). (Image courtesy of Mariya Miteva, MD.)

pediatric population, CCCA should not be forgotten in this age group to prevent further disease progression.

Genodermatoses
Finally, a number of rare genodermatoses can present with cicatricial alopecia, including but not limited to chondrodysplasia punctata or Conradi-Hünermann syndrome, keratosis follicularis spinulosa decalvans, incontinentia pigmenti, focal dermal hypoplasia or Goltz syndrome, and ectodermal dysplasias.[7]

The diseases aforementioned of patchy pediatric alopecia are summarized in Table 19.2.

DIFFUSE ALOPECIA IN CHILDHOOD
There are a limited number of etiologies presenting with diffuse pediatric alopecia. The most common cases are reviewed; hair shaft disorders can present as diffuse hypotrichoses; however, they will be reviewed in a subsequent section.

Telogen Effluvium
Telogen effluvium manifests as diffuse hair thinning and shedding, precipitated by an identifiable physical or emotional stressor occurring approximately 3 months before the onset of symptoms. Telogen effluvium is a relatively common cause of alopecia in childhood. In a study of 210 children, ages 2 months to 16 years, presenting with the chief complaint of hair loss, approximately 17% of cases were attributable to telogen effluvium.[2] The most common cause in this series was due to preceding illness with high-grade fever, followed by iron-deficiency anemia.[2] Clinical examination reveals diffuse alopecia without discrete alopecic patches. Dermoscopic examination of acute telogen effluvium may show empty follicles and short regrowing hairs of normal thickness.[38] A hair pull test is positive and is indicative of active shedding. Microscopic examination will show telogen hairs that are characteristically club-shaped, without pigment, and having uniform shaft diameters. The diagnosis can be suspected by a history of an identifiable illness, hospitalization, or trigger in combination with characteristic clinical and dermoscopic findings. Spontaneous regrowth is expected within several months after removal of the offending precipitant. Telogen effluvium is further discussed in detail in Chapter 6.

TABLE 19.2
Diagnosis of Patchy Alopecia in Childhood[17]

	History	Clinical Findings	Trichoscopic Findings
Alopecia areata	Waxing and waning course	Alopecic patch/patches Ophiasis Alopecia totalis/universalis	Exclamation mark hairs Yellow dots Black dots Broken hairs Short regrowing hairs
Aplasia cutis congenita	Present since birth	Atrophic alopecic patch	Radially arranged elongated hair bulbs at the periphery of lesion Translucent and vascular skin in the center
Trichotillomania	Self-manipulation of lesions	Irregular patch/patches with variable hair length Tonsure pattern	Broken hairs V-sign Tulip hairs Flame hairs
Temporal triangular alopecia	Present since birth	Localized alopecic patch in the frontotemporal area	Central vellus hairs Terminal hairs on the periphery
Tinea capitis	Recent onset	Inflammatory alopecic patche/patches, scaling, +/– lymphadenopathy	Comma hairs Corkscrew hairs Zigzag hairs Broken hairs
Traction alopecia	Predisposing hairstyles that exert pressure	Peripheral Marginal band like alopecia Patchy non-marginal alopecia	Broken hairs Hair casts

Anagen Effluvium

Anagen effluvium occurs when there is an interruption to the anagen or predominant growth phase of the hair. As most hair follicles are in the anagen phase at one time, the clinical presentation manifests as diffuse and abrupt shedding of the entire scalp. Anagen effluvium is caused by a variety of etiologies including most commonly drugs, such as chemotherapy, in addition to radiation, toxin exposure, and infection. Other hair-bearing sites may similarly be affected. In a review of pediatric patients with a recent diagnosis of lymphoma and leukemia, anagen effluvium was the most common cutaneous manifestation diagnosed on dermatologic examination, occurring in 74% of pediatric patients after induction chemotherapy.[39] On examination of these patients, a hair pull test will reveal "pencil-point" hairs with proximal tips that taper to a point; a hair pull test late in the disease will yield exclusively the spared telogen hairs.[40] Therapy rests on discontinuation of the inciting etiology.

Of note, **permanent alopecia after chemotherapy** has been described in children. Bresters et al. examined patients who underwent hematopoietic stem cell transplantation before 19 years of age, and who were at least

2 years after transplant, and found that approximately 15% of patients suffered from permanent alopecia.[41] All patients had diffuse alopecia, and they additionally discovered an association with use of busulfan in the conditioning regimen before transplantation.[41] Another study, performed on 159 pediatric patients who had also undergone chemotherapy followed by hematopoietic stem cell transplantation, discovered that 12% of patients experienced permanent alopecia and were strongly associated with the use of the alkylating medication, thiotepa.[42] These studies demonstrate the importance of counseling about this realistic side effect that may be encountered in this select patient population.

Loose Anagen Syndrome

Loose anagen syndrome (LAS) presents clinically with diffuse hair loss due to abnormal anchorage of the hair shaft to the follicle. A retrospective chart review of 37 cases of LAS concluded that the disease is more common in Caucasian females with blonde hair; the mean age of presentation was 5 years.[43] LAS is typically sporadic or autosomal dominant in presentation but may also be associated with certain genetic syndromes

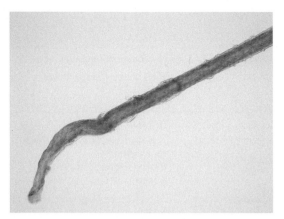

FIG. 19.6 Microscopic examination of the hair in loose anagen syndrome displays anagen hairs devoid of external root sheaths and proximal ruffling of the cuticle. (Image courtesy of Mariya Miteva, MD.)

including Noonan syndrome and Noonan-like syndrome.[44] Scalp examination demonstrates reduced density and short hair, as the hair is readily removed by minimal trauma. Parents may complain that their child's hair simply does not grow long. A hair pull test is usually positive, unless they have immediately combed the hair before the visit; microscopic examination exhibits characteristic findings with anagen hairs devoid of external root sheaths and proximal ruffling of the cuticle (Fig. 19.6).[43] Trichoscopy in LAS reveals rectangular granular structures, presumed to correspond to the rectangular shape of an anagen follicle, and solitary yellow dots, indicative of follicular openings filled with sebum or keratin.[45]

Hair pull test

Hair pull test results in LAS show more than 3, and often more than 10 loose anagen hairs, compared with the pull test findings of normal children, which usually show 1 or 2 loose anagen hairs.[46]

Treatment involves reassurance and gentle hairstyles; the condition may improve with age.

Short Anagen Syndrome

Short anagen syndrome is a hair cycle disorder caused by an idiopathic short anagen phase with a reduced duration of approximately 4–10 months and clinically presents with a maximum hair length of approximately 6 cm.[47–49] The patients present with increased shedding and complain of hair that will not grow long. A positive hair pull test demonstrates the characteristic microscopic findings of short telogen hairs with tapered ends. The main differential diagnosis includes LAS; however,

LAS will present with unique microscopic findings as previously discussed. Treatment consists of reassurance of the benign etiology and gentle hair practices; some may improve with puberty.[48] Topical minoxidil has been use to help prolong the anagen phase and thus increase the hair length, while minimizing episodes of telogen effluvium; parents must be reminded that this topical option is not FDA approved and requires daily maintenance therapy.[50,51]

The diseases aforementioned of diffuse pediatric alopecia are summarized in Table 19.3.

HAIR SHAFT DISORDERS
Hair Shaft Disorders With Increased Fragility

Only the most common hair shaft disorders are discussed here. Trichoscopy is an invaluable tool for the diagnosis, particularly in children.[52]

Monilethrix

Monilethrix is an autosomal dominant hair shaft defect, manifesting as short hair with a characteristic "beaded" appearance and most frequently involves the occipital scalp. The hair is short because of breakage of the hair shaft as it emerges due to narrowed hair shaft segments.[7] The hair is usually normal at birth; however, within weeks, the affected hairs become brittle and dull, leading to breakage at lengths of approximately 0.5–2.5 cm. Surrounding follicular hyperkeratosis of the scalp, face, and extremities may be appreciable, as well as koilonychia on clinical examination. Microscopy of the beaded appearance demonstrates nodes that represent the normal hair and the intervening narrower portions that are the sites of fracture. Characteristic mutations in the hair keratins K81 (hHb1) or K86 (hHb6) on chromosome 12 lead to the inherent pathology. Autosomal recessive presentations have been demonstrated because of mutations on chromosome 18, affecting desmoglein 4 that leads to alterations of the hair shaft desmosomes.[7] The prognosis is favorable as the disease improves with age, especially in girls, perhaps due to the hormonal influence.[53]

Trichorrhexis invaginata (Netherton syndrome)

Trichorrhexis invaginata (TI), also known as "bamboo hair," is characterized by an abnormal hair shaft that wraps around a distal firmer shaft, creating the appearance of a shallow invagination of the distal hair shaft into the proximal hair shaft, forming a ball-and-socket configuration microscopically. TI is a specific finding for Netherton syndrome, an autosomal recessive genodermatosis that manifests by the triad of atopy, ichthyosis

TABLE 19.3
Diagnosis of Diffuse Alopecia in Childhood

	History	Clinical Findings	Microscopic Findings
Telogen effluvium	Preceding illness or stressful event	Diffuse alopecia	Club-shaped telogen hairs
Anagen effluvium	Chemotherapy, radiation, toxin exposure, or infection	Diffuse to total alopecia	Telogen hairs on the hair pull test with tapered proximal tips
Loose anagen syndrome	Caucasian female complaining of hair that will not grow long	Diffuse alopecia with short hair length	Anagen hairs devoid of external root sheaths Proximal ruffled cuticle Positive pull test
Short anagen syndrome	Female complaining of hair that will not grow long	Diffuse alopecia with short hair length	Short telogen hairs with tapered ends Positive pull test

linearis circumflexa, and TI.[10] Netherton syndrome is caused by a mutation in SPINK5, a serine protease inhibitor, on chromosome 5.[10] Affected patients present with fragile, short, and dull hair; the scalp, eyebrows, eyelashes, and hair of the trunk and extremities may be affected.[34] Changes in the eyebrows may precede scalp involvement. It is imperative to remember that only a few shafts may exhibit these alterations; thus, a thorough search of affected hair-bearing regions should be performed and put into context with the clinical presentation. The hair will remain short, brittle, and easily susceptible to trauma throughout the patient's lifetime.

Bubble hair

Bubble hair is an acquired hair shaft abnormality due to numerous trapped air bubbles within the hair and is typically due to increased heat damage from practices such as hair drying and hair straightening. Dry heating can widen hair medulla, causing cortex dilations that appear as bubbles; the hair shafts can then break off at their widest ballooning segments.[7] Clinical examination demonstrates broken, dry hair with patchy alopecia due to increased fragility. Microscopy is diagnostic, revealing multiple air-filled spaces within the hair shaft; it may be associated with other acquired hair shaft defects such as trichorrhexis nodosa (TN) and trichoptilosis, also known as splaying of the hair shaft or split ends.[54] Treatment includes cessation of thermal injury to the hair.

Pili torti

Pili torti is characterized by hair shafts that are flattened and twisted on their own axis. Trichoscopy exhibits hair shafts that are irregularly bent at acute angles on low magnification and characteristic 180-degree twists of flattened hair on higher magnification.[34] Pili torti may be seen in Menkes syndrome, an X-linked recessive genodermatosis due to an ATP7A mutation, leading to a copper deficiency.[10,55] These patients present with short "steel wool" hair in infancy; the hair is light-colored and dry, breaking at different lengths. Patients with Menkes syndrome experience significant neurologic deterioration, and unfortunately, most do not survive beyond several years of life. Pili torti is also associated with Björnstad syndrome, which has similar features to Menkes; however, these patients experience sensorineural hearing loss and have a normal life expectancy. Pili torti may also be seen in association with Bazex syndrome, Beare-Stevenson syndrome, Crandall syndrome, or nutritional deficiencies such as anorexia nervosa or can be acquired with systemic retinoid therapy.[7,34]

Trichothiodystrophy

Trichothiodystrophy (TTD) is an autosomal recessive neuroectodermal disorder caused by several functionally related gene defects that lead to clinical findings of fragile hair, thinning and longitudinal ridging of the nails, and additional cutaneous findings such as photosensitivity, ichthyosis, erythroderma, or generalized fine scaling at birth.[55] Patients may also have developmental abnormalities, decreased fertility, and cognitive deficits. Clinically, the hair of the scalp, eyebrows, and eyelashes may be short and brittle because of low sulfur content. Light microscopy highlights flattened hair shafts with clean, transverse fractures or trichoschisis, whereas polarized light highlights the unique finding of alternating dark and light bands, known as "tiger-tail" banding.[7] Liang et al. examined 14 patients with TTD and found that all demonstrated tiger-tail banding, among a myriad of other findings including trichoschisis, TN-like defects, ribboning, and surface irregularities.[56] Trichoscopy is not characteristic except for trichoschisis; hair shafts may show the spotted tiger-like structures, alternating dark and light bands, and weaving contours.[7] Hair abnormalities are persistent and are a vital clue to the diagnosis.

Trichorrhexis nodosa

TN refers to the presence of nodules or fractures on the hair shafts and is represented microscopically with the hair shaft fracture splaying out, producing an appearance analogous to the ends of two brushes pushed together.[7] The defect causes the hair to be fragile and break spontaneously or with trauma. TN may be inherited as an autosomal dominant trait or found in association with argininosuccinic aciduria; however, it is most commonly acquired because of external injury from hair dryers, hair straighteners, or chemical treatments.[10] Trichoscopy at low magnification shows intermittent white nodules or gaps along the hair shaft, and higher magnification will reveal the sites of fracture with numerous fibrils facing each other.[34] The pull test is positive, and the hair breaks off readily at the nodule sites.[7] Treatment for acquired TN involves the avoidance of harsh hair treatments including repetitive exposure to heat, chemical treatments, and excessive physical forces.

Hair Shaft Disorders Without Increased Fragility

Pili trianguli et canaliculi (uncombable hair syndrome)

Uncombable hair syndrome manifests as unruly, dry, and light-colored hair in children that is impossible to comb and characteristically described as *"spun glass hair."* The hair is frizzy and stands away from the scalp. The hair is usually normal in length and tensile strength. Hair shafts differ from the usual cylindrical shape and are described as *pili trianguli et canaliculi* because of the aberrant triangular shape.[57] A cross-sectional view of the hair shaft on scanning electron microscopy demonstrates the triangular shape, which is due to the presence of channels along the longitudinal axis.[7] However, this longitudinal grooving can be seen in other syndromes including progeria, Hay-Wells syndrome, oral facial digital syndrome, ectrodactyly ectodermal dysplasia, and hypohidrotic ectodermal dysplasia.[10] Uncombable hair syndrome is an uncommon diagnosis with less than 100 cases in the literature, and both autosomal dominant and recessive patterns have been described.

Pili annulati

Pili annulati refers to alternating bright and dark bands, with the bright areas corresponding to light scattered from clusters of air-filled cavities within the cortex.[34] Pili annulati is also known as ringed hair because of the alternating dilations of the medulla that produce the banded appearance.[7] Pili annulati can be sporadic or inherited as an autosomal dominant trait and is merely of cosmetic concern as the associated hair is not fragile. Scanning electron microscopy exhibits longitudinal folding in bands of the abnormal areas, possibly because of the evaporation of air in the corresponding spaces.[10] Transmission electron microscopy demonstrates multiple holes within the cortex. Pili annulati is usually an autosomal dominant disorder or seen occasionally in alopecia areata.[34]

Woolly hair

Woolly hair presents as curly, soft, and thin hair and may present diffusely as an inherited condition, localized as in a woolly hair nevus, or may be acquired in both patchy and diffuse presentations.[7] Dermoscopic features described have included a "crawling snake" appearance as short intervals of close undulations along affected hair shafts.[58] Woolly hair is significant given the numerous associations including ocular abnormalities, Noonan syndrome, giant axonal neuropathy, and epidermal nevi.[10] One must be particularly cognizant of a child presenting with woolly hair and palmoplantar keratoderma, given the association with cardiomyopathy in both Naxos disease and Carvajal syndrome. A search for associated conditions is warranted, and the hair manifestations are lasting. Surgical excision is an option for a localized patch; however, this option is considered solely for cosmetic appearances and is generally not recommended.

REFERENCES

1. Bernardis E, Nukpezah J, Li P, Christensen T, Castelo-Soccio L. Pediatric severity of alopecia tool. *Pediatr Dermatol.* 2018;35(1):e68–e69.
2. Al-Refu K. Hair loss in children: common and uncommon causes; clinical and epidemiological study in Jordan. *Int J Trichology.* 2013;5(4):185.
3. Lenane P, Pope E, Krafchik B. Congenital alopecia areata. *J Am Acad Dermatol.* 2005;52(2 suppl 1):8–11.
4. Mohan GC, Silverberg JI. Association of vitiligo and alopecia areata with atopic dermatitis: a systematic review and meta-analysis. *JAMA Dermatol.* 2015;151(5):522–528.
5. Sorrell J, Petukhova L, Reingold R, et al. Shedding light on alopecia areata in pediatrics: a retrospective analysis of comorbidities in children in the National Alopecia Areata Registry. *Pediatr Dermatol.* 2017;34(5):e271–e272.

6. Patel D, Li P, Bauer AJ, Castelo-Soccio L. Screening guidelines for thyroid function in children with alopecia areata. *JAMA Dermatol.* 2017;153(12):1307–1310.

7. Ferrando J, Grimalt R. *Pediatric Hair Disorders: An Atlas and Text.* 3rd ed. Boca Raton, FL: CRC Press; 2017:1–85.

8. Craiglow BG, Liu LY, King BA. Tofacitinib for the treatment of alopecia areata and variants in adolescents. *J Am Acad Dermatol.* 2017;76(1):29–32.

9. Wang E, Lee JS, Tang M. Current treatment strategies in pediatric alopecia areata. *Indian J Dermatol.* 2012;57(6):459–465.

10. Schachner LS, Hansen RC. Hair disorders. In: Krafchik BR, Lucky AW, Paller AS, Rogers M, Torrelo A, eds. *Pediatric Dermatology.* 4th ed. China: Mosby Elsevier; 2011:768–793.

11. Tay YK, Levy ML, Metry DW. Trichotillomania in childhood; case series and review. *Pediatrics.* 2004;113(5):e494–e498.

12. Rakowska A, Slowinska M, Olszewska M, Rudnicka L. New trichoscopy findings in trichotillomania: flame hairs, V-sign, hook hairs, hair powder, tulip hairs. *Acta Derm Venereol.* 2014;94(3):303–306.

13. Miteva M, Romanelli P, Tosti A. Pigmented casts. *Am J Dermatopathol.* 2014;36(1):58–63.

14. Yamazaki M, Irisawa R, Tsuboi R. Temporal triangular alopecia and a review of 52 past cases. *J Dermatol.* 2010;37(4):360–362.

15. Kim HJ, Park KB, Yang JM, Park SH, Lee ES. Congenital triangular alopecia in phakomatosis pigmentovascularis: report of 3 cases. *Acta Derm Venereol.* 2000;80(3):215–216.

16. Campos JG, Oliveira CM, Romero SA, Klein AP, Akel PB, Pinto GM. Use of dermoscopy in the diagnosis of temporal triangular alopecia. *An Bras Dermatol.* 2015;90(1):123–125.

17. Rakowska A, Maj M, Zadurska M, et al. Trichoscopy of focal alopecia in children – new trichoscopic findings: hair bulbs arranged radially along hair-bearing margins in aplasia cutis congenita. *Skin Appendage Disord.* 2016;2(1–2):1–6.

18. Commens C, Rogers M, Kan A. Heterotropic brain tissue presenting as bald cysts with a collar of hypertrophic hair. The 'hair collar' sign. *Arch Dermatol.* 1989;125(9):1253–1256.

19. Bassi A, Greco A, de Martino M. Aplasia cutis with 'hair collar sign'. *Arch Dis Child.* 2014;99(11):1003.

20. Chien MM, Chen KL, Chiu HC. The "hair-collar" sign. *J Pediatr.* 2016;168:246.

21. Drolet BA, Clowry Jr L, McTigue MK, Esterly NB. The hair collar sign: marker for cranial dysraphism. *Pediatrics.* 1995;96(2 Pt 1):309–313.

22. Neri I, Savoia F, Giacomini F, Raone B, Aprile S, Patrizi A. Usefulness of dermatoscopy for the early diagnosis of sebaceous nevus and differentiation from aplasia cutis congenita. *Clin Exp Dermatol.* 2009;34(5):e50–e52.

23. Amer M, Helmy A, Amer A. Trichoscopy as a useful method to differentiate tinea capitis from alopecia areata in children at Zagazig University Hospitals. *Int J Dermatol.* 2017;56(1):116–120.

24. Hughes R, Chiaverini C, Bahadoranp W, et al. Corkscrew hair: a new dermoscopic sign for diagnosis of tinea capitis in black children. *Arch Dermatol.* 2011;147(3):355–356.

25. Slowinska M, Rudnicka L, Schwartz RA, et al. Comma hairs: a dermatoscopic marker for tinea capitis: a rapid diagnostic method. *J Am Acad Dermatol.* 2008;59(5 suppl):S77–S79.

26. Bennassar A, Grimalt R. Management of tinea capitis in childhood. *Clin Cosmet Investig Dermatol.* 2010;3:89–98.

27. Wright DR, Gathers R, Kapke A, Johnson D, Joseph CL. Hair care practices and their association with scalp and hair disorders in African American girls. *J Am Acad Dermatol.* 2011;64(2):253–262.

28. Fox GN, Stausmire JM, Mehregan DR. Traction folliculitis: an underreported entity. *Cutis.* 2007;79(1):26–30.

29. Samrao A, Price VH, Zedek D, Mirmirani P. The "fringe sign"-a useful clinical finding in traction alopecia of the marginal hair line. *Dermatol Online J.* 2011;17(11):1.

30. Hantash BM, Schwartz RA. Traction alopecia in children. *Cutis.* 2003;71(1):18–20.

31. Tosti A, Miteva M, Torres F, Vincenzi C, Romanelli P. Hair casts are a dermoscopic clue for the diagnosis of traction alopecia. *Br J Dermatol.* 2010;163(6):1353–1355.

32. Khokhar RS, Baaj J, Alhazmi HH, Dammas FA, Aldalati AM. Pressure-induced alopecia in pediatric patients following prolonged urological surgeries: the case reports and a review of the literature. *Anesth Essays Res.* 2015;9(3):430–432.

33. Atarquine H, Hocar O, Hamdaoui A, Akhdari N, Amal S. Frontal fibrosing alopecia: report on three pediatric cases. *Arch Pediatr.* 2016;23(8):832–835.

34. Lencastre A, Tosti A. Role of trichoscopy in children's scalp and hair disorders. *Pediatr Dermatol.* 2013;30(6):674–682.

35. Moises-Alfaro C, Berrón-Pérez R, Carrasco-Daza D, Gutiérrez-Castrellón P, Ruiz-Maldonado R. Discoid lupus erythematosus in children: clinical, histopathologic, and follow-up features in 27 cases. *Pediatr Dermatol.* 2003;20(2):103–107.

36. Christensen KN, Lehman JS, Tollefson MM. Pediatric lichen planopilaris: clinicopathologic study of four new cases and a review of the literature. *Pediatr Dermatol.* 2015;32(5):621–627.

37. Eginli AN, Dlova NC, McMichael A. Central centrifugal cicatricial alopecia in children: a case series and review of the literature. *Pediatr Dermatol.* 2017;34(2):133–137.

38. Miteva M, Tosti A. Hair and scalp dermatoscopy. *J Am Acad Dermatol.* 2012;67(5):1040–1048.

39. Cardoza-Torres MA, Liy-Wong C, Welsh O, et al. Skin manifestations associated with chemotherapy in children with hematologic malignancies. *Pediatr Dermatol.* 2012;29(3):264–269.

40. Sperling LC. Evaluation of hair loss. *Curr Probl Dermatol.* 1996;8(97).

41. Bresters D, Wanders DCM, Louwerens M, et al. Permanent diffuse alopecia after hematopoietic stem cell transplantation in childhood. *Bone Marrow Transplant.* 2017;52(7):984–988.

42. Choi M, Kim MS, Park SY, et al. Clinical characteristics of chemotherapy-induced alopecia in childhood. *J Am Acad Dermatol.* 2014;70(3):499–505.

43. Swink SM, Castelo-Soccio L. Loose anagen syndrome: a retrospective chart review of 37 cases. *Pediatr Dermatol.* 2016;33(5):507–510.

44. Ferrero GB, Picco G, Baldassarre G, et al. Transcriptional hallmarks of Noonan syndrome and Noonan-like syndrome with loose anagen hair. *Hum Mutat.* 2012;33(4):703–709.

45. Rakowska A, Zadurska M, Czuwara J, et al. Trichoscopy findings in loose anagen hair syndrome: rectangular granular structures and solitary yellow dots. *J Dermatol Case Rep.* 2015;9(1):1–5.

46. Olsen EA, Bettencourt MS, Coté NL. The presence of loose anagen hairs obtained by hair pull in the normal population. *J Investig Dermatol Symp Proc.* 1999;4(3):258–260.

47. Antaya RJ, Sideridou E, Olsen EA. Short anagen syndrome. *J Am Acad Dermatol.* 2005;53(2):S130–S134.

48. Giacomini F, Starace M, Tosti A. Short anagen syndrome. *Pediatr Dermatol.* 2011;28(2):133–134.

49. Herskovitz I, de Sousa IC, Simon J, Tosti A. Short anagen hair syndrome. *Int J Trichology.* 2013;5(1):45–46.

50. Cheng Y-P, Chen Y-S, Lin S-J, Hsiao C-H, Chiu H-C, Chan J-YL. Minoxidil improved hair density in an Asian girl with short anagen syndrome: a case report and review of literature. *Int J Dermatol.* 2016;55(11):1268–1271.

51. Jung HD, Kim JE, Kang H. Short anagen syndrome successfully controlled with topical minoxidil and systemic cyclosporine. *J Dermatol.* 2011;38(11):1108–1110.

52. Miteva M, Tosti A. Dermatoscopy of hair shaft disorders. *J Am Acad Dermatol.* 2013;68(3):473–481.

53. Gebhart M, Fischer T, Claussen U, et al. Monilethrix-improvement by hormonal influences? *Pediatr Dermatol.* 1999;16(4):297–300.

54. Savitha A, Sacchidanand S, Revathy T. Bubble hair and other acquired hair shaft anomalies due to hot ironing on wet hair. *Int J Trichology.* 2011;3(2):118–120.

55. Paller AS, Mancini AJ. Disorders of hair and nails. In: *Hurwitz Clinical Pediatric Dermatology.* 5th ed. Canada: Elsevier; 2016:136–164.

56. Liang C, Kraemer KH, Morris A, et al. Characterization of tiger-tail banding and hair shaft abnormalities in trichothiodystrophy. *J Am Acad Dermatol.* 2005;52(2):224–232.

57. Calderon P, Otberg N, Shapiro J. Uncombable hair syndrome. *J Am Acad Dermatol.* 2009;61(3):512–515.

58. Rakowska A, Slowinska M, Kowalska-Oledzka E, et al. Trichoscopy in genetic hair shaft abnormalities. *J Dermatol Case Rep.* 2008;2:14–20.

CHAPTER 20

Hair and Scalp Infections

GISELLE MARTINS, MD • MARIYA MITEVA, MD

INTRODUCTION

Infections of hair and scalp are common in the hair practice and can be associated with hair loss. Several groups of infections affect the scalp: bacterial (impetigo, syphilis, folliculitis decalvans), fungal (seborrheic dermatitis [SD], piedra, tinea capitis [TC]), viral (herpes simplex and herpes zoster), and parasitic (pediculosis, demodicosis). In some infectious disease, hair can be secondarily involved and/or show abnormal features (for example, hair changes in human immunodeficiency virus infection [HIV] and alopecia universalis as a side effect in the treatment of hepatitis C infection).

Only primary scalp and hair infections are discussed here.

TINEA CAPITIS

Etiology

TC is a dermatophytic infection of the scalp hair follicles. There are two main causative pathogens in TC: *Trichophyton* (anthropophilic) and *Microsporum* (zoophilic). The type of hair invasion is classified as ectothrix, endothrix, or favus. Ectothrix anthropophilic infections potentially spread rapidly, whereas endothrix and favic infections are less contagious.[1] TC is a common dermatophytic infection affecting prepubertal children. In the United States, TC most commonly occurs in female children (59% girls vs. 41% boys) and 95% of patients are infected with *Trichophyton tonsurans*.[2,3] It is spread most commonly via direct contact with an infected child or indirectly via infected fomites, but also via a contact with an asymptomatic adult carrier.[4] The second most common cause of TC is *Microsporum canis*, and it is the predominant causative organism in many countries of the Mediterranean basin. The carriers of this dermatophyte are cats and dogs as well pet puppies, kittens, and rabbits.[4]

Clinical Presentation

Four patterns have been described:
- *Noninflammatory black dot pattern*: characterized by well-demarcated areas of hair loss, associated with the characteristic appearance of black dots on the alopecic patch. This occurs because the hairs break off at or below the scalp surface. Cell-mediated immunity to fungal antigen skin test is usually negative, and adenopathy is often absent[4] (Fig. 20.1)
- *Noninflammatory SD type*: diffuse or patchy, fine, white, adherent scale affecting the scalp. This is the most difficult to diagnose because it resembles dandruff.[4]
- *Kerion celsi or inflammatory TC*: there are one or multiple tender, inflamed, alopecic nodules with pustules on their surface (Fig. 20.2A and B). Fever, occipital adenopathy, leukocytosis, and even a diffuse, morbilliform rash may occur.[4] Kerion celsi has the potential to cause scarring alopecia. Some cases may be indistinguishable from dissecting cellulitis of the scalp (TC mimicking dissecting cellulitis) (Fig. 20.2C).
- *Favus* (caused by *Trichophyton schoenleinii*): rare type of inflammatory TC characterized by typical honey-colored, cup-shaped, follicular crusts called scutula, which can cause scarring alopecia too.[4] The scalp has unpleasant "mousy" odor.

Dermoscopy

The trichoscopy features of TC include comma hairs, corkscrew hairs, and broken hairs[5] (Fig. 20.3A and B). Comma hairs are specific for TC and are reported in both Caucasians and African-Americans, whereas corkscrew hairs can be seen in ectodermal dysplasia as well and are exclusive to African-Americans. Other

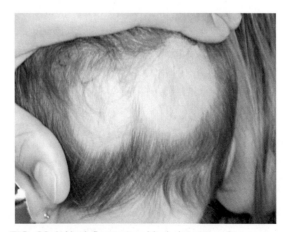

FIG. 20.1 Noninflammatory black dot pattern in a young girl characterized by well-demarcated areas of hair loss.

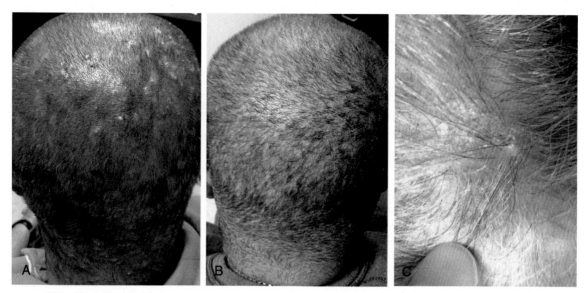

FIG. 20.2 **(A)** Inflammatory tinea capitis in a young man in his 30s misdiagnosed and treated with oral antibiotics for folliculitis. The patient had lymphadenopathy and used to take pain medication to be able to sleep. **(B)** The same patient after a course of prednisone and oral terbinafine with complete resolution of the infection. **(C)** An elderly woman in her 80s with individual pustules and boggy inflamed areas on the scalp treated with antibiotics for suppurative folliculitis. The correct diagnosis is inflammatory tinea capitis mimicking dissecting cellulitis (see the pathology in Fig. 20.3B). The diagnosis was made by a repeated fungal culture positive for *Trichophyton* spp.

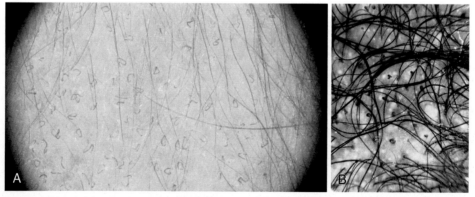

FIG. 20.3 **(A)** Comma hairs on dermoscopy in a Caucasian child with noninflammatory tinea capitis. **(B)** Comma hairs on dermoscopy in an African-American child.

described trichoscopic findings include barcode-like hairs and zigzag hairs. Comma hairs help to differentiate TC from other common scalp diseases in children such as alopecia areata and trichotillomania.

Pathology

In TC caused by ectothrix infection, the hyphae and spores cover the outside surface of the hair shaft, which results in destruction of the cuticle.

In TC caused by endothrix infection, the inside of the hair shaft is invaded only by rounded and box-like arthrospores and not by hyphae (Fig. 20.4A). In inflammatory TC (kerion), there is dense mixed cell inflammatory infiltrate of neutrophils, plasma cells, eosinophils, lymphocytes, and histiocytes as well as giant cells (suppurative granulomatous folliculitis) (Fig. 20.4B). The special stains may be falsely negative in up to half of the cases.

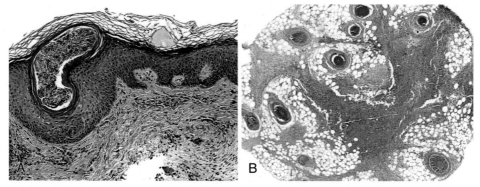

FIG. 20.4 **(A)** Tinea capitis: Endothrix infection is characterized by hair shafts loaded with spores but no hyphae (hematoxylin and eosin, ×10). **(B)** Inflammatory tinea capitis: On horizontal sections, there is an abscess-like dense mixed cell infiltrate among the bulbs that extends up to the infundibulum (hematoxylin and eosin, ×4).

Culture

The diagnosis of TC is based on microscopic examination of infected hairs by KOH preparation and confirmatory culture. The material for culture is obtained by scraping scales and hair with a No. 15 scalpel blade or by plucking hairs from the scalp (a needleholder can be used for that purpose). Other methods include using toothbrushes, hairbrushes, wet gauze, and adhesive tape to collect material. Mycologic culture is fundamental for the identification of the causative organism. Wood's lamp examination is a useful tool for the diagnosis in some cases, for example, green fluorescence in *Microsporum* spp. and none in *Trichophyton* spp.

Management

TC must be treated with systemic antifungal therapy because topical agents do not penetrate the hair shaft. Randomized clinical trials have confirmed that griseofulvin, terbinafine, and fluconazole have equal effectiveness. The current options are summarized in Table 20.1. However, a concomitant topical treatment, for example, 1% or 2.5% selenium sulfide shampoo or 2% ketoconazole shampoo should be used for several weeks because it may reduce transmission, and family members should be using it as well.[6,7] We usually leave patients on an antifungal shampoo for a year after the infection has been resolved. If the infection recurs, family members (usually siblings) should be evaluated for an asymptomatic carriage of *Trichophyton* spp.

In conclusion, terbinafine and fluconazole have shorter treatment courses.[8–11] Terbinafine may be superior to griseofulvin for *Trichophyton* species, whereas griseofulvin may be superior to terbinafine for the less common *Microsporum* species.[11,12]

PEDICULOSIS CAPITIS

Etiology

Pediculosis capitis (PC) is an ectoparasitic disease caused by infestation of the scalp with head lice (*Pediculus humanus capitis*). It is a ubiquitous disease in pediatric population in the age group of 6–12 years and is especially frequent in poor communities in developing countries.[13–19] The prevalence of PC is around 40%.[15–18] Girls are 2–4 times more frequently infested than boys, especially in rural and developing areas owing to the long hair length.[20]

The life cycle of the head louse has three stages: egg, nymph, and adult. Eggs are laid by an adult fertile female and are cemented at the base of the hair shaft nearest the scalp. The egg hatches to release a single nymph. The adult louse is about the size of 2–4 mm, has six legs (each with claws), and is tan to gray-white. The claw at the distal end is for clutching the hair shaft (Fig. 20.5).

Clinical Presentation

The main symptom of PC is pruritus of the scalp, but excoriations, impetiginization, and cervical lymphadenopathy may also be present.[17,18] Transmission occurs by intimate head-to-head contact, and the other routes of transmission such as sharing fomites (hairbrushes, combs, towels, and bedding) remain a matter of debate.[21,22] On examination, one can see nits that are firmly attached to hair shaft within 6 mm from the scalp skin.[20] The occipital and retroauricular areas of the head are easier to detect the adults and the nits. Repeated scratching by the affected individual leads to loss of skin integrity with secondary bacterial infection, impetignization, and cervical and

TABLE 20.1
Oral Antifungals Used in the Treatment of Tinea Capitis (TC)

TERBINAFINE

Route: oral

Dosage: 3–6 mg/kg/day based on weight

<55 lb: 125 mg once daily

55–78 lb: 185.5 mg once daily

>78 lb: 250 mg once daily

Duration: 2–6 weeks, longer for *Microsporum* infections

Side effects: gastrointestinal discomfort and headache

Age: 4 years and older

GRISEOFULVIN

Route: oral

Dosage: 20–25 mg/kg/day for microsized formulation and 10–15 mg/kg/day for ultramicrosized formulation

Duration: 6–12 weeks

Side effects: gastrointestinal discomfort and headache

Age: 2 years and older

ITRACONAZOLE

Route: oral

Dosage: 3–5 mg/kg/day in capsules

Duration: 2–4 weeks continuously or 1-week pulses for 2–3 months

Side effects: gastrointestinal discomfort and headache

Age: not FDA approved for treatment of TC; safety and efficacy not established in children younger than 3 years

FLUCONAZOLE

Route: oral

Dosage: 6 mg/kg/day

Duration: 3–6 weeks continuously or 1-week pulses for 2–3 months

Side effects: gastrointestinal discomfort and headache

Age: not FDA approved for treatment of TC, but approved for use in children older than 6 months

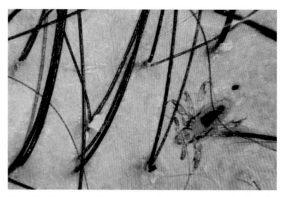

FIG. 20.5 The adult louse has six legs (each with claws) and is tan to grayish-white in color.

Dermoscopy

The term nit refers to either a louse egg or a louse nymph. They are hard to see without a dermoscopic device and are often confused with dandruff, hair casts, or hair sprays. However, these nits cannot be moved along the hair shaft in contrast to pseudonits. The dermoscopy can detect the head lice and the nits fixed on the hair shaft. An opaque structure with a convex free ending separated by millimeters from the hair shaft means a viable nit (Fig. 20.6A), and a translucent structure with fissured free ending that is more than 1 cm away from the scalp means an empty egg[23] (Fig. 20.6B).

Pathology

Pathology is not useful in the diagnosis of PC.

Treatment

The treatment includes topical pediculicidal agents, wet combing, and oral therapy (Table 20.2). All pediculicidal agents should be rinsed after prescribed time limit with cool water over a sink. Rinsing with warm water can increase systemic absorption because of vasodilation of scalp vasculature.[20,25]

Wet combing is a manual procedure of removing the nits with a fine-tooth comb.[24] Prior priming of nit-infested hair with vinegar (4% acetic acid) for 3 min dissolves the cementing substance that attaches the nits to hair shaft and can make combing easier. The combing procedure is done on wet hair with added lubricant (hair conditioner or coconut oil/vegetable oil) and continued until no lice are found (15–30 min per session or longer for long, thick hair). Combing is repeated once every 2–3 days for several weeks and should continue for 2 weeks after any session in which an adult louse is found.[20,24]

occipital lymphadenopathy.[20] Some patients have innumerable nits and live lice and can present with a tangled mass of infested hair shafts (plica polonica/plica neuropathica).

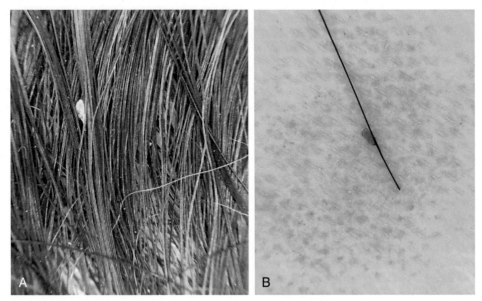

FIG. 20.6 **(A)** Pediculosis capitis: This opaque structure with a convex free ending is a viable nit. **(B)** Pediculosis capitis: a translucent empty nit.

In conjunction with medical treatment, disinfestation of surrounding household environment is necessary to prevent relapse. All clothing, towels, and bed linens used by an infested child within 2 days before diagnosis should be washed in hot water at about 50°C or machine dried at the highest heat setting for at least 30 min.[20]

Systemic therapy of pediculosis acts as an adjuvant therapy in conjunction with topical treatment.[20,26]

Patients can be also referred to specialized lice treatment clinics for more expedited and professional treatment.

PIEDRA

Etiology

Superficial mycoses are fungal infections of the skin, hair, and nail that invade only the stratum corneum and the superficial layers of the skin. Piedra spp. cause superficial mycosis because they neither invade living tissue nor provoke an immune response by the host. Two varieties may be seen: one is called black piedra and the other one white piedra. Black piedra is typically caused by the fungi *Piedraia hortae* and *Trichosporon ovoides*. It is mostly found in warm and humid tropical countries in South America and Southeast Asia.[27] On the other hand, white piedra, caused by other *Trichosporon* species, occurs in semitropical and temperate countries. *Trichosporon* genus is subdivided into six

distinct human pathogenic species of which *T. ovoides*, *Trichosporon inkin*, *Trichosporon mucoides*, and *Trichosporon asahii* are linked to white piedra.[28] *T. ovoides*, which are involved in causing both types of piedra, are found in soil, lake water, and plants and can occasionally be detected as normal flora of the human skin and mouth.[29] The fact that they select hair as substratum is possibly because of their keratinophilic affinity.[29] Infection does not seem to be related to personal hygiene or exposure to an infected person, but it is suggested that its spread can be prevented by not sharing brushes, combs, and other hair accessories.[30]

Clinical Presentation

Piedra is an asymptomatic fungal infection of the hair shaft, resulting in the formation of nodules of different hardness on the infected hair.

Black piedra usually affects the scalp and is characterized by the presence of firm black, hard, gritty nodules that are actually concretions of fungus cells on the hair shaft. They cause disintegration and breakage in the hair fiber. These stone hard black nodules are usually localized to the scalp but may also be seen on hairs of the beard, pubic hair, and mustache.

White piedra is characterized by white to light brown nodules that may surround the entire hair shaft. Nodules are soft, and the fungal mass can easily be detached from the hair. It usually affects body hairs (mustache, axillary hair, eyebrows, and eyelashes).

TABLE 20.2
Treatment Options for Pediculosis Capitis

PERMETHRIN 1%

Route: topical

Forms: topical shampoo

Duration: apply on day 1 and 8 on clean and dry hair for 10 min

PERMETHRIN 5%

Route: topical

Forms: topical cream

Duration: apply on day 1 and 8 on clean hair overnight

Side effects: gastrointestinal discomfort and headache

Age: 2 months and older

MALATHION 0.5%

Route: topical

Forms: topical cream

Duration: apply on day 1 and 8 on clean hair for 8–12 h

Side effects: burning, stinging sensation on eroded skin

Age: 2 months and older

IVERMECTIN

Route: oral

Forms: tablets 3 mg, 6 mg

Dosage: 200 μg/kg of body weight

Duration: two oral doses of the medication 7–10 days apart

Side effects: gastrointestinal discomfort

Age: not recommended below 5 years of age and in pregnancy and lactation

ALBENDAZOLE

Route: oral

tablets 400 mg

Dosage: 400 mg either as a single oral dose or repeated daily for 3 days

Duration: single dose or three doses

Side effects: gastrointestinal discomfort

Age: not recommended below 5 years of age and in pregnancy and lactation

LEVAMIZOLE

Route: oral

tablets 400 mg

Dosage: 400 mg as either a single oral dose or repeated daily for 3 days

Duration: single dose or three doses

Side effects: gastrointestinal discomfort

Age: not recommended below 5 years of age and in pregnancy and lactation

Dermoscopy

Encapsulated arthroconidia or blastoconidia with polygonal appearance are observed under dermoscopy or direct microscopic examination (Fig. 20.7A and B).

Culture

Culture in agar Mycosel for 2 weeks produces a wrinkled white-to-cream yeastlike colony.

Treatment

The most effective therapy for white and black piedra is cutting and shaving the hairs. Topical antifungals are

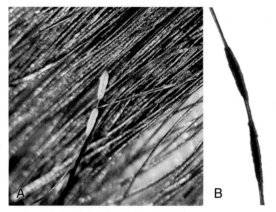

FIG. 20.7 **(A)** On dermoscopy, white piedra is characterized by white to light brown nodules that may surround the entire hair shaft. **(B)** Microscopic examination of hair shafts in white piedra shows the light brown nodules around the hair shaft. In Brazil, white piedra is reported commonly to affect the scalp.

also recommended, and the application of clotrimazole cream alone or after shampooing with ketoconazole proved to be a good therapeutic treatment for white piedra.[31]

SYPHILIS

Etiology

Syphilis, also known as "the great imitator," can present with various cutaneous manifestations. Syphilis is a systemic infectious disease caused by *Treponema pallidum*, which can disseminate to any organ shortly after infection. Syphilitic alopecia (SA) is an uncommon clinical manifestation of secondary syphilis with an incidence of 2.9%–11.2%.[32,33]

Clinical Presentation

SA is manifestation of secondary syphilis. This can be the only sign of the disease, or it can be associated with systemic manifestations such as malaise, low-grade fever, lymphadenopathies, asthenia, and anorexia. Mucosal and cutaneous manifestations, as generalized nonpruritic papulosquamous rash predominantly affecting the trunk, palmoplantar lesions with Biett collarettes, ulceration of the oral mucosa, and condylomata lata, can be seen. SA may clinically mimic a wide range of hair disorders, including alopecia areata, trichotillomania, lichen planopilaris, TC, and telogen effluvium.

According to its clinical appearance, SA is classified into two forms: (1) *symptomatic SA* that presents with skin lesions on the scalp, usually in the form of papulosquamous lesions (Fig. 20.8A), and (2) *essential SA*,

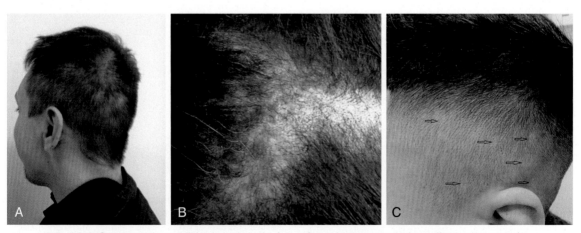

FIG. 20.8 Symptomatic syphilitic alopecia in the form of papulosquamous lesions affecting the scalp (A and B). Essential syphilitic alopecia presenting with moth-eaten patches. Note the very discrete moth-eaten pattern (arrows) (C). Image courtesy of Susana Ruiz-Tagle, MD and Letty Pincay Cedeño, MD.)

characterized by hair loss with no other visible syphilitic lesions on the scalp.

Essential SA has three patterns[34,35]:

1. Moth-eaten or patchy alopecia, characterized by small alopecic patches irregularly distributed over the scalp (Fig. 20.8C)
2. Diffuse alopecia, characterized by diffuse hair loss
3. Mixed form (i.e., combination of diffuse hair loss and alopecic moth-eaten patches)

Scarring alopecia is rarely described in the literature as a manifestation of secondary syphilis; however, it has been described in patients with tertiary syphilis.[36]

The diagnostic workup of SA includes trichoscopy, serologic tests, and scalp biopsy. The serologic tests are a rapid plasma reagin (RPR) test and a *T. pallidum* hemagglutination test.

Dermoscopy

Scalp dermoscopy can help in diagnosing SA. The trichoscopic findings of moth-eaten SA are black dots, focal atrichia, hypopigmentation of hair shaft, and yellow dots in the center of the alopecic patches along with few black dots at the periphery.[37] Some patients have reduction in the number of terminal hairs and presence of empty hair follicles, vellus hairs, red-brown background, and irregularly dilated capillaries with small blood extravasation.[38] In fact, one study found that trichoscopy of the "moth-eaten" areas showed alopecia mainly because of reduction in the number of terminal hairs[38] (Fig. 20.9). Tapering hairs can be detected at the periphery of the moth-eaten patches as single or double bending.[39]

Pathology

Scalp biopsy from the moth-eaten alopecic patches in secondary syphilis demonstrates reduced number of anagen follicles and an increased number of catagen and telogen follicles, which corresponds to the dermoscopy showing reduced number of terminal follicles and/or black dots. Of note, the pathology can be indistinguishable from that of acute stage alopecia areata, as presence of peribulbar lymphocytic infiltrate, widened infundibular ostia, and pigment casts have been observed in both (Fig. 20.10). Presence of plasma cells in the infiltrate is not a sustainable finding for the diagnosis, as they may be absent in more than half of the cases or missed.

Treatment

The treatment of SA is the same as for secondary syphilis. The drug of choice is penicillin G benzathine 2.4 millions UI intramuscular, once a week, total of two doses.

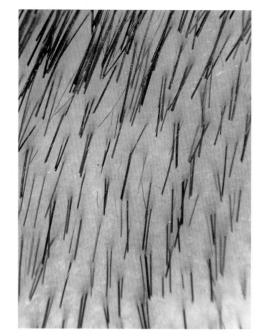

FIG. 20.9 Dermoscopy of a moth-eaten alopecic patch reveals decreased number of terminal hairs and some vellus hairs. (Image courtesy of Susana Ruiz-Tagle, MD and Letty Pincay Cedeño, MD.)

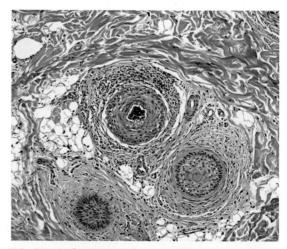

FIG. 20.10 Scalp biopsy from an alopecic moth-eaten patch reveals features similar to those of acute stage alopecia areata because of the increased number of telogen follicles, peribulbar lymphocytic infiltrate, and trichomalacia (hematoxylin and eosin, ×10).

Alternative drugs include (1) doxycycline 100 mg twice daily for 15 days; (2) tetracycline 500 mg every 6 h for 15 days; (3) procaine penicillin 2.4 millions UI + probenecide 500 mg for 14 days; and (4) Ceftriaxone 250 mg IM/IV q.d. for 10–14 days.

DEMODEX FOLLICULITIS

Etiology

Demodex spp. are tiny parasitic mites that live within or near the hair follicles of mammals. There are two species, *Demodex folliculorum* and *Demodex brevis*, typically found on humans. Infestation with *Demodex* is common, with prevalence in healthy adults varying between 23% and 100%.[40] *Demodex* infestation usually remains asymptomatic, although occasionally skin symptoms may occur because of imbalance in the immune mechanisms.

The adult *D. folliculorum* mites are 0.3–0.4 mm in length, and those of *D. brevis* are slightly shorter of 0.15–0.2 mm length, with females somewhat shorter and rounder than males.[40] This makes them invisible to the naked eye, but under the microscope, their structure is clearly visible as a semitransparent, elongated body that consists of two fused segments.

Clinical Presentation

Demodex is an ectoparasite of the pilosebaceous follicle and sebaceous gland, typically found on the face including cheeks, nose, chin, forehead, temples, eyelashes, brows, and also scalp, neck, and ears. Demodicidosis of the scalp can cause dryness, follicular scaling, superficial vesicles, and pustules. The patient can complain of burning and pruritic sensation.

Dermoscopy

Dermoscopic examination reveals *Demodex* tails and *Demodex* follicular openings, considered specific features for demodicidosis of face.[41] Sometimes in the scalp, only yellowish perifollicular scaling and multiple arborizing vessels are seen (Fig. 20.11).

Pathology

The mite is usually found as an incidental finding in scalp biopsies, for example, from androgenetic alopecia (Fig. 20.12), and is particularly better appreciated within the hair canal in horizontal sections at the level of the infundibulum.

Treatment

Various therapeutic regimens have been proposed to treat demodicidosis including those with ivermectin,

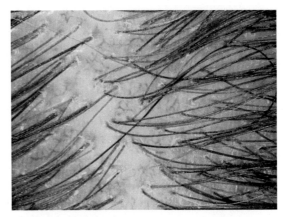

FIG. 20.11 Demodex infestation of scalp. Note the yellowish perifollicular scaling and multiple arborizing vessels on dermoscopy.

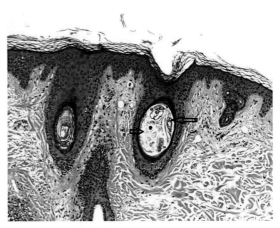

FIG. 20.12 Scalp biopsy of androgenetic alopecia: On horizontal sections, *Demodex* mites (*long arrow*) are found within the infundibular canal (*short arrow*) (hematoxylin and eosin, ×10).

permethrin, crotamiton, and lindane. Some data from ophthalmology suggest that topical tea tree oil can be helpful to reduce the counts of *Demodex* in ocular itching due to *Demodex* blepharitis.[42]

SEBORRHEIC DERMATITIS

Etiology

SD is a chronic and recurrent superficial dermatitis with a prevalence of 1%–3% in the general population.[43] However, SD is more prevalent in patients with immunodeficiencies and neurologic conditions, such as HIV/ AIDS or Parkinson's disease.[44]

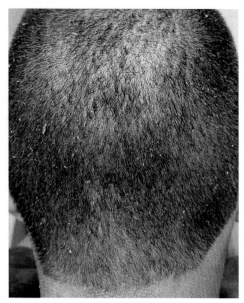

FIG. 20.13 Seborrheic dermatitis with numerous white flakes on the scalp visible to the naked eye.

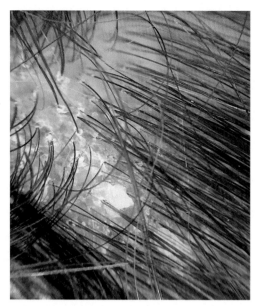

FIG. 20.14 Seborrheic dermatitis shows on dermoscopy yellowish perifollicular scaling and diffuse erythema.

The etiopathogenesis has not been fully elucidated; many factors such as *Malassezia* spp. colonization, sebum production, and individual immune response are thought to play an important role in its pathogenesis.[44]

Dandruff (pityriasis simplex capitis) is a mild presentation of the disease, resulting in fine scaling of the scalp. SD occurs most often on the face, scalp, and chest.

Clinical Presentation

Clinical lesions of SD are characterized by yellowish moist, greasy scales, erythema, and pruritus over the scalp and over oily areas such as eyebrows, beard, nasolabial and postauricular creases. Dandruff is marked by white-grayish tiny flakes that can accumulate and fall from the scalp onto the shoulders (Fig. 20.13). Usually the scalp is neither inflamed nor pruritic.

Dermoscopy

The trichoscopy features of scalp SD include yellowish perifollicular scaling and multiple thin arborizing vessels[45,46] (Fig. 20.14).

Pathology

SD on pathology is characterized by peri-infundibular (shoulder-like) parakeratosis, dilated sebaceous canals, and hyperplastic sebaceous glands. There is usually mild spongiosis of the epidermis and the follicular epithelium at the isthmus and infundibular level as well as a nonspecific inflammatory infiltrate in the dermis (Fig. 20.15).

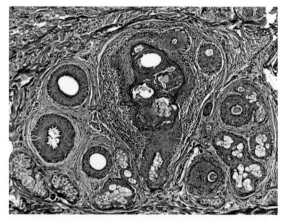

FIG. 20.15 Seborrheic dermatitis: On horizontal sections at the level of the isthmus, there are follicular parakeratosis (*black arrow*), dilated sebaceous canals (*yellow arrow*), and hyperplastic sebaceous glands. There are usually mild spongiosis and nonspecific inflammatory infiltrate in the dermis (*blue arrow*) (hematoxylin and eosin, ×10).

Treatment

Treatment options for SD are summarized in Table 20.3.

Treatment choice depends on many factors including type of hair, processed versus natural hair, age, race, and location on the body (see also Chapter 27). Topical

TABLE 20.3
Treatment Options for Seborrheic Dermatitis

Antiseborrheic shampoos: ketoconazole 1%–2%, ciclopirox, selenium sulfide, zinc pyrithione, or coal tar

Topical low-potency steroids (e.g., hydrocortisone, betamethasone)

Topical antifungal medications (e.g., miconazole or ketoconazole)

Topical calcineurin inhibitors (e.g., tacrolimus, pimecrolimus)

Topical keratolytics (salicylic acid or urea)

ORAL REGIMENS[44]:

Ketoconazole 200 mg daily for 4 weeks

Itraconazole 200 mg/d for the first week of the month followed by 200 mg/d on the first 2 days for 2–11 months

Terbinafine 250 mg/d either as a continuous (4–6 weeks) or as an intermittent regimen (12 days per month) for 3 months

Fluconazole 50 mg/d for 2 weeks or 200–300 mg weekly for 2–4 weeks

agents that reduce inflammation and scale production have been shown to be effective in the management of SD. These include either symptomatic keratolytic agents or etiologic therapies, e.g., antifungal medications and corticosteroids. Topical antifungal treatments reduce *Malassezia* spp. proliferation and the resulting inflammation, thus leading to improvement of SD.[47] Corticosteroid treatments are generally used to reduce inflammation.

As there is no cure for SD, patients must be made aware that this is a relapsing condition that may require maintenance treatment.

REFERENCES

1. Ilkit M, Demirhindi H. Asymptomatic dermatophyte scalp carriage: laboratory diagnosis, epidemiology and management. *Mycopathologia.* 2008;165(2):61–71. Epub 2007 Nov 23.
2. Bournerias I, De Chauvin MF, Datry A, et al. Unusual *Microsporum canis* infections in adult HIV patients. *J Am Acad Dermatol.* 1996;35(5 Pt 2):808–810.
3. Bronson DM, Desai DR, Barsky S, Foley SM. An epidemic of infection with *Trichophyton tonsurans* revealed in a 20-year survey of fungal infections in Chicago. *J Am Acad Dermatol.* 1983;8(3):322–330.
4. Bennassar A, Grimalt R. Management of tinea capitis in childhood. *Clin Cosmet Investig Dermatol.* 2010;3:89–98.
5. Sandoval AB, Ortiz JA, Rodrigues JM, Vargas AG, Quintero DG. Dermoscopic pattern in tinea capitis. *Rev Iberoam Micol.* 2010;27(3):151–152.
6. Ali S, Graham TA, Forgie SE. The assessment and management of tinea capitis in children. *Pediatr Emerg Care.* 2007;23(9):662–665.
7. Chen C, Koch LH, Dice JE, et al. A randomized, double-blind study comparing the efficacy of selenium sulfide shampoo 1% and ciclopirox shampoo 1% as adjunctive treatments for tinea capitis in children. *Pediatr Dermatol.* 2010;27(5):459–462.
8. Deng S, Hu H, Abliz P, et al. A random comparative study of terbinafine versus griseofulvin in patients with tinea capitis in Western China. *Mycopathologia.* 2011;172(5):365–372.
9. Elewski BE, Cáceres HW, DeLeon L, et al. Terbinafine hydrochloride oral granules versus oral griseofulvin suspension in children with tinea capitis: results of two randomized, investigator-blinded, multicenter, international, controlled trials. *J Am Acad Dermatol.* 2008; 59(1):41–54.
10. González U, Seaton T, Bergus G, et al. Systemic antifungal therapy for tinea capitis in children. *Cochrane Database Syst Rev.* 2007;(4):CD004685.
11. Gupta AK, Adam P, Dlova N, et al. Therapeutic options for the treatment of tinea capitis caused by *Trichophyton* species: griseofulvin versus the new oral antifungal agents, terbinafine, itraconazole, and fluconazole. *Pediatr Dermatol.* 2001;18(5):433–438.
12. Tey HL, Tan AS, Chan YC. Meta-analysis of randomized, controlled trials comparing griseofulvin and terbinafine in the treatment of tinea capitis. *J Am Acad Dermatol.* 2011;64(4):663–670.
13. Nutanson I, Steen CJ, Schwartz RA, Janniger CK. Pediculus humanus capitis: an update. *Acta Dermatovenerol Alp Pannonica Adriat.* 2008;17(4):147–154.
14. Suleman M, Jabeen N. Head lice infestation in some urban localities of NWFP. *Pak Ann Trop Med Parasitol.* 1989;83:539–547.
15. Heukelbach J, Wilcke T, Winter B, Feldmeier H. Epidemiology and morbidity of scabies and pediculosis capitis in resource-poor communities in Brazil. *Br J Dermatol.* 2005;153:150–156.
16. Catalá S, Junco L, Vaporaky R. Pediculus capitis infestation according to sex and social factors in Argentina. *Rev Saude Publica.* 2005;39:438–443.
17. Bachok N, Nordin RB, Awang CW, Ibrahim NA, Naing L. Prevalence and associated factors of head lice infestation among primary schoolchildren in Kelantan, Malaysia. *Southeast Asian J Trop Med Public Health.* 2006;37:536–543.
18. Falagas ME, Matthaiou DK, Rafailidis PI, Panos G, Pappas G. Worldwide prevalence of head lice. *Emerg Infect Dis.* 2008;14:1493–1494.
19. Bloomfield D. Head lice. *Pediatr Rev.* 2002;23:34–35.
20. Madke B, Khopkar U. Pediculosis capitis: an update. *Indian J Dermatol Venereol Leprol.* 2012;78:429–438.

21. Janniger CK, Kuflik AS. Pediculosis capitis. *Cutis.* 1993;51:407–408.

22. Mumcuoglu KY, Klaus S, Kafka D, Teiler M, Miller J. Clinical observations related to head lice infestation. *J Am Acad Dermatol.* 1991;25:248–251.

23. Slowinska M, Rudnicka L, Schwartz RA, et al. Comma hairs: a dermoscopic marker of tinea capitis: a rapid diagnostic method. *J Am Acad Dermatol.* 2008;59(5 suppl):S77–S79.

24. Neira PE, Molina LR, Correa AX, Américo Muñoz NR, Oschilewski DE. Metal microchanelled fine-toothed comb use in the diagnosis of pediculosis. *An Bras Dermatol.* 2009;84:615–621.

25. Dodd CS. Interventions for treating headlice. *Cochrane Database Syst Rev.* 2001;2:CD001165.

26. Ameen M, Arenas R, Villanueva-Reyes J, et al. Oral ivermectin for treatment of pediculosis capitis. *Pediatr Infect Dis J.* 2010;29:991–993.

27. Magalhaes AR, Mondino SSB, Silva M, Nishikawa MM. Morphological and biochemical characterization of the aetiological agents of white piedra. *Mem Inst Oswaldo Cruz.* 2008;103(8):786–790.

28. Chagas-Neto TC, Chaves GM, Colombo AL. Update on the genus *Trichosporon. Mycopathologia.* 2008;166:121–132.

29. Saxena S, Uniyal V, Bhatt RP. Inhibitory effect of essential oils against *Trichosporon ovoides* causing Piedra hair infection. *Braz J Microbiol.* 2012;43(4):1347–1354.

30. Gip L. Black Piedra: the first case treated with terbinafine (Lamisil). *Br J Dermatol.* 1994;130:26–28.

31. Kubec K, Dvorak R, Alsaleh QA. Trichosporosis (white piedra) in Kuwait. *Int J Dermatol.* 1998;37:186–187.

32. Vafaie J, Weinberg JM, Smith B, Mizuguchi RS. Alopecia in association with sexually transmitted disease: a review. *Cutis.* 2005;76:361–366.

33. Hira SK, Patel JS, Bhat SG, Chilikima K, Mooney N. Clinical manifestations of secondary syphilis. *Int J Dermatol.* 1987;26:103–107.

34. Bi MY, Cohen PR, Robinson FW, Gray JM. Alopecia syphilitica- report of a patient with secondary syphilis presenting as moth- eaten alopecia and a review of its common mimickers. *Dermatol Online J.* 2009;15:6.

35. Hernandez-Bel P, Unamuno B, Sánchez-Carazo JL, Febrer I, Alegre V. Alopecia sifilitica: presentacion de 5 casos y revision de la literatura. *Actas Dermosifiliogr.* 2013;104:512–517.

36. Jordaan HF, Louw M. The moth-eaten alopecia of secondary syphilis. A histopathological study of 12 patients. *Am J Dermatopathol.* 1995;17:158–162.

37. Ye Y, Zhang X, Zhao Y, et al. The clinical and trichoscopic features of syphilitic alopecia. *J Dermatol Case Rep.* 2014;3:78–80.

38. Piraccini BM, Broccoli A, Starace M, et al. Hair and scalp manifestations in secondary syphilis: epidemiology, clinical features and trichoscopy. *Dermatology.* 2015;231(2):171–176.

39. Tognetti L, Cinotti E, Perrot J-L, Campoli M, Rubegni P. Syphilitic alopecia: uncommon trichoscopic findings. *Dermatol Pract Concept.* 2017;7(3):55–59.

40. Rather PA, Hassan I. Human *Demodex* mite: the versatile mite of dermatological importance. *Indian J Dermatol.* 2014;59(1):60–66.

41. Friedman P, Sabban EC, Cabo H. Usefulness of dermoscopy in the diagnosis and monitoring treatment of demodicidosis. *Dermatol Pract Concept.* 2017;7(1):35–38.

42. Gao YY, Xu DL, Huang lJ, Wang R, Tseng SC. Treatment of ocular itching associated with ocular demodicosis by 5% tea tree oil ointment. *Cornea.* 2012;31(1):14–17.

43. Mameri ACA, Carneiro S, Mameri LMA, Telles da Cunha JM, Ramos-E-Silva M. History of seborrheic dermatitis: conceptual and clinico-pathologic evolution. *Skinmed.* 2017;15(3):187–194.

44. Gupta AK, Bluhm R. Seborrheic dermatitis. *J Eur Acad Dermatol Venereol.* 2004;18:13–26.

45. Kim GW, Jung HJ, Ko HC, et al. Dermoscopy can be useful in differentiating scalp psoriasis from seborrheic dermatitis. *Br J Dermatol.* 2011;164(3):652–656.

46. Ross EK, Vincenzi C, Tosti A. Videodermoscopy in the evaluation of hair and scalp disorders. *J Am Acad Dermatol.* 2006;55(5):799–806.

47. Stefanaki I, Katsambas A. Therapeutic update on seborrheic dermatitis. *Skin Ther Lett.* 2010;15(5):1–4.

CHAPTER 21

The Itchy Scalp

NAYOUNG LEE, MD • GIL YOSIPOVITCH, MD

INTRODUCTION

Scalp pruritus is a clinical feature that is shared by a vast array of medical conditions and a common chief complaint of patients presenting to the dermatology clinic. According to a US survey of 735 people, scalp pruritus was reported in up to 50%.[1] This symptom can have a profound and significant negative impact on quality of life.[2] Chronic scalp pruritus is especially prevalent in the aging population.[3,4] The scalp is a location consisting of complex neural and vasculature networks. It is highly innervated by branches of the trigeminal nerve as well as the cervical plexus.[5,6] Depending on the etiology, scalp pruritus can pose a diagnostic and/or therapeutic challenge. Scalp pruritus can be initially divided into two broad categories: (1) pruritus associated with a primary cutaneous disease and (2) pruritus without primary cutaneous findings. The first category includes inflammatory, infectious, and neoplastic processes. The latter category can be further subdivided into scalp pruritus due to an underlying systemic disease, neurologic disorders, and psychiatric conditions. This chapter will focus on diseases primarily localized to the scalp or with prominent involvement of the scalp, with a particular focus on treatment strategies tailored to the specific etiologies.

DERMATOLOGIC PRURITUS

Physical examination may reveal a primary dermatologic condition affecting the scalp. Skin conditions that can cause scalp pruritus consist of diseases that have a predilection for the scalp and diseases without a particular predilection but can present on the scalp (Table 21.1).

PRIMARY CUTANEOUS DISEASES
Inflammatory
Seborrheic dermatitis
The most common cause of scalp pruritus is seborrheic dermatitis,[7] an inflammatory disease attributed to *Malassezia* spp. The scalp, rich in sebaceous glands, provides the ideal environment to host the obligate lipophilic *Malassezia* spp. Seborrheic dermatitis is easily recognized, characterized by erythema of the scalp with overlying greasy, yellow interfollicular scale. Sixty-six percent of patients with seborrheic dermatitis complain of pruritus.[1] Available treatments include antifungal shampoos containing ingredients with activity against *Malassezia*, such as pyrithione zinc, ciclopirox, selenium sulfide, and ketoconazole, and keratolytic agents, such as salicylic acid. Evidenced-based Danish guidelines recommend azole antifungals as the first-line treatment.[8] Two recent Cochrane reviews reported that the antifungal agents, such as ketoconazole 1%–2% and ciclopirox 1%, and topical corticosteroids, such as 0.1%–1% hydrocortisone, 0.05%–0.1% betamethasone, 0.05% clobetasol, 0.1% mometasone, and 0.01% fluocinolone acetonide, were effective in decreasing scaling and pruritus in seborrheic dermatitis of the scalp. However, they noted that the effects of these treatments on scalp pruritus specifically were difficult to ascertain because of the lack of an adequate scale for measuring this symptom.[9,10] Potent topical corticosteroids can be used for severe cases, as well as oral antifungal agents. Itraconazole 200 mg daily for 1 week followed by 200 mg daily for the first 2 days of every month for 3 months has been shown to improve pruritus.[11] Patients receiving itraconazole had a lower recurrence rate compared with those receiving placebo, suggesting that itraconazole may be beneficial as maintenance therapy. In another study, fluconazole failed to demonstrate statistically significant efficacy in reducing pruritus and scaling.[12]

While antifungal agents, keratolytics, and topical corticosteroids aim at decreasing pruritus by reducing scaling, an alternative approach to improving the perception of pruritus may be to target histamine. Interestingly, higher concentrations of histamine have been found in the scalp stratum corneum in patients with seborrheic dermatitis compared with those without, suggesting a role for antihistamines in the treatment of pruritus in these patients.[13]

TABLE 21.1
Etiologies of Scalp Pruritus

Primary cutaneous disease	Inflammatory	Seborrheic dermatitis Scalp psoriasis Atopic dermatitis Dermatomyositis Scarring alopecias (such as lichen planopilaris and central centrifugal cicatricial alopecia) Allergic contact dermatitis Lichen simplex chronicus Bullous pemphigoid Epidermolysis bullosa acquisita Cicatricial pemphigoid, Brunsting-Perry variant Linear scleroderma, en coup de sabre
	Infectious	Tinea capitis Pediculosis Folliculitis Scabies
	Neoplastic	Leukemia Lymphoma Polycythemia vera Cutaneous T-cell lymphoma Basal cell carcinoma
Pruritus without cutaneous findings	Underlying systemic disease	Diabetes mellitus Chronic renal failure Cholestatic liver disease Drug-induced pruritus Endocrine disorders (i.e., thyroid disease) Eosinophilic arteritis of the scalp
	Neurologic disorders	Postherpetic neuralgia Migraine headache Atypical facial neuralgia Scalp dysesthesia Spinal cord injury Cervical spinal stenosis Wallenberg syndrome Brain tumors Trigeminal trophic syndrome
	Psychiatric disorders	Obsessive-compulsive disorders Anxiety disorders Somatoform and dissociative disorders Tactile hallucinations Delusions of parasitosis Schizophrenia Depression Substance abuse
	Miscellaneous	Pruritus of advanced aging

Scalp psoriasis

A condition that can sometimes be difficult to clinically distinguish from seborrheic dermatitis is scalp psoriasis, another inflammatory cause of pruritus. Scalp involvement is common in psoriasis and can be the only sign of their disease in some patients.[14] In a survey of 195 patients with psoriasis, 58% reported scalp pruritus.[15] A separate Italian survey of 90 patients with moderate-to-severe psoriasis reported the scalp to be the most common site with pruritus.[16] Pruritus was localized to the affected areas on the scalp in 70% of the cases.[16]

Treatment of scalp pruritus in these patients involves treatment of their underlying psoriasis. There are few topical agents available for scalp psoriasis. Topical corticosteroids are more effective than vitamin D analogues, such as calcipotriene or calcipotriol, though adding vitamin D analogues may be helpful in the long-term in reducing symptoms.[17,18] There is no current consensus on the most effective topical corticosteroid and the preferred vehicle of delivery, such as shampoo, solution, lotion, or foam. Betamethasone valerate foam 0.12% or clobetasol foam 0.05% is typically used.[19–21]

Other topical agents that have been reported to have efficacy in scalp psoriasis, albeit lower efficacy than topical corticosteroids, include coal tar and salicylic acid. Because of its antiproliferative and antipruritic properties, coal tar is still considered the first-line agent in many parts of the world.[22,23] Salicylic acid in concentrations greater than 5% is a potent keratolytic agent and is useful for descaling thick psoriatic plaques.[24] Owing to its skin-softening effect, salicylic acid facilitates penetration of other topical agents and enhances their efficacy.[25] Salicylic acid also has a direct antipruritic effect and has been shown to reduce pruritus in scalp psoriasis.[26–28] Side effects are mild, although acute telogen effluvium has been noted in patients treated with salicylic acid for scalp psoriasis.[27] Combination therapy with topical corticosteroid and salicylic acid appears to be more effective than monotherapy with either agent alone.[29,30] In conclusion, salicylic acid can be helpful as an adjunctive therapy along with topical corticosteroids, especially when there is thick scaling.

Of note, various neurogenic mediators are proposed to be involved in propagating pruritus in scalp psoriasis. Increased intraepidermal nerve fiber density has been observed in scalp psoriasis plaques compared with nonlesional skin.[31] Compared with nonlesional skin, psoriatic plaques have been shown to be highly innervated in the epidermis and the papillary dermis, with higher numbers of perivascular nerve fibers containing substance P, a known mediator of pruritus, and increased expression of nerve growth factor and its receptor.[32] This same study also showed mast cell degranulation in the papillary dermis in lesional skin. Thus, it stands to reason that topical agents targeting cutaneous nerves, such as the compounded formulation of ketamine 10%, amitriptyline 5%, and lidocaine 5% in a foam vehicle, may have a role in reducing pruritus in these patients.

This compounded formulation is thought to function by inhibiting N-methyl-D-aspartate receptor and sodium channels, thereby decreasing Aδ- and C-nerve fiber hypersensitivity.[33]

Oral antihistamines may also be helpful in combination with other therapies.

In refractory cases of pruritus associated with scalp psoriasis, topical pramoxine, applied three to four times per day, may be beneficial.[34] Phototherapy with a narrowband UVB comb three times a week and excimer laser therapy twice weekly have been shown to be helpful.[35,36]

Systemic therapies, such as methotrexate, cyclosporine, biologic agents, and small molecule immune modulators, are typically reserved for patients with lesions on also the body, and few have been assessed for their efficacy in scalp psoriasis specifically. The anti-TNF-α agents, infliximab, etanercept, and adalimumab, and anti-IL-12/IL-23 drugs are thought to be similarly effective for scalp psoriasis, with resultant reduction in scalp pruritus, although there are no randomized controlled trials focusing on the scalp in particular. The anti-IL-17 agents have proven to be particularly effective for reducing psoriatic pruritus. Secukinumab, a monoclonal antibody targeting IL-17A, has been shown to significantly improve scalp scaling and pruritus when administered at 300 mg monthly, compared with 150 mg monthly or placebo.[37] It has been shown to have greater efficacy in reducing pruritus after 16 weeks of treatment compared with ustekinumab, an anti-IL-12/IL-23 drug, in a head-to-head trial.[38] Similarly, ixekizumab, another anti-IL-17A agent, has also been shown to be effective, and results of a phase III trial suggest that ixekizumab may have more success than etanercept for scalp psoriasis.[39] In vivo mouse studies have found that scalp psoriasis had a Th1/Th17 activation profile, similar to skin psoriasis, but with more Th1 and less Th22 activation, providing a possible explanation for the success of biologic agents targeting the Th17/IL-17 pathway, such as ixekizumab and secukinumab, in the treatment of scalp lesions in psoriasis patients.[40]

Newer oral agents have also demonstrated efficacy in scalp psoriasis. Patients treated with apremilast, a phosphodiesterase-4 inhibitor, reported a significant improvement in scalp pruritus just after two weeks of treatment.[41] FDA-approved for the treatment of rheumatoid arthritis, tofacitinib is an oral janus kinase inhibitor that is currently under investigation for use in various conditions, including psoriasis. A randomized controlled trial demonstrated improvement in pruritus in more than 87% of patients, and the effect of this medication on scalp pruritus in particular remains to be seen.[42]

Atopic dermatitis

Although the main symptom of atopic dermatitis is pruritus, scalp pruritus is not a profound symptom in adult atopic dermatitis patients as it is in pediatric patients. Topical corticosteroids and calcineurin inhibitors have been traditionally used and can reduce itch. A newer topical agent is crisaborole, a phosphodiesterase-4 inhibitor, which has been shown to significantly reduce pruritus by day 14 of therapy.[43,44] Crisaborole is indicated for patients older than two years and has not shown to induce skin atrophy or malignancies.[45,46] However, crisaborole was not used on the scalp in any of the studies on atopic dermatitis because of difficulty in application onto hair-bearing areas. A novel biologic agent targeting the α subunit of interleukin-4 receptor (IL-4R), dupilumab, has recently gained FDA approval for the treatment of moderate-to-severe atopic dermatitis. Dupilumab is effective for recalcitrant patients who do not respond to topical steroids or calcineurin inhibitors. Its role in reducing itchy scalp in atopic dermatitis remains to be investigated.

Dermatomyositis

A pruritic and psoriasiform rash on the scalp is a common finding in the classic presentation of adult dermatomyositis.[47] A recent study showed that scalp pruritus is more common in anti-TIF-1γ antibody–positive patients. As anti-TIF-1γ antibodies are associated with malignancy, scalp pruritus in dermatomyositis may be a marker for underlying malignancy.[48] Severity of pruritus has been shown to correlate with the severity of cutaneous disease, and therefore, treatment of pruritus in these patients should be aimed at reducing disease activity.[49] Topical calcineurin inhibitors have been shown to be useful for itch in dermatomyositis.[50-52] For systemic therapy, hydroxychloroquine 200–400 mg daily is first line and is effective in 80% of patients.[53] Quinacrine 100 mg twice a day can be added or hydroxychloroquine can be switched to chloroquine 250–500 mg daily if the response is inadequate. Patients should be counseled, however, that they have a higher risk of cutaneous adverse reactions to antimalarials.[54] Methotrexate 15–35 mg weekly or mycophenolate mofetil (MMF) 1–1.5 g twice daily may be beneficial, given that they are used to treat cutaneous dermatomyositis and they have demonstrated antipruritic effects in primary biliary cirrhosis and atopic dermatitis, respectively.[55,56] However, their role in ameliorating pruritus specifically associated with dermatomyositis is not yet clear.

Recent studies suggest that scalp pruritus in dermatomyositis may be of neuropathic etiology. Scalp biopsies in these patients revealed alterations in the epidermal and dermal nerve fibers, with increased percentage of neuropeptide-containing nerves compared with control biopsies.[57] This mechanism may provide an explanation for the authors' successful experience with topical ketamine 10%, amitriptyline 5%, and lidocaine in foam formulation for the treatment of scalp pruritus in dermatomyositis.

Scarring alopecias

Inflammatory disorders leading to scarring alopecia of the scalp are commonly associated with pruritus of the affected area. In a case series of 29 patients with lichen planopilaris (LPP), scalp pruritus was the most commonly reported symptom[58] and is thought to signal disease activity.[59] Treatment of pruritus in these patients is aimed at treating the underlying inflammation. Monotherapy with topical corticosteroids or topical calcineurin inhibitors is often insufficient and many require systemic therapies.[60] The first-line agent used in LPP is hydroxychloroquine 6.5 mg/kg/day or 200 mg twice a day, with a response rate of 55%, which peaks 12 months after initiation of therapy. Although the efficacy of hydroxychloroquine in halting the progression of hair loss has been debated, it appears to decrease symptoms of LPP, including scalp pruritus, burning, and pain.[61] Cyclosporine has also been found to be helpful in reducing pruritus after three to five months.[62] Patients who fail to respond to hydroxychloroquine or cyclosporine can be tried on MMF. Sixteen patients with refractory LPP were treated with MMF 500 mg twice daily for four weeks, then 1 g twice daily for at least 20 weeks, and 83% of the patients improved with therapy. Those that responded to MMF all did so within six months of drug initiation.[63]

Scalp pruritus, in addition to tenderness, can also be present in central centrifugal cicatricial alopecia (CCCA), a common cause of scarring alopecia in African-American women.[64] Given that these symptoms may signal disease activity, treatment of the underlying disease, as well as discouraging damaging hair-grooming practices, is crucial in CCCA.[65] Currently there are no prospective controlled studies to evaluate the efficacies of various therapies for CCCA. For mild disease, first-line therapy includes high-potency steroids daily until the disease is stable, then with reduced frequency, such as three times weekly, for maintenance.[66] Intralesional corticosteroids up to 10 mg/mL can be injected monthly for at least 6 months, then as needed for symptom control thereafter. A recent retrospective chart review of 15 patients suggested that topical corticosteroids with intralesional corticosteroid injections might prevent disease progression, though this was not a statistically significant result.[67] Tetracyclines can be used for at least 6 months in active disease because of their anti-inflammatory properties.[68] Bin Saif et al. showed that the severity of cowhage-induced pruritus correlated with the severity of CCCA, suggesting a role of drugs targeting protease-activated receptor (PAR)-2, a receptor for cowhage, in the treatment of the symptoms associated with CCCA.[6] PAR-2 is a known mediator of chronic pruritus and is expressed in the inner root sheath in the human hair follicle.[69] Interestingly, tetracycline decreases PAR-2 signaling, which may explain the reported efficacy of this antibiotic for this condition. Washing the hair at least once a week and using medicated shampoos containing ketoconazole or zinc pyrithione can decrease scaling in this inflammatory scalp disorder and improve pruritus.[70] Other systemic treatments that have been tried in this condition include hydroxychloroquine, thalidomide, cyclosporine, and MMF. All treatments should be tried for at least 6 months and can be gradually tapered and discontinued after 1 year of remission.[66]

Allergic contact dermatitis

The most common allergens for contact dermatitis of the scalp are chemicals found in hair dyes, hair treatments, and hair care products. Paraphenylenediamine, found in black hair dye, is a potent sensitizer. Withdrawal of the allergen and symptomatic treatment with topical corticosteroids and oral antihistamines are used to reduce pruritus.

Infectious
Tinea capitis

Several infections have a predilection for the scalp and present with scalp itching. The most common in the prepubertal population is tinea capitis. *Trichophyton tonsurans* is the most common causal organism of tinea capitis, representing greater than 90% of cases, followed by *Microsporum canis*.[71] Inflammatory tinea capitis presents with pustules and abscesses, and severe cases may present with a kerion, which is a boggy, purulent, tender nodule. Noninflammatory tinea capitis can have a more subtle presentation with patches of alopecia, often with fine scaling, accompanied by cervical or postauricular lymphadenopathy. Sebum has an inhibitory effect on the growth of dermatophytes, and the lack of mature sebaceous glands increases the susceptibility of prepubertal scalp to this scalp infection.[71] Therefore, tinea capitis is an important entity to consider in the investigation of scalp itching in pediatric patients in particular.

Treatment depends on the offending species. A randomized controlled trial demonstrated a higher cure rate for *T. tonsurans* tinea capitis with terbinafine than griseofulvin.[72] A separate meta-analysis revealed a higher cure rate of 50.9% for griseofulvin versus 34.7% with terbinafine for the treatment of tinea capitis attributed to *Microsporum* spp.[73]

Pediculosis capitis

Yet another condition that is more often seen in the pediatric population is pediculosis capitis caused by infestation of the scalp by the obligate parasitic head louse, *Pediculus humanus capitis*. Extremely contagious via close contact and fomites, head lice are typically seen in children who attend daycare or school. Caucasian and Asian hair is more susceptible to infestation than African-American hair because the organisms are unable to readily grip curly hair.[74] Head lice feed on the blood of human hosts every four to six hours, and the inflammatory response to the saliva and feces leads to intense pruritus, especially in the postauricular and occipital scalp. The diagnosis is confirmed by visualization of the adult louse or the nits adherent to hair shafts with the naked eye. Secondary cutaneous findings, such as erythema, excoriations, and superimposed impetigo, can be seen. The simplest treatment is to cut the hair. In 62 patients with confirmed head lice infestation, topical ivermectin lotion 1% had a higher cure rate than oral ivermectin and led to faster resolution of scalp pruritus.[75]

Neoplastic

Primary cutaneous malignancies, such as basal cell carcinoma (BCC) and squamous cell carcinoma (SCC) localized on the scalp, can be pruritic. A survey of 268 patients with scalp cutaneous malignancies, including BCC, SCC, and melanoma, revealed that itch was present in 37% of patients, mostly those with nonmelanoma skin cancer.[76] In cutaneous T-cell lymphoma (CTCL), pruritus is a prominent symptom and is particularly severe in patients with the folliculotropic variant, which is often associated with alopecia when present on the scalp. Gabapentin has also been used with good results in combination with low-dose mirtazapine 7.5–15 mg nightly for pruritus associated with CTCL.[77] Aprepitant, a neurokinin-1 receptor antagonist that is typically prescribed for its antiemetic properties, has also demonstrated efficacy in patients with pruritus attributed to Sezary syndrome.[78]

In addition, hematologic malignancies, such as lymphomas and leukemias, can present with scalp pruritus.[79] Treatment of pruritus involves the treatment of its underlying malignancy, which will not be reviewed here. Butorphanol 3–4 mg daily, prednisone, and thalidomide 200 mg daily have been reported to be effective for refractory pruritus due to Hodgkin lymphoma.[80,81]

PRURITUS WITHOUT ASSOCIATED SKIN FINDINGS

Neuropathic

Diabetes mellitus

A survey of geriatric patients with chronic pruritus revealed that there was a high prevalence of type 2 diabetes mellitus (DM2) in these patients, and the scalp was one of the most common locations affected by pruritus.[3] 40% of patients with DM2 reported scalp pruritus, as opposed to 17.5% of patients without DM2.[3] Increased frequency of pruritus localized to the scalp in DM2 could perhaps be attributed to diabetic neuropathy.[3] Scalp pruritus in diabetes mellitus has been shown to resolve with adequate blood glucose control.[82]

Postherpetic neuralgia

Although often painful, postherpetic neuralgia (PHN) can also be pruritic, especially if it occurs in the head and neck area in the V1 trigeminal nerve distribution.[83]

Cervical spine disease

In a retrospective study of 15 patients with scalp pruritus and burning, 14 of these patients were found to have cervical spine disease on imaging, with degenerative disk disease at the C5–C6 levels being the most common abnormality.[84]

Treatment for neuropathic pruritus

The compounded formulation of ketamine 10%, amitriptyline 5%, and lidocaine 5% in a lipoderm base has been shown to be effective for reducing neuropathic pruritus, as mentioned earlier.[33] A foam formulation is more easily applied onto the scalp and can be used up to three times daily. In general, agents that suppress glutamate release from presynaptic neurons, such as gabapentin and pregabalin, are helpful in the treatment of neuropathic pruritus, as glutamate is a major excitatory neurotransmitter.[85,86] Topical gabapentin 6% has demonstrated efficacy in various pruritic conditions, including PHN and trigeminal trophic syndrome.[87,88] In the authors' experience, topical gabapentin foam in concentrations up to 12% is only mildly effective for neuropathic itch on the scalp.

Underlying Systemic Disease

Various underlying systemic diseases are associated with intractable pruritus without any primary cutaneous findings. The pruritus may involve the scalp but is typically more generalized. The treatments are varied depending on the etiologies and are beyond the scope of this chapter.

Pruritus in the Elderly

Chronic pruritus is a common complaint in the elderly, and the scalp is frequently affected. The etiology is often multifactorial. Xerosis due to loss of skin barrier function, decreased sebaceous glands, increased skin pH, neuropathic changes, such as damage to the central or peripheral nerves secondary to aging and/or various comorbidities such as diabetes and nerve compression, and polypharmacy all contribute to the development of chronic pruritus in this population.[4] Furthermore, the immune system in the aging skin undergoes a process called immunosenescence. This phenomenon is characterized by alterations in the population of immune cells, with higher numbers of terminally differentiated T cells that preferentially produce IFN-γ and TNF-α, which serve to promote a proinflammatory environment.[89] Of note, lichen simplex chronicus is common in the elderly.

In addition to the aforementioned therapies aimed at treating the various etiologies of pruritus, topical interventions to reduce scalp pruritus should aim to promote an acidic pH in the skin. Patients should be advised to bathe in lukewarm water and to avoid using soap-based cleansers that can raise the skin pH. Acidic agents, such as salicylic acid, may be helpful.[4] For the neuropathic component of scalp pruritus in the elderly, topical ketamine, amitriptyline, and lidocaine, topical capsaicin, a desensitizer of peripheral nerves, and topical pramoxine, a local anesthetic, may be helpful.

Psychiatric Conditions

Trichotillomania

Trichotillomania is a habit-tic disorder characterized by a sense of tension before pulling the hair, followed by relief after completing the act.[90] Patients may have an urge to scratch a perceived sense of itch. A helpful intervention is habit reversal training (HRT), a psychologic technique that attempts to replace negative behaviors with neutral actions.[91] Selective serotonin reuptake inhibitors, clomipramine, and N-acetylcysteine 1200–2400 mg daily have also demonstrated benefit.[92]

Stress and scalp itch

In general, psychologic stress has been shown to aggravate pruritus in patients with underlying pruritic dermatoses as well as scalp itch.[93] Various psychologic interventions can be helpful in mitigating the symptom of itch in these patients. HRT attempts to replace negative behaviors with neutral actions and has shown efficacy not only in disorders with obsessive behaviors, such as prurigo nodularis and trichotillomania, but also in atopic dermatitis.[94,95] Relaxation techniques, including progressive muscle relaxation (PMR) and autogenic training, have also shown to be helpful in atopic dermatitis. PMR involves repeated intervals of tensing different muscle groups followed by a period of relaxation. PMR twice daily for 4 weeks significantly reduced itch intensity as well as sleep quality in atopic dermatitis patients.[96] Autogenic training uses suggestive phrases to induce certain body sensations. Other psychologic interventions, such as cognitive behavioral therapy and mindfulness-based stress reduction, could be useful in reducing chronic pruritus.[97] However, these interventions may only be effective in patients who remain open-minded about the efficacy of these methods.

REFERENCES

1. Elewski BE. Clinical diagnosis of common scalp disorders. *J Investig Dermatol Symp Proc.* 2005;10(3):190–193.
2. Tan J, Thomas R, Wang B, et al. Short-contact clobetasol propionate shampoo 0.05% improves quality of life in patients with scalp psoriasis. *Cutis.* 2009;83(3):157–164.
3. Valdes-Rodriguez R, Mollanazar NK, Gonzalez-Muro J, et al. Itch prevalence and characteristics in a hispanic geriatric population: a comprehensive study using a standardized itch questionnaire. *Acta Derm Venereol.* 2015;95(4): 417–421.
4. Valdes-Rodriguez R, Stull C, Yosipovitch G. Chronic pruritus in the elderly: pathophysiology, diagnosis and management. *Drugs Aging.* 2015;32(3):201–215.
5. Bin Saif GA, Ericson ME, Yosipovitch G. The itchy scalp–scratching for an explanation. *Exp Dermatol.* 2011;20(12):959–968.
6. Bin Saif GA, McMichael A, Kwatra SG, Chan YH, Yosipovitch G. Central centrifugal cicatricial alopecia severity is associated with cowhage-induced itch. *Br J Dermatol.* 2013;168(2):253–256.
7. Pierard-Franchimont C, Hermanns JF, Degreef H, Pierard GE. From axioms to new insights into dandruff. *Dermatology.* 2000;200(2):93–98.
8. Hald M, Arendrup MC, Svejgaard EL, et al. Evidence-based Danish guidelines for the treatment of *Malassezia*-related skin diseases. *Acta Derm Venereol.* 2015;95(1):12–19.
9. Kastarinen H, Okokon EO, Verbeek JH. Topical anti-inflammatory agents for seborrheic dermatitis of the face or scalp: summary of a Cochrane Review. *JAMA Dermatol.* 2015;151(2):221–222.
10. Okokon EO, Verbeek JH, Ruotsalainen JH, Ojo OA, Bakhoya VN. Topical antifungals for seborrhoeic dermatitis. *Cochrane Database Syst Rev.* 2015;(5):CD008138.
11. Ghodsi SZ, Abbas Z, Abedeni R. Efficacy of oral itraconazole in the treatment and relapse prevention of moderate to severe seborrheic dermatitis: a randomized, placebo-controlled trial. *Am J Clin Dermatol.* 2015;16(5):431–437.
12. Comert A, Bekiroglu N, Gurbuz O, Ergun T. Efficacy of oral fluconazole in the treatment of seborrheic dermatitis: a placebo-controlled study. *Am J Clin Dermatol.* 2007;8(4):235–238.
13. Kerr K, Schwartz JR, Filloon T, et al. Scalp stratum corneum histamine levels: novel sampling method reveals association with itch resolution in dandruff/seborrheic dermatitis treatment. *Acta Derm Venereol.* 2011;91(4):404–408.
14. Farber EM, Nall L. Natural history and treatment of scalp psoriasis. *Cutis.* 1992;49(6):396–400.
15. O'Neill JL, Chan YH, Rapp SR, Yosipovitch G. Differences in itch characteristics between psoriasis and atopic dermatitis patients: results of a web-based questionnaire. *Acta Derm Venereol.* 2011;91(5):537–540.
16. Prignano F, Ricceri F, Pescitelli L, Lotti T. Itch in psoriasis: epidemiology, clinical aspects and treatment options. *Clin Cosmet Investig Dermatol.* 2009;2:9–13.
17. Klaber MR, Hutchinson PE, Pedvis-Leftick A, et al. Comparative effects of calcipotriol solution (50 micrograms/ml) and betamethasone 17-valerate solution (1 mg/ml) in the treatment of scalp psoriasis. *Br J Dermatol.* 1994;131(5):678–683.
18. Schlager JG, Rosumeck S, Werner RN, et al. Topical treatments for scalp psoriasis. *Cochrane Database Syst Rev.* 2016;(2):CD009687.
19. Andreassi L, Giannetti A, Milani M, Scale Investigators G. Efficacy of betamethasone valerate mousse in comparison with standard therapies on scalp psoriasis: an open, multicentre, randomized, controlled, cross-over study on 241 patients. *Br J Dermatol.* 2003;148(1):134–138.
20. Lassus A. Local treatment of psoriasis of the scalp with clobetasol propionate and betamethasone-17,21-dipropionate: a double-blind comparison. *Curr Med Res Opin.* 1976;4(5):365–367.
21. Katz HI, Lindholm JS, Weiss JS, et al. Efficacy and safety of twice-daily augmented betamethasone dipropionate lotion versus clobetasol propionate solution in patients with moderate-to-severe scalp psoriasis. *Clin Ther.* 1995;17(3):390–401.
22. Roelofzen JH, Aben KK, Khawar AJ, Van de Kerkhof PC, Kiemeney LA, Van Der Valk PG. Treatment policy for psoriasis and eczema: a survey among dermatologists in The Netherlands and Belgian Flanders. *Eur J Dermatol.* 2007;17(5):416–421.

23. van de Kerkhof PC, Franssen ME. Psoriasis of the scalp. Diagnosis and management. *Am J Clin Dermatol.* 2001; 2(3):159–165.

24. Lebwohl M. A clinician's paradigm in the treatment of psoriasis. *J Am Acad Dermatol.* 2005;53(1 suppl 1):S59–S69.

25. Chan CS, Van Voorhees AS, Lebwohl MG, et al. Treatment of severe scalp psoriasis: from the medical board of the National Psoriasis Foundation. *J Am Acad Dermatol.* 2009;60(6):962–971.

26. Yosipovitch G, Sugeng MW, Chan YH, Goon A, Ngim S, Goh CL. The effect of topically applied aspirin on localized circumscribed neurodermatitis. *J Am Acad Dermatol.* 2001;45(6):910–913.

27. Dawn A, Yosipovitch G. Treating itch in psoriasis. *Dermatol Nurs.* 2006;18(3):227–233.

28. Kircik L. Salicylic Acid 6% in an ammonium lactate emollient foam vehicle in the treatment of mild-to-moderate scalp psoriasis. *J Drugs Dermatol.* 2011;10(3):270–273.

29. Nolting S, Hagemeier HH. Therapy of erythrosquamous dermatoses. Betamethasone dipropionate plus salicylic acid in comparison with betamethasone dipropionate solution. *Fortschr Med.* 1983;101(37):1679–1683.

30. Elie R, Durocher LP, Kavalec EC. Effect of salicylic acid on the activity of betamethasone-17,21-dipropionate in the treatment of erythematous squamous dermatoses. *J Int Med Res.* 1983;11(2):108–112.

31. Kim TW, Shim WH, Kim JM, et al. Clinical characteristics of pruritus in patients with scalp psoriasis and their relation with intraepidermal nerve fiber density. *Ann Dermatol.* 2014;26(6):727–732.

32. Nakamura M, Toyoda M, Morohashi M. Pruritogenic mediators in psoriasis vulgaris: comparative evaluation of itch-associated cutaneous factors. *Br J Dermatol.* 2003;149(4):718–730.

33. Lee HG, Grossman SK, Valdes-Rodriguez R, et al. Topical ketamine-amitriptyline-lidocaine for chronic pruritus: a retrospective study assessing efficacy and tolerability. *J Am Acad Dermatol.* 2017;76(4):760–761.

34. Stull C, Grossman S, Yosipovitch G. Current and emerging therapies for itch management in psoriasis. *Am J Clin Dermatol.* 2016;17(6):617–624.

35. Taneja A, Racette A, Gourgouliatos Z, Taylor CR. Broadband UVB fiber-optic comb for the treatment of scalp psoriasis: a pilot study. *Int J Dermatol.* 2004;43(6):462–467.

36. Morison WL, Atkinson DF, Werthman L. Effective treatment of scalp psoriasis using the excimer (308 nm) laser. *Photodermatol Photoimmunol Photomed.* 2006;22(4):181–183.

37. Kircik L, Fowler J, Weiss J, Meng X, Guana A, Nyirady J. Efficacy of secukinumab for moderate-to-severe head and neck psoriasis over 52 weeks: pooled analysis of four phase 3 studies. *Dermatol Ther.* 2016;6(4):627–638.

38. Thaci D, Blauvelt A, Reich K, et al. Secukinumab is superior to ustekinumab in clearing skin of subjects with moderate to severe plaque psoriasis: CLEAR, a randomized controlled trial. *J Am Acad Dermatol.* 2015;73(3): 400–409.

39. Reich K, Leonardi C, Lebwohl M, et al. Sustained response with ixekizumab treatment of moderate-to-severe psoriasis with scalp involvement: results from three phase 3 trials (UNCOVER-1, UNCOVER-2, UNCOVER-3). *J Dermatolog Treat.* 2017;28(4):282–287.

40. Ruano J, Suarez-Farinas M, Shemer A, Oliva M, Guttman-Yassky E, Krueger JG. Molecular and cellular profiling of scalp psoriasis reveals differences and similarities compared to skin psoriasis. *PLoS One.* 2016;11(2):e0148450.

41. Sobell JM, Foley P, Toth D, et al. Effects of apremilast on pruritus and skin discomfort/pain correlate with improvements in quality of life in patients with moderate to severe plaque psoriasis. *Acta Derm Venereol.* 2016;96(4):514–520.

42. Mamolo CM, Bushmakin AG, Cappelleri JC. Application of the itch severity score in patients with moderate-to-severe plaque psoriasis: clinically important difference and responder analyses. *J Dermatolog Treat.* 2015;26(2):121–123.

43. Paller AS, Tom WL, Lebwohl MG, et al. Efficacy and safety of crisaborole ointment, a novel, nonsteroidal phosphodiesterase 4 (PDE4) inhibitor for the topical treatment of atopic dermatitis (AD) in children and adults. *J Am Acad Dermatol.* 2016;75(3):494–503.e494.

44. Draelos ZD, Stein Gold LF, Murrell DF, Hughes MH, Zane LT. Post hoc analyses of the effect of crisaborole topical ointment, 2% on atopic dermatitis: associated pruritus from phase 1 and 2 clinical studies. *J Drugs Dermatol.* 2016;15(2):172–176.

45. Zane LT, Chanda S, Jarnagin K, Nelson DB, Spelman L, Gold LS. Crisaborole and its potential role in treating atopic dermatitis: overview of early clinical studies. *Immunotherapy.* 2016;8(8):853–866.

46. Jarnagin K, Chanda S, Coronado D, et al. Crisaborole topical ointment, 2%: a nonsteroidal, topical, anti-inflammatory phosphodiesterase 4 inhibitor in clinical development for the treatment of atopic dermatitis. *J Drugs Dermatol.* 2016;15(4):390–396.

47. Callen JP, Wortmann RL. Dermatomyositis. *Clin Dermatol.* 2006;24(5):363–373.

48. Fiorentino DF, Kuo K, Chung L, Zaba L, Li S, Casciola-Rosen L. Distinctive cutaneous and systemic features associated with antitranscriptional intermediary factor-1gamma antibodies in adults with dermatomyositis. *J Am Acad Dermatol.* 2015;72(3):449–455.

49. Robinson ES, Feng R, Okawa J, Werth VP. Improvement in the cutaneous disease activity of patients with dermatomyositis is associated with a better quality of life. *Br J Dermatol.* 2015;172(1):169–174.

50. Yosipovitch G, Tan A, LoSicco K, et al. A comparative study of clinical characteristics, work-up, treatment, and association to malignancy in dermatomyositis between two tertiary skin centers in the USA and Singapore. *Int J Dermatol.* 2013;52(7):813–819.

51. Quain RD, Werth VP. Management of cutaneous dermatomyositis: current therapeutic options. *Am J Clin Dermatol.* 2006;7(6):341–351.

52. Lampropoulos CE, D' Cruz DP. Topical tacrolimus treatment in a patient with dermatomyositis. *Ann Rheum Dis.* 2005;64(9):1376–1377.

53. Woo TY, Callen JP, Voorhees JJ, Bickers DR, Hanno R, Hawkins C. Cutaneous lesions of dermatomyositis are improved by hydroxychloroquine. *J Am Acad Dermatol.* 1984;10(4):592–600.

54. Pelle MT, Callen JP. Adverse cutaneous reactions to hydroxychloroquine are more common in patients with dermatomyositis than in patients with cutaneous lupus erythematosus. *Arch Dermatol.* 2002;138(9):1231–1233. Discussion 1233.

55. Giljaca V, Poropat G, Stimac D, Gluud C. Methotrexate for primary biliary cirrhosis. *Cochrane Database Syst Rev.* 2010;(5):CD004385.

56. Jackson JM, Fowler Jr JF, Callen JP, Lorenz DJ. Mycophenolate mofetil for the treatment of chronic dermatitis: an open-label study of 16 patients. *J Drugs Dermatol.* 2010;9(4):356–362.

57. Hurliman E, Groth D, Wendelschafer-Crabb G, et al. Small-fibre neuropathy in a patient with dermatomyositis and severe scalp pruritus. *Br J Dermatol.* 2017;176(1):209–211.

58. Cevasco NC, Bergfeld WF, Remzi BK, de Knott HR. A case-series of 29 patients with lichen planopilaris: the Cleveland Clinic Foundation experience on evaluation, diagnosis, and treatment. *J Am Acad Dermatol.* 2007;57(1):47–53.

59. Chiang C, Sah D, Cho BK, Ochoa BE, Price VH. Hydroxychloroquine and lichen planopilaris: efficacy and introduction of Lichen Planopilaris Activity Index scoring system. *J Am Acad Dermatol.* 2010;62(3):387–392.

60. Whiting DA. Cicatricial alopecia: clinico-pathological findings and treatment. *Clin Dermatol.* 2001;19(2):211–225.

61. Donati A, Assouly P, Matard B, Jouanique C, Reygagne P. Clinical and photographic assessment of lichen planopilaris treatment efficacy. *J Am Acad Dermatol.* 2011;64(3):597–598. Author reply 598–599.

62. Mirmirani P, Willey A, Price VH. Short course of oral cyclosporine in lichen planopilaris. *J Am Acad Dermatol.* 2003;49(4):667–671.

63. Cho BK, Sah D, Chwalek J, et al. Efficacy and safety of mycophenolate mofetil for lichen planopilaris. *J Am Acad Dermatol.* 2010;62(3):393–397.

64. McMichael AJ. Hair and scalp disorders in ethnic populations. *Dermatol Clin.* 2003;21(4):629–644.

65. Fu JM, Price VH. Approach to hair loss in women of color. *Semin Cutan Med Surg.* 2009;28(2):109–114.

66. Gathers RC, Lim HW. Central centrifugal cicatricial alopecia: past, present, and future. *J Am Acad Dermatol.* 2009;60(4):660–668.

67. Eginli A, Dothard E, Bagayoko CW, Huang K, Daniel A, McMichael AJ. A retrospective review of treatment results for patients with central centrifugal cicatrical alopecia. *J Drugs Dermatol.* 2017;16(4):317–320.

68. Summers P, Kyei A, Bergfeld W. Central centrifugal cicatricial alopecia – an approach to diagnosis and management. *Int J Dermatol.* 2011;50(12):1457–1464.

69. Steinhoff M, Corvera CU, Thoma MS, et al. Proteinase-activated receptor-2 in human skin: tissue distribution and activation of keratinocytes by mast cell tryptase. *Exp Dermatol.* 1999;8(4):282–294.

70. Callender VD, McMichael AJ, Cohen GF. Medical and surgical therapies for alopecias in black women. *Dermatol Ther.* 2004;17(2):164–176.

71. Elewski BE, Hughey LC, Sobera JO, Hay R. Fungal diseases. In: Bolognia JL, Jorizzo JL, Schaffer JV, eds. *Dermatology.* Elsevier; 2012.

72. Elewski BE, Caceres HW, DeLeon L, et al. Terbinafine hydrochloride oral granules versus oral griseofulvin suspension in children with tinea capitis: results of two randomized, investigator-blinded, multicenter, international, controlled trials. *J Am Acad Dermatol.* 2008;59(1):41–54.

73. Chen X, Jiang X, Yang M, et al. Systemic antifungal therapy for tinea capitis in children. *Cochrane Database Syst Rev.* 2016;(5):CD004685.

74. Burkhart CN, Burkhart CG. Head lice: scientific assessment of the nit sheath with clinical ramifications and therapeutic options. *J Am Acad Dermatol.* 2005;53(1):129–133.

75. Ahmad HM, Abdel-Azim ES, Abdel-Aziz RT. Assessment of topical versus oral ivermectin as a treatment for head lice. *Dermatol Ther.* 2014;27(5):307–310.

76. Yosipovitch G, Mills KC, Nattkemper LA, et al. Association of pain and itch with depth of invasion and inflammatory cell constitution in skin cancer: results of a large clinicopathologic study. *JAMA Dermatol.* 2014;150(11):1160–1166.

77. Demierre MF, Taverna J. Mirtazapine and gabapentin for reducing pruritus in cutaneous T-cell lymphoma. *J Am Acad Dermatol.* 2006;55(3):543–544.

78. Duval A, Dubertret L. Aprepitant as an antipruritic agent? *N Engl J Med.* 2009;361(14):1415–1416.

79. McCrary WJ, Hurst MD, Hiatt KM, Singh ZN, Wirges ML. Acute alopecia with underlying pruritic erythema. *J Am Acad Dermatol.* 2015;73(5):893–894.

80. Wang H, Yosipovitch G. New insights into the pathophysiology and treatment of chronic itch in patients with end-stage renal disease, chronic liver disease, and lymphoma. *Int J Dermatol.* 2010;49(1):1–11.

81. Goncalves F. Thalidomide for the control of severe paraneoplastic pruritus associated with Hodgkin's disease. *Am J Hosp Palliat Care.* 2010;27(7):486–487.

82. Scribner M. Diabetes and pruritus of the scalp. *JAMA.* 1977;237(15):1559.

83. Oaklander AL, Bowsher D, Galer B, Haanpaa M, Jensen MP. Herpes zoster itch: preliminary epidemiologic data. *J Pain.* 2003;4(6):338–343.

84. Thornsberry LA, English 3rd JC. Scalp dysesthesia related to cervical spine disease. *JAMA Dermatol.* 2013;149(2):200–203.

85. Cevikbas F, Steinhoff M, Ikoma A. Role of spinal neurotransmitter receptors in itch: new insights into therapies and drug development. *CNS Neurosci Ther*. 2011;17(6): 742–749.

86. Tey HL, Wallengren J, Yosipovitch G. Psychosomatic factors in pruritus. *Clin Dermatol*. 2013;31(1):31–40.

87. Brid T, Sacristan de Lama MP, Gonzalez N, Baamonde A. Topical gabapentin as add-on therapy for trigeminal neuralgia. A case report. *Pain Med*. 2017;18(9):1824–1826.

88. Hiom S, Patel GK, Newcombe RG, Khot S, Martin C. Severe postherpetic neuralgia and other neuropathic pain syndromes alleviated by topical gabapentin. *Br J Dermatol*. 2015;173(1):300–302.

89. Arnold CR, Wolf J, Brunner S, Herndler-Brandstetter D, Grubeck-Loebenstein B. Gain and loss of T cell subsets in old age–age-related reshaping of the T cell repertoire. *J Clin Immunol*. 2011;31(2):137–146.

90. Kuhn H, Mennella C, Magid M, Stamu-O'Brien C, Kroumpouzos G. Psychocutaneous disease: clinical perspectives. *J Am Acad Dermatol*. 2017;76(5):779–791.

91. Bloch MH, Landeros-Weisenberger A, Dombrowski P, et al. Systematic review: pharmacological and behavioral treatment for trichotillomania. *Biol Psychiatry*. 2007;62(8): 839–846.

92. Grant JE, Odlaug BL, Kim SW. N-acetylcysteine, a glutamate modulator, in the treatment of trichotillomania: a double-blind, placebo-controlled study. *Arch Gen Psychiatry*. 2009;66(7):756–763.

93. Yamamoto Y, Yamazaki S, Hayashino Y, et al. Association between frequency of pruritic symptoms and perceived psychological stress: a Japanese population-based study. *Arch Dermatol*. 2009;145(12):1384–1388.

94. Azrin NH, Nunn RG. Habit-reversal: a method of eliminating nervous habits and tics. *Behav Res Ther*. 1973; 11(4):619–628.

95. Noren P, Melin L. The effect of combined topical steroids and habit-reversal treatment in patients with atopic dermatitis. *Br J Dermatol*. 1989;121(3):359–366.

96. Bae BG, Oh SH, Park CO, et al. Progressive muscle relaxation therapy for atopic dermatitis: objective assessment of efficacy. *Acta Derm Venereol*. 2012;92(1):57–61.

97. Schut C, Mollanazar NK, Kupfer J, Gieler U, Yosipovitch G. Psychological interventions in the treatment of chronic itch. *Acta Derm Venereol*. 2016;96(2):157–161.

CHAPTER 22

Scalp Psoriasis

LAILA EL-SHABRAWI-CAELEN, MD

PSORIASIS OF THE SCALP AND PSORIASIFORM ALOPECIA: INTRODUCTION

Given the high frequency of psoriasis of the scalp, psoriasiform alopecia has drawn little attention in the literature.[1,2] There are, however, some peculiar changes attached to this disorder where the answers are still missing:

- Why is there such a degree of sebaceous gland atrophy?
- Why do some patients experience only temporary hair loss, whereas others suffer from a permanent scarring alopecia?
- Can we clearly differentiate true psoriasis of the scalp from tumor necrosis factor (TNF) α blocker–induced psoriasiform alopecia?

Let us dig into these subjects and try to answer some of these questions!

The prevalence of psoriasis lies between 2% and 5% of the general population, and the scalp is a site of predilection being involved in up to 80% of patients.[3] Typical psoriatic scaly plaques may develop all over the scalp, and extension beyond the hairline with advancing edges into the retroauricular area, neck, and face is common. Trichograms of plucked hair show an increased telogen rate, dystrophic hairs, and a higher number of vellus-like hairs.[4]

CLINICAL PATTERNS

Different types of alopecia can occur in the setting of psoriasis:

1. Patchy or diffuse hair loss in areas of psoriasis
2. Telogen effluvium
3. Scarring alopecia

The most common presentation (75%) is circumscribed hair loss within psoriatic plaques affecting not only the scalp (Fig. 22.1A and B) but also other body parts (Fig. 22.1C).[1] Fifty percent of patients have acute hair loss, whereas 10% show a chronic relapsing course.[1] The hair loss can be widespread and diffuse if larger areas are involved by psoriasis (25% of patients) and can coincide with the beginning of topical treatment

(30% of patients).[1] Local therapy induces desquamation of scales, and telogen hairs are increasingly shed with the scales. Friction- and therapy-induced manipulation enhances hair loss in affected areas.

This type of alopecia should not be confused with genuine telogen effluvium, which can be induced by antipsoriatic drugs, such as methotrexate, retinoids, and others.

In up to one-third of patients, the hair loss is the initial and sole manifestation of psoriasis and especially in such a circumstance dermatoscopy is helpful.

On **dermatoscopy** the observation of red dots and globules, twisted red loops, and glomerular vessels is highly suggestive of scalp psoriasis, whereas seborrheic dermatitis of the scalp, as the main differential diagnosis, commonly features an arborizing and atypical vascular pattern.[5]

COURSE AND PROGNOSIS

Forty percent of patients with psoriatic alopecia reveal a chronic clinical course of symptoms. An accurate and prompt therapy, however, is highly recommended, because some individuals may develop permanent, scarring alopecia, being observed in 12% of cases.[1,2,6–8] The destructive and permanent course of psoriatic alopecia is likely to be attributed to a long-standing and severe course of the disease, because the inflammation in psoriasis does not primarily target the vulnerable isthmic area, as is the case in, for example, lichen planopilaris. Inflammation in psoriatic alopecia is found mainly around the infundibulum. It is unlikely that the inflammation per se is the primary event that leads to scarring alopecia in psoriasis.[9,10]

The mechanism of scarring in psoriatic alopecia is poorly understood. The role of the sebaceous glands should be reconsidered, because on histopathology there is one striking phenomenon: sebaceous glands disappear. A pronounced atrophy and even loss of sebaceous glands is observed (see Fig. 22.1F). In up to 80% of cases with scalp psoriasis, sebaceous glands are diminished in size with 50%

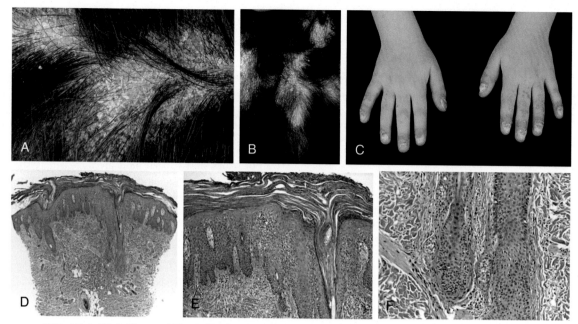

FIG. 22.1 **(A)** A 10-year-old boy with patchy alopecia and prominent white scales within areas of psoriasis. **(B)** Multiple areas of lesional alopecia on the scalp in the 10-year-old boy. **(C)** The same boy with psoriasis on the back of the hands, fingers, and advanced psoriasiform nail changes and underlying psoriasiform arthritis. **(D)** Hematoxylin and eosin stained slide 40× with typical features of psoriasis: psoriasiform epidermal hyperplasia with hypogranulosis, intracorneal and intraepidermal microabscess formation, and parakeratosis. **(E)** Higher power view ×100 reveals slight spongiosis, hypogranulosis, serum crusts with parakeratosis above follicular infundibula (lipping), and intracorneal and intraepidermal pustules. **(F)** Two non-anagen follicles with rudimentary sebaceous glands; note that the latter could be partly due to the physiologic prepubertal hypoplasia of sebaceous glands.

of these cases revealing a marked reduction or even loss of sebaceous glands.[9] An identical observation with dramatic sebaceous gland hypoplasia has been made in psoriatic lesions from body sides other than the scalp.[10]

Given the fact that sebum exerts an antimicrobial function, pronounced reduction of sebum is likely to be associated with an increased risk of bacterial infection. Bacterial superinfections therefore may play a role in the development of cicatricial alopecia in some individuals.[6] As we know from studies with asebia mice, loss of sebaceous gland function leads to elongation of follicles, their rupture, and eventual scarring. Sebum is required for an orderly separation of the inner root sheath from the hair shaft.[11] A default detachment of the hair shaft from the inner root sheath inhibits the shaft to grow outward. Instead hair shafts grow downward and may eventually rupture the follicular epithelium eliciting a foreign body reaction. Indeed hair follicles are significantly longer in psoriatic plaques compared with nonlesional areas of psoriasis.[10] In summary, scarring alopecia in psoriasis is likely a sequela of severe and/or long-standing psoriasis and should not be regarded as a primary cicatricial alopecia.

What Are the Driving Forces Behind Such a Degree of Sebaceous Hypoplasia?

Is the sebostasis pathogenically involved in the development of psoriasis or is the sebaceous hypoplasia a consequence of psoriasis? Transforming growth factor (TGF) β regulates sebaceous gland production by maintaining sebaceous glands in an undifferentiated state.[12] In mouse models TGF-β overexpression leads to a psoriasis-like eruption.[13] These observations indicate that overproduction of TGF-β in psoriasis could be one of the driving forces of the sebaceous gland hypoplasia. In addition, it could explain the paradox development of psoriasiform alopecia in patients under anti–TNF-α agents, who previously did not suffer from psoriasis. TNF-α blockers trigger the production of TGF-β in macrophages.[14] This may underline the hypothesis that increased levels of TGF-β induce hypoplasia of sebocytes.

Alopecia can also occur in the setting of pustular and erythrodermic psoriasis and is commonly due to a therapy-induced telogen effluvium.[15] There are also descriptions of the development of alopecia universalis in patients with generalized pustular psoriasis type, Zumbusch psoriasis, underlining the complex immunologic overlap between psoriasis and alopecia areata.[16] The association of alopecia areata and psoriasis has been noted, as well as remission of alopecia areata within psoriatic plaques, also known as the Renbök phenomenon, which in general describes the fading of one disease with the appearance of another disorder.[17,18]

HISTOPATHOLOGY

The interfollicular epidermis reveals typical feature of psoriasis, such as psoriasiform epidermal hyperplasia, hypogranulosis, thinning of suprapapillary plates, and parakeratosis with microabscess formation (Fig. 22.1D and E). The epidermis may show spongiosis, and at times it can be difficult to differentiate psoriasis from seborrheic dermatitis, because parakeratosis around follicular orifices (lipping) is a feature found in both diagnoses (Fig. 22.1E). If patients are pretreated topically, epidermal changes can be subtle or absent. The inflammation is usually superficial, involving the superficial plexus, the infundibulum, and at times the upper isthmus. An extension around the follicular bulbs and within follicular stelae has been observed in psoriasiform alopecia but should prompt a critical exclusion of an associated alopecia areata or TNF-α blocker–induced psoriasiform alopecia.[19] The lymphocytic infiltrate is predominantly lymphocytic but can house a few eosinophils and plasma cells. If these cells are present, they usually lie within upper dermis (Fig. 22.2E). The detection of deep eosinophils or plasma cells is unusual. The overall amount of follicles is more or less preserved. The telogen rate, however, is markedly increased. Up to 80% of follicles shift into catagen and telogen.[1] One of the most intriguing signs of psoriasiform alopecia is atrophy or complete loss of sebaceous gland. Even in areas of psoriasis without alopecia, sebaceous gland atrophy has been observed.[9] Sometimes sebaceous glands shrink to islands of basophilic keratinocytes. These structures can be misinterpreted as telogen germinal units.[19] Occasionally, isolated follicles rupture and naked hair shafts are extruded into the dermis where they elicit a foreign body reaction. These findings, especially when focal, are not necessarily associated with a scarring outcome.[19]

TREATMENT

Treatment with tar, salicylic acid formulations, vitamin D analogs, and high-potency topical steroids usually control the symptoms of scalp psoriasis, although thick scaly plaques may require intralesional injections of triamcinolone. Hair loss may be initially enhanced during topical therapy, but hair regrowth is to be expected, especially when therapy is promptly started and adequate. In advanced cases, systemic treatment with steroids and biologics (especially with ustekinumab) may be necessary. Methotrexate may be problematic, because it can induce telogen effluvium. Cyclosporine, known to increase hair growth, should be used with caution, especially in those patients who underwent extensive ultraviolet treatment, where the development of nonmelanoma skin cancer is likely.

The most important **differential diagnoses** include seborrheic dermatitis, tinea capitis, and TNF-α blocker–induced psoriasiform alopecia.

It is sometimes a challenge to differentiate psoriasis from *seborrheic dermatitis* because of considerable clinical and histopathologic overlap, especially when the scalp is the sole site of manifestation. Dermoscopy may be utterly useful in such instance revealing red dots and globules, twisted red loops, glomerular vessels in scalp psoriasis, and arborizing and atypical vessels in seborrheic dermatitis.[5] Psoriasis should be suspected when following features are detected on histopathologic grounds: psoriasiform epidermal hyperplasia with thinning of suprapapillary plates, increased mitoses within the basal layer, spongiform pustules, and microabscess formation within mounds of parakeratosis. Seborrheic dermatitis usually shows uneven epidermal hyperplasia, more pronounced spongiosis, follicular plugging, and prominent exocytosis of lymphocytes.[20] *Tinea capitis* can be ruled out via fungal cultures and with a periodic acid–Schiff staining histologically and does not reveal sebaceous hypoplasia.

TNF-α blocker–induced psoriasiform alopecia is an entity increasingly observed not only in adults, but also in children, where it is commonly misdiagnosed as tinea capitis.[21-25] Many of these patients receive the anti-TNF treatment for an underlying inflammatory bowel disease or for a rheumatoid disorder, such as ankylosing spondylitis and rheumatoid arthritis, and do not have a positive personal or family history of psoriasis (Figs. 22.2–22.4). Most of the patients received therapy with infliximab and adalimumab and were suffering from Crohn disease. The incidence rate of anti-TNF blocker–induced psoriasiform skin lesions in general (also outside the scalp) is almost 5%.[26] Smoking (active or a history of smoking) is one

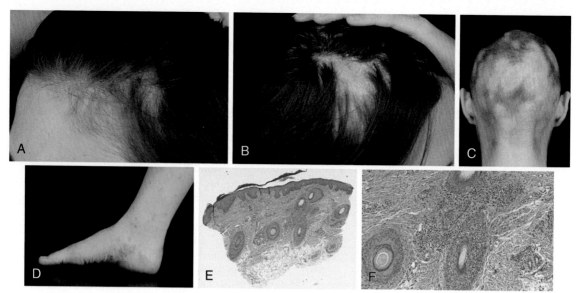

FIG. 22.2 A 34 year old woman with ankylosing sponylitis with infiiximab-induced psoriasiform alopecia. Note the rapid evolution of widepread alopecia (Compare **A**, **B** and **C**). **(D)** In addition, she developed recalcitrant pustular psoriasis on the feet. **(E)** Hematoxylin and eosin (HE) stained slide ×40: apart from the psoriasiform epidermal hyperplasia one can observe a superficial and deep peri- and intrafollicular eosinophil-rich infiltrate and catagen follicles. **(F)** Close-up (HE ×100) shows two catagen follicles and a mixed peri- and intrafollicular infiltrate with numerous eosinophils.

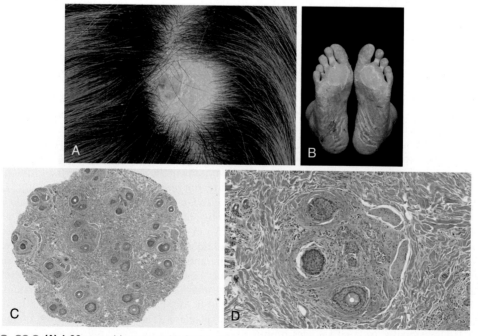

FIG. 22.3 **(A)** A 38-year-old woman with Crohn disease and a solitary slightly scaly patch of infliximab-induced psoriasiform alopecia. Note some prominent vessels within the area of alopecia. **(B)** The same patient with plantar involvement. **(C)** Low-power view (HE-stained slide ×40) shows features reminiscent of alopecia areata, namely pronounced follicular miniaturization and increase in non-anagen follicles. Unlike genuine alopecia areata, however, note the pronounced sebaceous hypoplasia. **(D)** Higher power view (HE ×200) through the isthmic region demonstrates the rudimentary sebaceous gland and small follicles.

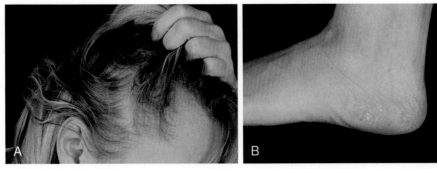

FIG. 22.4 **(A** and **B)** A 45-year-old woman with ankylosing spondylitis under infliximab therapy developed telogen effluvium and pustular plantar psoriasis.

of the main risk factor being detected in up to 80% of patients.[26] The onset of eruption varies largely. Rapid onsets within weeks and long-standing intervals of several years have been noted. Patients present with psoriasiform plaques with or without alopecia (Fig. 22.2). A thorough clinical examination commonly reveals psoriasiform lesions outside the scalp. Check palms and soles for palmoplantar pustulosis (Figs. 22.2D, 22.3B, and 22.4B); the intertriginous regions for scaly papules and plaques, retroauricular scales, and fissures; and the nails for pitting, onycholysis, and subungual hyperkeratosis. The severity and activity of the underlying disorder and the extent of the scalp lesions should guide treatment options. If standard topical therapy is insufficient to control symptoms, a switch to another biologic or a cessation of the TNF-α blocker may be necessary. According to a study in 40% of patients, the TNF blocker was ultimately withdrawn.[27] Scarring alopecia is a possible severe side effect; thus treatment should be prompt and effective.[21] Ustekinumab, an anti-interleukin (IL) 12/IL-23 antibody, seems to be a treatment option in therapy-resistant cases.[26] TNF-α blocker–induced psoriasiform alopecia shares many histologic features with genuine psoriasiform alopecia, such as psoriasiform epidermal hyperplasia, hypogranulosis, and prominent tortuous vessels within the papillary dermis (Fig. 22.2E). Even microabscess formation within the stratum corneum and epidermis, as well as sebaceous gland hypoplasia may be found. There is also a marked increase in catagen and telogen follicles (Fig. 22.3C and D). Unlike ordinary psoriasiform alopecia, the infiltrate in TNF-α blocker–induced psoriasiform alopecia often houses numerous eosinophils and plasma cells and extends deep into the dermis and may be found around the bulbs (Fig. 22.2F). The infiltrates contain Th17 and Th1 cells.[26]

Genuine alopecia areata may occur during the treatment of TNF-α blockers and should be differentiated from TNF-α blocker–induced psoriasiform alopecia.[28-31]

REFERENCES

1. Runne U, Kroneisen-Wiersma P. Psoriatic alopecia: acute and chronic hair loss in 47 patients with scalp psoriasis. *Dermatology.* 1992;185(2):82–87.
2. Shuster S. Psoriatic alopecia. *Br J Dermatol.* 1972;87(1): 73–77.
3. van de Kerkhof PC, Steegers-Theunissen RP, Kuipers MV. Evaluation of topical drug treatment in psoriasis. *Dermatology.* 1998;197(1):31–36.
4. George SM, Taylor MR, Farrant PB. Psoriatic alopecia. *Clin Exp Dermatol.* 2015;40(7):717–721.
5. Kim GW, Jung HJ, Ko HC, et al. Dermoscopy can be useful in differentiating scalp psoriasis from seborrhoeic dermatitis. *Br J Dermatol.* 2011;164(3):652–656.
6. Bardazzi F, Fanti PA, Orlandi C, Chieregato C, Misciali C. Psoriatic scarring alopecia: observations in four patients. *Int J Dermatol.* 1999;38(10):765–768.
7. Wright AL, Messenger AG. Scarring alopecia in psoriasis. *Acta Derm Venereol.* 1990;70(2):156–159.
8. Kretzschmar L, Biel K, Luger TA, Goerdt S. Generalized granuloma annulare or diffuse dermal histiocytosis? *Hautarzt.* 1995;46(8):561–567.
9. Headington JT, Gupta AK, Goldfarb MT, et al. A morphometric and histologic study of the scalp in psoriasis. Paradoxical sebaceous gland atrophy and decreased hair shaft diameters without alopecia. *Arch Dermatol.* 1989;125(5):639–642.
10. Rittie L, Tejasvi T, Harms PW, et al. Sebaceous gland atrophy in psoriasis: an explanation for psoriatic alopecia? *J Invest Dermatol.* 2016;136(9):1792–1800.
11. Sundberg JP, Boggess D, Sundberg BA, et al. Asebia-2J (Scd1(ab2J)): a new allele and a model for scarring alopecia. *Am J Pathol.* 2000;156(6):2067–2075.

12. McNairn AJ, Doucet Y, Demaude J, et al. TGFbeta signaling regulates lipogenesis in human sebaceous glands cells. *BMC Dermatol.* 2013;13:2.

13. Zhang Y, Meng XM, Huang XR, Wang XJ, Yang L, Lan HY. Transforming growth factor-beta1 mediates psoriasis-like lesions via a Smad3-dependent mechanism in mice. *Clin Exp Pharmacol Physiol.* 2014;41(11):921–932.

14. Szondy Z, Pallai A. Transmembrane TNF-alpha reverse signaling leading to TGF-beta production is selectively activated by TNF targeting molecules: therapeutic implications. *Pharmacol Res.* 2017;115:124–132.

15. Guillhou JM, Malbos S, Meynadier J. Oral treatment of severe psoriasis with a new aromatic retinoid (Ro 10-9359) (author's transl). *Ann Dermatol Venereol.* 1978;105(10): 813–818.

16. Miyazaki Y, Yamamoto T, Watanabe K, Katayama I, Nishioka K. Alopecia universalis associated with Zumbusch-type generalized pustular psoriasis. *Dermatology.* 2002;204(4):308–309.

17. Ganor S. Diseases sometimes associated with psoriasis. II. Alopecia areata. *Dermatologica.* 1977;154(6):338–341.

18. Happle R, Van Der Steen P, Perret C. The Renbök phenomenon: an inverse Köebner reaction observed in alopecia areata. *Eur J Dermatol.* 1991;(1):39–40.

19. Sperling LC. *An Atlas of Hair Pathology with Clinical Correlations;* 2012.

20. Park JH, Park YJ, Kim SK, et al. Histopathological differential diagnosis of psoriasis and seborrheic dermatitis of the scalp. *Ann Dermatol.* 2016;28(4):427–432.

21. El Shabrawi-Caelen L, La Placa M, Vincenzi C, Haidn T, Muellegger R, Tosti A. Adalimumab-induced psoriasis of the scalp with diffuse alopecia: a severe potentially irreversible cutaneous side effect of TNF-alpha blockers. *Inflamm Bowel Dis.* 2010;16(2):182–183.

22. Manni E, Barachini P. Psoriasis induced by infliximab in a patient suffering from Crohn's disease. *Int J Immunopathol Pharmacol.* 2009;22(3):841–844.

23. Papadavid E, Gazi S, Dalamaga M, Stavrianeas N, Ntelis V. Palmoplantar and scalp psoriasis occurring during anti-tumour necrosis factor-alpha therapy: a case series of four patients and guidelines for management. *J Eur Acad Dermatol Venereol.* 2008;22(3):380–382.

24. Perman MJ, Lovell DJ, Denson LA, Farrell MK, Lucky AW. Five cases of anti-tumor necrosis factor alpha-induced psoriasis presenting with severe scalp involvement in children. *Pediatr Dermatol.* 2012;29(4):454–459.

25. Osorio F, Magro F, Lisboa C, et al. Anti-TNF-alpha induced psoriasiform eruptions with severe scalp involvement and alopecia: report of five cases and review of the literature. *Dermatology.* 2012;225(2):163–167.

26. Tillack C, Ehmann LM, Friedrich M, et al. Anti-TNF antibody-induced psoriasiform skin lesions in patients with inflammatory bowel disease are characterised by interferon-gamma-expressing Th1 cells and IL-17A/IL-22-expressing Th17 cells and respond to anti-IL-12/IL-23 antibody treatment. *Gut.* 2014;63(4):567–577.

27. Rahier JF, Buche S, Peyrin-Biroulet L, et al. Severe skin lesions cause patients with inflammatory bowel disease to discontinue anti-tumor necrosis factor therapy. *Clin Gastroenterol Hepatol.* 2010;8(12):1048–1055.

28. Le Bidre E, Chaby G, Martin L, et al. Alopecia areata during anti-TNF alpha therapy: nine cases. *Ann Dermatol Venereol.* 2011;138(4):285–293.

29. Posten W, Swan J. Recurrence of alopecia areata in a patient receiving etanercept injections. *Arch Dermatol.* 2005;141(6):759–760.

30. Chaves Y, Duarte G, Ben-Said B, Tebib J, Berard F, Nicolas JF. Alopecia areata universalis during treatment of rheumatoid arthritis with anti-TNF-alpha antibody (adalimumab). *Dermatology.* 2008;217(4):380.

31. Pelivani N, Hassan AS, Braathen LR, Hunger RE, Yawalkar N. Alopecia areata universalis elicited during treatment with adalimumab. *Dermatology.* 2008;216(4):320–323.

CHAPTER 23

Hair Weathering

DÉBORA C. DE FARIAS, MD

DEFINITION

Hair weathering is an acquired progressive degeneration of hair from root to tip due to a variety of environmental and cosmetic factors. It can cause hair loss due to hair breakage and hair appearance that is shaggy and hard to manage.

HAIR ANATOMY

The hair shaft is a complex structure, with multiple layers that can be disrupted by environmental or cosmetic damage. There are two distinct structures when we talk about hair: hair follicle and hair shaft. The hair follicle is the portion located in the dermis and subdermis. The hair shaft is the visible hard filamentous portion that extends above the skin surface and varies in diameter and shape according to ethnicity. It is composed of proteins, which form 65%–95% of the hair by weight.[1,2] The greatest mass of the hair shaft is the cortex, where the melanin granules are located (constitutes about 3% of hair fiber weight). The cortex is protected by the cuticle, a protective layer of overlapping, keratinized scales, which can account for 10% of the hair fiber weight.[3] The healthy cuticles have a regular formation and hydrophobic surface; they provide hair with good texture, alignment, and appearance.

Under very high trichoscopy magnifications, such as 700×, and scanning electron microscopy (SEM), the outer layer has a fish scale appearance due to the overlapping layers of cuticle that cover underlying layers (Fig. 23.1). Loss of the cuticle layer allows underlying layers to lose structure and form ridges, fissures, and nodules (Fig. 23.2). Damage in the cortex only occurs after damage in the cuticle.

To maintain a hair surface healthy, it is known that the fatty acid 18-MEA (methyl eicosanoic acid) plays an important role. This lipid is covalently bound to the cuticle surface and provides lubrication and smooth alignment as well as contributes to the fine luster of hair fiber.[4–7]

Water content is also important in relation to physical and cosmetic properties of hair. The healthy hair shaft has natural hydrophobic properties. When it is impregnated with water, the process of absorption is very rapid. 75% of the maximum possible amount of water is absorbed within 4 min, and its weight increases from 12% to 18%.[3]

We usually notice this "weathering" in scalp hair, but body hair can be similarly damaged by environmental factors and by hard scratching with fingernails.

CAUSES OF WEATHERING

Sunlight

Sunlight exposure can damage hair. Dryness, reduced strength, rough surface texture, loss of color, decreased luster, and brittleness of hair are caused by sun exposure.

Photochemical degradation of hair results in attack on both hair proteins and melanin.

By sunlight exposure, the amino acids of the cuticle are more altered than those of the cortex because the outer layers of the hair shaft receive higher intensities of radiation. This sunlight exposure can lead to rupture and detachment of the cuticle layers of the hair. Ultraviolet (UV) radiation absorbed hair amino acids produce free radicals that can break the disulfide bonds.[1–8]

Blonde and red hair

Studies have shown that sunlight-induced hair color changes increase with the decrease in hair melanin content.[3,8,9] In blonde and red hair, the pheomelanin is very sensitive to damage by UVA and visible rays and produces superoxides; thus, color change and hair damage are more readily seen in blonde and red hair.

Dark hair

In dark hair, photobleaching of eumelanin occurs.

Dark hairs have more melanin and more photosensitive amino acids than light hairs. Melanin can attribute photoprotection to hair proteins but only in the cortex. As dark hairs have more photosensitive amino acids than light hairs, they can show a greater protein loss in the cuticle region.[10] In the cortex, dark hair has more melanin to absorb the UV radiation.[8] However, in the process of protecting the hair proteins from light,

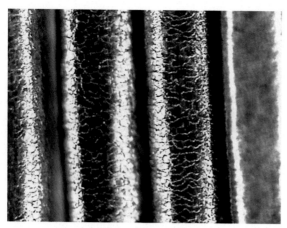

FIG. 23.1 The healthy cuticle has a fish scale appearance. Dry trichoscopy, 700x magnification.

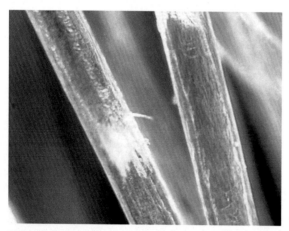

FIG. 23.2 Tricorrhexis nodosa. Loss of the cuticle integrity with multiple small fibers protruding out of the hair fiber. Dry trichoscopy, 700× magnification.

the pigments are degraded or bleached.[8,9,11,12] The protein degradation is caused by UV light–induced oxidation of the sulfur-containing molecules within the hair shaft. The total amount of amino acids more susceptible to photodegradation (tryptophan, cysteine, tyrosine, and histidine) depends on hair type.[1–8]

Gray hair

The highest tryptophan concentrations are found in gray and white hairs.[10] Nogueira et al. showed that white hair photobleaches after exposure to UV and visible radiations and photoyellows after infrared radiation. Yellowness changes are related to amino acid damage, mainly that of tryptophan.[9]

Excessive Wetting

Excessive wetting and shampooing, mainly with hot water and surfactant solutions, damage the hair, causing the growth of cavities in the endocuticle and displacement, cracking, and cleavage of cuticle cells. The holes in the endocuticle are caused by dissolution of proteins during shampooing. Excessive wetting and shampooing also cause cavities in the intermacrofibrillar cement, in the cell membrane complex, and around the melanin granules in the cortex. Changes in hair color may occur.[13,14] There is difficulty in untangling the strands and the frizz effect.

Studies showed that internal lipids are extracted by surfactants during extensive washing.[1] Wiesche et al. demonstrated significant changes in the lipid composition and water resorption after approximately 100 middle European summer days (equivalent to 50 cycles of shampooing, blow-drying, and sunlight exposure).[15]

The hardness of the water, determined by the amount of salts (calcium carbonate and magnesium sulfate), used for washing is commonly believed to cause fragility of hair. Srinivasan et al. compared tensile strength and elasticity of the hair treated in hard water and distilled water in 15 volunteers and found that the hardness of water does not interfere with the tensile strength and elasticity of hair.[16]

Another study by the same group used SEM to study the surface of 15 hair samples treated with hard and soft water and concluded that hair treated with hard water has a higher mineral deposition, which can lead to irregularity of the surface and decreased thickness of hair over a period of time.[17]

Alahmmed et al compared structural differences and relative deposition of calcium and magnesium salts on the hair shaft surface using SEM between hair shaft samples from 20 healthy volunteers treated with hard and soft water and found no statistically significant difference between the study and control group as far as surface changes under SEM and relative deposition of calcium was concerned. However, analysis of magnesium deposition showed a higher level of magnesium in the samples washed with hard water.[18]

A bigger study by Luqman et al., with 76 volunteers, suggested that tensile strength might be affected by the hardness of water. In this study, the tensile strength of hair was significantly reduced in hair treated with hard water compared with that treated with soft water. It has been postulated that long-term deposition of salts on the hair shaft may lead to an abrasive action on the hair shaft, causing surface damage, water loss, and eventually decreased thickness.[19]

To minimize hair weathering and preserve beauty, patients should avoid excessive wetting and

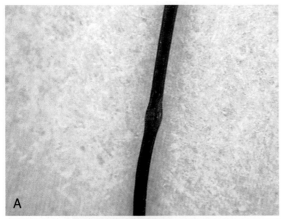

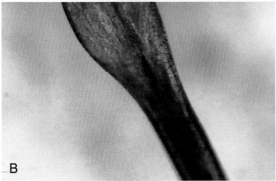

FIG. 23.3 Bubble hair: single bubble in the hair shaft. Dry trichoscopy (**A**, 30× magnification. **B**, 700× magnification).

shampooing (mainly with hot water and surfactant solutions), particularly with hard water. Conditioners should be used to decrease friction, detangle the hair, minimize frizz, and improve combability.[20]

Physical Damage

Friction and physical hair shaft injury caused by hard combing and brushing, braiding, and cornrowing are significant causes of weathering.[21] Cosmetic overheating procedures, such as those with blow-dryers, flat irons, and hot combs, can cause bubbles or cavities that often distend the shaft (Fig. 23.3). Exposure of wet hair to excessive heat causes sudden evaporation of water with formation of cavities filled with steam, resulting in bubble hair. The bubble areas are fragile, and the hair shaft easily breaks in these areas.[22]

Hair extensions

Hair extensions are strands of synthetic or human hair that are attached to existing hair fibers by means of glue, braids, sewing, or clips (Fig. 23.4A and B). Hair extensions are added to both straighter and natural hair. Hair extensions may cause traction alopecia and hair loss due to hair shaft breakage (Fig. 23.5). Traction alopecia is initially nonscarring but may lead to scarring alopecia.

Braided hairstyles are plaits of varying lengths that have human or synthetic hair braided in seamlessly with natural scalp hair. Breakage of hair shaft and traction alopecia may appear because of continuous unidirectional traction and very tight braided pattern.

Weaves refer to a style where entire hair is braided in cornrows close to the scalp. Once the braids are made, a needle is used to sew extensions (human or synthetic hair) into the braids. Adhesives may also be used.

To maintain healthy scalp hair, the braided or weave-in styles must be done with as little traction as possible and the braid direction must be changed with time.

Considerable longitudinal traction performed experimentally causes surface cells of the cuticle to lift up and away from underlying cells and transverse cuticular fissure. However, in vivo, similar pulling forces generally remove hair from scalp before significant damage has occurred.[23]

Chemical Damage

Studies suggested that procedures such as bleaching, dyeing, hair straightening, permanent waving, hair curling, and the use of degreasing shampoos can "weather" the hair.[24–27]

Hair dye

Temporary hair coloring techniques do not damage the hair because their particle size is too large to penetrate through the cuticle. This not only minimizes damage but also accounts for their temporary nature, as they are removed in one shampooing.

Permanent hair coloring damages hair cuticle. To alter natural hair color, hair cosmetics need to get through the cuticle into the inner part of the hair shaft. Ammonia or other alkaline substances are used to open the cuticle layer so that the developer and colorants together penetrate into the cortex. In this process colorless dye precursors (primary intermediates: *p*-phenylenediamines, *p*-toluenediamine, and *p*-aminophenols, etc.) chemically react with hydrogen peroxide inside the hair shaft to produce colored molecules (oxidation process). After that they are exposed to couplers (resorcinol, 1-naphthol, *m*-aminophenol, etc.) to result in a variety of dyes.

Higher concentrations of hydrogen peroxide can bleach melanin; thus, the oxidizing step functions both in color production and in bleaching.

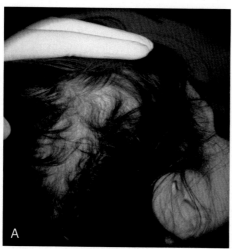
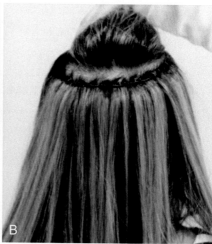

FIG. 23.4 **(A** and **B)** Sew-in hair extensions in Caucasian patients.

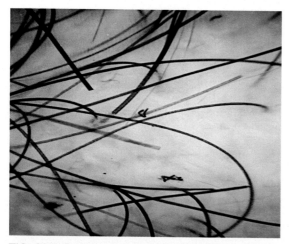

FIG. 23.5 Broken hair shafts in a patient wearing hair extensions. Dry trichoscopy, 30× magnification.

Wiesche et al. proved that bleaching process removes hair shaft surface lipids and increases water resorption.[15] Reduction of 18-MEA has been reported in bleached hair.[28-33]

Under SEM, Kaliyadan et al, showed that hair shafts submitted to hair dye and/or bleaching developed a range of changes from irregular overlay of the cuticle without cracks or holes to severe lift up the cuticle with cracks but without exposure of the cortex, and partial exposure of the cortex in some shafts.[25]

Dyeing the hair the same color as the natural hair is the best to minimize damage and cover gray hair.[34]

Hair straightening

Hair straightening products are formulated in very high pH (8.5–12) causing hair damage. Intercellular material loss occurs. The neutralization process is not able to correct the damage of the cuticle, which results in loss of elasticity, traction resistance, and swelling. During the straightening process, damages are not limited to elasticity loss and traction resistance, but they also include the fiber swelling. The hair develops cleavages along the thread that makes the breakage easier.[35]

Alkaline straighteners contain 1%–10% sodium hydroxide (lye-based straighteners), lithium hydroxide, calcium hydroxide, or a combination of these ingredients such as guanidine carbonate and calcium hydroxide (no lye relaxers).[20] These reagents cause lanthionization of hair and irreversible hair straightening. Disulfide bonds undergo rearrangement until 35% of cysteine of the hair is converted to lanthionine. The difference between the cysteine and lanthionine is the loss of one sulfur atom. The hair fiber loses its strength after lanthionization.[20,26,35] The alkaline pH (9.0–14.0) of the lotion opens the cuticle scales and allows the alkaline agent to penetrate under the cuticle into the cortex. In contact with the cortex, the straightening product reacts with keratin, breaking and rearranging disulfide bridges. The spiral keratin molecule softens and can stretch to take up the shape the patient desires.[1,26] There is no need to use external forces or heat (such as flat iron or blow-dryer) because of the phenomena called "supercontraction" that provides enough stress to straighten the fiber in a permanent basis.[20] For hair to come back to the physiologic pH value (pH 4–6), acid shampoos are used (pH 4.5–6).

Ammonium thioglycolate is another nonlye relaxer that can cause swelling of the fiber but causes less supercontraction than the alkaline relaxers that go through lanthionization. The disulfide bonds are converted to sulfhydryl groups to allow the mechanical relaxation of the protein structure of hair fibers. After relaxation, free sulfhydryl groups are reoxidized (neutralized) to reform the disulfide bonds, thus acquiring the desired conformation.[34] It is the same reaction used for waving hair. To finish the reaction, a neutralizing agent (acid pH) is used, which closes the cuticle scales and fixes the new shape of hair fibers. As they act with high pH, these straightening agents cause considerable damage to hair, for instance, making it dry and brittle. Thioglycolate causes less protein loss than hydroxides.[20]

The addition of conditioning agents to the straightening emulsion with ammonium thioglycolate benefits the hair fiber, thus diminishing protein loss, protecting the hair thread, and improving the resistance to breakage. Jojoba oil and lauryl PEG/PPG-18/18 methicone are conditioning agents that present the best results. Straightening emulsions with ammonium thioglycolate containing aqua (and) cystine bis-PG-propyl silanetriol and cyclopentasiloxane (and) PEG-12 dimethicone cross-polymer provide higher breakage resistance of the thread.[35,36]

Hydroxides and thioglycolate are incompatible with each other (Fig. 23.6) and both are incompatible with bleached hair.

Considerations:

- Thicker hair with longer diameter of cortex, as well as hair with high grade of sulfur and higher amount of keratin, demands a longer processing time.
- When the cuticle scales are in a narrow overlap, this slows the straightening ingredient penetration.
- Straightening ingredient rapidly penetrates into the thread and reaches the cortex when the hair is damaged (porous). It demands a shorter processing time.
- Thin hair has less mass, which allows a faster saturation with the straightening product. A shorter processing time is demanded. Exception occurs when the cuticle layer is very resistant.[37]

Brazilian keratin treatment (BKT) is very popular in Brazil and all around the world. BKT is compatible with other hair treatments such as bleaching, permanent dyes, and hair relaxers.[20] BKT ingredients are

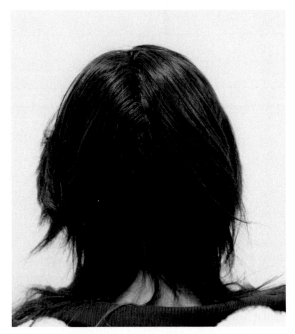

FIG. 23.6 Clinical picture of a patient with broken hair shafts after the use of two incompatible hair straighteners. Note the different hair shaft lengths in a disorganized pattern.

based on formaldehyde releasers such as methylene glycol or glyoxylic acid. Both substances are capable of releasing formaldehyde when heated during blow-dry and hot iron application. The formaldehyde or other aldehydes are not hair straightening products. The hair is remodeled straight because water breaks hydrogen bonds of the keratin molecule, followed by blow-dry and flat iron. The newly redesigned keratin is then kept in this shape because the formaldehyde cross-links the keratin filaments in such a perfect alignment that the hair is then set straight.[20] The light that reaches the hair shaft reflects from the very well-reorganized keratin filaments, showing the desired bright shiny hair.

In Brazil, formaldehyde is prohibited in concentrations above 0.2% for cosmetics and 5% for nail polish. Exposure to it is known to cause eye irritation, eczema-like psoriasiform skin reaction, burning of the throat, allergic skin reaction in those who are sensitive to it, and irritation of the respiratory tract. It has also been shown to cause cancer in animals and may cause cancer in humans.[20,38]

Boga et al. performed SEM to compare hair fiber treated with basic solution plus iron with hair fiber treated with glyoxylic acid straightening and with that

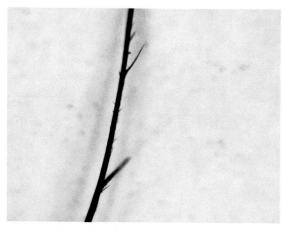

FIG. 23.7 Hair shaft with loss of the cuticle and cortex exposure from a patient who underwent multiple Brazilian keratin treatments. Dry trichoscopy, 50× magnification.

of a control group. The group of hair fiber treated with basic solution and then ironed showed a surface less regular when compared with controls, indicating a damage at the cuticle after basic solution and thermal stress. The group subjected to glyoxylic acid showed the surface to be almost regular, similar to the control sample. It was also shown that the treatment with glyoxylic acid produced the major conformational rearrangements within the hair fiber rather than in cuticle.[38]

Leite et al. studied mechanical properties of curly hair after formaldehyde and glyoxylic acid treatment. Analysis of the SEM images revealed that the hair treated with formaldehyde presented great surface irregularity and the glyoxylic acid group presented absence of cuticle. Formaldehyde decreased mechanical properties of the hair under the tensile tests, indicating that it causes great damage to hair structure. Hair treated with glyoxylic acid showed decreased mechanical properties compared with that treated with formaldehyde. The decrease of water sorption was also observed in both groups.[39]

In conclusion, although the hair looks glossy and beautiful after formaldehyde and glyoxylic acid treatment, both of them damage the cuticle (Fig. 23.7).[44,45]

The companies that market keratin treatment suggest that keratin treatment leaves hair healthier. Currently there is no scientific evidence that support this theory.

Age
As hair ages and naturally "weathers," the cuticle scales become jagged and break off. Takahashi et al. showed

that there is an age-dependent resistance to daily grooming stresses, such as shampooing and blow-drying.[41] After the grooming process, the loss of cuticle increases with aging. The hair follicle can produce cuticles of constant size for some decades, but on the other hand, the constituents of these cuticles deteriorate and become fragile with aging.[41-43] It was revealed that aging also causes loss of 18-MEA, especially in the age range older than 40 years. The surface cuticles of the subjects older than 40 years are prone to be broken, and this phenomenon is promoted by aging.[40]

DIAGNOSIS
Hair has no nerve connections and thus cannot give one a feeling of pain when it is damaged. As many environmental and cosmetic factors play a role in life, it may be difficult to blame one factor responsible for hair weathering. A physician, with special expertise in hair loss, can assist a patient in identifying and avoiding factors that cause hair to appear "weathered." In rare instances, a genetic condition may contribute to breakage and frazzling of the hair shaft. The hair expert will rule out the presence of any of these genetic conditions during the full medical and scalp examination.

CLINICAL EXAMINATION
The weathered hair appears dry and brittle.

Water retention index (WRI) test may be helpful in studies that want to prove the hair shaft damage. Owing to chemical degradation of protein that generates hydrophilic groups, the WRI is higher in bleached and damaged hair. Day by day, aging causes significant reduction of the natural hydrophobic properties of virgin hair.[15,42]

Trichoscopy can be helpful, as it allows to better recognize hair shaft damage during the office visit.[43] It is an easy, fast, and affordable tool that every dermatologist should consider using. I also believe that it is a very important tool to show and educate the patient about hair damage.

SEM and transmission electron microscopy are the ultimate tools to demonstrate hair shaft damage, including early and subtle hair shaft damage.[11,33]

Hair Weathering Findings
Trichorrhexis nodosa
The outer fibers bulge outward, causing a segmental increasing in hair diameter. Under naked eye, small and white nodules located along hair shaft can be noted.

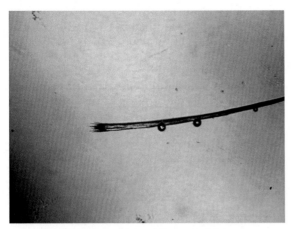

FIG. 23.8 Hair shaft with brushlike ends. Trichoscopy with immersion fluid, 50× magnification.

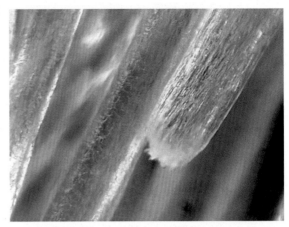

FIG. 23.10 Trichorrhexis nodosa. Hair shaft end at the breaking point in trichorrhexis nodosa. Dry trichoscopy, 700× magnification.

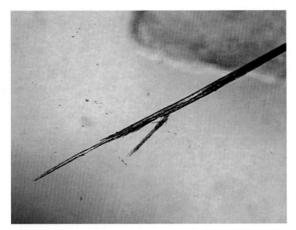

FIG. 23.9 Trichoptilosis. Longitudinal splitting of the hair shaft. Trichoscopy with immersion fluid, 50× magnification.

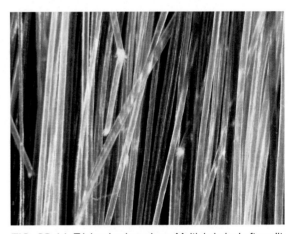

FIG. 23.11 Trichorrhexis nodosa. Multiple hair shafts split longitudinally into numerous small fibers, resembling the ends of two brushes aligned in opposition.

Hairs eventually break at these points, leaving brush-like ends (Fig. 23.8). The hair appears dry and brittle, and the hair shaft splits longitudinally into many small fibers (Fig. 23.9). Proximal trichorrhexis nodosa occurs in Afro-Caribbean tightly curled hair. Distal trichorrhexis nodosa occurs in other, straighter racial hair type. Trichoscopy of trichorrhexis nodosa will depend on the magnifications and presence of immersion fluid. At low magnifications, trichoscopy reveals nodular thickenings along hair shafts, and these thickenings appear lighter in the dark hair shafts. At these sites, the hair bends and eventually breaks, leaving a slightly thickened rounded hair shaft end (Fig. 23.10). At higher magnifications, trichoscopy reveals numerous small fibers, producing a picture that resembles two brushes aligned in opposition (Fig. 23.11). To better visualize trichorrhexis nodosa, the hairs should be evaluated with dry trichoscopy.

Trichoptilosis
It is the longitudinal splitting of the hair shaft into two or more fibrils. Trichoscopy allows the physician to better recognize it (Fig. 23.12).

Trichoclasis
It is a transverse fracture of the hair shaft partly surrounded by intact cuticle. Cuticle, cortex, and sulfur content are normal.[3]

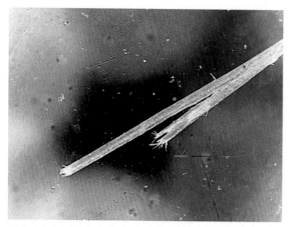

FIG. 23.12 Trichoptilosis. Longitudinal splitting of the hair shaft. Dry trichoscopy, 700× magnification.

Trichoschisis

It is a transverse fracture of the hair shaft through cuticle and cortex associated with localized loss of cuticular cells. Probably, there is a decrease in the high-sulfur matrix protein content and particularly a similar decrease in the exocuticle and a layer of cuticular cells. It may be prominent in the sulfur syndromes.[3]

Bubble hair

The hair shaft becomes coarse. Trichoscopy shows segmental areas with increased hair shaft diameter that corresponds to the bubbles (Fig. 23.3). They are found as single or multiple, and either adjacent or separate. Under SEM large cavities or a reticulated Swiss cheese appearance is seen in the hair shaft.

TREATMENT

The main treatment consists of avoiding exposure to sunlight and grooming techniques that can damage hair, such as excessive wetting and shampooing, blow-drying and other overheating procedures, excessive hair combing, bleaching, dyeing, hair straightening, and hair curling.

The use of oils and conditioners has been recommended to reduce the hair shaft cuticular damage and to reduce the hair comb friction to already damaged hair. Some studies suggest that regular oiling of the scalp with various oils such as coconut oil, mineral oil, sunflower oil, olive oil, argan oil, or Cupuacu butter may prevent hair shaft damage, either naturally occurring or secondary to hair treatments.[44,45]

The coconut oil, when used as a prewash conditioner, has a protective effect on undamaged hair and also on heat exposed, chemically treated and UV-treated hair.[45]

Head scarves and hats have protective effect against environmental damage on hair such as sun exposure. There are sunscreen products made to be applied to the hair to prevent weathering. These products can be helpful if the patient spend a lot of time under sunlight. Chemically treated hair, particularly after bleaching and perming, needs sun protection to prevent further damage.

REFERENCES

1. Robbins CR. *Chemical and Physical Behavior of Human Hair.* 5th ed. New York: Springer-Verlag; 2012.
2. Draelos ZD. The biology of hair care. *Dermatol Clin.* 2000;18:651–658.
3. Dawber R. Hair: structure and response to cosmetics. *Clin Dermatol.* 1996;14:105–112.
4. Swift JA. Human hair cuticle: biologically conspired to the owner's advantage. *J Cosmet Sci.* 1999;50:23–47.
5. Tate ML, Kamath YK, Ruetsch SB. Quantification and prevention of hair damage. *J Soc Cosmet Chem.* 1993;44: 347–371.
6. Rogers GE. Electron microscope studies of hair and wool. *Ann N Y Acad Sci.* 1959;83:378–399.
7. Robbins C. The cell membrane complex: three related but different cellular cohesion components of mammalian hair fibers. *J Cosmet Sci.* 2009;60:437–465.
8. Nogueira ACS, Joekes I. Hair color changes and protein damage caused by ultravioleta radiation. *J Photochem Photobiol B Biol.* 2004;74:109–117.
9. Nogueira AC, Richena M, Dicelio LE, Joekes I. Photo yellowing of human hair. *J Photochem Photobiol B.* 2007;88 (2–3):119–125.
10. Bertazzo A, Biasiolo M, Costa CVL, Stefani EC, Allegri G. Tryptophan in human hair: correlation with pigmentation. *Il Farmaco.* 2000;55:521–525.
11. Tolgyesi E. Weathering of hair. *Cosmet Toilet.* 1983;98: 29–33.
12. Hoting E, Zimmermann M, Hilterhaus-Bong S. Photochemical alterations on human hair. Part I: artificial irradiation and investigations of hair proteins. *J Soc Cosmet Chem.* 1995;46:85–99.
13. Scanavez C, Silveira M, Joekes I. Human hair: color changes caused by daily care damages on ultra structure. *Colloids Surf B Biointerfaces.* 2003;28:39–52.
14. Gould JG, Sneath RL. Electron microscopy image analysis: quantification of ultrastructural changes in hair fiber cross sections as a result of cosmetic treatment. *J Soc Cosmet Chem.* 1985;36:53–59.
15. Wiesche ES, Körner A, Schäfer K, Wortmann FJ. Prevention of hair surface aging. *J Cosmet Sci.* 2011;62(2):237–249.

16. Srinivasan G, Srinivas CR, Mathew AC, Duraiswami D. Effects of hard water on hair. *Int J Trichology*. 2013;5(3):137–139.

17. Srinivas CR. Scanning electron microscopy of hair treated in hard water. *Int J Dermatol*. 2016;55(6):e344–e346.

18. Alahmmed LM, Alibrahim EA, Alkhars AF, Almulhim MN, Ali SI, Kaliyadan F. Scanning electron microscopy study of hair shaft changes related to hardness of water. *Indian J Dermatol Venereol Leprol*. 2017;83:740.

19. Luqman MW, Ali R, Khan Z, Ramzan MH, Hanan F, Javaid U. Effect of topical application of hard water in weakening of hair in men. *J Pak Med Assoc*. 2016;66(9):1132–1136.

20. Dias MFG. Hair cosmetics: an overview. *Int J Trichology*. 2015;7(1):2–15.

21. Martin AM, Sugathan P. Localised acquired trichorrhexis nodosa of the scalp hair induced by a specific comb and combing habit – a report of three cases. *Int J Trichology*. 2011;3(1):34–37.

22. McMichael AJ, Roseborough IE. Hair care practices in African-American patients. *Semin Cutan Med Surg*. 2009;28:103–108.

23. Dawber R. Cosmetic and medical causes of hair weathering. *J Cosmet Dermatol*. 2000;1:196–201.

24. Ali N, Zohra RR, Qader SA, Mumtaz M. Scanning electron microscopy analysis of hair index on Karachi's population for social and professional appearance enhancement. *Int J Cosmet Sci*. 2015;37(3):312–320.

25. Kaliyadan F, Gosai BB, Al Melhim WN, et al. Scanning electron microscopy study of hair shaft damage secondary to cosmetic treatments of the hair. *Int J Trichology*. 2016;8(2):94–98.

26. Miranda-Vilela AL, Botelho AJ, Muehlmann LA. An overview of chemical straightening of human hair: technical aspects, potential risks to hair fibre and health and legal issues. *Int J Cosmet Sci*. 2014;36(1):2–11.

27. Joo KM, Kim AR, Kim SM, et al. Metabolomic analysis of aminoacids and lipids in human hair altered by dyeing, perming and bleaching. *Exp Dermatol*. 2016;25(9):729–731.

28. Okamoto M, Ishikawa K, Tanji N, et al. Investigation of the damage on the outermost hair surface using ToF-SIMS and XPS. *Surf Interface Anal*. 2012;44:736–739.

29. Breakspear S, Smith JR, Luengo G. Effect of the covalently linked fatty acid 18-MEA on the nanotribology of hair's outermost surface. *J Struct Biol*. 2005;149:235–242.

30. Jones LN, Rivett DE. The role of 18-methyleicosanoic acid in the structure and formation of mammalian hair fibres. *Micron*. 1997;28:469–485.

31. Okamoto M, Tanji N, Habe T, et al. ToF-SIMS characterization of the lipid layer on the hair surface. II: effect of the 18-MEA lipid layer on surface hydrophobicity. *Surf Interface Anal*. 2011;43:298–301.

32. Smith JR, Swift JA. Maple syrup urine disease hair reveals the importance of 18-methyleicosanoic acid in cuticular delamination. *Micron*. 2005;36:261–266.

33. Habe T, Tanji N, Inoue S, et al. ToF-SIMS characterization of the lipid layer on the hair surface. I: the damage caused by chemical treatments and UV radiation. *Surf Interface Anal*. 2011;43:410–412.

34. Feughelman M. A note on the permanent setting of human hair. *J Soc Cosmet Chem*. May/June 1990;41:209–212.

35. Syed AN, Ayoub H, Kuhajda A. Recent advances in treating excessively curly hair. *Cosmet Toilet*. 1998;113:47–56.

36. Dias TCS, Baby AR, Kaneko TM, Velasco MVR. Protective effect of conditioning agents on Afro-ethnic hair chemically treated with thioglycolate-based straightening emulsion. *J Cosmet Dermatol*. 2008;7(2):120–126.

37. Obukowho P, Birman M. Alisantes para cabelos–avaliação da função, da química e da produção. *Cosmet Toilet Ed Port*. 1996;8:44–49.

38. Boga C, Taddei P, Micheletti G, et al. Formaldehyde replacement with glyoxylic acid in semipermanent hair straightening: a new and multidisciplinary investigation. *Int J Cosmet Sci*. 2014;36(5):459–470.

39. Leite MGA, Maia Campos PMBG. Mechanical characterization of curly hair: influence of the use of nonconventional hair straightening treatments. *Skin Res Technol*. 2017;23(4):539–544.

40. Takahashi T, Mamada A, Breakspear S, Itou T, Tanji N. Age-dependent changes in damage processes of hair cuticle. *J Cosmet Dermatol*. 2015;14(1):2–8.

41. Rogers GE. Hair follicle differentiation and regulation. *Int J Dev Biol*. 2004;48:163–170.

42. Rogers G, Koike K. Laser capture microscopy in a study of expression of structural proteins in the cuticle cells of human hair. *Exp Dermatol*. 2009;18:541–547.

43. Miteva M, Tosti A. Dermatoscopy of hair shaft disorders. *J Am Acad Dermatol*. 2013;68:473–481.

44. Rele AS, Mohile RB. Effect of mineral oil, sunflower oil, and coconut oil on prevention of hair damage. *J Cosmet Sci*. 2003;54:175–192.

45. Faria PM, Camargo LN, Carvalho RS, Paludetti LA, Velasco MVR, da Gama RM. Hair protective effect of Argan oil (*Argania spinosa* Kernel Oil) and Cupuassu butter (*Theobroma grandiflorum* seed butter) post treatment with hair dye. *J Cosmet Dermatol Sci Appl*. 2013;3:40–44.

CHAPTER 24

Hair Changes due to Drugs

BIANCA M. PIRACCINI, PHD • MICHELA STARACE, MD •
AURORA ALESSANDRINI, MD

INTRODUCTION

Many chemical agents can interfere with the follicular cycle inducing mainly an anagen effluvium or a telogen effluvium.[1]

In anagen effluvium, hair loss usually occurs within a few days to several weeks of drug administration, whereas in telogen effluvium hair loss becomes evident 2–4 months after starting treatment. When there is a temporal association between the onset of hair loss and intake of a medication, the drug is commonly thought to have caused the hair loss. The frequency and the gravity of the alopecia depend both on the type of chemical and on the individual predisposition. Drug-induced alopecia is usually reversible after withdrawal.

The clinical evaluation of a patient with hair problems is a fundamental step for the correct diagnosis, as it gives important information and helps in choosing the diagnostic tools that should be used to confirm the clinical suspicion.[2] Scalp dermoscopy or "trichoscopy" will afterward add additional data that can be further increased by scalp biopsy for histopathology and/or by other more specific tests. Trichoscopy is a valuable, noninvasive technique, used routinely, for the evaluation of patients with hair loss that allows for magnified visualization of the hair and scalp. This method is simple, quick, and easy to perform; reduces the need for scalp biopsy; is well accepted by patients; and is useful for monitoring treatment and follow-up.

Pathophysiology

Drugs can interfere with the follicular cycle by two mechanisms: (1) producing an abrupt cessation of mitotic activity of the cells of the matrix (*anagen effluvium*); (2) interrupting the anagen phase and inducing a premature transition of the follicle from growth phase to the phase of rest (*telogen effluvium*). Follicles in the scalp are at different stages of the cycle, so their response to pathogenic insults is closely related to their mitotic activity, which varies in the different subphases of anagen. For this reason, the same drug could cause an anagen effluvium in some follicles and a telogen effluvium in others.

HAIR AND DRUGS

Antineoplastic Agents

Classic-traditional antimitotic drugs

Hair loss is the most common cutaneous side effect of antineoplastics, and it is more frequent and severe in combination chemotherapy. In the majority of patients, an anagen hair loss occurs, starting around 2 weeks after the drug administration, and it is complete by 8 weeks. This kind of alopecia is generally reversible and hair regrows typically after 3–6 months. Associated loss of telogen hair is usually observed. Weekly chemotherapy generally results in slower and occasionally incomplete hair loss, whereas high-dose chemotherapy causes rapid and complete hair loss.

The pathogenic mechanism of chemotherapy-induced alopecia (CIA) involves the matrix keratinocytes, which are the main targets of anticancer drugs. They are proliferative during anagen phase, becoming sensitive to toxins and drugs.[3] Catagen and telogen follicles are not affected because they are in mitotically inactive phases, but when hair is in late anagen phase, with a lower mitotic rate, chemotherapy accelerates the normal transition to telogen.

The scalp is the most affected area because 90% of scalp follicles are normally in anagen phase.

The estimated incidence is 65% among patients undergoing treatment,[4] even if the degree of hair loss is dependent on the agent, dose, route, and individual response (Table 24.1).

According to Rossi et al.,[5] the reported incidence of alopecia with antimicrotubule agents is 80%, 60%–100% with topoisomerase inhibitors, >60% with alkylators, and 10%–50% with antimetabolites. Hair side effects cause significant psychologic distress to the patient, with negative influence on body image and self-esteem and, unfortunately, treatment options are still limited. For some patients, the fear of CIA may be so severe as to lead to refusing or delaying this essential treatment.

Clinical presentation. The clinical pattern of chemotherapy-induced hair loss is a balance with the treatment-related aspects, such as drug type or dosage;

TABLE 24.1
Drugs Responsible of Hair Loss

Classic-traditional antimitotic drugs	Leflunomide
Antitarget drugs	Maprotiline
Angiotensin-converting enzyme inhibitors	Mesalazine
Anticoagulants	Methysergide
β-blockers	Nitrofurantoin
Tricyclic antidepressants	Octreotide
Androgens	Piroxicam
Antiepileptics	Potassium thiocyanate
Antipsychotics	Pyridostigmine
Indinavir	Risperidone
Interferons	Salicylates
Levodopa	Serotonin reuptake inhibitors (fluoxetine, paroxetine)
Lithium	
Radiation	
Retinol (vit. A)	Terbinafine
Retinoids	Sulphasalazine
Analgesics/anti-inflammatories	Tamoxifen
Amiodarone	Terfenadine
Antithyroid drugs	Thiamphenicol
Minoxidil	Vasopressin
Oral contraceptives	Triazoles
Benzimidazoles	Spironolactone
Bromocriptine	Allopurinol
Buspirone	Mesalazine
Chloramphenicol	Piroxicam
Cimetidine	Cholestyramine
Clotrimazole	Cidofovir
Diazoxide	
Dixyrazine	
Danazol	
Ethambutol	
Ethionamide	
Glatiramer acetate	
Glibenclamide	
Haloperidol	
Immunoglobulins	

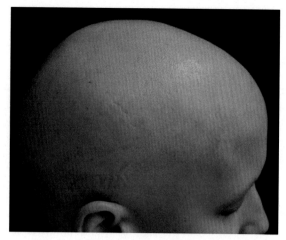

FIG. 24.1 Total alopecia due to chemotherapy.

administration type and modality; chemotherapy alone or with radiotherapy; the patient-related aspects, such as age and gender; and local or systemic comorbidities. Very important is the clinical hair pattern before starting the chemotherapy; the presence of androgenetic alopecia, especially in the crown region and sides of head above the ear that is the first affected area due to chemotherapy, predisposes to development of evident hair thinning. At the beginning, the hair shedding starts as a diffuse or patchy alopecia to became a total alopecia over time (Fig. 24.1), which is the most common clinical manifestation. Because of the great insult to the follicles in anagen, hair shedding is characterized by dystrophic anagen hairs with pigmented hair shafts (Fig. 24.2). When the follicles are in telogen, the hair shedding is characterized by dystrophic catagen/telogen hairs with depigmented hair shaft. Another effect of chemotherapy includes thinning of the hair shaft at the time of maximal chemotherapy effect, resulting in Pohl-Pinkus constriction: the hair shaft may break at the follicular ostium during the resting phase of the hair cycle. There is an increase in hair shedding diffusely over the scalp, which results in a thinner hair density until new anagen growth can replace the shed hair.

Loss of beard, eyebrows, and eyelashes, as well as axillary and pubic hair, is variable and depends on the percentage of hairs in anagen phase and may occur after the last dose of chemotherapy.

Hair regrowth after chemotherapy is often characterized by changes in the hair color, texture, and shape, with darker and curler hair compared with their original form. These alterations can be expected in more than 60% of patients.[6] Hair regrowth is generally more rapid on the other affected sites of the body than on the scalp.

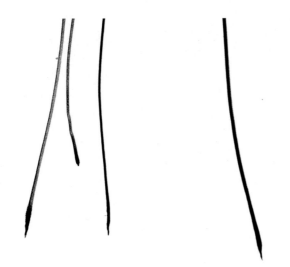

FIG. 24.2 Dystrophic hair shafts obtained by pull test in a patient on chemotherapy.

Trichoscopy. The dermoscopic aspects of chemotherapy-induced hair loss reflect the different clinical patterns: in the early stage, in case of acute damage of anagen follicles, the presence of black dots and short hairs of different lengths are the most frequent features; a possible worsening of androgenetic alopecia, with hair miniaturization and empty follicles, usually occurs in patients where androgenetic alopecia was present before starting chemotherapy; another possible manifestation is an aspect similar to that of alopecia areata incognita, with the presence of numerous empty follicles and yellow dots with or without the presence of short vellus hairs.

Presence of only empty follicles on the scalp is the final presentation of total alopecia.

Management of chemotherapy-induced alopecia. No drugs are actually approved to prevent hair loss, but some molecules have been studied. Soref et al.[7] studied the role of topical epinephrine/norepinephrine in preventing radiotherapy-induced alopecia and CIA in 10-day-old rats, with good results and no side effects, based on the concept that the induction of hypoxia signaling could help hair follicle stem cells to maintain their function and that vasoconstriction may reduce the drug dose reaching hair follicle. Another instrument proposed as preventive therapy for alopecia is scalp cooling, which acts probably with the same mechanism of vasoconstriction, decreasing local concentration of chemotherapy and cellular uptake at the hair follicle and reducing metabolic uptake. A recent meta-analysis reported that it significantly reduces CIA.[8] As reviewed by Rossi et al.,[4]

the best results have been described for alopecia induced by doxorubicin, epirubicin, and docetaxel, whereas scalp cooling is not recommended in hematologic malignancies because of the risk of scalp skin metastasis. During chemotherapy, some basic advice can be given to the patient, such as the use of a gentle shampoo, protection of the scalp from sun, or the application of a wig.

After chemotherapy, the goal is to accelerate hair regrowth: the most promising agent is calcitriol (1,25-dihydroxyvitamin D3), which has several effects on keratinocytes, such as inhibition of DNA synthesis, inhibition of Ki67 expression, a marker of cycling cells, and inhibition of the growth of a multiplicity of other cell types.[9] Other interesting possibilities include topical minoxidil and N-acetylcysteine, but more studies are necessary.

Antitarget drugs

Vemurafenib is a selective *BRAF* kinase inhibitor, used in previously untreated, unresectable, BRAF V600 mutation B-Raf proto-oncogene serine/threonine kinase–positive stage IIIC or stage IV melanoma. In the literature, hair changes are reported in 8%–36% of patients. A recent study[10] focused on hair changes in patients with melanoma undergoing vemurafenib therapy; five of six patients experienced hair problems, including mainly acute telogen effluvium, with two patients also shedding eyelashes, axillary, pubic, and limb hair. Authors believed that BRAF-mediated acute interruption of anagen phase in the matrix cell of the hair bulb may occur, leading anagen follicles into regression with apoptosis, followed by telogen. In one patient hair shape changes were also noted, with curly and wirelike hair, probably caused by elastic fiber damage due to the paradoxic activation of the Ras pathway. The study was then expanded[11] with the examination of 24 patients on target therapy for metastatic melanoma (vemurafenib, dabrafenib, and combination of dabrafenib and trametinib): hair changes due to vemurafenib and dabrafenib were frequently noted, with the most common hair side effect being acquired hair kinking (80% and 60%, respectively), often associated with pigmentation of grey hair.

The active multitargeted tyrosine kinase inhibitor (TKI) sorafenib causes diffuse and reversible alopecia in up to 50% of patients, with the regrown hair usually more brittle and curly or, occasionally, more pigmented than before treatment.[10-12]

Alopecia has also been described in patients treated with vismodegib, an orally active agent approved for advanced basal cell cancer.[13] It is a sonic hedgehog pathway inhibitor (the sonic hedgehog pathway is important for the normal hair follicle morphogenesis).

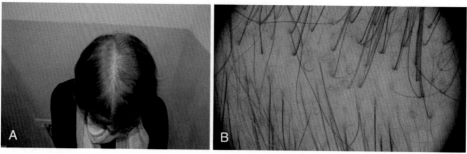

FIG. 24.3 Clinical picture of telogen effluvium due to vemurafenib leading to diffuse hair thinning of the entire scalp **(A)**; trichoscopy showing a decrease of hair density and numerous empty follicles appearing as *yellow dots* **(B)**.

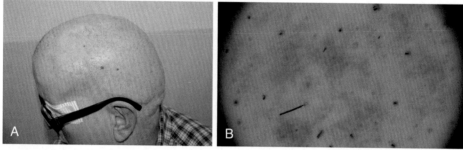

FIG. 24.4 Clinical picture of diffuse alopecia involving total hair body in a patient during therapy with vemurafenib **(A)**; trichoscopy showing acute phase of alopecia characterized by the presence of *black dots* and *yellow dots* **(B)**.

Fifteen percent of patients treated with palbociclib, an orally active inhibitor of cyclin-dependent kinase 4 and 6 used in advanced hormone receptor–positive breast cancer in combination with hormone therapy, showed mild alopecia, and the same drug effect has been described for the related agent ribociclib.[14,15]

Epidermal growth factors inhibitors have also been associated with hair changes, such as slower growth of hair of the scalp, trichomegaly of eyelashes, and hypertrichosis of the facial hair.[16] Drugs such as bevacizumab and ranibizumab can induce hair kinking.[17]

Pazopanib, sunitinib, and dasatinib, which are **multitargeted receptor TKIs**, can cause reversible hair depigmentation.[18,19] In particular, hair depigmentation on the scalp, eyebrows, eyelashes, or body hair is reversible, dose-dependent, and is reported in 7%–14% of patients (dosage of 50 mg daily) and in up to 64% of patients on higher doses. Alopecia occurs in 6% of patients receiving sunitinib, and the regrowing hair is usually more brittle, curly, and pigmented than the original hair.[20]

Imatinib, a TKI approved for the treatment of chronic myeloproliferative disease, has been associated with reversible hair lightening and darkening, with onset of hair changes occurring after a median time of 4 weeks after starting therapy.

Clinical presentation

- The clinical pattern is usually a diffuse non-scarring alopecia but a scarring alopecia mimicking folliculitis decalvans has occasionally been described.[21-23] Nonscarring alopecia is typical of vemurafenib, with an initial telogen effluvium leading to evident diffuse hair thinning involving the entire scalp (Fig. 24.3A and B) and eyelashes, axillary, pubic, and limb hair (Fig. 24.4A and B). The pull test result is positive with telogen roots.[24] In a few cases, a massive scalp scaling is associated with diffuse follicular hyperkeratosis and yellow adherent hair casts along the hair shafts. Total hair regrowth can be seen after drug withdrawal or with therapy with steroids (Fig. 24.5A and B).
- Other possible antitarget drug–induced hair changes are diffuse hair kinking, characterized by a progressive change in the texture of the hair, which become curlier, and development of diffuse woolly and

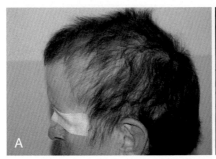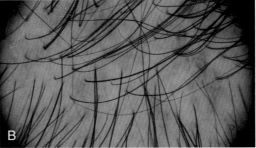

FIG. 24.5 Clinical picture **(A)** and trichoscopy **(B)** of total hair regrowth after vemurafenib withdrawal and steroid therapy.

lusterless hair, difficult to comb and slowly growing.[25] These hair shaft alterations involve 30%–100% of the scalp and may appear during therapy or during hair regrowth phase. Hair kinking is also a possible side effect of epidermal growth factor receptor (EGFR) inhibitors, due to keratinization of the inner root sheath, causing the altered texture and shape of the hair shaft.[17]

- Scarring alopecia is typical of epidermal growth factor inhibitors, such as erlotinib and gefitinib.[21–23] Clinically, the pattern is characterized by tufted hair folliculitis and diffuse perifollicular pustules. A great inflammation may also be present with a reticular and elongated vascular pattern at trichoscopy. Pathologically, this pattern corresponds to chronic folliculitis and perifolliculitis with a mixed infiltrate of lymphocytes, plasma cells, eosinophils, and neutrophils.
- Hair color change, another possible clinical pattern, is a consequence of interference with signals controlling melanogenesis, reversible during regrowth.

Trichoscopy. In telogen effluvium, trichoscopy shows a decrease of hair density and numerous empty follicles appearing as yellow dots (Fig. 24.3B) and in acute phases possible observation of black dots (Fig. 24.4B); in hair kinking it shows thin and irregular twisting hair shafts; in case of scalp scaling the major feature is represented by perifollicular hyperkeratosis and yellow hair casts along the hair shafts. Trichoscopy of folliculitis decalvans shows the presence of tufted hairs, where more than six hairs are grouped together and emerge from the same follicular ostium. The number of hairs can reach >15. Because of the traction of high number of hairs, the capillaries are directed to the follicular ostium and appear elongated and stretched. Presence of pustules is also typical of this scarring alopecia.

Radiation Therapy

Radiation-induced alopecia is common and develops following radiation therapy of neoplasms. Severity of radiation-induced alopecia depends on the dose, total duration, interval between each irradiation, size of area irradiated, angle of irradiation, and patient-related factors. In addition, a great number of drugs have also been reported to increase radiosensitivity.

Radiotherapy of brain tumors often produces scarring alopecia. X-ray dosages >700 Gy in fact permanently destroy the hair follicle. Patchy alopecia resembling alopecia areata is another possible side effect of neurosurgical operations with fluoroscopic procedures.[26] It is benign and self-limiting. Complete hair regrowth generally occurs within 2–4 months after irradiation, and no treatment or preventive measures appear to be generally effective.

Clinical presentation. Pathogenesis of radiation-induced temporary alopecia involves acute damage to actively dividing matrix cells of anagen follicles, causing immediate loss of dystrophic anagen hairs (anagen effluvium), and premature entry of some anagen hair follicles into catagen and then into telogen phase, resulting in delayed onset of hair shedding (telogen effluvium). It is characterized by patches of nonscarring alopecia confined to the area of radiation, usually asymptomatic without signs of scalp inflammation. Hair pull test is positive at the periphery of the alopecic patch with telogen hairs extracted. Hair loss mostly occurs within 1–3 weeks after radiation exposure with spontaneous regrowth of hair within 2–4 months.

Total or partial destruction of hair follicle stem cell is responsible for permanent alopecia due to radiation (Fig. 24.6A). Lately, the use of fluoroscopic procedures permits reducing the area involved by surgery and limits the size of the alopecia.

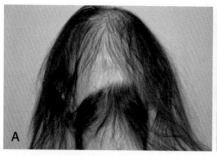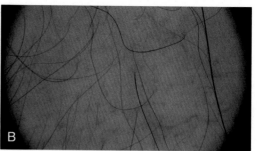

FIG. 24.6 Permanent alopecia due to radiation **(A)**. *Yellow dots* and thin shafts as the only signs on trichoscopy **(B)**.

Trichoscopy. Dermoscopic examination of the alopecic area due to fluoroscopic procedures shows a pattern of alopecia areata with mostly yellow dots, black dots, short vellus hairs, and blue-grey dots in a target pattern around yellow dots and follicles.[26] In permanent alopecia due to radiation, yellow dots and thin shafts are the only signs (Fig. 24.6B).

Anticoagulants

These drugs include heparin and its derivates, coumarins, warfarin, and phenindione. They can induce a telogen effluvium, generally correlated to the dosage, with an unknown mechanism of action.

Nevertheless, both heparins and coumarins determine a similar pattern of alopecia, so it can be stated that they share a mechanism related to the anticoagulant activity that causes a change on the vasculature of the scalp. According to Watras et al.,[27] the database of the World Health Organization (WHO)-Uppsala Monitoring Centre (UMC) VigiBase has received 877 reports of alopecia related to warfarin, 105 to acenocoumarol, 2 to phenindione, and 134 to heparins. The published data suggest that alopecia is reversible on cessation of the drug and reappears on challenge. In particular, for warfarin and heparin, hair loss generally begins after 3 months of drug intake, but the time range is wide. Women are more affected than men but maybe because a diagnosis of male androgenetic alopecia is wrongly made.

The WHO also registered 143 reports of alopecia for rivaroxaban, 215 for dabigatran, 47 for apixaban, and none for edoxaban, which are the novel oral anticoagulants.

Clinical presentation. Acute telogen effluvium appears after few weeks of drug intake because of a premature transformation of growing hair follicles into the resting phase. The pull test is positive with telogen hair roots, but hair thinning is usually absent. In fact, there is a great interindividual variability in baseline daily hair loss and in density of telogen scalp hair, which dictates whether the increase in rate of loss will lead to cosmetically compromising alopecia.[27]

Trichoscopy. The dermoscopic pattern of acute telogen effluvium is characterized by the presence in the scalp of diffusely short hair with the same length, which reflects the time of the shedding. Another possible feature is the presence of empty follicles not only in the androgen-dependent area but also diffusely.

Antihypertensive Agents

Both angiotensin-converting enzyme inhibitors (mainly captopril) and β-blockers, in particular metoprolol and propranolol, can cause a severe telogen effluvium.[28–30]

A case of lisinopril-induced alopecia in a 53-year-old male has recently been described: in particular, lisinopril was discontinued and switched to an angiotensin-receptor blocker (losartan potassium) with alopecia resolution after 4 weeks.[31]

Telogen effluvium is a possible side effect of timolol eye drops; only few reports have been published.[32] As stated by Diggory et al.[33] ophthalmic β-adrenergic blockers enter the blood stream through the lacrimal and conjunctival system, and the blood levels of β-adrenergic blockers increase inducing systemic reactions even with ophthalmic usage. According to the authors, two drops of 0.5% timolol eyedrops can cause blood concentrations equivalent to those of 10 mg oral timolol.

Clinical presentation. Telogen effluvium is the typical clinical pattern in alopecia due to antihypertensive agents.[34]

Trichoscopy. As in acute telogen effluvium, trichoscopy confirms the absence of miniaturization, typical of androgenetic alopecia.

Interferons

The combination of pegylated interferon α (PEG–IFN-α) and ribavirin (RBV) for chronic hepatitis C has been associated with many systemic and cutaneous side effects, such as psoriasis, sarcoidosis, vitiligo, and specific drug eruptions. Hair disorders associated with this drug combination have been reported in 19% of patients[35] and include not only diffuse thinning of the hair but also trichomegaly of eyelashes, hypertrichosis, hair curling, and hair repigmentation.[36]

In the scalp, three types of alopecia can occur: telogen effluvium, alopecia areata, or localized transient alopecia at the injection site.[37] Occurrence of this type of alopecia is considered unpredictable.

Typically, there is no correlation between the severity of the telogen effluvium and the dosage, and in some patients, it can regress without interrupting the drugs.

A case of dystrophic anagen effluvium has been described in a patient affected by rheumatoid arthritis and Hashimoto thyroiditis treated with PEG-IFN-α-2a/ribavarin therapy for chronic hepatitis C.[38] This type of alopecia presented with patchy hair loss that had started 9 months after beginning IFN therapy and was cured 4 months after stopping the therapy. The authors stated that dystrophic anagen effluvium might have been caused by the insult of increased cytotoxic T cells to anagen hair follicles.

Alopecia areata has also been described with the combination of IFN/RBV for hepatitis C[38] and with IFN-α prescribed for melanoma.[39] Alopecia universalis (AU) has also been reported[40] and according to the authors is benign and reversible, so it is not an indication for stopping the therapy. Interestingly, the authors proposed the hypothesis that PEG-IFN modifies the immune response in AU, leading to the synthesis of Th1 cytokines, such as interleukin 1 (IL-1), IL-2, and IFN-γ. When the cytokine IFN-α2b is also involved, it may induce the production of antibodies directed against the follicular epithelium. A case of irreversible AU during treatment with PEG-IFN/RBV for hepatitis C has also been described and reviewed.[42]

Clinical presentation. According to the degree of toxicity, there are three possible clinical patterns of hair loss due to IFN:

- In telogen effluvium, the clinical presentation is characterized by diffuse hair thinning and loss; the pull test usually however is negative.

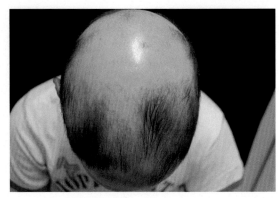

FIG. 24.7 Alopecia areata in a patient in treatment with interferon/ribavirin for hepatitis C.

- In alopecia areata, the clinical presentation varies from well-circumscribed patches in the scalp to the loss of all the scalp hair, as alopecia areata totalis, or the body hair, as alopecia areata universalis (Fig. 24.7A). The last form is the most frequent. The hair shedding is copious a few weeks after the therapy. The pull test is strongly positive for dystrophic hairs with tapered ends, visible through the microscope.[40,41]
- Only one case of irreversible AU has been reported in the literature. The hair loss involved all the body hair, with a significant amount of fallen hair after 1 month of the completion of the combined antiviral therapy and a complete AU by the end of the third month. The irreversible pattern of alopecia was confirmed by skin biopsy, with the absence of terminal hair follicles.[42]

Trichoscopy

- There is no hair shaft variability despite the diffuse hair thinning and reduced hair density.
- Trichoscopy shows the typical signs of acute alopecia areata in the initial phase, such as black dots, cadaverized hair, dystrophic hair, exclamation point hair, whereas the chronic signs are present after hair shedding, such as yellow dots.
- The dermoscopic pattern of AU is characterized by the presence of only yellow dots.

Retinol (Vitamin A) and Retinoids

Even if this vitamin is often prescribed for hair diseases, a prolonged administration can cause a mild hair loss, involving pubic hair, axillary hair, and vellus hair. An increased hair shaft fragility can often be observed. In our experience, the contemporary administration of vitamin E increases vitamin A toxicity.

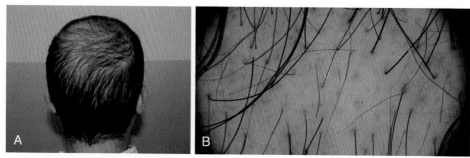

FIG. 24.8 Alopecia involving more than 50% of the scalp producing hair thinning during therapy with retinoids for acne vulgaris **(A)**. Diffuse hair miniaturization and empty follicles with yellowish discoloration visible through trichoscopy **(B)**.

Acitretin, etretinate, and isotretinoin cause hair loss with visible alopecia in up to 20% of patients.[43] Premature teloptosis is probably the main mechanism for retinoid-induced hair loss. The side effect is dose-related and may affect body hairs as well.

Clinical presentation. Diffuse hair shedding is present with reduced hair density until a new anagen replaces the last telogen. Alopecia rarely involves more than 50% of the scalp producing hair thinning[44] (Fig. 24.8A). Hair kinking is often associated. Hair repigmentation has been reported with acitretin and etretinate.[45–47]

Trichoscopy. Diffuse hair miniaturization over the entire scalp is the most frequent dermoscopic pattern. Trichoscopy shows an androgenetic alopecia pattern not only in the androgen-dependent area but also over the entire scalp and possible empty follicles with yellowish discoloration (Fig. 24.8B).

Antiretrovirals

Severe telogen effluvium and patchy hair loss resembling alopecia areata are common side effects of antiretroviral therapy, occurring in up to 10% of patients. Body hair can also be involved.

The protease inhibitor class, in particular indinavir, is the most commonly reported cause of hair loss, followed by the nucleoside reverse transcriptase inhibitor (NRTI), lamivudine. In a recent review of the literature,[48] scalp alopecia was the most frequently reported side effect, with a median time of onset of 2.5 months and a partial reversal in half the cases at the discontinuation of the drug within 1–3 months.

Alopecia areata associated with abacavir therapy, an NRTI used in combination with other retroviral, has been reported.[49]

Oral Contraceptives

A change in or a withdrawal of any oral contraceptive can cause telogen hair shedding[50] typically after 2–3 months, probably because under the effect of the estrogen hormones, the follicles prolong their cycle and undergo physiologic synchronization (extension of anagen). Discontinuation of treatment with oral contraceptives determines the entry into resting phase of all those follicles that have extended their cycle. Even changing the oral contraceptive can precipitate a telogen effluvium. Oral contraceptives containing an androgenic progestin and hormonal replacement therapy with high-dose progesterone can cause telogen hair shedding with or without patterned alopecia.[51]

Clinical presentation and trichoscopy. Both clinically and dermoscopically the pattern of hair shedding due to oral contraceptives is an acute telogen effluvium with no visible reduction in hair density over the crown and no signs of androgenetic alopecia, but the presence of short hair all over the scalp, with a positive pull test.

In patients with associated androgenetic alopecia, the use of progesterone-based preparations may induce or worsen the condition.

Drugs Acting on the Nervous System

Telogen effluvium is a frequent side effect of a lithium therapy and becomes evident a few months after the beginning of the treatment.[52] This may also be a consequence of lithium-induced hypothyroiditis. It is not correlated with the dosage and is more frequent in females. Hair straightening has also been associated with lithium intake.

Valproic acid and/or divalproex precipitates alopecia in up to 12% of patients and is dose-dependent. These drugs can also change hair color and structure, inducing kinky hair or bleaching/darkening of the hair.[20,53] Carbamazepine has been reported to induce alopecia in 6% of the patients. Tricyclic antidepressants, such as maprotiline, trazodone, haloperidol, olanzapine, risperidone, and clonazepam, and virtually all the new generation of antidepressants may less commonly induce alopecia, except for neuroleptics, benzodiazepines, or barbiturates and selected antihistamines. Discontinuation of the medication or reduction of dosage leads to complete hair regrowth.[54] Hair loss is commonly observed in patients taking fluoxetine or paroxetine.[55]

Hair loss occurring during dopaminergic therapy for Parkinson disease is possible: in particular, the reported cases in the literature include levodopa and both ergot alkaloid and nonergot alkaloid dopamine receptor agonists.[56] The pathophysiologic relationship between these drugs and hair loss remains unclear, as well as why female patients are more affected than males. The prognosis is good.

Clinical presentation. The clinical presentation of alopecia because of lithium is hair thinning that usually occurs 4–6 months after starting the medication. Because of an unknown mechanism of action, these drugs induce an increase in telogen shedding. This shedding is typical of chronic telogen effluvium also because it occurs few months to sometimes even a year after starting the medication and the patient notices hair loss several years after the drugs.

Trichoscopy. The dermoscopic aspect is similar to androgenetic alopecia with hair miniaturization not only in the androgen-dependent areas but also diffusely in the scalp but without empty follicles. Most of the hair is diffusely thinned.

Azathioprine

Azathioprine is an antimetabolite that interferes with cellular DNA synthesis used as an immunosuppressive drug in several autoimmune disorders. In the literature, few reports of azathioprine-induced anagen effluvium are described.[57]

Clinical presentation. The clinical pattern of anagen effluvium is characterized by diffuse and copious hair loss leading to generalized hair thinning.

Trichoscopy. Trichoscopy reveals intact follicular openings and absence of yellow dots or exclamation mark hair, which excludes hair anagen shedding due to acute alopecia areata. Hair shaft microscopy

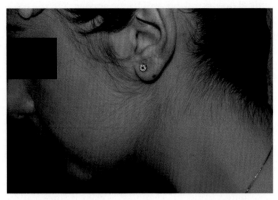

FIG. 24.9 Hypertrichosis due to minoxidil application for androgenetic alopecia.

reveals a few dystrophic hair shafts with tapered, irregular, and pigmented hair that suggest anagen hair and a few telogen hairs.[57]

Minoxidil

A withdrawal of a treatment with systemic or topic minoxidil can cause a telogen effluvium occurring after 2–3 months, because of the abrupt transition in telogen of all the follicles that extend their growth phase under the effect of minoxidil. Some patients present with a telogen effluvium at the beginning of the treatment with minoxidil; this might be because of the fact that initiation of anagen induced by minoxidil stimulates teloptosis.

Topical minoxidil often causes hypertrichosis of the face and neck due to contamination or incorrect use (Fig. 24.9). Some patients using 5% topical minoxidil develop diffuse hypertrichosis, which is probably due to systemic absorption of the drug.

Clinical presentation and trichoscopy. The typical telogen effluvium after discontinuation of minoxidil is characterized by relevant hair shedding with a positive pull test of telogen hairs. Trichoscopy shows diffusely a great number of short vellus hairs of similar length over the entire scalp.

Strontium Ranelate

Strontium ranelate is indicated for the treatment of postmenopausal osteoporosis. The onset of alopecia during this therapy has been reported with diffuse hair loss pattern or even alopecia areata universalis.[58–60] Improvement occurred in most cases after discontinuation of the drug and the exclusion of other possible causes.

Clinical presentation and trichoscopy. On the basis of the type of hair loss, the clinical manifestation and trichoscopy can be consistent with telogen effluvium or alopecia areata.

Thallium

Thallium is a heavy metal whose salts are colorless, tasteless, and odorless. It has been historically used as a lethal poison or is used in the manufacture of optical lenses, semiconductors, low-temperature switching devices, green-colored fireworks, imitation jewelry, and as a chemical catalyst.[61]

Thallium is highly toxic to humans, and a fatal dose is estimated to be 10–15 mg/kg,[62] even if intoxication is usually chronic due to repeated exposure. Thallium poisoning is manifested by neurologic, gastrointestinal, and dermatologic signs.

In particular, an anagen effluvium is a typical sign of thallium poisoning. Typically, hair loss starts after 2 weeks and affects scalp, arms, legs, eyebrows, and eyelashes.[63]

Clinical presentation. Acute and diffuse hair shedding of scalp and the lateral part of the eyebrow is the typical clinical presentation of intoxication by thallium. The pull test is positive with hair roots showing tapered pigmented hair bulb covered by a triangular root sheath consistent with anagen dystrophic hair.

Trichoscopy. Examination of the hair by dermoscopy and polarized light microscopy may show a characteristic dystrophic anagen hair with dark pigmentation in the hair bulb, disorganized cortex, and intermittent dark transverse bands in the hair shaft as a result of the accumulation of gaseous inclusions that diffract the light. These changes are characteristic of, but not specific to, thallium intoxication. Study under a polarized light microscope revealed black pigmentation in the hair bulb and multiple dark transverse bands in the hair follicle.[63]

Cyclosporin A

The major side effect of systemic cyclosporin A (CsA) is nephrotoxicity, but hair disorders such as hypertrichosis and trichomegaly have also been reported.[64,65] Reversible hypertrichosis is common and most frequently affects the face and back. It is dose-related, occurring in up to 50% of patients taking high dosages of the drugs after transplantation.

An interesting case of CsA ophthalmic emulsion–induced hypertrichosis has been described.[66] Concerning the pathogenesis, the factors that regulate the

TABLE 24.2
Drugs Inducing Eyelash Trichomegaly

Latanoprost, bimatoprost
Cetuximab, panitumumab
Erlotinib, gefitinib
Interferon-α2b
Zidovudine
Minoxidil
Phenytoin
Acetazolamide
Cyclosporine
Tacrolimus
Topiramate
Psoralens
Corticosteroids
Streptomycin
Penicillamine

growth cycle of the eyelash hair follicles remain unclear. CsA could induce telogen follicles to enter the anagen phase, implying a role of CsA in regulating the hair follicle immune system and its cellular components, releasing inhibitory/stimulatory cytokines.

Prostaglandin Analogs

Several prostaglandin F2-α analogs used for the topical treatment of glaucoma produce darkening of the eyelashes and acquired trichomegaly.[67] These include mainly latanoprost and bimatoprost.

Thanks to the conversion from telogen to anagen phase of the hair follicles, a cosmetic effect can be obtained. The Food and Drug Administration approved bimatoprost 0.03% solution for treatment of patients with hypotrichosis of the eyelashes.[68] Drugs inducing eyelashes trichomegaly are listed in Table 24.2.

Chloroquine

This drug is an antimalarial approved for the treatment of lupus erythematosus and rheumatoid arthritis. Reversible hair discoloration is a typical symptom described with chloroquine treatment. In more detail, hair lightening starts 3–4 months after the beginning of treatment and typically affects the hair scalp, whereas eyelashes, eyebrows, and body hair are less frequently affected.[20] Hair discoloration is due to a toxic effect of chloroquine on pheomelanin synthesis

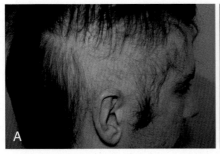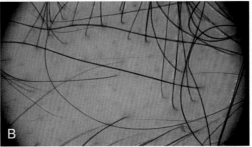

FIG. 24.10 Permanent alopecia in a pattern with diffuse hair loss and residual sparse and short hair, more evident in the parietal region in a patient treated with high dose of chemotherapy with busulfan **(A)**. Trichoscopy shows visible hair thinning with a reduced number of follicles **(B)**.

with accumulation of nonmelanized or poorly melanized melanosomes, and it is in fact more common in patients with blond, light brown, or red hair.

Hair hypopigmentation has also been described with hydroxychloroquine.[69]

Clinical presentation and trichoscopy. Brightening of any hair color leading to whitening is present during a treatment with chloroquine. Hair lightening is also shown with trichoscopy as an alternation of hair darker and lighter all around the scalp.

Permanent Alopecia due to Chemotherapy

In specific cases, hair regrowth after chemotherapy is not complete and a permanent alopecia, defined as an absence of or incomplete hair regrowth at 6 months after chemotherapy, can persist.

High dose of chemotherapy with busulfan, cyclophosphamide, thiotepa, and hematopoietic cell transplantation[70-72] are associated with permanent alopecia.

However, in the literature, there are a number of case reports of permanent alopecia after standard-dose chemotherapy for breast cancer (particularly with docetaxel, which is dose- and duration-dependent)[73,74] and germ cell tumors.[75]

Fonia et al.[76] proposed a clinicopathologic model of hair follicles destruction resulting in permanent alopecia in 10 patients after taxane chemotherapy and adjuvant hormonal therapy.

As mentioned, taxane induces an anagen effluvium attacking the hair bulb. After this step, the authors noted the disrupted peribulbar area of immune privilege loss with bulbar antigen exposure triggering alopecia areata–like features, including peribulbar lymphoid cell infiltrate, shift out of anagen with "inflammatory" telogen effluvium, and miniaturization. The residual hair follicles with underlying obliterated end-stage

fibrous tracts had "arrested" in a status of "follicular inertia," and the following adjuvant antiestrogen hormonal therapy had caused hair miniaturization with a female pattern hair loss. Long-term use of small molecule EGFR inhibitors, such as gefitinib and erlotinib, can also cause permanent alopecia.[23,77]

Clinical presentation. Patterns of permanent alopecia due to chemotherapy are divided into three groups[76]:
1. Diffuse hair loss with residual sparse and short hair (Fig. 24.10);
2. Diffuse hair alopecia with accentuation on the vertex of the scalp;
3. Diffuse and patchy alopecia.

Trichoscopy. Visible hair thinning is appreciated in all cases with a reduced number of follicles in the scalp, such as in a diffuse pattern, and an increased number of vellus hair is noted with the decreased hair density. On the basis of the different clinical manifestations, it is possible to observe androgenetic alopecia pattern with an accentuation of one specific site, such as vertex, with absence of scarring alopecia but a diffuse, mark, and thinned hair of the scalp.

This pattern is also confirmed by pathologic observation of nonscarring alopecia with a preserved number of follicular units and lack of fibrosis.

CONCLUSIONS

Anything that interrupts the normal hair cycle can cause a diffuse hair loss. The evaluation of a patient with hair problems is a fundamental step for the correct diagnosis of disease, as it gives important information and helps in choosing the diagnostic tools that should be used to confirm the clinical suspicion. Telogen effluvium and anagen effluvium are the most common types of diffuse hair shedding due to drugs, but dermatologists should remember that drugs may be responsible also for changes in hair texture and color. The evaluation includes a clinical history and patient examination and is followed by invasive and noninvasive tests. Often, only clinical examination permits correct diagnosis of the hair disease and evaluation of its severity and progression. For this reason, time should be spent to obtain all necessary anamnestic data and to carefully examine the patient.

Hair loss has psychologically negative effects on life, with loss of self-esteem and confidence, loss of virility for men, and loss of beauty for women. In most cases, hair loss due to chemicals is generally reversible with the chemical's withdrawal, with a good prognosis. Cases of permanent alopecia after chemotherapy are not as rare as in the past. The knowledge of side effects of the drugs that we prescribe is crucial for better management of the patient.

REFERENCES

1. Mounsey AL, Reed SW. Diagnosing and treating hair loss. *Am Fam Physician*. 2009;80(4):356–362.
2. Piraccini BM. Evaluation of hair loss. *Curr Probl Dermatol*. 2015;47:10–20.
3. Paus R, Haslam IS, Sharov AA, Botchkarev VA. Pathobiology of chemotherapy-induced hair loss. *Lancet Oncol*. 2013;14:e50–e59.
4. Trüeb RM. Chemotherapy-induced hair loss. *Skin Ther Lett*. 2010;15(7):5–7. Review.
5. Rossi A, Fortuna MC, Caro G, et al. Chemotherapy-induced alopecia management: clinical experience and practical advice. *J Cosmet Dermatol*. 2017;16(4).
6. Yun SJ, Kim SJ. Hair loss pattern due to chemotherapy-induced anagen effluvium: a cross-sectional observation. *Dermatology*. 2007;215:36–40.
7. Soref CM, Fahl WE. A new strategy to prevent chemotherapy and radiotherapy-induced alopecia using topically applied vasoconstrictor. *Int J Cancer*. 2015;136:195–203.
8. Hyoseung S, Seong JJ, Do HK, Ohsang K, Seung-Kwon M. Efficacy of interventions for prevention of chemotherapy-induced alopecia: a systematic review and meta-analysis. *Int J Cancer*. 2015;136:E442–E454.
9. Wang J, Lu Z, Au JL. Protection against chemotherapy-induced alopecia. *Pharm Res*. 2006;23:2505–2514.
10. Autier J, Escudier B, Wechsler J, et al. Prospective study of the cutaneous adverse effects of sorafenib, a novel multikinase inhibitor. *Arch Dermatol*. 2008;144:886.
11. Escudier B, Eisen T, Stadler WM, et al. Sorafenib in advanced clear-cell renal-cell cancer. *N Engl J Med*. 2007;356:125.
12. Robert C, Mateus C, Spatz A, Wechsler J, Escudier B. Dermatologic symptoms associated with the multikinase inhibitor sorafenib. *J Am Acad Dermatol*. 2009;60:299–305.
13. Chang AL, Solomon JA, Hainsworth JD, et al. Expanded access study of patients with advanced basal cell carcinoma treated with the Hedgehog pathway inhibitor, vismodegib. *J Am Acad Dermatol*. 2014;70:60.
14. Finn RS, Martin M, Rugo HS, et al. Palbociclib and letrozole in advanced breast cancer. *N Engl J Med*. 2016;375:1925.
15. Hortobagyi GN, Stemmer SM, Burris HA, et al. Ribociclib as first-line therapy for HR-positive, advanced breast cancer. *N Engl J Med*. 2016;375:1738.
16. Robert C, Soria JC, Spatz A, et al. Cutaneous side-effects of kinase inhibitors and blocking antibodies. *Lancet Oncol*. 2005;6:491–500.
17. Macdonald JB, Macdonald B, Golitz LE, LoRusso P, Sekulic A. Cutaneous adverse effects of targeted therapies: Part I: inhibitors of the cellular membrane. *J Am Acad Dermatol*. 2015;72(2):203–218. Quiz 219–220.
18. Routhouska S, Gilliam AC, Mirmirani P. Hair depigmentation during chemotherapy with a class III/V receptor tyrosine kinase inhibitor. *Arch Dermatol*. 2006;142:1477–1479.
19. Fujimi A, Ibata S, Kanisawa Y, et al. Reversible skin and hair depigmentation during chemotherapy with dasatinib for chronic myeloid leukemia. *J Dermatol*. 2016;43(1):106–107.
20. Ricci F, De Simone C, Del Regno L, Peris K. Drug-induced hair colour changes. *Eur J Dermatol*. 2016;26(6):531–536.
21. Graves JE, Jones BF, Lind AC, et al. Non scarring alopecia associated with epidermal growth factor receptor inhibitor gefitinib. *J Am Acad Dermatol*. 2006;55:349–353.
22. Donovan JC, Ghazarian DM, Shaw JC. Scarring alopecia associated with the use of the epidermal growth factor receptor inhibitor gefitinib. *Arch Dermatol*. 2008;144:1524–1525.
23. Hepper DM, Wu P, Anadkat MJ. Scarring alopecia associated with the epidermal growth factor receptor inhibitor erlotinib. *J Acad Ermatol*. 2011;64:996–998.
24. Piraccini BM, Patrizi A, Fanti PA, et al. RASopathic alopecia: hair changes associated with vemurafenib therapy. *J Am Acad Dermatol*. 2015;72(4):738–741.
25. Dika E, Patrizi A, Ribero S, et al. Hair and nail adverse events during treatment with targeted therapies for metastatic melanoma. *Eur J Dermatol*. 2016;26(3):232–239.
26. Ounsakul V, Iamsumang W, Suchonwanit P. Radiation-induced alopecia after endovascular embolization under fluoroscopy. *Case Rep Dermatol Med*. 2016;2016:8202469.
27. Watras MM, Patel JP, Arya R. Traditional anticoagulants and hair loss: a role for direct oral anticoagulants? A review of the literature. *Drugs Real World Outcomes*. 2016;3(1):1–6.
28. Mubki T, Rudnicka L, Olszewska M, Shapiro J. Evaluation and diagnosis of the hair loss patient: part I. History and clinical examination. *J Am Acad Dermatol*. 2014;71:415. e411–e415.
29. Patel M, Harrison S, Sinclair R. Drugs and hair loss. *Dermatol Clin*. 2013;31(1):67–73.
30. Steckelings UM, Artuc M, Wollschläger T, Wiehstutz S, Henz BM. Angiotensin-converting enzyme inhibitors as inducers of adverse cutaneous reactions. *Acta Derm Venereol*. 2001;81(5):321–325. Review.

31. Kataria V, Wang H, Wald JW, Phan YL. Lisinopril-Induced Alopecia: A Case Report. *J Pharm Pract.* 2017 Oct;30(5):562–566.

32. Muramatsu K, Nomura T, Shiiya C, Nishiura K, Tsukinaga I. Alopecia induced by timolol eye-drops. *Acta Derm Venereol.* 2017;97(2):295–296.

33. Diggory P, Franks W. Glaucoma: systemic side effects of topical medical therapy – a common and under recognized problem. *J R Soc Med.* 1994;87:575–576.

34. Gilmore S, Sinclair R. Chronic telogen effluvium is due to reduction in the variance of anagen duration. *Australas J Dermatol.* 2010;51:163–167.

35. Wright M, Forton D, Main J, et al. Treatment of histologically mild hepatitis C virus infection with interferon and ribavirin: a multicentre randomized controlled trial. *J Viral Hepat.* 2008;12:58–66.

36. Mistry N, Shapero J, Crawford RI. A review of adverse cutaneous drug reactions resulting from the use of interferon and ribavirin. *Can J Gastroenterol.* 2009;23(10):677–683. Review.

37. Lang AM, Norland AM, Shuneman RL, Tope WD. Localized interferon alpha-2b-induced alopecia. *Arch Dermatol.* 1999;135:1126–1128.

38. Agesta N, Zabala R, Diaz-Perez JL. Alopecia areata during interferon alpha-2b/ribavirin therapy. *Dermatology.* 2002;205:300–301.

39. Radny P, Bauer J, Caroli UM, et al. Alopecia areata induced by adjuvant treatment with alpha-interferon in malignant melanoma? *Dermatology.* 2004;209:249–250.

40. Verma P, Dayal S, Jain VK, Amrani A. Alopecia universalis as a side effect of pegylated interferon α-ribavirin combination therapy for hepatitis C: a rare case report. *J Chemother.* 2016:1–3.

41. Turker K, Tas B, Ozkaya M, Tas E, Caglar A, Tetikkurt US. Dystrophic-anagen effluvium occurring during pegylated interferon-α-2a/ribavirin therapy. *Hepat Mon.* 2015;15(3):e24804.

42. Omazzi B, Prada A, Borroni G, Sacrini F. Irreversible alopecia universalis during treatment with pegylated interferon-ribavirin for chronic hepatitis C virus infection: case report and published work review. *Hepatol Res.* 2012;42(12):1248–1251.

43. Berth-Jones J, Shuttleworth D, Hutchinson PE. A study of etretinate alopecia. *Br J Dermatol.* 1990;122:751–755.

44. Olsen EA. Chemotherapy-induced alopecia: overview and methodology for charactering hair changes and regrowth. In: Oliver IN, ed. *The MASCC Textbook of Cancer Supportive Care and Survivoeship.* New York, NY: Springer; 2011:381–388.

45. Clarke JT, Price H, Clarke S, George R, Miller JJ. Acquired kinking of the hair caused by acitretin. *J Drugs Dermatol.* 2007;6(9):937–938.

46. Seckin D, Yildiz A. Repigmentation and curling of hair after acitretin therapy. *Australas J Dermatol.* 2009;50(3):214–216.

47. Ward PD, Miller HL, Shipman AR. A case of repigmentation and curling of hair on acitretin therapy. *Clin Exp Dermatol.* 2014;39(1):91–92.

48. Woods EA, Foisy MM. Antiretroviral-related alopecia in HIV-infected patients. *Ann Pharmacother.* 2014;48(9):1187–1193.

49. Kim HS, Shin HS. Alopecia areata associated with abacavir therapy. *Infect Chemother.* 2014;46(2):103–105.

50. Tosti A, Pazzaglia M. Drug reactions affecting hair: diagnosis. *Dermatol Clin.* 2007;25:223–231.

51. Harrison S, Bergfeld W. Diffuse hair loss: its triggers and management. *Cleve Clin J Med.* 2009;76(6):361–367.

52. Paquet P, Claessens N, Piérard-Franchimont C, Piérard GE. Cutaneous adverse effects of lithium. *Rev Med Liege.* 2005;60(11):885–887. Review.

53. Caneppele S, Mazereeuw-Hautier J, Bonafé JL. Sodium valproate-induced kinky hair. *Ann Dermatol Venereol.* 2001;128(2):134–135.

54. Mercke Y, Sheng H, Khan T, Lippmann S. Hair loss in psychopharmacology. *Ann Clin Psychiatry.* 2000;12(1):35–42. Review.

55. Gautam M. Alopecia due to psychotropic medications. *Ann Pharmacother.* 1999;33(5):631–637. Review.

56. Miwa H, Kondo T. Hair loss induced by dopamine agonist: case report and review of the literature. *Parkinsonism Relat Disord.* 2003;10(1):51–52. Review.

57. Sonthalia S, Daulatabad D. Azathioprine-associated anagen effluvium. *Indian J Dermatol Venereol Leprol.* 2016;82(3):322–324.

58. Sainz M, del Pozo JG, Arias LH, Carvajal A. Strontium ranelate may cause alopecia. *BMJ.* 2009;338:b1494.

59. Lee YY, Yang CH, Chen CH, Hwang JS. Alopecia associated with strontium ranelate use in a 62-year-old woman. *Osteoporos Int.* 2013;24(3):1127–1129.

60. García Llopis P, Vicente Valor MI, Martínez Cristóbal A. Alopecia areata universalis due to strontium ranelate. *Med Clin (Barc).* 2012;138(5):229.

61. Zhao G, Ding M, Zhang B, et al. Clinical manifestations and management of acute thallium poisoning. *Eur Neurol.* 2008;60(6):292–297.

62. Moore D, House I, Dixon A. Thallium poisoning: diagnosis may be elusive but alopecia is the clue. *BMJ.* 1993;306:1527–1529.

63. Curto-Barredo L, Segura S, Martín-Ezquerra G, Lloveras B, Gallardo F, Pujol RM. Anagen effluvium due to thallium poisoning derived from the intake of Chinese herbal medicine and rodenticide containing thallium salts. *J Dermatol.* 2015;42(10):1027–1029.

64. Krupp P, Timonen O, Gülich A. Side effects and safety of sandimmun in long-term treatment of transplant patients. In: Schindler R, ed. *Cyclosporin in Autoimmune Disease.* Berlin: Springer Verlag; 1985:43–49.

65. Akgül S, Balcı YI, Ünal Ş, Alikaşifoğlu A, Gürgey A. Hypertrichosis: the possible side effect of cyclosporin in an infant with hemophagocytic lymphohistiocytosis receiving HLH-2004 chemotherapy protocol. *Turk J Haematol.* 2009;26(3):154–156.

66. Lei HL, Ku WC, Sun MH, Chen KJ, Lai JY, Sun CC. Cyclosporine a eye drop-induced elongated eyelashes: a case report. *Case Rep Ophthalmol.* 2011;2(3):398–400.

67. Kaur S, Mahajan BB. Eyelash trichomegaly. *Indian J Dermatol*. 2015;60(4):378–380.

68. Mechcatie E. Bimatoprost approved for eyelash lengthening. *Skin Allergy News*. 2009;40:10.

69. Meller S, Gerber PA, Homey B. Clinical image: blonde by prescription. *Arthritis Rheum*. 2008;58:2286.

70. Machado M, Moreb JS, Khan SA. Six cases of permanent alopecia after various conditioning regimens commonly used in hematopoietic stem cell transplantation. *Bone Marrow Transplant*. 2007;40:979.

71. Palamaras I, Misciali C, Vincenzi C, et al. Permanent chemotherapy-induced alopecia: a review. *J Am Acad Dermatol*. 2011;64:604.

72. Miteva M, Misciali C, Fanti PA, Vincenzi C, Romanelli P, Tosti A. Permanent alopecia after systemic chemotherapy: a clinicopathological study of 10 cases. *Am J Dermatopathol*. 2011;33(4):345–350.

73. Tallon B, Blanchard E, Goldberg LJ. Permanent chemotherapy-induced alopecia: case report and review of the literature. *J Am Acad Dermatol*. 2010;63:333.

74. Kluger N, Jacot W, Frouin E, et al. Permanent scalp alopecia related to breast cancer chemotherapy by sequential fluorouracil/epirubicin/cyclophosphamide (FEC) and docetaxel: a prospective study of 20 patients. *Ann Oncol*. 2012;23:2879.

75. de Jonge ME, Mathôt RA, Dalesio O, et al. Relationship between irreversible alopecia and exposure to cyclophosphamide, thiotepa and carboplatin (CTC) in high-dose chemotherapy. *Bone Marrow Transplant*. 2002;30:593.

76. Fonia A, Cota C, Setterfield JF, Goldberg LJ, Fenton DA, Stefanato CM. Permanent alopecia in patients with breast cancer after taxane chemotherapy and adjuvant hormonal therapy: clinicopathologic findings in a cohort of 10 patients. *J Am Acad Dermatol*. 2017;76(5):948–957.

77. Toda N, Fujimoto N, Kato T, et al. Erosive pustular dermatosis of the scalp-like eruption due to gefitinib: case report and review of the literature of alopecia associated with EGFR inhibitors. *Dermatology*. 2012;225:18.

CHAPTER 25

Novel Treatment Modalities for Hair Loss

ARON G. NUSBAUM, MD • SUCHISMITA PAUL, MD

INTRODUCTION

Hair loss is a common complaint in the dermatology practice, with androgenetic alopecia (AGA) being the most common in the daily routine. Currently there are only three Food and Drug Administration–approved treatment options for AGA, including the 5-α reductase inhibitor finasteride, the topical medication minoxidil, and a low-level laser device. However, patients' expectations and interest in new treatment modalities for hair loss has grown exponentially in the last years, especially as we live in times of easy access to an expanding variety of antiaging and beauty preserving cosmetic procedures. In this chapter, we review the current literature about the most common novel treatment options for alopecia, including platelet-rich plasma, microneedling, mesotherapy, low-level laser therapy, and adipose-derived fat stem cell therapy.

PLATELET-RICH PLASMA

Autologous platelet-rich plasma (PRP) has gained increasing notoriety in various aspects of regenerative medicine and as a potential treatment for several etiologies of hair loss. This is performed as an in-office procedure and involves drawing varying volumes of the patient's blood, which is then added to an anticoagulant substance and subsequently centrifuged to separate the platelet-rich fraction. The PRP is injected into the affected areas of the scalp at the level of the follicular bulb in small aliquots, with approximately 5 mm between injection sites. Several preparation kits are commercially available claiming different levels of platelet concentration. Variations in technique include concomitant use of microrollers at the time of injection to both presumably activate the Wnt pathway and promote platelet lysis, addition of pharmacologic activators to the PRP preparation prior to injection, or just injecting the inactivated PRP fraction with the thought that trauma from the injection needle is sufficient to cause platelet activation. The use of local anesthesia as a ring block prior to injection is an option to decrease pain during the procedure.

Possible Mechanism of Action

The therapeutic effect of PRP is presumably mediated by platelet release of growth factors and cytokines such as platelet-derived growth factor (PDGF), transforming growth factor (TGF), vascular endothelial growth factor (VEGF), insulin-like growth factor (IGF), epidermal growth factor, fibroblast growth factor, and interleukin 1. The initial evidence supporting the use of this modality for alopecia stems from the finding that transplanted follicular unit hair grafts submerged in PRP resulted in an increased follicular density of 15% as compared to saline.[1] In addition, in vitro evidence demonstrates that PRP induces the proliferation of dermal papilla cells and upregulation of Wnt pathway components.[2] The use of PRP for hair loss is likewise supported by in vivo animal studies demonstrating a faster telogen to anagen transition in mice injected with PRP,[2] as well as an increase in the number of newly formed follicles and earlier hair formation in grafted murine epidermal and dermal papilla cells exposed to human PRP.[3] These findings have led to a number of clinical trials investigating the potential benefits of PRP as a therapeutic option for alopecia.

Studies

At present, the majority of studies evaluating the effects of PRP in patients with androgenetic alopecia (AGA) suggest some degree of positive effect. When interpreting these results, it is important to note that there are several variations among studies, such as the use and type of control groups, platelet concentration and preparation, study population, methods of localization of treatment sites, and tools for assessment, among others.

The largest trial consisted of a single treatment arm of 64 patients who underwent two sessions of PRP injections separated by a 3-month interval.[4] A microroller was applied to the treatment area immediately before injection of leukocyte-rich PRP with added concentrated plasmacytic proteins (platelet concentration 4× baseline). The addition of plasmacytic proteins and fibrin presumably served to prolong release of platelet-derived growth factors. Patients were evaluated by global photographic assessment, with two evaluators observing a "clinically important difference" in 40.6% and 54.7% of the subjects at 6 months.

In a study of 26 men and women with pattern hair loss, PRP alone was compared with PRP combined with dalteparin and protamine microparticles (PRP-DP) as a carrier for controlled release of growth factors.[5] A PRP concentration of approximately 6× was used and five treatments were administered at 2- to 3-week intervals with evaluation at 12 weeks. Both preparations increased hair shaft diameter, with a greater effect seen in the PRP-DP group. Target areas were localized by landmarks rather than a tattoo, which should be taken into account when interpreting these results.

Alves and Grimalt evaluated the effects of PRP versus placebo in a half-head paired comparison study of 22 patients with AGA (equal numbers of men and women).[6] Three treatments were administered at monthly intervals to two symmetric areas on each side of the scalp with either saline or activated PRP (3× concentration). Phototrichogram assessments of tattooed target areas were obtained at baseline, 3 and 6 months. Compared with baseline, PRP resulted in a significant increase in total hair density and terminal hair density at 6 months, yet only terminal hair density was found to be significantly increased (just below 10%) when PRP was compared with placebo.

In a randomized controlled study of 20 males with AGA, three PRP treatments were performed at 1 month intervals, with assessment of tattooed sites performed via TrichoScan analysis.[7] At 3 months, PRP resulted in a significant improvement in mean hair counts and hair density as compared with both baseline and placebo. In addition, immunohistochemistry revealed an increase in number of follicles as well as Ki67+ basal keratinocytes and hair follicle bulge cells. Of note, PRP and placebo treatment areas varied anatomically based on individual AGA patterns rather than being standardized to left and right symmetric target sites.

Gniki performed a noncontrolled study of 20 patients (18 men and 2 women) treated with three sessions of PRP (5× concentration) injected at 3 week intervals and followed for a total of 1 year.[8] Photomicrographs of treatment sites localized by measured landmarks showed an increased hair density from baseline of 20% at 3 months. The effect, however, was not sustained as at 6 and 12 months, the improvement diminished to 9% and 7%, respectively.

In a series of 10 male patients, Cervelli administered three monthly treatments of PRP (1.5×10^6 concentration) versus saline placebo.[9] Trichoscan evaluation of tattooed treatment sites demonstrated a significant increase in mean hair count and hair density (approximately 20%) at 14 weeks. Histologic evaluation of PRP-treated areas showed an increase in cell proliferation via Ki67 keratinocytes in the epidermis and HF bulge cells, as well as a slight increase in small blood vessels around hair follicles.

Studies failing to demonstrate a therapeutic effect of PRP in AGA include a placebo controlled trial of 26 women treated with PRP (approximately 3× concentration), which showed no difference in hair counts or hair mass index at 26 weeks,[10] and a study of 17 males where PRP showed no effectiveness as compared with saline placebo.[11]

Conclusions and Unmet Goals

1. Larger, well-controlled studies are needed to evaluate PRP as a therapy for not only AGA but also other hair loss conditions, such as telogen effluvium, alopecia areata, and scarring alopecias.
2. Study protocols should standardize the method of PRP preparation as numerous systems are currently available.
3. Another variable to be investigated is whether platelets should be activated or not, and what agent (calcium gluconate, thrombin, etc.) should be used for this purpose.
4. In addition, the optimal volume of PRP per injection, distance between injection sites, proper depth, as well as ideal treatment intervals need to be determined.
5. It should be recognized that PRP may be useful not only as monotherapy but also as an adjunct to other established therapies. PRP may also be optimized by the addition of biologic constituents, such as extracellular matrix or stem cells.

In summary, PRP shows promise as an addition to the current armamentarium for the treatment of alopecia[12] (Fig. 25.1A and B). It is possible that platelet constituents such as cytokines and growth factors, rather than platelets themselves are the active agents needed to achieve efficacy. Following this principle, emerging therapies may consist of preparations containing only purified bioactive molecules.

LOW-LEVEL LASER/LIGHT THERAPY

The ability of laser light to stimulate hair growth in mice as described by Mester in 1967[13] along with more recent reports of paradoxical hair growth in patients undergoing laser hair removal[14] provided a basis for evaluating low-level laser/light therapy (LLLT) as a treatment for alopecia.

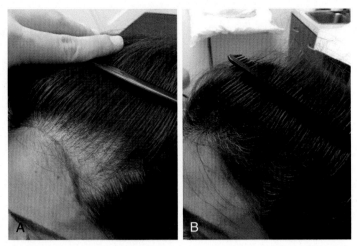

FIG. 25.1 **(A and B)** Significant improvement in a female with androgenetic alopecia at 5 months after treatment with platelet-rich plasma and ACell.

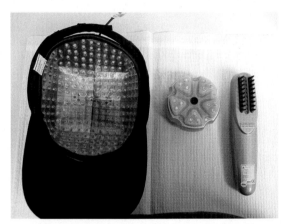

FIG. 25.2 Examples of low-level laser devices for home use. Left to right: Lasercap (Capillus), x5 Hair laser (Spencer Forrest), Hairmax laser comb (Lexington International).

Possible Mechanism of Action

The underlying mechanism of action of LLLT is presumably the absorption of photons by cytochrome oxidase in the mitochondrial respiratory chain, resulting in increased oxygen consumption and ATP production.[15] In addition, it has been shown that LLLT may stimulate hair growth by facilitating a telogen to anagen transition, increasing the duration of anagen, as well as exerting antiinflammatory effects.[16,17] Several devices are available emitting a wavelength of 630–680 nm (Fig. 25.2). Some are available as in-office systems resembling hair salon dryer hoods, yet most patients use in-home devices in the form of specialized combs, caps, helmets, or head bands. Although treatment protocols are empirical, typically treatments are administered every other day for varying durations depending on power of the device. In general, a minimum of 4 months of treatment is necessary prior to determining efficacy.

LLLT has an excellent safety profile with minimal adverse effects. These are limited to temporary telogen effluvium at the initiation of therapy, headache, and heat or burning sensation. It has yet to be determined whether the wavelength emitted from these devices has any therapeutic effect on seborrheic dermatitis or scalp psoriasis, yet they offer a therapeutic alternative for patients with these conditions in whom topical applications may be irritating.

Studies

The Hairmax laser comb (Lexington International) received FDA 510K clearance in 2005 and was evaluated by Leavitt in 2009 in a sham-controlled study of 110 male patients with AGA.[18] A 9-laser 655 nm device was administered three times per week for 26 weeks and resulted in a significant increase in mean terminal hair density as compared with control. The Hairmax was also used by Jimenez in a study of 269 patients (128 men, 141 women) treated three times per week for 26 weeks.[19] Treatment with devices containing 7, 9, or 12 lasers all resulted in an equivalent significant increase in terminal hair density as compared with a sham control.

Kim evaluated 40 patients with AGA (26 men, 14 women) using a helmet-type device containing various LEDs emitting between 630 and 650 nm versus a sham control.[20] Treatment was administered daily for 6 months. Hair density and mean hair diameter were significantly increased as compared with control.

In two separate sham-controlled studies,[21,22] Lanza-fame assessed the effects of a helmet-type device with both 655 nm LEDs and laser diodes used every other day for 4 months. In 44 men and 47 women with AGA, increases in hair counts of 35% and 37% were achieved, respectively.

Conclusions

As with all other treatments for AGA, results achieved with LLLT vary greatly among individuals. Although this modality has not been studied as concomitant therapy, it is possible that it may have additive or synergistic effects when used in combination with other approved treatments for AGA. In addition, further well-controlled studies are needed to determine the optimal frequency, power, and treatment times for treating AGA with LLLT.

MESOTHERAPY

Mesotherapy entails the use of superficial injections of pharmaceuticals and vitamin compounds into the scalp with agents that presumably have efficacy to treat AGA via the oral or topical route.

Possible Mechanism of Action

The rationale for its use is based on delivery of therapeutic agents directly to the level of the hair follicle, avoiding both the systemic side effects of oral administration as well as the reduced compliance encountered with daily topical applications.

Although there are no established treatment protocols, typically weekly injections are administered initially, followed by longer intervals so that maintenance treatments may be performed as infrequently as every 2–3 months. Multiple, small volume injections (0.02–0.05 mL) are equally spaced approximately 5 mm apart to cover the involved alopecic area (Fig. 25.3). Compounds used include minoxidil, finasteride, dutasteride, biotin, tretinoin, pantothenic acid, pyridoxine, procaine, and other vitamins and minerals. Although there is a paucity of data on the use of mesotherapy for hair loss, the majority of the studies in the literature evaluated dutasteride for this purpose.

Studies

In a study of 90 men with AGA, injections with dutasteride 0.005% (D), dutasteride 0.005% + D-panthenol + biotin + pyridoxine (D+), or saline control were administered over 5 months.[23] Only in the D+ treated group was there a statistically significant increase in

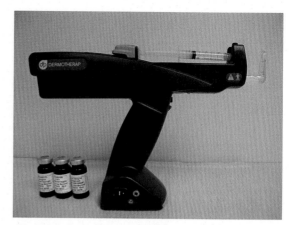

FIG. 25.3 Power injector to enhance ergonomics of mesotherapy. These devices provide depth control as well as metered injections.

anagen hair and anagen-telogen ratio. Both the D and D+-treated groups showed a significant increase in hair shaft diameter as compared with baseline. Interestingly, no changes in sperm parameters were observed in the study, as this is a known concern with orally administered dutasteride, especially in the younger male population.

In regard to the treatment of female AGA, 126 women were treated with either a combination of dutasteride + D-panthenol + biotin + pyridoxine or saline over 4 months.[24] Photographic improvement was seen in 63% of patients treated with dutasteride + additives as compared with 17.5% with control. Minimal side effects were reported.

Conclusions and Caveats

In general, mesotherapy for alopecia is well tolerated, although pain during injections and mild headache for about 24 h posttreatment frequently occur.[24] Scalp abscesses and subsequent fat necrosis were reported in one patient after injections of a "vitamin" cocktail, and cases of patchy alopecia have occurred after injections with dutasteride combinations, homeopathic agents, and mesoglycan.[25,26] Although in some patients the alopecia resolved, in others, permanent scarring alopecia ensued.

MICRONEEDLING

Microneedling is a minimally invasive procedure in which small channels are created through the epidermis using fine needles. The most commonly used devices include manual rollers and automated electrical

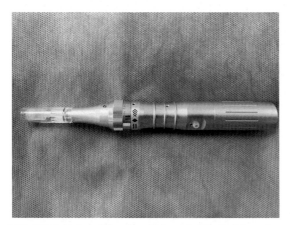

FIG. 25.4 Eclipse MicroPen (Eclipse Aesthetics) for automated microneedling.

micropens (Fig. 25.4). Although this modality is often used for enhanced topical drug delivery, microwounds themselves induce tissue remodeling and the wound healing cascade that is shown to be beneficial in a number of dermatologic conditions.

Possible Mechanism of Action

Microneedling appears to be a novel, safe, and effective treatment modality for alopecia, and it has been shown to induce hair growth by various mechanisms.[27,28] Microneedling causes stimulation of the dermal papilla and activation of stem cells in the hair follicle bulge area. It also increases blood supply to the hair follicles. In mice, Kim et al. demonstrated that repeated microneedle stimulation promotes hair growth via overexpression of hair growth–related genes, such as VEGF, B catenin, Wnt3a, and Wnt10b.[28] Microneedling also causes increased release of PDGF and epidermal growth factors through platelet activation and the skin wound regeneration mechanism.

Studies

The first human study to demonstrate the success of microneedling as a treatment modality for AGA was published in 2013 by Dhurat et al.[29] One hundred patients were treated with 5% minoxidil lotion twice daily with or without weekly microneedling using a dermaroller. At 12 weeks, treatment with minoxidil and microneedling resulted in a statistically significant improvement in hair counts, global photography, and patient assessment of hair growth as compared with the minoxidil-only control group.

Dhurat et al. also reported new hair follicle formation with microneedling in four patients with AGA

who had previously shown stabilization of their hair loss but no regrowth after 2–5 years of minoxidil and finasteride therapy.[30] This study also included a modified microneedling protocol to reduce frequent patient visits. The patients were initially treated with microneedling weekly for four sessions and then every 2 weeks for a subsequent 11 sessions over 6 months while they continued treatment with minoxidil and finasteride. New hairs were noticed after 3 months of initiation of microneedling treatment, and significant scalp coverage was noticed after 6 months. Three patients reported more than 75% improvement and one patient reported more than 50% improvement based on patients' subjective hair growth assessment scale. Results were sustainable during the 18-month follow-up period.

As discussed earlier, microneedling with PRP has also been shown to be safe and effective for the management of AGA.[4,31] In two cases of resistant alopecia areata, Chandrashekar et al. demonstrated successful treatment using microneedling with a dermaroller consisting of 192 needles of 1.5 mm length each, followed by topical application of triamcinolone acetonide at 3 week intervals for a total of three sessions.[32]

Conclusions

Although microneedling appears to be a promising treatment modality for alopecia, it is important to note that only a limited number of studies exist. Further well-controlled clinical trials are needed to investigate the efficacy of microneedling for alopecia, as well as to optimize needle size, treatment frequency, and duration.

ADIPOSE-DERIVED STEM CELL THERAPY

In most studies involving mesenchymal stem cells, they are derived from the bone marrow; however, mesenchymal stem cells can also be found in adipose tissues. Adipose-derived stem cells (ADSCs) are adult stem cells isolated from fat tissues during procedures such as liposuction, abdominoplasty, or breast reduction and can be used to promote skin and hair growth.

Possible Mechanism of Action

ADSCs are a promising treatment modality in cosmetic dermatology, especially in skin aging, based on their ability to produce several growth factors, such as VEGF, hepatocyte growth factor, basic fibroblast growth factor, PDGF, keratinocyte growth factor, TGF-β1, IGF-binding protein precursors, fibronectin, and superoxide dismutase.[33] Recent studies have supported the use of ADSCs to promote hair growth via secretion of several of the growth factors mentioned earlier.[34,35] In addition, several studies have demonstrated that ADSC-conditioned medium, when harvested under hypoxic conditions, contains these growth factors and can also be used to stimulate hair growth.[36] Adipose-derived stem cell protein extract is a commercially available form of this conditioned media developed by Prostemics Co, Ltd (Seoul, Korea).

Studies

In a study by Fukuoka et al., ADSC-derived proteins injected by mesotherapy techniques led to successful hair growth in 12 women and 13 men with alopecia evaluated by a visual analog scale.[37] ADSC-conditioned media was harvested under hypoxic conditions and combined with buflomedil, cysteine, coenzyme Q10, and vitamins and then the protein solution was applied during four treatment sessions performed within 3–4 months.

Fukuoka et al. further demonstrated the successful use of adipose-derived stem cell–conditioned medium in 11 men and 11 women with AGA.[38] ADSC-conditioned medium was intradermally injected every 3–5 weeks for a total of six sessions and resulted in a significant increase in hair numbers based on trichograms. Increased hair density and thickness has also been demonstrated after treatment with ADSC-conditioned media in a study of female pattern hair loss.[39]

Anderi et al. reported successful hair regrowth with transplantation of autologous ADSCs in a clinical trial involving 20 patients.[40] Patients were treated with autologous ADSCs (instead of ADSC conditioned media), and 6 months later, there was an increase in hair diameter, improvement of hair density, and decrease in hair pull test. This study confirmed that this treatment modality for alopecia was safe and effective. The proposed mechanism through which ADSCs are effective for the treatment of alopecia includes not only release of growth factors but also vascularization and improved blood supply to the scalp.

Aside from ADSCs, recent studies have also shown that *autologous bone marrow–derived mononuclear cells* are safe, tolerable, and effective for the treatment of alopecia areata and AGA.[41] In an open label, phase 1/phase 2 study by Li et al., stem cell educator therapy was used in nine patients with severe alopecia areata and clinical data suggested improved hair regrowth and quality of life.[42] This method involves separation of mononuclear cells from the whole blood from patients and allows the cells to briefly interact with adherent human cord blood–derived multipotent stem cells. The "educated" autologous stem cells are then returned to the patient's circulation.

Conclusions

The most common adverse effect of ADSC treatment includes pain that can be avoided with local anesthetics. Contraindications for ADSC include local skin inflammation or infection, autoimmune disease, pregnancy, cancer, and current anticoagulant therapy.[38] Based on recent studies, ADSCs appear to be safe and tolerable for the treatment of alopecia; however, further studies are needed to confirm the long-term effects of this modality.

REFERENCES

1. Uebel CO, da Silva JB, Cantarelli D, Martins P. The role of platelet plasma growth factors in male pattern baldness surgery. *Plast Reconstr Surg.* 2006;118(6):1458–1466; discussion 1467.
2. Li ZJ, Choi HI, Choi DK, et al. Autologous platelet-rich plasma: a potential therapeutic tool for promoting hair growth. *Dermatol Surg.* 2012;38(7 Pt 1):1040–1046.
3. Miao Y, Sun YB, Sun XJ, Du BJ, Jiang JD, Hu ZQ. Promotional effect of platelet-rich plasma on hair follicle reconstitution in vivo. *Dermatol Surg.* 2013;39(12):1868–1876.
4. Schiavone G, Raskovic D, Greco J, Abeni D. Platelet-rich plasma for androgenetic alopecia: a pilot study. *Dermatol Surg.* 2014;40(9):1010–1019.
5. Takikawa M, Nakamura S, Nakamura S, et al. Enhanced effect of platelet-rich plasma containing a new carrier on hair growth. *Dermatol Surg.* 2011;37(12):1721–1729.
6. Alves R, Grimalt R. A randomized placebo-controlled, double-blind, half-head study to assess the efficacy of platelet-rich plasma on the treatment of androgenetic alopecia. *Dermatol Surg.* 2016.
7. Gentile P, Garcovich S, Bielli A, Scioli MG, Orlandi A, Cervelli V. The effect of platelet-rich plasma in hair regrowth: a randomized placebo-controlled trial. *Stem Cells Transl Med.* 2015;4(11):1317–1323.
8. Gkini MA, Kouskoukis AE, Tripsianis G, Rigopoulos D, Kouskoukis K. Study of platelet-rich plasma injections in the treatment of androgenetic alopecia through an one-year period. *J Cutan Aesthet Surg.* 2014;7(4):213–219.
9. Cervelli V, Garcovich S, Bielli A, et al. The effect of autologous activated platelet rich plasma (AA-PRP) injection on pattern hair loss: clinical and histomorphometric evaluation. *Biomed Res Int.* 2014;2014:760709.
10. Puig CJ, Reese R, Peters M. Double-Blind, placebo-controlled pilot study on the use of platelet-rich plasma in women with female androgenetic alopecia. *Dermatol Surg.* 2016;42(11):1243–1247.
11. Mapar MA, Shahriari S, Haghighizadeh MH. Efficacy of platelet-rich plasma in the treatment of androgenetic (male-patterned) alopecia: a pilot randomized controlled trial. *J Cosmet Laser Ther.* 2016;18(8):452–455.
12. Valente Duarte de Sousa IC, Tosti A. New investigational drugs for androgenetic alopecia. *Expert Opin Investig Drugs.* 2013;22(5):573–589.

13. Mester E. Effect of laser on hair growth in mice. *Kiserl Orvostud*. 1967;19:628–631.
14. Bernstein EF. Hair growth induced by diode laser treatment. *Dermatol Surg Off Publ Am Soc Dermatol Surg*. 2005;31(5):584–586.
15. Farjo N. An interview with professor Michael Hamblin. *Hair Transpl Forum Int*. 2010;20(3):83.
16. Wikramanayake TC, Rodriguez R, Choudhary S, et al. Effects of the Lexington LaserComb on hair regrowth in the C3H/HeJ mouse model of alopecia areata. *Lasers Med Sci*. 2012;27(2):431–436.
17. Mafra de Lima F, Villaverde AB, Salgado MA, et al. Low intensity laser therapy (LILT) in vivo acts on the neutrophils recruitment and chemokines/cytokines levels in a model of acute pulmonary inflammation induced by aerosol of lipopolysaccharide from *Escherichia coli* in rat. *J Photochem Photobiol B*. 2010;101(3):271–278.
18. Leavitt M, Charles G, Heyman E, Michaels D. HairMax LaserComb laser phototherapy device in the treatment of male androgenetic alopecia: a randomized, double-blind, sham device-controlled, multicentre trial. *Clin Drug Investig*. 2009;29(5):283–292.
19. Jimenez JJ, Wikramanayake TC, Bergfeld W, et al. Efficacy and safety of a low-level laser device in the treatment of male and female pattern hair loss: a multicenter, randomized, sham device-controlled, double-blind study. *Am J Clin Dermatol*. 2014;15(2):115–127.
20. Kim H, Choi JW, Kim JY, Shin JW, Lee SJ, Huh CH. Low-level light therapy for androgenetic alopecia: a 24-week, randomized, double-blind, sham device-controlled multicenter trial. *Dermatol Surg*. 2013;39(8):1177–1183.
21. Lanzafame RJ, Blanche RR, Bodian AB, Chiacchierini RP, Fernandez-Obregon A, Kazmirek ER. The growth of human scalp hair mediated by visible red light laser and LED sources in males. *Lasers Surg Med*. 2013;45(8):487–495.
22. Lanzafame RJ, Blanche RR, Chiacchierini RP, Kazmirek ER, Sklar JA. The growth of human scalp hair in females using visible red light laser and LED sources. *Lasers Surg Med*. 2014;46(8):601–607.
23. Sobhy N, Aly H, El Shafee A, El Deeb M. Evaluation of the effect of injection of dutasteride as mesotherapeutic tool in treatment of androgenetic alopecia in males. *Our Dermatol Online*. 2013;4(1):40–45.
24. Moftah N, Abd-Elaziz G, Ahmed N, Hamed Y, Ghannam B, Ibrahim M. Mesotherapy using dutasteride-containing preparation in treatment of female pattern hair loss: photographic, morphometric and ultrastructural evaluation. *J Eur Acad Dermatol Venereol JEADV*. 2012.
25. Duque-Estrada B, Vincenzi C, Misciali C, Tosti A. Alopecia secondary to mesotherapy. *J Am Acad Dermatol*. 2009;61(4):707–709.
26. El-Komy M, Hassan A, Tawdy A, Solimon M, Hady MA. Hair loss at injection sites of mesotherapy for alopecia. *J Cosmet Dermatol*. 2017.
27. Jeong K, Lee Y, Kim J, Park Y, Kim B, Kang H. Repeated microneedle stimulation induce the enhanced expression of hair-growth-related genes. *Int J Trichol*. 2012;4:117.
28. Kim YS, Jeong KH, Kim JE, Woo YJ, Kim BJ, Kang H. Repeated microneedle stimulation induces enhanced hair growth in a murine model. *Ann Dermatol*. 2016;28(5):586–592.
29. Dhurat R, Sukesh M, Avhad G, Dandale A, Pal A, Pund P. A randomized evaluator blinded study of effect of microneedling in androgenetic alopecia: a pilot study. *Int J Trichol*. 2013;5(1):6–11.
30. Dhurat R, Mathapati S. Response to microneedling treatment in men with androgenetic alopecia who failed to respond to conventional therapy. *Indian J Dermatol*. 2015;60(3):260–263.
31. Shah KB, Shah AN, Solanki RB, Raval RC. A comparative study of microneedling with platelet-rich plasma plus topical minoxidil (5%) and topical minoxidil (5%) alone in androgenetic alopecia. *Int J Trichol*. 2017;9(1):14–18.
32. Chandrashekar B, Yepuri V, Mysore V. Alopecia areata-successful outcome with microneedling and triamcinolone acetonide. *J Cutan Aesthet Surg*. 2014;7(1):63–64.
33. Park BS, Jang KA, Sung JH, et al. Adipose-derived stem cells and their secretory factors as a promising therapy for skin aging. *Dermatol Surg*. 2008;34(10):1323–1326.
34. Won CH, Yoo HG, Kwon OS, et al. Hair growth promoting effects of adipose tissue-derived stem cells. *J Dermatol Sci*. 2010;57(2):134–137.
35. Festa E, Fretz J, Berry R, et al. Adipocyte lineage cells contribute to the skin stem cell niche to drive hair cycling. *Cell*. 2011;146(5):761–771.
36. Fukuoka H, Narita K, Suga H. Hair regeneration therapy using proteins secreted by adipose-derived stem cells. *Curr Stem Cell Res Ther*. 2017.
37. Fukuoka H, Suga H. Hair regeneration treatment using stem cell conditioned medium. *Am J Cosmet Surg*. 2012;29:273–282.
38. Fukuoka H, Suga H. Hair regeneration treatment using adipose-derived stem cell conditioned medium: follow-up with trichograms. *Eplasty*. 2015;15:e10.
39. Shin H, Ryu HH, Kwon O, Park BS, Jo SJ. Clinical use of conditioned media of adipose tissue-derived stem cells in female pattern hair loss: a retrospective case series study. *Int J Dermatol*. 2015;54(6):730–735.
40. Anderi R, Makdissy N, Rizk F, Hamade A. Hair quality improvement in alopecia patients following adipose-derived stem cell treatment. *JPRAS*. 2017.
41. Ibrahim ZA, Elmaadawi IH, Mohamed BM, et al. Stem cell therapy as a novel therapeutic intervention for resistant cases of alopecia areata and androgenetic alopecia. *J Dermatol Treat*. 2016:1–30.
42. Li Y, Yan B, Wang H, et al. Hair regrowth in alopecia areata patients following Stem Cell Educator therapy. *BMC Med*. 2015;13:87.

CHAPTER 26

Clinical Trials and Hair Loss

JOSE A. JALLER, MD • FLOR MACQUHAE, MD • ANNA J. NICHOLS, MD, PHD

BURDEN OF DISEASE IN ALOPECIA

Hair loss is a common and distressing condition. More than 150 trials are currently being conducted to understand alopecia and develop better treatments. According to the American Hair Loss Association, by the age of 35, two-thirds of American men will have some degree of appreciable hair loss, and by the age of 50, approximately 85% of men will have significant hair thinning.[1] Some studies have estimated the prevalence of female pattern hair loss to be 6% in women less than 50 years of age and 38% in those more than 70; however, other studies have shown a prevalence as high as 32% in women more than 20 years of age.[2,3] The global alopecia market was valued at over $7.3 billion United States dollars (USD) in 2015, with almost USD 2.5 billion spent in the United States alone.[4] The surgical hair restoration worldwide market has been estimated to be nearly USD 2.5 billion in 2014, and more than 1 million patients sought either surgical or nonsurgical treatments in that same year.[5]

Hair is an essential aspect of human appearance and can have a significant impact on a person's perceived attractiveness and self-esteem.[6] Many people who experience hair loss will experience some degree of psychosocial impact. As an example, most patients suffering hair loss following chemotherapy have reported that hair loss is the most traumatic side effect associated with chemotherapy.[7] In a telephone survey with 1536 randomly chosen 18- to 45-year-old male participants, 47% reported hair loss, 70% reported hair to be an important part of personal attractiveness, and 62% believed that hair loss could affect self-esteem. In the survey, 21% of participants who reported hair loss acknowledged feelings of depression.[8] These data serve to highlight the importance of developing better treatments for hair loss disorders.

Hair loss disorders comprise an extensive group of conditions that can be classified as scarring and nonscarring alopecia. Primary scarring alopecia is caused by inflammatory diseases of the scalp that lead to the destruction of pilosebaceous structures and replacement of the pilosebaceous structures with scar tissue, leading to irreversible hair loss. Primary scarring alopecias directly affect the hair follicles, whereas secondary scarring alopecias target the dermis and consequently destroy the follicles.[9] Lichen planopilaris (LPP), central centrifugal cicatricial alopecia (CCCA), discoid lupus erythematosus, and folliculitis decalvans are associated with irreversible scarring alopecia. Nonscarring alopecias include some of the most common types of hair loss disorders and are characterized by minimal or absent inflammation. In contrast to scarring alopecia, in nonscarring alopecia, there is no destruction of the hair follicles. Therefore, some degree of hair regrowth is expected after the condition has been stabilized. Androgenetic alopecia, telogen effluvium, trichotillomania, alopecia areata, early stages of traction alopecia, and tinea capitis are included among others in this group.[10]

Because multiple factors play a role in the pathophysiology of hair loss, management of these conditions can be very complex. Therapeutic targets can be divided into four groups: therapies that increase blood flow to dermal papillae, treatments that reduce inflammation, therapies that modulate hormonal balance, and surgical or procedural interventions. Despite the large size of the global market and high demand for effective therapies, at this time very little high-quality evidence supports the effectiveness of the available treatments (Table 26.1). Well-designed clinical trials are urgently needed to establish the actual efficacy of currently available therapies and those novel therapies that are on the horizon.

DRUGS

The U.S. Food and Drug Administration (FDA) defines a drug as a substance, other than food or device, intended to affect structure or function in a human or animal. A variety of drugs are used to treat the different types of alopecia. Despite the high prevalence of hair loss and its social and economic impact, only androgenetic alopecia has FDA-approved drugs for its management: minoxidil for women and minoxidil and finasteride for men. At this point, all other therapies used for the various types of alopecia are used off-label. This fact

TABLE 26.1
Level of Evidence of Therapies Commonly Used in Nonscarring (Light Gray) and Scarring (Dark Gray) Alopecia

AGA	AA	CTE	Traction
Minoxidil—A	Minoxidil—A	Minoxidil—B	Minoxidil—E
Low-level laser therapy—A	Topical/IL steroids—A		
Platelet-rich plasma—A	Platelet-rich plasma—A		
Finasteride/dutasteride—A	Topical immunotherapy—A		
Fractional laser—D	Excimer laser—C		
Spironolactone—D	Pulsed infrared diode laser—C		
	Methotrexate—D		
	Tofacitinib—D		
	Apremilast—E		
	Ruxolitinib—E		
	Fractional laser—E		

LPP	CCCA	Dissecting Cellulitis	Folliculitis Decalvans
Hydroxychloroquine—B	Topical/IL steroids—D	Oral antibiotics—D	Oral antibiotics—D
Dutasteride—B (for FFA)		Isotretinoin—D	Isotretinoin—D
Topical/IL steroids—C		Pulsed diode laser—E	Photodynamic therapy—D
Minoxidil—E		Topical/IL steroids—E	Topical/IL steroids—E
Low-level laser therapy—E		Radiation therapy—E	Long pulsed laser—E
Cyclosporine—E		Adalimumab—E	Radiation therapy—E
Mycophenolate mofetil—E		Infliximab—E	Adalimumab—E
		Zinc—E	Infliximab—E
		Compression therapy—E	Fusidic acid + zinc—E

AA, alopecia areata; *AGA,* androgenetic alopecia; *CCCA,* central centrifugal cicatricial alopecia; *CTE,* chronic telogen effluvium; *FFA,* frontal fibrosing alopecia; *IL,* intralesional; *LPP,* lichen planopilaris.
Evidence Levels: A, double-blind study; B, clinical trial ≥ 20 subjects; C, clinical trial < 20 subjects; D, series ≥ 5 subjects; E, anecdotal case reports.

highlights the unmet need for well-designed clinical trials for hair loss disorders that would ultimately lead to approved therapies.

Vasodilator: Minoxidil

Minoxidil is a potassium channel opener that hyperpolarizes cell membranes, causing vascular muscle dilation and a consequent increase in blood flow. It is approved for both men and women for the treatment of androgenetic alopecia as a topical solution and topical foam. It has also been used as an adjuvant therapy in other forms of alopecia. Table 26.2 summarizes the most representative clinical trials examining minoxidil for androgenetic

alopecia. The discovery and approval process of this medication is reviewed in the section *Androgenetic Alopecia: An Illustrative Example* later in this chapter.

5α-Reductase Inhibitors: Finasteride and Dutasteride

Finasteride and dutasteride are 5α-reductase (5AR) inhibitors that block the conversion of testosterone to dihydrotestosterone. Finasteride is a type 2 5AR inhibitor, whereas dutasteride is both a type 1 and type 2 5AR inhibitor. Type 2 AR is found mainly in male genitalia and hair follicles, and type 1 AR is primarily located in the skin, hair follicles, and sebaceous

TABLE 26.2
Clinical Trials of Minoxidil for Androgenetic Alopecia

References	Intervention(s)	Primary Outcome	Secondary Outcome(s)	Improvement From Baseline	# Subjects
Kreindler[11]	Arm 1: 2% minoxidil solution Arm 2: 3% minoxidil solution Arm 3: placebo, then 3% minoxidil	Nonvellus hair count	Vellus hair count, total hair count, subjective evaluation by investigator, hair growth rate	Not enough information	150 (males)
Rietschel and Duncan[12]	Arm 1: 2% minoxidil solution Arm 2: 3% minoxidil solution Arm 3: placebo then 3% minoxidil	Hair count	Change from baseline, terminal hair count	38.74% 49.34% 36.46%	149 (not provided)
Jacobs et al.[13]	Arm 1: 2% minoxidil solution Arm 2: placebo	Change from baseline of nonvellus TAHC	Subjective visible new hair growth by investigator and patient. Subjective degree of hair shedding	24.21% 13.66%	346 (females)
DeVillez et al.[14]	Arm 1: 2% minoxidil solution Arm 2: placebo	Nonvellus hair count	Subjective visible new hair growth by investigator and patient. Subjective degree of hair shedding	16.16% 7.28%	308 (females)
Price et al.[15]	Arm 1: 5% minoxidil solution Arm 2: 2% minoxidil solution Arm 3: placebo Arm 4: no intervention	Mean percentage change in hair weight	Mean percentage change in hair count	Not enough information	33 (males)
Olsen et al.[16]	Arm 1: 5% minoxidil solution Arm 2: 2% minoxidil solution Arm 3: placebo	Nonvellus hair count	Patient and investigator assessments of hair growth using questionnaire	Not enough information	393 (males)
Vexiau et al.[17]	Arm 1: 2% minoxidil solution Arm 2: cyproterone	Change in number of hairs >40 μm in diameter	Total number of hairs, number of hairs in anagen, number of hairs in telogen	9.1% Not enough information	66 (females)
Berger et al.[18]	Arm 1: 1% pyrithione zinc shampoo Arm 2: 5% minoxidil solution+placebo shampoo	Significant total hair count increase	Hair diameter, patient and investigator global assessment of hair growth	Not enough information	200 (males)

Continued

TABLE 26.2
Clinical Trials of Minoxidil for Androgenetic Alopecia—cont'd

References	Intervention(s)	Primary Outcome	Secondary Outcome(s)	Improvement From Baseline	# Subjects
Lucky et al.[19]	Arm 1: 5% minoxidil solution Arm 2: 2% minoxidil solution Arm 3: placebo shampoo Arm 4: 1% pyrithione zinc shampoo + 5% minoxidil solution	Change from baseline nonvellus hair count	Patient and investigator assessment of hair growth/scalp coverage	Not enough information	381 (females)
Olsen et al.[20]	Arm 1: 5% minoxidil foam Arm 2: placebo	Change from baseline on vertex TAHC	Subject assessment of improvement of hair growth using a questionnaire, global photographic review	13.40% 3.40%	352 (males)
Tsuboi et al.[21]	Arm 1: 1% minoxidil solution Arm 2: placebo	Mean change of nonvellus hair from baseline	Investigator and patient assessment	Not enough information	280 (females)
Tsuboi et al.[22]	Arm 1: 5% minoxidil solution Arm 2: 1% minoxidil solution	Nonvellus hair count	Investigator (dermatologist) photograph evaluation with 5-point scale, patient self-assessment with 5-point scale	20.30% 16.18%	300 (males)
Blume-Peytavi et al.[23]	Arm 1: 5% minoxidil foam Arm 2: 2% minoxidil solution	Change from baseline of nonvellus TAHC	TAHW, global photographic review	16.20% 13.80%	113 (females)
Hillmann et al.[24]	Arm 1: 5% minoxidil foam Arm 2: placebo	Change from baseline frontotemporal TAHC	Change from baseline vertex TAHC, frontotemporal and vertex TAHW change, global expert panel and subjective rating of scalp coverage	4.20% 1.06%	70 (males)
Hu et al.[25]	Arm 1: oral finasteride Arm 2: 5% minoxidil solution Arm 3: oral finasteride + 5% minoxidil solution	Hair growth	None	Not enough information	428 (males)

TAHC, target area hair count; *TAHW*, target area hair width.

glands.[26] These two medications are used in androgenetic alopecia, either as monotherapy or as combination therapy with minoxidil.[27] However, only finasteride 1 mg daily is approved by the FDA for men with androgenetic alopecia. Recent studies have suggested that 5AR inhibitors may be beneficial in frontal fibrosing alopecia.[28] Table 26.3 includes some of the pivotal clinical trials that have led to the approval of this class of medications.

Immunomodulators

Corticosteroids, either topical, intralesional, or systemic, are frequently used in conditions where excessive inflammation is the primary cause of hair loss. They have proven efficacy in the treatment of alopecia areata in multiple randomized controlled trials (RCTs).[39] Their use in less common conditions such as LPP and CCCA has been reported in case series.[40,41]

TABLE 26.3
Clinical Trials of Finasteride or Dutasteride for Androgenetic Alopecia

References	Intervention	Primary Outcome	Secondary Outcome(s)	Improvement From Baseline	Subjects (#)
Kaufman et al.[29]	Arm 1: finasteride 1 mg	Hair count and patient self-assessment	Investigator assessment and global photographic assessment	11%	1553 (males)
	Arm 2: placebo			−2.70%	
Leyden et al.[30]	Arm 1: finasteride 1 mg	Hair counts in target area scanned with macrophotography	Patient, investigator and global assessment	9.60%	326 (males)
	Arm 2: placebo			−2.00%	
Roberts et al.[31]	Pilot. Arm 1: finasteride 5 mg	Change from baseline, hair count in target area	Patient, investigator, and global assessment	11%	693 (males)
	Pilot. Arm 2: placebo			−2%	
	Dose range. Arm 1: finasteride 1 mg			9%	
	Dose range. Arm 2: finasteride 0.2 mg			7%	
	Dose range. Arm 3: finasteride 0.01 mg			−2%	
	Dose range. Arm 4: placebo			Not available	
Price et al.[32]	Arm 1: finasteride 1 mg	Hair counts in target area scanned with macrophotography	Patient, investigator, and global assessment	−5.76%	137 (females)
	Arm 2: placebo			−4%	
Van Neste et al.[33]	Arm 1: finasteride 1 mg	Total and anagen hair counts in target area scanned with macrophotography	Not available	Total: 3.7%. Anagen: 14.54%	212 (males)
	Arm 2: placebo			Total: −4.9%. Anagen: −7.39%	
Price et al.[34]	Arm 1: finasteride 1 mg	Target area hair weight	Target area hair count, laboratory measurements	20.40%	66 (males)
	Arm 2: placebo			−5.20%	

Continued

TABLE 26.3
Clinical Trials of Finasteride or Dutasteride for Androgenetic Alopecia—cont'd

References	Intervention	Primary Outcome	Secondary Outcome(s)	Improvement From Baseline	Subjects (#)
Olsen et al.[35]	Arm 1: dutasteride 0.05 mg	Change from baseline of hair count in target area determined by macrophotography	Exploratory assessment of hair count. Panel, investigator, and subject assessment. Stage of male pattern hair loss using the modified Hamilton-Norwood classification	Not available	416 (males)
	Arm 2: dutasteride 0.1 mg			8.64%	
	Arm 3: dutasteride 0.5 mg			10.19%	
	Arm 4: dutasteride 2.5 mg			11.28%	
	Arm 5: finasteride 5 mg			8.38%	
	Arm 6: placebo			−3.50%	
Price et al.[36]	Arm 1: finasteride 1 mg	Target area hair weight after three study extensions (4 years in total)	Target area hair count, laboratory measurements	21.60%	22 (males)
	Arm 2: placebo			−24.50%	
Eun et al.[37]	Arm 1: dutasteride 0.5 mg	Hair count using macrophotographic phototrichogram on vertex at 6 months	Hair count at 3 months. Subject and investigator hair growth assessment	8.23%	153 (males)
	Arm 2: placebo			3.25%	
Olsen et al.[38]	Trial 1. Arm 1: finasteride 1 mg	Global photographic assessment of vertex	Global photographic assessment of anterior/mid, frontal, and temporal scalp regions	Not available	1977 (males)
	Trial 1. Arm 2: placebo				
	Trial 2. Arm 1: finasteride 1 mg				
	Trial 2. Arm 2: placebo				
Gubelin Harcha et al.[26]	Arm 1: dutasteride 0.02 mg	Change from baseline in target area hair count in the vertex at 24 weeks using macrophotography	Change from baseline of hair width and terminal hair. Panel global assessment, investigator assessment, and change in androgenetic alopecia stage according to Norwood-Hamilton scale	Not available	917 (males)
	Arm 2: dutasteride 0.1 mg				
	Arm 3: dutasteride 0.5 mg				
	Arm 4: finasteride 1 mg				
	Arm 5: placebo				
Hu et al.[25]	Arm 1: oral finasteride	Global photographic evaluation	None	Not available	428 (males)
	Arm 2: 5% minoxidil Solution				
	Arm 3: oral finasteride and 5% minoxidil solution				

Other immunomodulators such as methotrexate, tofacitinib, and ruxolitinib have resulted in hair growth in alopecia areata in some cohort studies and case reports. However, future controlled studies are necessary to confirm these initial findings.[42–47]

Diuretics/Antiandrogen Therapies

Spironolactone is a potassium-sparing diuretic that has been used to treat androgenetic alopecia because of its antiandrogenic effect: It reduces adrenal androgen production and inhibits free testosterone from binding to the androgen receptors. Despite having a mechanism of action that should be effective in theory and reports of effectiveness in a retrospective analysis of 19 patients,[48] spironolactone showed no benefit in females with androgenetic alopecia compared with baseline in the only clinical trial conducted with this medication to date.[49]

Prostaglandin Agonists

Latanoprost and bimatoprost are prostaglandin agonists that have been studied only minimally for the treatment of androgenetic alopecia and alopecia areata. Latanoprost resulted in increased hair growth in androgenetic alopecia compared with placebo in one RCT, but the sample size was small.[50] Results in alopecia areata have been contradictory, with one study concluding no significant difference compared with placebo and another study demonstrating significant hair growth compared with baseline.[51,52]

DEVICES

The FDA uses the term device to denote an instrument, apparatus, implement, machine, contrivance, implant, in vitro reagent, or other similar or related article intended for use in the diagnosis, cure, mitigation, treatment, or prevention of disease. Most results are based on case reports and case series; however, some devices have undergone more rigorous testing in clinical studies.

Microneedling is a procedure that consists of the use of fine needles to create hundreds of small puncture wounds in the skin. The purported mechanisms for hair growth include stimulation of wound regeneration mechanisms activated by microinjury, release of multiple growth factors through platelet activation, and enhanced drug absorption. One RCT of microneedling combined with minoxidil compared with minoxidil alone showed a significant increase in hair counts in the microneedling plus minoxidil group. Microneedling combined with minoxidil also resulted in significantly increased hair counts compared with baseline

hair counts in patients with AGA.[53] This procedure, combined with topical steroids, has been reported to result in significant hair growth in alopecia areata in two patients in India, where a high dose of triamcinolone (10 mg/mL) was applied topically before and immediately after the microneedling procedure.[54]

The excimer laser is a device that emits a 308-nm ultraviolet wavelength light that induces apoptosis, hence its potential efficacy in cutaneous inflammatory conditions. It has shown positive results in alopecia areata, in both adults and children, although only reported in case series.[55,56] It was also reported to be beneficial in 10 patients with LPP.[57] RCTs are necessary to confirm these promising initial observations.

Low-level laser light therapy is another technology that delivers light through different types of combs. Every device has a different number of beams and a specific target wavelength. Although its exact hair growth mechanism remains unknown, it is thought to accelerate mitosis and stimulate the activation of follicular keratinocytes. This therapy has shown significant efficacy in randomized, sham device–controlled studies in both men and women with androgenetic alopecia.[58,59] In 2007, HairMax LaserComb received FDA clearance for the treatment of men with androgenetic alopecia. The HairMax LaserBand received FDA clearance for the treatment of androgenetic alopecia in both men and women in 2014.

DIETARY SUPPLEMENTS AND NUTRACEUTICALS

Dietary supplements are defined as products that contain nutrients derived from food; they are not considered a drug but a subcategory of food. However, it is important to note that although the term nutraceutical is used to denote nutrients that have pharmaceutical properties, this term is not officially recognized by the FDA.[60] In response to the high demand and lack of efficacious hair growth drugs, multiple dietary supplements for hair loss have been introduced to the market during the past decades. A small number of clinical trials have been performed to validate their use, and most supplements have no or low-quality data to support their use. Vitamin A was one of the first supplements associated with hair growth because of results observed in a trial of topical tretinoin for androgenetic alopecia; however, excessive vitamin A is associated with hair shedding.[61] Most hair growth multivitamins contain vitamin A, yet no trials support its efficacy. Supplementation with omega 3 and omega 6 fatty acids is among the only supplements with data from a RCT. These

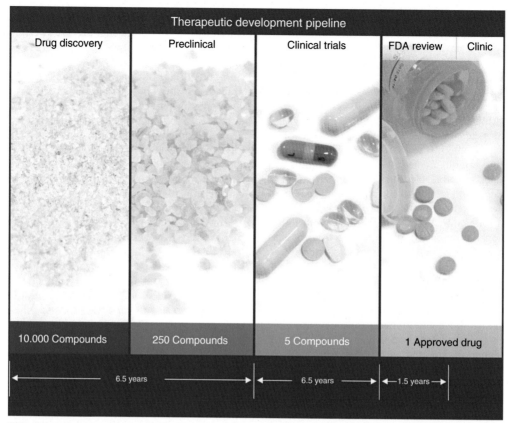

FIG. 26.1 Representation of the number of substances identified as potential drugs, compounds that reach preclinical and clinical testing and those that ultimately obtain FDA approval. (Modified form Eaglstein WH. The FDA Approval Process and Drug Development. The FDA for Doctors. Switzerland: Springer; 2014.)[65]

supplements improved hair density and reduced telogen percentage compared with placebo in 120 healthy female volunteers with androgenetic alopecia.[62] Also, a supplement composed of vitamin C, zinc, horsetail, flax seed extract, and AminoMar marine complex (containing shark and mollusk powder) reported a significant increase in total hair count, total hair density, and terminal hair density after 180 days of treatment compared with placebo.[63]

DRUG DEVELOPMENT AND THE FDA APPROVAL PROCESS

The process of developing a drug and taking it through the approval process is extremely time consuming and costly, as illustrated above. This at least partially explains why only two medications have been approved for the treatment of any alopecia. Initial in vitro studies need to be performed before a drug can be tested in animals. Once evaluated in animals, preclinical analysis takes place before the drug can be tested for the first time in humans. Most compounds that are selected as potential drugs never receive approval, and in fact, most never get tested in humans (Fig. 26.1).

Preclinical Testing

Preclinical testing or preclinical research refers to any study of a potential drug performed before testing it in humans. It is usually executed by basic scientists in laboratories following good laboratory practices, a set of minimum requirements that regulate and oversee this type of research. Some of the crucial aspects of these requirements include general provisions, organization and personnel, facilities, equipment, testing facilities operation, test and control articles, and protocols for the conduct of nonclinical laboratory studies.[64] Thousands of substances are evaluated by scientists to determine which ones have the potential to become a drug. When a potential drug is identified, multiple processes, referred as Chemistry, Manufacturing, and Control processes, will determine the specific chemical structure of the substance, its solubility, and its stability over time. After this information is obtained, in vitro and animal studies are performed to establish the chemical's bioactivity, metabolism, and mechanism of action.[65]

Generally, preclinical studies are not very extensive. Nevertheless, these studies are necessary to generate vital information about drug dosing and toxicity. Following the acquisition of this information, researchers then determine whether the drug should be tested in humans.

Clinical Testing

According to the FDA, there are four sequential clinical research study phases that proceed after preclinical testing: phase 1, phase 2, phase 3, and phase 4 studies. The drug approval process can be very arduous, and most of the investigational drugs never achieve FDA approval. The probability of success of a phase 1 study to proceed to a phase 2 study is 63.2%. The probability of a phase 2 study to proceed to a phase 3 study is 30.7%. The probability of a phase 3 study proceeding to a new drug application (NDA) is 58.1%. Approximately 85.3% of NDAs are eventually approved. Thus, the overall probability of a new investigational drug being ultimately approved has been estimated to be only 9.6%.[66]

Phase 1 Clinical Studies

The purpose of phase 1 studies is to determine frequent and severe adverse events related to the investigational new drug (IND). These studies must also generate adequate pharmacokinetic, pharmacodynamic, and safety data to enable the design of phase 2 controlled trials. Phase 1 studies are conducted in a small population, usually less than 100 subjects. These studies typically enroll healthy volunteers as subjects but may enroll volunteers with the disease or condition of interest.

Phase 2 Clinical Studies

Phase 2 studies enroll subjects with the disease or condition of interest. The ultimate purpose of phase 2 studies is to gather preliminary data on effectiveness, while simultaneously evaluating safety. These studies typically have a control group that may be a placebo, an active comparator, or standard of care treatment. Pilot studies are included in this category and are used to confirm the drug concept and predict possible dosing for future studies. Efficacy endpoints are usually very broad in phase 2 studies.

Phase 3 Clinical Studies

Phase 3 studies collect additional information about safety and efficacy by studying different populations and doses while monitoring closely for adverse events. These studies enroll a much larger number of subjects compared with phase 1 and phase 2 studies; typically 300–3000 volunteers who have the disease or condition of interest participate in these trials. Phase 3 trials are the most expensive part of the drug development and approval process. The results of these studies are ultimately submitted to the FDA as part of an NDA.

Phase 4 Clinical Studies

Phase 4 studies are postmarketing studies. These studies are conducted following the FDA approval of a drug and are crucial for the identification of a drug's side effects. They include several thousand volunteers who have the disease or condition of interest, and they are designed to gather information about drug safety, efficacy, and optimal use.[67] Additionally, phase 4 studies are sometimes used to obtain labeling approval for a new indication.

Investigational New Drug

An IND is a drug that is studied for a new indication or in a new population not yet been approved by the FDA.[67] Federal law requires that a drug is approved for marketing before it can be transported and distributed across states. Because a sponsor (pharmaceutical company) needs to ship the drug to different sites for clinical investigations, the IND status becomes the exemption through which the sponsor obtains FDA permission to do this. To receive IND status, the investigator has to submit an IND application to the FDA.[68] The FDA reviews the IND application to ensure that adequate preclinical testing in animals has been conducted to support further testing in humans. The application must address three key points for approval. First, it must include animal pharmacology and toxicology studies. Second, it has to detail the composition, stability, and control of the drug. Third, protocols of clinical studies need to be submitted with the application.

Investigational Device Exemption

Medical devices require an investigational device exemption (IDE) to be used in a clinical study designed to test safety and effectiveness. The IDE approval process depends on the level of risk that the device may present to the study subject. Significant risk devices require both FDA and Institutional Review Board (IRB) approval before the initiation of a clinical study. This is in contrast to nonsignificant risk devices, which only require IRB approval. The classification of a product as a drug or a device can be challenging.

New Drug Application

INDs must progress through various clinical trial phases to accumulate the necessary data needed to apply for an NDA. An NDA is a vehicle through which drug sponsors formally request that the FDA approve a new pharmaceutical for sale and marketing in the United States. This application includes information regarding whether the drug is safe and effective for the proposed use, whether its benefits outweigh the associated risks, whether the label is appropriate, and whether the methods used in manufacturing preserve the drug's identity, strength, quality, and purity.[68]

Clinical Study Design

A clinical study is a clinical trial where patients are assigned to receive an intervention so that biomedical and health outcomes of the intervention can be obtained. The study type defines the inherent nature of the study, and each type of study will generate different types of conclusions.

Prepost studies evaluate an outcome before and after an intervention. They have limited validity because they do not control other variables that can influence the outcome. RCTs are studies where subjects are divided into two groups by chance, leading to comparable groups. They are the most common type of clinical trial and have multiple subtypes. The trial can be conducted with a placebo or an active comparator (often standard of care) as the control group. If both the subject and the investigator are aware of what each group is receiving, the study is said to be open-label. These studies are associated with multiple levels of bias; however, some interventions are impossible to mask, so this becomes the only option in such instances. If the subject is not aware of the treatment type, but the investigator is, the study is single-blind. These studies are associated with observer bias, where higher expectations lead to increased performance. If neither the patient nor the investigator knows the treatment, the study is double-blind. Double-blind studies are the most rigorous study design because they are associated with less inherent risk of bias. In crossover RCTs, subjects receive sequential treatments in different phases of the study. This design can correct an unsuccessful randomization, demonstrate treatment reversibility, and enable a more efficient investigation because subjects will be randomized into more than one treatment arm within one

study.[69] Tables 26.4 and 26.5 list all of the current clinical trial listed on clinicaltrials.gov for alopecia areata and androgenetic alopecia, respectively. Scarring alopecia has very few treatment options, and research for the development of new therapies is urgent. Presently, there is only one active interventional clinical trial for any form of scarring alopecia. This trial is being done in the United States and is investigating the efficacy of a biocellular mixture of emulsified adipose-derived tissue with high-density platelet-rich plasma via intravenous infusion for the treatment of scarring alopecia and alopecia areata.[70]

ANDROGENETIC ALOPECIA: AN ILLUSTRATIVE EXAMPLE

Androgenetic alopecia is the only hair loss disorder that has FDA approved treatments: topical minoxidil for both men and women and oral finasteride for men. We will discuss the history of minoxidil as an illustrative example of the long process that ultimately leads to FDA approval. In 1960, the compound N, N-diallylmelamine (DAM) demonstrated reduced gastric acidity in rats, and this was thought to be due to an anticholinergic mechanism. An in vivo study in dogs contradicted this proposed mechanism. However, an interesting side effect was noted: There was a prolonged reduction in blood pressure. DAM N-oxidase (DAMN-O) was identified as the active metabolite, and direct peripheral vasodilation was suggested as the new mechanism of action. This compound was tested in a 30-day trial, but severe side effects such as hemorrhagic lesions in the right atrium, tachycardia, and salt and water retention resulted. A safer analogue of DAMN-O was then identified as minoxidil. An IND for oral minoxidil was submitted in 1968 and was initially tested for severe, refractory hypertension. In 1971, Gottlieb et al. reported hypertrichosis in five of eight patients treated with oral minoxidil for more than 2 months. At this point, a topical solution was created. Six years later, in 1977, an IND for topical minoxidil was submitted to the FDA.[71]

Kreindler published the first RCT of topical minoxidil in androgenetic alopecia.[11] The study population included 150 men with an average age of 36 years. The trial was composed of three arms: minoxidil 2% solution, minoxidil 3% solution, and placebo. At 4 months, subjects applying the active medication had a significant increase in nonvellus hair growth compared with placebo; however, total hair count was comparable in the three arms during the 12 months of the trial. Additional trials, in both males and

TABLE 26.4

Clinical Trials in Alopecia Areata Listed on clinicaltrials.gov[70] (October 2017)

Clinical Trial Title	Intervention(s)	Phase	# Subjects	Status
Vytorin in the Treatment of Alopecia Areata	Arm 1: Vytorin	Phase 1	29	Completed
Stem Cell Educator Therapy in Alopecia Areata	Arm 1: stem cell educator device	Phase 1/2	30	Unknown
Evaluation of the Efficacy and Tolerability of Treatment With Interleukin-2 in Severe and Resistant Alopecia Areata	Arm 1: interleukin-2	Phase 1/2	10	Unknown
A Study of Secukinumab for the Treatment of Alopecia Areata	Arm 1: secukinumab Arm 2: placebo	Phase 2	11	Terminated
Study to Evaluate the Efficacy of Tofacitinib in Moderate to Severe Alopecia Areata, Totalis and Universalis	Arm 1: tofacitinib	Phase 2	15	Active, not recruiting
Pilot Study to Evaluate the Efficacy of Ruxolitinib in Alopecia Areata	Arm 1: ruxolitinib	Phase 2	12	Completed
A Clinical Trial to Evaluate the Efficacy of Abatacept in Moderate to Severe Alopecia Areata	Arm 1: abatacept Arm 2: placebo	Phase 2	0	Withdrawn
Excimer Light for Alopecia Areata	Arm 1: UVB excimer saser device	Phase 2	18	Unknown
An Open-Label Single-Arm Clinical Trial to Evaluate the Efficacy of Abatacept in Moderate to Severe Patch Type Alopecia Areata	Arm 1: abatacept	Phase 2	15	Active, not recruiting
A Pilot Study of Tralokinumab in Subjects With Moderate to Severe Alopecia Areata	Arm 1: tralokinumab Arm 2: placebo	Phase 2	30	Recruiting
A Study With INCB018424 Phosphate Cream Applied Topically to Subjects With Alopecia Areata (AA)	Arm 1: placebo cream Arm 2: INCB018424 phosphate cream	Phase 2	90	Active, not recruiting
Study to Evaluate the Efficacy and Safety Profile of PF-06651600 and PF-06700841 in Subjects With Alopecia Areata	Arm 1: PF-06651600 Arm 2: PF-06700841 Arm 3: placebo	Phase 2	132	Recruiting
LEO 124249 Ointment in the Treatment of Alopecia Areata	Arm 1: LEO 124249 Arm 2: placebo (vehicle)	Phase 2	31	Completed
Safety and Efficacy Study of SHAPE Gel in Alopecia Areata	Arm 1: SHAPE Gel	Phase 2	40	Not yet recruiting
Adrenal Function and Use of Intralesional Triamcinolone Acetonide 10 mg/mL (Kenalog-10) in Patients With Alopecia Areata	Arm 1: triamcinolone acetonide 10 mg/mL (Kenalog-10)	Phase 2	18	Completed with results
Study to Evaluate the Safety and Efficacy of CTP-543 in Adult Patients With Moderate to Severe Alopecia Areata	Arm 1: CTP-543 Arm 2: placebo	Phase 2	90	Recruiting
Topical Tofacitinib for the Treatment of Alopecia Areata and Its Variants	Arm 1: tofacitinib ointment	Phase 2	10	Active, not recruiting

Continued

TABLE 26.4
Clinical Trials in Alopecia Areata Listed on clinicaltrials.gov[70] (October 2017)—cont'd

Clinical Trial Title	Intervention(s)	Phase	# Subjects	Status
Tofacitinib for the Treatment of Alopecia Areata and Variants	Arm 1: tofacitinib	Phase 2	30	Completed with results
Phase II Randomized Bilateral Comparison of Topical Targretin Gel 1% in Alopecia Areata	Arm 1: Targretin gel 1%	Phase 2/3	46	Completed
Study of LH-8 in Paediatric Alopecia Areata	Arm 1: LH-8 Arm 2: placebo	Phase 2/3	100	Not yet recruiting
Topical Garlic Concentrate for Alopecia Areata in Children	Arm 1: garlic concentrate	Phase 3	20	Recruiting
A Trial of Clobetasol Propionate Versus Hydrocortisone in Children With Alopecia Areata	Arm 1: hydrocortisone 1% Arm 2: clobetasol propionate 0.05%	Phase 3	41	Completed
TREg Activation in the Treatment of the PELADE (Alopecia Areata)	Arm 1: interleukin-2 Arm 2: placebo	Phase 3	56	Recruiting
The Efficiency of the Methotrexate at Patients Affected By Grave Pelade	Arm 1: methotrexate Arm 2: placebo	Phase 3	90	Recruiting
Plaquenil for Alopecia Areata, Alopecia Totalis	Arm 1: hydroxychloroquine	Phase 4	16	Completed
Intralesional Steroids in the Treatment of Alopecia Areata	Arm 1: IL triamcinolone 2.5 mg/mL Arm 2: IL triamcinolone 5 mg/mL Arm 3: IL triamcinolone 10 mg/mL Arm 4: placebo (IL saline)	Phase 4	68	Recruiting
Comparison of Topical Latanoprost Versus Topical Corticosteroid in Treatment of Localized Alopecia Areata	Arm 1: topical latanoprost 0.005% Arm 2: topical betamethasone 0.05%	Phase 4	50	Completed
Response of Topical Capsaicin in Alopecia Areata	Arm 1: capsaicin	Phase 4	24	Completed
Aldara for the Treatment of Extensive Alopecia Areata	Arm 1: Aldara cream 5%	Phase 4	20	Completed
Characteristics of T Cells From Alopecia Areata Scalp Skin Before and After Treatment With Aldara 5%	Arm 1: Aldara cream 5%	Phase 4	20	Completed
Safety and Efficacy of Clobetasol Propionate 0.05% E Foam in Alopecia	Arm 1: clobetasol 0.05% Foam	Phase 4	30	Unknown
Safety and Efficacy of Oral Mega Pulse Methylprednisolone in Severe Therapy Resistant Alopecia Areata	Arm 1: methylprednisolone sodium succinate	Phase 4	42	Completed

IL, intralesional.

TABLE 26.5
Phase 2 and Phase 3 Clinical Trials for Androgenetic Alopecia Listed on clinicaltrials.gov[70] (October 2017)

Clinical Trial Title	Intervention(s)	Phase	# Subjects	Status
A Study of SM04554 Applied Topically to the Scalp of Male Subjects With Androgenetic Alopecia Analyzed by Biopsy of the Scalp Prior To and Post Dosing	Arm 1: topical SM04554 solution 0.15% Arm 2: topical SM04554 solution 0.25% Arm 3: topical vehicle solution	Phase 2	49	Completed
Treatment of Androgenetic Alopecia in Males With Theradome LH80 PRO	Arm 1: LH80 PRO Arm 2: sham device	Phase 2	80	Active, not recruiting
The Effect of Platelet-Rich Plasma in Subjects With Androgenetic Alopecia	Arm 1: platelet-rich plasma Arm 2: placebo (sterile saline)	Phase 2	30	Not yet recruiting
Effectiveness and Safety of Minoxidil Foam Versus Placebo Foam for Androgenetic Alopecia	Arm 1: minoxidil 5% foam Arm 2: vehicle	Phase 2	70	Completed
A Study of the Safety, Tolerability, and Efficacy of Topical SM04554 Solution in Male Subjects With Androgenetic Alopecia (AGA)	Arm 1: topical SM04554 solution 0.15% Arm 2: topical SM04554 solution 0.25% Arm 3: topical vehicle solution	Phase 2	310	Completed
A Phase 2 Study to Evaluate the Safety and Efficacy of CB-03-01 Solution, a Comparator Solution and Vehicle Solution in Males With Androgenetic Alopecia	Arm 1: CB-03-01 solution Arm 2: minoxidil 5% solution Arm 3: placebo solution	Phase 2	95	Completed
Dose-Ranging Efficacy Study of Topical Tetrapeptide Aldehyde Proteasome Inhibitor (NEOSH101) to Treat Male Pattern Hair Loss	Arm 1: NEOSH101 2% Arm 2: NEOSH101 1% Arm 3: NEOSH101 0.5% Arm 4: placebo	Phase 2	140	Unknown
Efficacy Study of Topical NEOSH101 to Treat Male Pattern Hair Loss	Arm 1: NEOSH101 2% Arm 2: minoxidil 5% Arm 3: placebo	Phase 2	180	Completed
Treatment of Male Pattern Baldness With Botulinum Toxin	Arm 2: botulinum toxin A intramuscular injections	Phase 2		Completed
Efficacy of Nutrition Supplement for Treatment of Men With Hair Loss	Arm 1: HCap formula Arm 2: placebo	Phase 2	33	Completed
Topical AS101 for Treatment of FAGA (Female Androgenetic Alopecia) in Menopause Women	Arm 1: AS101	Phase 2	40	Unknown
The Efficacy and Safety of Topical Valproic Acid in Preventing Hair Loss	Arm 1: valproic acid solution Arm 2: placebo	Phase 2	40	Completed
Topical Bimatoprost Effect on Androgen Dependent Hair Follicles	Arm 1: bimatoprost Arm 2: placebo	Phase 2	33	Completed

Continued

TABLE 26.5
Phase 2 and Phase 3 Clinical Trials for Androgenetic Alopecia Listed on clinicaltrials.gov[70] (October 2017)—cont'd

Clinical Trial Title	Intervention(s)	Phase	# Subjects	Status
Phase 2A Study of Setipiprant Tablets in Androgenetic Alopecia in Males	Arm 1: setipiprant Arm 2: placebo	Phase 2	169	Active, not recruiting
Adipose Tissue Derived Stem Cell Based Hair Restoration Therapy for Androgenetic Alopecia	Arm 1: stem cells Arm 2: platelet-rich plasma	Phase 2	88	Not yet recruiting
STYLE—A Trial of Cell Enriched Adipose for Androgenetic Alopecia	Arm 1: fat + high-dose adipose-derived regenerative cells (ADRCs) Arm 2: fat + low-dose ADRCs Arm 3: fat alone Arm 4: no fat control	Phase 2	70	Active, not recruiting
A Safety and Efficacy Study of Bimatoprost in Men With Androgenic Alopecia (AGA)	Arm 1: bimatoprost solution 1 twice daily Arm 2: bimatoprost solution 1 once daily Arm 3: bimatoprost solution 2 twice daily Arm 4: bimatoprost solution 2 once daily Arm 5: placebo	Phase 2	244	Completed
Safety and Efficacy Study of Bimatoprost in the Treatment of Men With Androgenic Alopecia	Arm 1: bimatoprost formulation A Arm 2: bimatoprost formulation B Arm 3: bimatoprost formulation C Arm 4: bimatoprost vehicle solution Arm 5: minoxidil 5% solution	Phase 2	307	Completed
A Study to Evaluate the Superiority, Efficacy and Tolerability of Combination Pantovigar With 2% Minoxidil Versus 2% Minoxidil in Women With Female Pattern Hair Loss	Arm 1: Pantovigar plus minoxidil 2% Arm 2: minoxidil 2% only	Phase 2	74	Completed
Dutasteride Versus Placebo and Finasteride in Men With Androgenetic Alopecia	Arm 1: finasteride 1 mg + dutasteride placebo Arm 2: dutasteride 0.02 mg + finasteride placebo Arm 3: dutasteride 0.1 mg + finasteride placebo Arm 4: dutasteride 0.5 mg + finasteride placebo Arm 5: finasteride placebo + dutasteride placebo	Phase 3	917	Completed
Efficacy and Safety Study to Compare Two Minoxidil Formulations on Women With Androgenetic Alopecia	Arm 1: 5% minoxidil topical foam Arm 2: 2% minoxidil topical solution	Phase 3	113	Completed

TABLE 26.5
Phase 2 and Phase 3 Clinical Trials for Androgenetic Alopecia Listed on clinicaltrials.gov[70] (October 2017)—cont'd

Clinical Trial Title	Intervention(s)	Phase	# Subjects	Status
Clinical Trial in Females for Female Pattern Hair Loss	Arm 1: 5% minoxidil topical foam Arm 2: vehicle topical foam	Phase 3	404	Completed
A Study to Evaluate the Effectiveness and Safety of 5% Minoxidil Foam in the Treatment of Male Pattern Hair Loss	Arm 1: 5% minoxidil topical foam	Phase 3	352	Completed
Effects of Finasteride on Serum Prostate-Specific Antigen (0906-111)	Arm 1: MK0906 + finasteride 1 mg Arm 2: placebo	Phase 3	355	Completed
Efficacy Study of Minoxidil Lotion Versus Combined Minoxidil and Finasteride Lotion to Treat Male Pattern Hair Loss	Arm 1: minoxidil 3% lotion Arm 2: minoxidil 3% + 0.1% finasteride lotion	Phase 3	40	Completed
Efficacy and Safety of Mesotherapy With Minoxidil 0.5%/2 mL for Androgenetic Alopecia in Female Patients	Arm 1: minoxidil 0.5%/2 mL Arm 2: saline	Phase 3	60	Unknown
A Study to Assess the Efficacy and Safety of Dutasteride 0.5 mg Once Daily for 6 Months in the Treatment Of Male Subjects With Androgenetic Alopecia	Arm 1: dutasteride 0.5 mg Arm 2: placebo	Phase 3	150	Completed
Sexual Function in Men Receiving Dutasteride for Androgenetic Alopecia	Arm 1: dutasteride 0.5 mg Arm 2: placebo	Phase 3	117	Completed
A Long-term Study to Determine Safety and Efficacy of Dutasteride in Male Subjects With Androgenetic Alopecia	Arm 1: dutasteride 0.5 mg	Phase 3	120	Completed
Study to Evaluate the Efficacy and Safety of P-3074 Topical Solution in the Treatment of Androgenetic Alopecia	Arm 1: P-3074 (finasteride 0.25% topical solution) Arm 2: oral finasteride 1 mg Arm 3: vehicle topical solution	Phase 3	450	Active, not recruiting
Clinical Trial in Females With Female Pattern Hair Loss	Arm 1: minoxidil 5% topical foam Arm 2: minoxidil 2% topical solution	Phase 3	322	Completed

females, would achieve their primary outcomes in the next 2 decades. In 1988, minoxidil 5% solution was approved for over-the-counter use for androgenetic alopecia in males. In 2002, Olsen et al. published a phase 2 RCT in 396 males showing that subjects who received either minoxidil solution 2% or 5% had a statistically significant higher nonvellus hair count compared with placebo.[16] Following these findings, a phase 3 RCT comparing minoxidil 5% foam versus placebo was studied. This study's primary endpoint was total hair count in the vertex of the scalp.[20] This study, together with two pharmacokinetic studies and one sensitization trial in healthy subjects, were submitted to the FDA in 2005 as an NDA, resulting in approval of minoxidil 5% foam for androgenetic alopecia in males the following year.[72] For women, minoxidil 2% solution was studied in two RCTs in the 1990s and was eventually approved for use in women in 1997.[13,14] In 2011, studies compared once-daily minoxidil 5% foam to twice-daily minoxidil 2%

solution in women. These studies showed noninferiority of once-daily minoxidil 5% foam, which lead to its approval for women in 2014.[23] Minoxidil has been extensively used and studied for different types of alopecia. More than 200 clinical trials have been conducted to assess its safety and efficacy for various indications.

CONCLUSIONS

Hair loss, independent of its etiology, is a distressing condition that significantly affects quality of life. Although it is disappointing that only androgenetic alopecia currently has FDA approved medications, the arduous process inherent to drug development makes this fact understandable. The development of new compounds and the rigorous testing of more effective interventions are urgently needed. Creating uniform standards for future clinical trials in hair loss disorders would help streamline part of this grueling new drug approval process by allowing more straightforward comparison of primary and secondary outcomes between studies.

REFERENCES

1. Mcandrews PJ. *Men's Hair Loss*. American Hair Loss Association. 2017. http://www.americanhairloss.org/men_hair_loss/introduction.asp. Access date: May 1, 2017.
2. Birch MP, Messenger JF, Messenger AG. Hair density, hair diameter and the prevalence of female pattern hair loss. *Br J Dermatol*. 2001;144(2):297–304.
3. Gan DC, Sinclair RD. Prevalence of male and female pattern hair loss in Maryborough. *J Investig Dermatol Symp Proc*. 2005;10(3):184–189.
4. *Alopecia Market Analysis by Treatment (Oral, Topical, Injectable), by Gender (Men, Women) and Segment Forecasts to 2024*. 2016.
5. Williams KJ, Moore HM, Davies AH. Haemodynamic changes with the use of neuromuscular electrical stimulation compared to intermittent pneumatic compression. *Phlebology*. 2015;30(5):365–372.
6. Stough D, Stenn K, Haber R, et al. Psychological effect, pathophysiology, and management of androgenetic alopecia in men. *Mayo Clin Proc*. 2005;80(10):1316–1322.
7. Cash TF. The psychosocial consequences of androgenetic alopecia: a review of the research literature. *Br J Dermatol*. 1999;141(3):398–405.
8. Alfonso M, Richter-Appelt H, Tosti A, Viera MS, Garcia M. The psychosocial impact of hair loss among men: a multinational European study. *Curr Med Res Opin*. 2005;21(11):1829–1836.
9. Rigopoulos D, Stamatios G, Ioannides D. Primary scarring alopecias. *Curr Probl Dermatol*. 2015;47:76–86.
10. Mubki T, Rudnicka L, Olszewska M, Shapiro J. Evaluation and diagnosis of the hair loss patient: part I. History and clinical examination. *J Am Acad Dermatol*. 2014;71(3):415.e411–415.e415.
11. Kreindler TG. Topical minoxidil in early androgenetic alopecia. *J Am Acad Dermatol*. 1987;16(3 Pt 2):718–724.
12. Rietschel RL, Duncan SH. Safety and efficacy of topical minoxidil in the management of androgenetic alopecia. *J Am Acad Dermatol*. 1987;16(3 Pt 2):677–685.
13. Jacobs JP, Szpunar CA, Warner ML. Use of topical minoxidil therapy for androgenetic alopecia in women. *Int J Dermatol*. 1993;32(10):758–762.
14. DeVillez RL, Jacobs JP, Szpunar CA, Warner ML. Androgenetic alopecia in the female. Treatment with 2% topical minoxidil solution. *Arch Dermatol*. 1994;130(3):303–307.
15. Price VH, Menefee E, Strauss PC. Changes in hair weight and hair count in men with androgenetic alopecia, after application of 5% and 2% topical minoxidil, placebo, or no treatment. *J Am Acad Dermatol*. 1999;41(5 Pt 1):717–721.
16. Olsen EA, Dunlap FE, Funicella T, et al. A randomized clinical trial of 5% topical minoxidil versus 2% topical minoxidil and placebo in the treatment of androgenetic alopecia in men. *J Am Acad Dermatol*. 2002;47(3):377–385.
17. Vexiau P, Chaspoux C, Boudou P, et al. Effects of minoxidil 2% vs. cyproterone acetate treatment on female androgenetic alopecia: a controlled, 12-month randomized trial. *Br J Dermatol*. 2002;146(6):992–999.
18. Berger RS, Fu JL, Smiles KA, et al. The effects of minoxidil, 1% pyrithione zinc and a combination of both on hair density: a randomized controlled trial. *Br J Dermatol*. 2003;149(2):354–362.
19. Lucky AW, Piacquadio DJ, Ditre CM, et al. A randomized, placebo-controlled trial of 5% and 2% topical minoxidil solutions in the treatment of female pattern hair loss. *J Am Acad Dermatol*. 2004;50(4):541–553.
20. Olsen EA, Whiting D, Bergfeld W, et al. A multicenter, randomized, placebo-controlled, double-blind clinical trial of a novel formulation of 5% minoxidil topical foam versus placebo in the treatment of androgenetic alopecia in men. *J Am Acad Dermatol*. 2007;57(5):767–774.
21. Tsuboi R, Tanaka T, Nishikawa T, et al. A randomized, placebo-controlled trial of 1% topical minoxidil solution in the treatment of androgenetic alopecia in Japanese women. *Eur J Dermatol*. 2007;17(1):37–44.
22. Tsuboi R, Arano O, Nishikawa T, Yamada H, Katsuoka K. Randomized clinical trial comparing 5% and 1% topical minoxidil for the treatment of androgenetic alopecia in Japanese men. *J Dermatol*. 2009;36(8):437–446.
23. Blume-Peytavi U, Hillmann K, Dietz E, Canfield D, Garcia Bartels N. A randomized, single-blind trial of 5% minoxidil foam once daily versus 2% minoxidil solution twice daily in the treatment of androgenetic alopecia in women. *J Am Acad Dermatol*. 2011;65(6):1126–1134.e1122.

24. Hillmann K, Garcia Bartels N, Kottner J, Stroux A, Canfield D, Blume-Peytavi U. A single-centre, randomized, double-blind, placebo-controlled clinical trial to investigate the efficacy and safety of minoxidil topical foam in frontotemporal and vertex androgenetic alopecia in men. *Skin Pharmacol Physiol.* 2015;28(5):236–244.

25. Hu R, Xu F, Sheng Y, et al. Combined treatment with oral finasteride and topical minoxidil in male androgenetic alopecia: a randomized and comparative study in Chinese patients. *Dermatol Ther.* 2015;28(5):303–308.

26. Gubelin Harcha W, Barboza Martinez J, Tsai TF, et al. A randomized, active- and placebo-controlled study of the efficacy and safety of different doses of dutasteride versus placebo and finasteride in the treatment of male subjects with androgenetic alopecia. *J Am Acad Dermatol.* 2014;70(3):489–498.e483.

27. Varothai S, Bergfeld WF. Androgenetic alopecia: an evidence-based treatment update. *Am J Clin Dermatol.* 2014;15(3):217–230.

28. Danesh M, Murase JE. Increasing utility of finasteride for frontal fibrosing alopecia. *J Am Acad Dermatol.* 2015;72(6):e157.

29. Kaufman KD, Olsen EA, Whiting D, et al. Finasteride in the treatment of men with androgenetic alopecia. Finasteride male pattern hair loss study group. *J Am Acad Dermatol.* 1998;39(4 Pt 1):578–589.

30. Leyden J, Dunlap F, Miller B, et al. Finasteride in the treatment of men with frontal male pattern hair loss. *J Am Acad Dermatol.* 1999;40(6 Pt 1):930–937.

31. Roberts JL, Fiedler V, Imperato-McGinley J, et al. Clinical dose ranging studies with finasteride, a type 2 5alpha-reductase inhibitor, in men with male pattern hair loss. *J Am Acad Dermatol.* 1999;41(4):555–563.

32. Price VH, Roberts JL, Hordinsky M, et al. Lack of efficacy of finasteride in postmenopausal women with androgenetic alopecia. *J Am Acad Dermatol.* 2000;43(5 Pt 1):768–776.

33. Van Neste D, Fuh V, Sanchez-Pedreno P, et al. Finasteride increases anagen hair in men with androgenetic alopecia. *Br J Dermatol.* 2000;143(4):804–810.

34. Price VH, Menefee E, Sanchez M, Ruane P, Kaufman KD. Changes in hair weight and hair count in men with androgenetic alopecia after treatment with finasteride, 1 mg, daily. *J Am Acad Dermatol.* 2002;46(4):517–523.

35. Olsen EA, Hordinsky M, Whiting D, et al. The importance of dual 5alpha-reductase inhibition in the treatment of male pattern hair loss: results of a randomized placebo-controlled study of dutasteride versus finasteride. *J Am Acad Dermatol.* 2006;55(6):1014–1023.

36. Price VH, Menefee E, Sanchez M, Kaufman KD. Changes in hair weight in men with androgenetic alopecia after treatment with finasteride (1 mg daily): three- and 4-year results. *J Am Acad Dermatol.* 2006;55(1):71–74.

37. Eun HC, Kwon OS, Yeon JH, et al. Efficacy, safety, and tolerability of dutasteride 0.5 mg once daily in male patients with male pattern hair loss: a randomized, double-blind, placebo-controlled, phase III study. *J Am Acad Dermatol.* 2010;63(2):252–258.

38. Olsen EA, Whiting DA, Savin R, et al. Global photographic assessment of men aged 18 to 60 years with male pattern hair loss receiving finasteride 1 mg or placebo. *J Am Acad Dermatol.* 2012;67(3):379–386.

39. Lenane P, Macarthur C, Parkin PC, et al. Clobetasol propionate, 0.05%, vs hydrocortisone, 1%, for alopecia areata in children: a randomized clinical trial. *JAMA Dermatol.* 2014;150(1):47–50.

40. Cevasco NC, Bergfeld WF, Remzi BK, de Knott HR. A case-series of 29 patients with lichen planopilaris: the Cleveland Clinic Foundation experience on evaluation, diagnosis, and treatment. *J Am Acad Dermatol.* 2007;57(1):47–53.

41. Eginli A, Dothard E, Bagayoko CW, Huang K, Daniel A, McMichael AJ. A retrospective review of treatment results for patients with central centrifugal cicatrical alopecia. *J Drugs Dermatol.* 2017;16(4):317–320.

42. Royer M, Bodemer C, Vabres P, et al. Efficacy and tolerability of methotrexate in severe childhood alopecia areata. *Br J Dermatol.* 2011;165(2):407–410.

43. Lim SK, Lim CA, Kwon IS, et al. Low-dose systemic methotrexate therapy for recalcitrant alopecia areata. *Ann Dermatol.* 2017;29(3):263–267.

44. Batalla A, Florez A, Abalde T, Vazquez-Veiga H. Methotrexate in alopecia areata: a report of three cases. *Int J Trichology.* 2016;8(4):188–190.

45. Liu LY, Craiglow BG, Dai F, King BA. Tofacitinib for the treatment of severe alopecia areata and variants: a study of 90 patients. *J Am Acad Dermatol.* 2017;76(1):22–28.

46. Mackay-Wiggan J, Jabbari A, Nguyen N, et al. Oral ruxolitinib induces hair regrowth in patients with moderate-to-severe alopecia areata. *JCI Insight.* 2016;1(15):e89790.

47. Alkhalifah A, Alsantali A, Wang E, McElwee KJ, Shapiro J. Alopecia areata update: part II. Treatment. *J Am Acad Dermatol.* 2010;62(2):191–202; quiz 203–204.

48. Famenini S, Slaught C, Duan L, Goh C. Demographics of women with female pattern hair loss and the effectiveness of spironolactone therapy. *J Am Acad Dermatol.* 2015;73(4):705–706.

49. Sinclair R, Wewerinke M, Jolley D. Treatment of female pattern hair loss with oral antiandrogens. *Br J Dermatol.* 2005;152(3):466–473.

50. Faghihi G, Andalib F, Asilian A. The efficacy of latanoprost in the treatment of alopecia areata of eyelashes and eyebrows. *Eur J Dermatol.* 2009;19(6):586–587.

51. El-Ashmawy AA, El-Maadawy IH, El-Maghraby GM. Efficacy of topical latanoprost versus minoxidil and beta-methasone valerate on the treatment of alopecia areata. *J Dermatol Treat.* 2017:1–10.

52. Roseborough I, Lee H, Chwalek J, Stamper RL, Price VH. Lack of efficacy of topical latanoprost and bimatoprost ophthalmic solutions in promoting eyelash growth in patients with alopecia areata. *J Am Acad Dermatol.* 2009;60(4):705–706.

53. Dhurat R, Sukesh M, Avhad G, Dandale A, Pal A, Pund P. A randomized evaluator blinded study of effect of microneedling in androgenetic alopecia: a pilot study. *Int J Trichology.* 2013;5(1):6–11.

54. Chandrashekar B, Yepuri V, Mysore V. Alopecia areata-successful outcome with microneedling and triamcinolone acetonide. *J Cutan Aesth Surg.* 2014;7(1):63–64.

55. Al-Mutairi N. 308-nm excimer laser for the treatment of alopecia areata. *Dermatol Surg.* 2007;33(12):1483–1487.

56. Al-Mutairi N. 308-nm excimer laser for the treatment of alopecia areata in children. *Pediatr Dermatol.* 2009;26(5):547–550.

57. Navarini AA, Kolios AG, Prinz-Vavricka BM, Haug S, Trueb RM. Low-dose excimer 308-nm laser for treatment of lichen planopilaris. *Arch Dermatol.* 2011;147(11): 1325–1326.

58. Jimenez JJ, Wikramanayake TC, Bergfeld W, et al. Efficacy and safety of a low-level laser device in the treatment of male and female pattern hair loss: a multicenter, randomized, sham device-controlled, double-blind study. *Am J Clin Dermatol.* 2014;15(2):115–127.

59. Leavitt M, Charles G, Heyman E, Michaels D. HairMax LaserComb laser phototherapy device in the treatment of male androgenetic alopecia: a randomized, double-blind, sham device-controlled, multicentre trial. *Clin Drug Investig.* 2009;29(5):283–292.

60. Eaglstein WH. *What Are Dietary Supplements and Nutraceuticals?* The FDA for Doctors. Switzerland: Springer; 2014.

61. Bazzano GS, Terezakis N, Galen W. Topical tretinoin for hair growth promotion. *J Am Acad Dermatol.* 1986;15(4 Pt 2):880–883, 890–893.

62. Le Floc'h C, Cheniti A, Connetable S, Piccardi N, Vincenzi C, Tosti A. Effect of a nutritional supplement on hair loss in women. *J Cosmet Dermatol.* 2015;14(1):76–82.

63. Ablon G. A 6-month, randomized, double-blind, placebo-controlled study evaluating the ability of a marine complex supplement to promote hair growth in men with thinning hair. *J Cosmet Dermatol.* 2016;15(4):358–366.

64. Satterwhite CL, Torrone E, Meites E, et al. Sexually transmitted infections among US women and men: prevalence and incidence estimates, 2008. *Sex Transmit Dis.* 2013;40(3):187–193.

65. Eaglstein WH. *The FDA Approval Process and Drug Development. The FDA for Doctors.* Switzerland: Springer; 2014.

66. Hay M, Thomas DW, Craighead JL, Economides C, Rosenthal J. Clinical development success rates for investigational drugs. *Nat Biotechnol.* 2014;32(1):40–51.

67. ClinicalTrials.gov. Glossary of Common Site Terms. Clinical Research Phase Study. ClinicalTrials.gov. US National Institute of Health.

68. Kaptchuk TJ, Friedlander E, Kelley JM, et al. Placebos without deception: a randomized controlled trial in irritable bowel syndrome. *PLoS One.* 2010;5(12):e15591.

69. Thiese MS. Observational and interventional study design types; an overview. *Biochem Med.* 2014;24(2):199–210.

70. NIH. *US National Library of Medicine*; 2017. http://www.clinicaltrials.gov/.

71. Zins GR. The history of the development of minoxidil. *Clin Dermatol.* 1988;6(4):132–147.

72. U.S. Department of Health and Human Services, Food and Drug Administration. *Statistical Review and Evaluation. Men's Rogaine Extra Strength Minoxidil 5% Topical Foam for Androgenetic Alopecia*; 2006.

CHAPTER 27

Hair Cosmeceuticals

GISELLE MARTINS, MD • MARIA FERNANDA REIS GAVAZZONI DIAS, MD, PHD

SHAMPOOS

Shampoos are typically composed of 10–30 ingredients, although products with as few as four ingredients are available. The components are grouped into the following:

1. Cleansing agents or surfactants;
2. Additives that contribute to the stability and comfort of the product;
3. Conditioning agents, which are intended to impart softness and gloss, to reduce flyaway and to enhance disentangling facility;
4. Special care ingredients, designated to treat specific problems, such as seborrheic dermatitis and psoriasis.

Surfactants

Surfactants are cleaning agents that substituted soap for hygiene (Table 27.1). They act through weakening of the physical-chemical adherence forces that bind impurities and residues to the hair. Surfactants dissolve these impurities, preventing them from binding to the shaft or the scalp.[1] Residues are nonsoluble fats (sebum) that do not dissolve with water. To be removed from the hair shaft, surfactants present a hydrophobic molecular portion, and another hydrophilic. The first will chemically bond with the fat, whereas the other will bond with the water. The surfactants are composed of a lipid chain of hydrocarbons with a polar extremity and a nonpolar one. The polar extremity is capable of giving this portion of the molecule hydrophilic traits that allow it to dissolve in water and wash away the residues. The surfactants in contact with the water attain the structural formation of a micelle. Their structure becomes spherical with a hydrophilic exterior, which can be rinsed with water, and a hydrophobic interior where the fats and residues are bonded.[1] Depending upon the electric charge of the polar extremity, the surfactants are classified into four groups: anionic, cationic, amphoteric, and nonionic. The main cleansing agents are anionic.[2] The soap, which is also an anionic detergent, in contact with water, leaves an alkaline residue that is very harmful to the hair and skin and that precipitates in the form of calcium salts, which accumulate in the hair shafts, leaving them opaque and tangled. Such effects do not happen with the new anionic surfactants that are derived from the sulfation of fatty acids and analogue polioxyethylenes (alkyl sulfates, alkyl ether sulfates), which are smooth cleansers and cosmetically superior. Some examples are sodium lauryl sulfate, ammonium lauryl sulfate, ammonium laureth sulfate, and α olefin sulfonate.[1,3,4] The current expression *"sulfate-free shampoo"* refers to a preparation without the anionic surfactant. An example of a surfactant with sulfate is the sodium lauryl sulfate. Cationic, amphoteric, and nonionic surfactants are added to some shampoo formulas to reduce the static electricity generating effects caused by the anionic surfactants. Because they carry the positive charge, cationic surfactants bond quickly with the negatively charged shafts by the use of anionic surfactants and reduce the frizz effect. Besides, they optimize the formation of foam and the viscosity of the final product. The static electricity after the use of shampoo is the exact result of the balancing out between the electric charges during the removal of sebum and residue. Negative charge of the hair fiber repels also the negative charge of the micelle. The repulsion of charges allows rinsing with water. However, the result is an increase of the preexisting negativity of the shafts and the formation of stable complexes that bond with the keratin, creating a repulsion between the shafts due to excessive static electricity. Although the cationic agents try to neutralize this effect, there is the interference of the shampoo pH, which can increase the static electricity and reduce charge neutralization.

Anionic Surfactants

Anionic surfactants are characterized by a negatively charged hydrophilic polar group. Examples of anionic surfactants are ammonium lauryl sulfate, sodium laureth sulfate, sodium lauryl sarcosinate, sodium myreth sulfate, sodium pareth sulfate, sodium stearte, sodium lauryl sulfate, α olefin sulfonate, and ammonium laureth sulfate.[1,2] Although very good in removing sebum and dirt, anionic surfactants are strong cleaners and may cause an increase in electrical negative charges on the hair surface and increase frizz and friction. To minimize damage, other surfactants called secondary surfactants, such as nonionic and amphoteric surfactants, are added to the formulation.

TABLE 27.1
Classification of Surfactants

SHAMPOO SURFACTANTS		
Class	**Example**	**Characteristics**
Anionic	Ammonium lauryl sulfate, sodium laureth sulfate, sodium lauryl sarcosinate, sodium myreth sulfate, sodium pareth sulfate, sodium stearate, sodium lauryl sulfate, α olefin sulfonate, ammonium laureth sulfate	Deep cleansing
Cationic	Trimethylalkylammonium chlorides and the chlorides or bromides of benzalkonium and alkylpyridinium ions	Hair softener Mild cleansing
Nonionic	Fatty alcohols, cetyl alcohol, stearyl alcohol, cetostearyl alcohol (consisting predominantly of cetyl and stearyl alcohols), and oleyl alcohol	Mild cleansing
Amphoteric	Alkyl iminopropionates and (amido) betaines	Do not irritate the eyes Moderate cleansing

Cationic Surfactants

Cationic surfactants have a positively charged hydrophilic end. Typical examples are trimethylalkylammonium chlorides and the chlorides or bromides of benzalkonium and alkylpyridinium ions.[1,2] All are examples of *quats*, so named because they all contain a quaternary ammonium ion. They tend to neutralize the negatively charged net of the hair surface and minimize frizz. They are often used as shampoo softeners.

Amphoteric Surfactants

For the amphoteric surfactants the charge of the hydrophilic part is controlled by the pH of the solution. This means that they can act as anionic surfactant in an alkaline solution or as cationic surfactant in an acidic solution. They are very mild and have excellent dermatologic properties. There are two types of amphoteric compounds: alkyl iminopropionates and (amido) betaines.[1]

Nonionic Surfactants

Nonionic surfactants have no electric charge. They do not ionize in aqueous solutions because their hydrophilic group is nondissociable. Many long-chain alcohols exhibit some surfactant properties. Prominent among these are the fatty alcohols, cetyl alcohol, stearyl alcohol, cetostearyl alcohol (consisting predominantly of cetyl and stearyl alcohols), and oleyl alcohol.

Conditioning Shampoos

It is common to use cationic ingredients in many shampoos' formulations with anionic surfactants to induce charge neutralization. Conditioning ingredients can promote different attributes of wet and dry hair. However, if a conditioning shampoo is applied to oily hair, it may have a negative effect and may cause build-up and oiliness. Bleached and chemically treated hair have the higher affinity to conditioning ingredients, because they have a low isoelectric point (higher concentration of negative sites) and are more porous than virgin hair. Functions of the conditioning agents are the following:

- improve combability
- imitate the hair natural lipid outer layer
- restore hydrofobicity
- seal the cuticle
- avoid or minimize frizz and friction: neutralize the negative charged net
- enhance shine, smoothness, and manageability

The conditioning ingredients that are normally added to shampoos are cationic surfactants (polyquaternium-7, polyquaternium-10, polyquaternium-44, polyquaternium-87, guar hydroxypropyltrimonium chloride), polymers, and polypeptides (such as hydrolyzed keratin of animal or vegetable origin).[1] They may be combined with silicone emulsions (called 2-in-1 shampoo), vegetable, and mineral oils.

Silicones are hybrid (inorganic-organic) inert, heat-resistant, and rubberlike polymers derived from crystal quartz. Silica (silicon dioxide) is common in sandstone and beach sand. Dimethicone is the most widely used silicone in hair care industry and entropy is important for its adsorption to the hair surface.[1,5] Other silicones include aminosilicones, siloxysilicates, anionic silicones, and so on. They differ by deposition and solubility in a water medium, therefore acting differently on the hair. Some silicones can enhance the shine of the hair fiber by reflecting the light. Dimethicone has the effect of protecting the hair shaft from abrasive actions, whereas siloxysilicates increase hair volume. Hydrophobic silicones are not rinsed by surfactants and may deposit to the hair fiber surface and under the cuticle scales leading to hair build-up.

Polysiloxane polymers may recement lifted cuticle scales and are believed to prevent damage from heat, although there is no scientific evidence. Dimethicones are hydrophobic, so they adsorb better on virgin hair and root rather than tips. To enhance the deposition of dimethicone on chemical-treated and damaged hair, the products use cationic bridging agents such as amino functional silicones, which increase the affinity between hair and the silicone.

Other polymers are polypeptides and proteins that are important for the hair because they have many ionic and polar sites for bonding and are large molecules to attach to the hair surface (van der Waals force). Small molecules can even diffuse into hair (smaller than 1000 Da), especially on damaged hair. Protein hydrolysates, in particular those with low-molecular-weight distribution, have been known to protect hair against chemical and environmental damage. Many types of protein hydrolysates from plants and animals have been used in hair and personal care, such as keratin hydrolysates obtained from nails, horns, and wool. A higher amount of protein is deposited on chemical-treated hair, especially bleached. As the hydrolyzed aminoacids are positively charged, it is possible that the negative charge of the damaged hair attracts the positively charged molecules, neutralizing the electrical charges and diminishing frizz and friction.

Keratin hydrolysates are usually prepared from keratin-containing animal parts, such as feathers, horns, hoofs, hair, and wool, collected from discarded materials. Some industries have developed products that use a complex of non–animal-free amino acids derived from wheat, corn, and soy proteins to mimic the natural composition of keratin. However, keratin is an irreplaceable protein in respect to its mechanical and protective properties and the using of aminoacids do not replace or restore the damaged molecule structure.

MINERAL AND VEGETABLE OILS

Oils play an important role in protecting hair from damage. Some oils can penetrate the hair and reduce the amount of water absorbed, thus reducing the swelling. This can result in lower hygral fatigue (repeated swelling and drying), a factor that can damage hair. The oil can fill the gap between the cuticle cells and prevent the penetration of the aggressive substances such as surfactants into the follicle. Applying oil on a regular basis can enhance lubrication of the shaft and help prevent hair breakage. The most used oils are mineral oil, coconut oil, and sunflower oil.[6-9] *Coconut oil* may reduce the protein loss for both undamaged and damaged

hair when used as a prewash and postwash grooming product.[10,11] Coconut oil, being a triglyceride of lauric acid (principal fatty acid), has a high affinity for hair proteins and, because of its low molecular weight and straight linear chain, is able to penetrate inside the hair shaft. *Sunflower oil* is a triglyceride of linoleic acid with a bulky structure and double bonds and has limited penetration to the fiber, not reaching the cortex.[11] The mineral oil and the sunflower oil may have a film effect and adsorb to the surface of the cuticle, enhancing shine and diminishing friction and for these, avoid hair damage.[11] The reduction of combing forces is a combination of water wetting and the lubricant effects of the oil on the fibers. The Brazilian nut, passion fruit seed, palm oil, buriti oil, and mineral oils produce combing force reduction. *Mineral oil* has no affinity to hair's proteins and is not able to diffuse in the fiber.[10,11] The main effects of mineral oil are its higher spreading capability on the hair surface, which improves gloss, combing ease, and reduction in split end formation.

Although coconut oil penetrates the fiber and mineral oil does not, there is equivalent reduction on water sorption for both oils.[11] Increasing the thickness of the oil layer on the fiber surface increases hair moisture regain. The oil that remains in the cuticle layer and not the oil that penetrates the cortex is the one responsible for the decrease in the water pick up.[10-12]

Marrocan argan oil has become very popular as a hair cosmetic main ingredient, referred as capable of keeping the hair moisturized and hydrophobic.[13,14] The argan tree (*Argania spinosa* [L.] Skeels) is an endemic tree in Morocco. The oil is rich in tocopherols and polyphenols, which are powerful antioxidants.[13-15] *Argan oil* is extracted from the kernels of argan fruits that have been sun-dried for either a few days or up to several weeks. The fruit drying time influences the quality of the extracted oil. Although there is scientific literature about the use of the marrocan oil for chronic conditions such as atherosclerosis and psoriasis because of its cardioprotective properties, there is a lack of data about the benefits for hair care.

SHAMPOO PH AND HAIR FRIZZ

The pH at which a protein or particle has an equivalent number of total positive and negative charges is called the isoionic point. The pH at which a protein or particle does not migrate in an electric field is the isoelectric point. The isoelectric point is around a 3.67 pH. The isoionic point is around 5.6. The hair reaches neutrality of charges when the pH is between 3.67 and 5.6.[1,3] Alkaline products may cause an increase in the negativity of the electric network of the hair, an increase in static electricity, and the repulsion between shafts: the so called "hair frizz." To reduce friction between fibers and to allow an adequate access for treatment of the scalp, a capillary cosmetic should not go beyond pH 5.5; this prevents a significant increase in static electricity and hair frizz. Pediatric shampoos, for example, usually have the "no tear" concept and therefore a pH around 7.0 and are not indicated for chemically treated hair without being followed by an antistatic hair conditioner.[1,3] Companies are not required to specify the pH of the shampoo. According to the work of Dias et al., most of the analyzed shampoos presented a pH higher than 5.5.

SHAMPOOS AND ALLERGY

Shampoos contain a wide spectrum of potential allergens, presenting a significant challenge for patients who have positive patch-test reactions to shampoo ingredients. Common allergens in shampoos include fragrance, cocamidopropyl betaine, Methylchloroisothiazolinone/methylisothiazolinone, formaldehyde-releasing preservatives, propylene glycol, vitamin E (tocopherol), parabens, benzophenones, iodopropynyl butyl carbamate, and methyldibromo glutaronitrile/phenoxyethanol.[4,16] Allergic contact dermatitis from shampoo can present as eyelid dermatitis, facial dermatitis, neck dermatitis, scalp dermatitis, and dermatitis of the upper back. Many of the relevant allergens are also irritants, which leads to possible false-positive results on patch testing. Although it is very difficult to find a hypoallergenic shampoo, owing to their transient contact of the shampoo with the skin surface, they are less likely to cause allergic contact dermatitis compared with leave-on products. Some of the ingredients such as fragrances are considered trade secrets, and companies are not required to list the specific chemicals. Therefore, patch-testing to a specific fragrance may be very difficult, leading to possible false-positive/-negative reactions. In case of doubt, a fragrance-free shampoo should be recommended first.

DIFFERENT TYPES OF COSMETIC SHAMPOOS

There are no scientific data about how shampoos are differently formulated regarding different types of hair and scalp. However, the market offers many types of shampoos apparently formulated differently according to hair type. The difference among them is in the concentration and type of surfactants and presence or absence of conditioning agents. Unfortunately, the percentage of those ingredients as well as the final shampoo pH is usually a trade secret, and the industry is not required to disclose the complete information.

In this chapter, we offer our practical hair care guidelines for different hair types.

Hair Care Guidelines for Different Hair Types
Oily hair and scalp
Oily virgin scalp and hair need daily shampoo with anionic surfactants as main ingredients. Shampoo must be reapplied. If the hair is short and virgin, there is no need for conditioning. If the hair is chemically treated or long, a light conditioner may be used without touching the scalp. There is no need for leave-in products or the hair will look dull.

Dry virgin hair
Shampooing may be daily or every other day. A shampoo with anionic surfactants combined with secondary surfactants and cationic polymers is indicated to avoid excess dryness of the fibers. The shampoo maybe repeated if needed. Conditioners with silicones must be used after shampoo and fully rinsed off. Leave-on products may be used for medium and long hair.

Normal hair
Needs a shampoo with anionic surfactants combined with secondary surfactants and cationic polymers to avoid excess dryness of the fibers. The shampoo maybe repeated if needed. Normal hair may be washed everyday in warm and humid weather, but less frequently in cold and dry weather. Medium to long hair will need a conditioner with silicones and oils to be used after every shampoo and a deep conditioner (mask) at least once a week. Leave-in product may be used if the hair is long and curly or wavy. In case the hair is chemically treated, the indicated shampoo may be alternated with a milder shampoo that contains secondary surfactants as the main ingredient (if the shampoo contains lauryl/laureth sodium sulfate, which comes last on the label, after all other surfactants) and cationic polymers. Long normal curly hair may need to be detangled while wet. In this case, combing may be done during conditioning. Start with the tips and work upward to the root. Rinse off thoroughly or the product will remain and lift the scales causing dullness. Clarifying shampoo must be used carefully at least once a month, followed by a deep moisturizing mask.

Oily scalp and dry hair

This is a very common problem for skin phototype III, of Hispanic and Asian ethnicity. The scalp needs a frequent and intense cleansing, but the fibers need conditioning and lubrication. The tips are usually dry, and trichoptilosis is frequently seen in chemically treated hair or due to harsh combing and grooming. Film-forming conditioners, quaternary ammonium compounds and silicones are necessary to minimize friction between the fibers and improve manageability. If high detergency is needed, the harsh effect of the shampoo will be neutralized by the moisturizer ingredients of the conditioner. In wet environment, the frizzing effect caused by humidity may be neutralized by a more frequent application of antifrizz conditioning ingredients either as an after-shampoo rinse-off conditioner/mask or as a leave-in product. The last one may be applied to dry or wet hair. If applied on a daily basis, without shampooing, it may lead to cuticle opening due to deposition of highly insoluble molecules (residues). Clarifying shampoos are needed at least once a month or whenever the hair begins to feel oily and dull, to remove excess of residues. A deep conditioner and a protein conditioner may be needed once a week.

Bleached hair

Bleaching is the most damaging procedure applied to the hair. Shampooing should be mild, with low-handling technique. Lubrication and increase of strength are both very necessary. Mild shampoos with low concentration of anionic surfactants and high levels of conditioning agents, such as silicones, quats, and oils, are needed after every shampoo. Cleansing frequency will depend on the level of scalp oiliness, but harsh shampoos are not indicated. For oily scalp, a daily cleansing may be necessary, if the environment is wet and humid. Dry environment needs less shampooing. The hair shaft is usually thinner on the tips, representing protein loss. Proteinaceous material cannot be replaced, but treatment with hydrolyzed aminoacids may, temporarily, increase the strength of the fiber and improve resistance to breakage. Lubrication is very important during every step of cleaning and grooming. If a hair dryer is used, it is important to protect the fiber with high substantive silicones that restore the broken cuticle and diffuse the heat through the hair length, minimizing heat damage. Finger combing with the help of a lubricating silicone serum, with or without heat, may avoid hair breakage. Low-pH products will neutralize negative electrical charges and improve manageability, as well as detangling. Baby shampoos

are too alkaline and not suitable for bleached hair, even though they carry mild surfactants. All 2-in-1 shampoos must be used with care, because they may not offer proper moisturization and lubrication. Bleached hair needs deep conditioning once or twice a week.

Seborrheic Dermatitis in Different Hair Types

The most used antidandruff substances are azoles, hydroxypyridones, zinc pyrithione, coal tar, salicylic acid, and selenium disulfide.

Oily hair

The use of antidandruff shampoos is not a problem for patients with oily hair and scalp. They usually tolerate well the most used substances, such as ketoconazole, salicylic acid, or zinc pyrithione. The antidandruff effect is highly dependent on the amount of active ingredient delivered to the scalp, and most of the shampoos also contain surfactants with a high cleansing property (anionic surfactants). Daily use of antidandruff shampoos are highly recommended and well accepted by patients with this type of hair. Damaged hair with oily and seborrheic scalp may use silicone-free, light, rinse-off conditioners.

Dry hair

The use of antidandruff shampoo may be restricted to two or three applications per week. Zinc pyrithione is better accepted than ketoconazole. In case of oily scalp, antidandruff shampoo may be alternated with normal scalp shampoo on a daily basis. Dry and curly hair may alternate with a mild surfactant shampoo. Light silicone conditioners may be used, but deep conditioners may increase seborrhea. Corticosteroids may be used in lotions. Alcoholic solutions should be avoided.

Chemically treated hair

Dry hair should be shampooed only two to three times a week, at least twice with antidandruff shampoo. If hair is too damaged, it is preferable to use lotions or nonalcoholic solutions containing antiseborrheic agents applied directly to the scalp, and in this case, shampoos may be used according to the suggestions made to dry hair without seborrheic dermatitis. Silicones conditioners and deep conditioners are needed but should not be applied to the scalp.

Natural African hair

In African hair, friction between hair fibers is increased by antidandruff shampoos. In this case, it is preferable to use lotions or nonalcoholic solutions containing antiseborrhea agents applied directly to the scalp every night until control of the symptoms is achieved. Antidandruff shampoos may be used once a week, but followed by deep conditioners and leave-in products. A mild regular shampoo may be alternated once a week.

Relaxed African hair

Relaxed textured hair has a better manageability than natural African hair; therefore, antidandruff shampoos may be applied to the scalp twice a week. Zinc pyrithione and salicylic acid are better tolerated than ketoconazole but direct application on the hair fiber should be avoided. If corticosteroids are needed, they must be prescribed in lotions or nonalcoholic solutions. Deep conditioners and leave-in conditioners may worsen the scalp desquamation if applied to the scalp. Mild regular shampoos may be alternated once a week.

Natural curly hair

Antidandruff shampoos may be used, but azoles are not so well tolerated as zinc pyrithione or salicylic acid. Mild regular shampoo may be alternated. Oily scalp may use it every other day. Dry scalp may use it two to three times a week followed by a silicone conditioner. Deep conditioner may be used less frequently, every 15 days.

Asian hair

Asian hair usually has oily scalp and therefore tolerates general antidandruff shampoos on a daily basis or every other day. Asian hair is course straight hair and needs a silicone conditioner to minimize tangling and friction between fibers. Conditioner should not be applied close to the scalp but remain at least 1 cm away from the scalp.

Shampoos for Special Scenarios
Oily straight Caucasian virgin hair

This type of hair usually needs to increase volume. Highly detergent surfactants are usually the choice for a fresh clean look, but excess washing without conditioning may cause hair damage by removing the 18-methyl eicosanoic acid (MEA) and cuticle scales. It is important to alternate with mild shampoos and use silicone-free conditioners. Leave-in products may weigh-down the hair.

Oily straight Caucasian virgin hair with dry tips

This type needs deep moisturization of the hair length without weighing down the whole hair. The use of high cleansing surfactants should be applied only to the scalp and in a very small quantity. A deep moisturizer with silicone has to be applied only to the tips (down from the middle of the hair). If the hair is combed while wet and before rinsing, conditioner may reach the scalp and increase oiliness. A silicone serum maybe applied to the tips during styling.

Wavy/curly virgin hair with dry tips and oily scalp

Oily scalp may be treated by increasing shampoo frequency with mild surfactants. The hair length may be first protected with a pool of vegetable oils or leave-in products to avoid contact of the shampoo with the shaft during rinsing. The oils may be applied overnight and rinsed next morning. Low-pH shampoos are mild products with a good performance. High pH shampoos must definitely be avoided because they increase frizz and impair tangling and fiber friction. Shampoos with silicones may increase scalp oiliness and should be used less frequently.

Relaxed African hair

Relaxed, straightened hair is a sensible fragile hair, very prone to breakage, which has suffered protein and 18-MEA loss during hair procedures.[17] Physical manipulation is one of the main causes of hair damage to textured hair. Shampoo may be applied as frequent as needed according to the necessity of hygiene. Detergency of the shampoo must be low, but for patients who wash the hair only once a week, it is necessary to use a more detergent surfactant shampoo. One way to diminish frizz caused by the use of anionic surfactants on African hair is the use of a second shampoo, this time a conditioning shampoo. This procedure may help if done before conditioning and allows a deeper removal of dirt and oiliness from the scalp. On the other hand, the frequent use of conditioning shampoos may lead to weigh down the hair and build up. In this case, the patient will need to use a clarifying shampoo at least every 6–8 weeks. Deep conditioners and protein conditioners are needed once a week and may be used separately or combined. To protect the fiber during washing, a combination of vegetable oils may be applied at least 20 min before shampoo or the night before washing. Another option would be the use of night repair leave-in products.

Bleached hair with Brazilian keratin treatment

This type should follow the instructions for bleached hair but need to increase shampoo frequency because of excess of scalp oiliness. Shampoos with pH higher than 5.5 should be avoided, because they may increase friction and frizz.[18] Direct application of conditioners, leave-in, and silicones on the scalp must be avoided.

Asian perm hair
Same instructions apply as for relaxed hair.

Wavy/curly relaxed hair with oily scalp and dry tips
This is the most common hair problem. The hair shaft is fragile and needs conditioning and lubrication but the scalp needs a medium to high detergent shampoo. The hair is too fragile with lack of lipids and protein loss. This hair needs treatments with silicones, oils, and aminoacids after every shampoo. Deep conditioners and concentrated hydrolyzed aminoacid serums may be applied once in every 15 days, for example, the first one at home and the latter at the salon. Shampoo must be applied three times a week with the proper care of low-handling grooming and combing. Hair should be protected with a silicone serum if blow-dried. Mild shampoos are preferable to deep cleansing shampoos but the latter may be used once a month to avoid residues.

Shampoos for Children
Straight Caucasian hair and Asian hair
Naturally straight hair, Caucasian or Asian, usually easily adapts to regular baby shampoos. Scalp may be washed daily and if the hair is long it may need a baby conditioner to help detangling and styling. There is no need for leave-in products except if combing is difficult. In this case moisturizing wet hair during grooming may help, but it can also make fine Caucasian hair look dull if used in excess.

Hair care in children with textured or curly/wavy/Hispanic hair
Textured and curly hair is difficult to comb after shampoo. Although the hair is virgin and the 18-MEA is intact, the curliness of the hair causes more frizz and fiber friction.[19-22] Baby shampoo has to be applied to damp scalp in small portions. The hair must be divided in at least four parts and shampoo applied separately to each region of the scalp, followed by a low-handling rubbing process, as if applying a cream to the skin. Washing should be thorough. Water is gently towel dried, followed by the application of a child shampoo. Course and full hair may need adult silicone conditioner to lubricate the fiber during next step: combing. Combing hair while wet can be made with care only if a moisturizer has been applied to the whole hair and the hair is divided in parts. Combing begins with the tips and moves upward toward the root. After the whole hair has been detangled, it should be rinsed thoroughly, avoiding the conditioner to touch the scalp. A leave-in product is only needed to thick coarse full hair.

Hair care with braids or dreadlocks
Hair care for children with curly and coarse hair is sometimes a challenge to the parents. This is one reason why sometimes the use of braids, locks, and weaves are considered the best choice for some children. Extended periods of time between hair cleansings instead of avoiding hair stress may increase hair damage and seborrheic dermatitis of the scalp, even in children. Dreadlocks are supposed to last longer, but braids should be removed at least every 3 months, with low-manipulation hair-handling.

If the child has irremovable braids and weaves or dreadlocks, a gentle child shampoo may be used and applied to the skin between the braids where the scalp can be seen and gently scrubbed. Scalp and hair must be rinsed in warm water before shampooing. Gently work the shampoo lather down the braids in a squeezing fashion. Shampoos can be transferred to squeeze bottles or applicators for precise placement between tracks along cornrow lines and braids extensions. Hair must be shampooed at least twice a week to avoid bad smell. After rinsing, gently pat dry the hair with a microfiber towel and allow the hair to air dry. A dryer set on low temperature may speed the process. However, there is always the risk of fungus infection if the hair is wet for too long or too moisturized. After rinsing thoroughly, there is no need for conditioning. Excess of conditioners may keep the tresses too moisturized and delay dryness. Sprays can reach the fiber better than creams or oils. Water with essential oils may be sprayed to the locks or the braids to moisturize the hair. The use of pomades or gels are sometimes necessary to restyle lose fibers, but greasy products should be avoided. Antidandruff shampoos with zinc pyrithione may be applied with the same technique. Start with a 1% Zinc pyrithione gentle shampoo. This procedure is the same as in adults, except that adults will need a protein-balancing treatment at least once a month. Protein-based sprays may enhance the hair strength, especially if the hair is chemically treated.

Children with curly or textured hair
Sometimes it is necessary to detangle curly hair before washing using a leave-in conditioner on to wet hair. The hair must be divided in parts: two parts on the front and two on the back of the head. Detangling the hair must begin with finger combing in a very gentle way. After the tightest knots are removed, a large teeth wooden comb may be used. The detangling process should begin with the tips and afterward climb up to the roots. Once the hair is combed, it must be damped in the shower and baby/children shampoo applied to

the scalp. A small amount of shampoo, the size of a penny coin, is applied to the scalp, first to the front, then to the sides, and last to the occipital region and gently until the entire scalp is covered. Shampoo must not be applied to the hair length, but it will reach the fibers during rinsing, from root to tips. Children shampoo has a no-tear property. Therefore, it has a pH of 7.0, just like the teardrops. This is very alkaline compared with the hair pH (3.67), and it has the capacity to open the cuticle scales and swallow the cortex.[21,22]The hair must be carefully towel dried before conditioning. Gentle adults shampoo may be used with care. Usually a child shampoo has the so-called "less-aggressive sulfate-free" surfactants, although there is no scientific data proving that sulfate-free surfactants are more gentle than sulfate surfactants. For children with natural hair, cationic polymers are especially helpful in reinforcing curl patterns and detangling. Children's virgin hair does not need nourishing or protein treatments. It only needs detangling and less frizz. A normal baby conditioner may be used for children before puberty, but if the hair is too coarse, an adult's conditioner with silicone and vegetable oils (coconut, jojoba, or castor oil) may be used. Extremely thick and full African or Hispanic hair may benefit from a regular adult rinse-out conditioner. If left to air dry, the coarse full hair may be better managed with a small amount of leave-in product before combing. Use the same combing process as before shampooing. Silicone or leave-in products should be used during styling.

Children with seborrheic dermatitis

If the child has seborrheic dermatitis and curly thick hair, even blond or red, there is a difficulty in applying a medical shampoo. Zinc pyrithione is the most acceptable antidandruff substance for curly hair, because it leads to less drying and stiffness. Avoid ketoconazole shampoo because it causes more friction between the fibers. Sometimes increasing the frequency of shampooing is enough to treat scalp desquamation, even with a regular product. If a medicated shampoo is needed, alternating regiments may be tried first: 1 day with zinc pyrithione and the next day with regular shampoo. It is necessary to apply a conditioner in both situations and rinse it thoroughly. In some countries, scalp solutions with zinc or salicylic acid are available and may be applied as a seborrheic dermatitis treatment instead of a shampoo. When corticosteroids are needed, lotions or creams are better choices than alcoholic solutions vehicles. Avoid conditioning shampoos for those who present with seborrheic dermatitis. The use of astringents or dry shampoos is popular in some countries and may be an option for those who wear hair locks or braids for long periods.

Although many curly and thick-hair individuals believe that their dry hair is caused by frequent shampooing, it actually may be due to inappropriate use of hair care products and regimens that are not ideal for their hair type. Cleansing with a shampoo that eliminates residues is recommended every 15 days for those who use leave-in products or heavy conditioners, even children.

Antiresidue Shampoos

Removing the residues without stripping the fiber is possible if antiresidue shampooing (laureth ammonium-sulfate) is followed by the application of a thick moisturizing hair mask preferably containing hydrolyzed aminoacids, silicones, and vegetable oils.[22] An antiresidue shampoo may be used each 10 shampooings, or even more frequently, depending on the need. Extremely highlighted hair is the most sensible to antiresidue formulations. In this type of hair, it may be used less frequently or not at all.

Considerations About the Hair Washing and Grooming Procedures

Shampoo must be applied on the scalp more than on the hair. The entire scalp has to be rubbed with the shampoo from the front to the back and small amounts of shampoo have to be applied on each region of the head under the hair. Applying the shampoo on the top of the head will increase hair friction and cause hair tangling. After full rinse of the shampoo, the hair must be gently towel dried and the conditioner should be applied on the hair length avoiding the scalp. Application of hair conditioners after shampoo will lower interfiber friction and reduce combing forces. If the hair is curly, leave-on products may be used during wet combing. The use of leave-on products on straight virgin hair may cause an oily look and make the hair dull. Gentle hair dealing actions (gentle shampooing, gentle towel drying, and gentle brushing or combing) are recommended. Many products may be used to lubricate and seal cuticle cells, such as silicones (dimethicone and aminoterminal silicones) and vegetable oils.

REFERENCES

1. Abraham LS, Moreira AM, Moura LH, Dias MF. Hair care: a medical overview (part 1). *Surg Cosmet Dermatol.* 2009;1(3):130–136.
2. O'lenick T. Anionic/cationic complexes in hair care. *J Cosmet Sci.* 2011;62:209–228.

3. Abraham LS, Moreira AM, Moura LH, Dias MF. Hair care: a medical overview (part 2). *Surg Cosmet Dermatol.* 2009;1(4):178–185.

4. Trüeb RM. Shampoos: composition and clinical applications. *Hautarzt.* 1998;49:895–901.

5. Bolduc C, Shapiro J. Hair care products: waving, straightening, conditioning, and coloring. *Clin Dermatol.* 2001; 19(4):431–436.

6. Draelos ZD. Shampoos, conditioners, and camouflage techniques. *Dermatol Clin.* 2013;31(1):173–178.

7. La Torre C, Bhushan B. Nanotribological effects of silicone type, silicone deposition level, and surfactant type on human hair using atomic force microscopy. *J Cosmet Sci.* 2006;57(1):37–56.

8. Nazir H, Lv P, Wang L, et al. Uniform-sized silicone oil microemulsions: preparation, investigation of stability and deposition on hair surface. *J Colloid Interface Sci.* 2011;364(1):56–64.

9. Nazir H, Wang L, Lian G, et al. Multilayered silicone oil droplets of narrow size distribution: preparation and improved deposition on hair. *Colloids Surf B Biointerfaces.* 2012;1(100):42–49.

10. Gode V, Bhalla N, Shirhhatis V, Mhaskar S, Kamath Y. Quantitative measurement of the penetration of coconut oil into human hair using radiolabeled coconut oil. *J Cosmet Sci.* 2012;63:27–31.

11. Rele AS, Mohile RB. Effect of mineral oil, sunflower oil, and coconut oil on prevention of hair damage. *J Cosmet Sci.* 2003;54(2):175–192.

12. Keis K, Huemmer CL, Kamath YK. Effect of oil films on moisture vapor absorption on human hair. *J Cosmet Sci.* 2007;58:135–145.

13. López LC, Cabrera-Vique C, Venegas C, et al. Argan oil-contained antioxidants for human mitochondria. *Nat Prod Commun.* 2013;8(1):47–50.

14. Harhar H, Gharby S, Kartah BE, El Monfalouti H, Charrouf Z, Guillaume D. Long argan fruit drying time is detrimental for argan oil quality. *Nat Prod Commun.* 2010;5(11):1799–1802.

15. El Abbassi A, Khalid N, Zbakh H, Ahmad A. Physicochemical characteristics, nutritional properties, and health benefits of argan oil: a review. *Crit Rev Food Sci Nutr.* 2014;54(11):1401–1414.

16. Shapiro J, Maddin S. Medicated shampoos. *Clin Dermatol.* 1996;14(1):123–128.

17. McMichael AJ. Hair breakage in normal and weathered hair: focus on the black patient. *J Invest Dermatol Sym Proc.* 2007;12:6–9.

18. Weathersby C, McMichael A. Brazilian keratin hair treatment: a review. *J Cosmet Dermatol.* 2013;12(2):144–148.

19. Syed AN. Ethnic hair care products. In: Johnson DH, ed. *Hair and Hair Care.* Vol. 17. New York: Marcel Dekker; 1997:235–259.

20. Khumalo NP, Doe PT, Dawber RP, Ferguson DJ. What is normal black African hair? A light and scanning electron-microscopic study. *J Am Acad Dermatol.* 2000;43:814–820.

21. Morelli JG, Weston WL. Soaps and shampoos in pediatric practice. *Pediatrics.* 1987;80:634–637.

22. Gavazzoni Dias MF, de Almeida AM, Cecato PM, Adriano AR, Pichler J. The shampoo pH can affect the hair: myth or reality? *Int J Trichology.* 2014;6(3):95–99.

CHAPTER 28

Hair Supplements

JANNETT NGUYEN, MD • DOROTA Z. KORTA, MD, PHD •
NATASHA A. MESINKOVSKA, MD, PHD

INTRODUCTION

The impact of nutrition on hair has been historically studied in the context of malnutrition and nutritional deficiency. For example, in states of severe protein malnutrition such as kwashiorkor, hairs are short, dull, decreased in diameter, and easily plucked.[1,2] Furthermore, diffuse hair loss may be an early sign of niacin deficiency or pellagra.[2,3] Although nutritional deficiencies are relatively rare in developed countries, high-risk groups include alcoholics, pregnant women, infants, and individuals with prior gastrointestinal surgeries or malabsorption disorders.[4] Given the known association between nutritional deficiency and hair health, it is not surprising that there are many dietary supplements on the market that claim to promote hair growth.

According to the United States Food and Drug Administration (FDA), a dietary supplement is a "product intended for ingestion that contains a 'dietary ingredient' intended to add further nutritional value to the diet." Dietary ingredients may include vitamins, minerals, herbs or botanicals, amino acids, concentrates, metabolites, constituents, or extracts.[5] In the United States, dietary supplements are considered "foods" and not "drugs" and as such are not subject to FDA review for safety or efficacy.

Because most hair supplements can be marketed without FDA approval, there are limited clinical studies evaluating their claims for efficacy and safety in treating hair conditions. We review the current evidence for the role of dietary supplements and their derivatives in the treatment of hair loss and provide recommendations regarding their use (Table 28.1).

MICRONUTRIENTS
Vitamins

Vitamins are common ingredients in over-the-counter hair supplements. Several studies have investigated the association between vitamin deficiency and alopecia and evaluated the efficacy of vitamins and their derivatives in the treatment of hair loss.

Vitamin A

Vitamin A is a fat-soluble group of compounds that includes retinol, retinal, retinoic acid, and β-carotenoids. These compounds play role in immune function, vision, reproduction, and cell growth and differentiation.[6] For example, in the skin, vitamin A promotes cell division, increases epithelial thickness, and stimulates dermal collagen and glycosaminoglycan synthesis.[7] In the diet, yellow-orange fruits and vegetables are rich in provitamin A carotenoids, and animal liver is rich in preformed retinol. Individuals with vitamin A deficiency may manifest with night blindness, dry eyes, and dry skin. Although uncommon in developed countries, vitamin A deficiency can result from inadequate dietary intake, conditions associated with fat malabsorption (e.g., cystic fibrosis), or excess alcohol intake, which depletes vitamin A stores in the liver.[6] Deficiency can be treated with dietary modification or oral supplementation. However, excess vitamin A has been linked to hair loss, seborrhea, generalized xerosis, and bone changes.[8]

Vitamin A and its derivatives are involved in the development and maintenance of many epithelial structures, including the hair follicle. For example, mice lacking vitamin A receptors have permanent hair loss due to follicle disintegration during catagen.[9] The role of vitamin A in alopecia is complex, and details involving its contribution to pathogenesis remain unclear. Dietary vitamin A appears to influence pathogenesis in mouse models of alopecia areata (AA) and cicatricial alopecia (CA), and precise levels influence disease development and severity.[9] In a mouse model of AA, high dietary vitamin A accelerated disease onset. However, a vitamin A–deficient diet resulted in gradual onset, but more severe disease over time.[10] In contrast, in a model of CA, mice fed excess levels of vitamin A (seven times the recommended level) developed less severe alopecia when compared with mice fed two times the recommended level of vitamin A.[11] The effects of dietary vitamin A in disease course or progression in humans with alopecia are unknown.

TABLE 28.1

Evidence and Recommendations for Oral or Topical Supplements for Treatment of Alopecia

Product	Mechanism of Action	Evidence of Clinical Efficacy and Treatment Recommendations
Biotin (vitamin B7)	Cofactor for carboxylase enzymes in the mitochondria. Role in hair unknown[19]	Studies investigating the benefits of oral biotin supplementation in the absence of deficiency are lacking.
Botanically derived phytosterols (β-sitosterol or phytosterol glycosides)	Inhibits 5α-reductase[67]	A RCT suggested that compared to placebo, there was clinical improvement in patients with AGA treated with β-sitosterol 50 mg and phytosterol glycosides (from saw palmetto extract) 200 mg twice daily.[68] Studies evaluating safety and efficacy of botanically derived 5-α-reductase inhibitors for treatment of alopecia are very limited. Practitioners should be aware that patients have access to these products over-the-counter.
Caffeine	Inhibits phosphodiesterase, increases cyclic adenine monophosphate, and decreases the effects of dihydrotestosterone on hair follicle[60]	Shampoo and lotion formulations of caffeine may increase hair tensile strength in patients with AGA.[62,63] The number of studies evaluating efficacy of topical caffeine is limited. There are no randomized clinical trials.
Fatty acids	Some unsaturated fatty acids may inhibit 5α-reductase.[57] Arachidonic acid may promote hair growth by inducing and prolonging anagen[58]	A RCT studying women with FPHL demonstrated that compared to placebo, 6-month oral supplementation with a combination of ω-3 and ω-6 fatty acids (fish and blackcurrant seed oils) and antioxidants (lycopene, vitamin C, vitamin E) increased hair density and reduced percentage of hairs in telogen, hair loss, and the proportion of miniaturized anagen hair.[59]
Iron	Cofactor in the rate-limiting step in DNA synthesis and is important in rapidly dividing cells.[47] Exact role in hair follicle cycling is unknown	Some studies suggest that iron deficiency may be more prevalent in patients with AA, AGA, TE, and diffuse hair loss, whereas others do not support this association.[48] Patients presenting with alopecia and relevant risk factors should be screened for iron deficiency. Patients with iron deficiency anemia should be treated with iron supplementation or dietary modifications. Ferritin level should be greater than 50 μg/L.[49] The role of iron supplementation in alopecia patients with iron deficiency without anemia is uncertain, although there is some evidence that iron supplementation in this setting could promote hair growth.[50]
Marine extracts	Enhances proliferation of dermal papilla cells and increases expression of alkaline phosphatase, a key marker of anagen[69]	Multiple RCTs have suggested that 3–6 month oral supplementation with marine extracts increases hair count and density and decreases hair shedding. Study populations include women with self-perceived hair loss[71,72] and men with AGA.[70] In current studies, marine protein supplements are well tolerated without adverse events.
Melatonin	Antiandrogenic and antioxidant effects mediated by signaling through the melatonin receptor at the hair follicle[64]	A RCT showed that compared to placebo, a 0.1% melatonin solution increased the number of anagen hairs in patients with AGA and diffuse hair loss.[65] A large nonrandomized prospective study suggested that topical melatonin may decrease the number of hairs pulled on pull test in patients with AGA.[66] The role of oral melatonin is unknown.

TABLE 28.1
Evidence and Recommendations for Oral or Topical Supplements for Treatment of Alopecia—cont'd

Product	Mechanism of Action	Evidence of Clinical Efficacy and Treatment Recommendations
Niacin (vitamin B3)	Signaling through niacin receptors on the skin stimulates the release of leptin, which has downstream effects involved in hair follicle cycling[17]	Niacin is not suitable for topical application because it causes intense vasodilation and has short residence time in the skin. Topical niacin derivatives, such as 0.5% octyl nicotinate and 5.0% tetradecyl nicotinate, may have utility in treating patients with FPHL, but the number of studies exploring this treatment is very limited[18]
Vitamin A (and derivatives)	Tretinoin may promote hair growth by increasing epithelial and vascular proliferation.[12] It also increases percutaneous permeability of minoxidil.[13]	Combination of 0.01% tretinoin and 5% minoxidil daily may achieve similar results as 5% minoxidil twice daily in patients with AGA.[14] The once-daily combination treatment may decrease the burden of twice-daily application of minoxidil.
Vitamin D	Vitamin D receptor is required for normal hair follicle cycling[27]	Topical calcipotriol cream or lotion may be a treatment option for patients with AA.[33,34] Role of oral vitamin D supplementation is unclear.
Vitamin E	Tocotrienols and tocopherols have antioxidant effects. Exact role in hair follicle is unknown	A RCT showed that compared to placebo, daily oral supplementation with mixed tocotrienols (100 mg capsule) increased the number of hairs in normal healthy volunteers without alopecia.[36] The role of oral supplementation of vitamin E in patients with alopecia is unclear.
Zinc	Exact role in hair follicle unknown	Daily oral supplementation with zinc 150 mg for 6–12 months may improve or cure hair loss in patients with zinc deficiency–related TE.[43] Daily oral zinc supplementation did not lead to clinical improvement in AA patients who were not zinc deficient.[44] Patients with zinc deficiency should receive supplementation. There is no evidence for benefits of supplementation in the absence of deficiency.
Zinc pyrithione	Releases zinc ions, which may have anti-inflammatory and antioxidant effects. Zinc ions also inhibit 5α-reductase in the skin.[45]	Zinc pyrithione shampoo alone increases hair count assessed by fiber microscopy but did not lead to global improvement.[45]

FPHL, female pattern hair loss; *RCT*, randomized controlled trial.

Although the role of oral supplementation is not established, topical forms of the vitamin A derivative tretinoin have been investigated as a treatment option alone and in combination with minoxidil for androgenetic alopecia (AGA). Tretinoin promotes hair growth by increasing epithelial and vascular proliferation.[12] In addition, tretinoin increases the permeability of the stratum corneum and increases percutaneous absorption of minoxidil threefold.[13] A randomized controlled trial (RCT) compared twice-daily application of 0.025% tretinoin solution alone and in combination with 5% minoxidil in 56 patients with AGA. After 1 year of treatment, 58% of patients receiving tretinoin alone had hair regrowth, compared to 66% of those receiving the combination.[12] Another RCT compared twice daily 5% minoxidil and once daily combined 5% minoxidil with 0.01% tretinoin in 31 male patients with AGA and found no difference in efficacy.[14] Thus, using a combination of minoxidil and tretinoin may allow patients to achieve similar outcomes without the burden of twice daily treatment.

Niacin (vitamin B3)
Niacin is a water-soluble vitamin that is also known as nicotinic acid or vitamin B3. Nicotinamide, the main

bioactive form of niacin, is used to form nicotinamide adenine dinucleotide (NAD) and nicotinamide adenine dinucleotide phosphate (NADP). NAD is a coenzyme necessary for catabolic energy processes (e.g., metabolism of carbohydrates, fatty acids, proteins), and NADP is involved in anabolic processes (e.g., fatty acid synthesis).[15] Dietary sources of niacin include meat, eggs, and legumes. Niacin can also be synthesized from tryptophan, vitamin B6, and thiamine, and thus, deficiencies of these substrates may also lead to niacin deficiency or pellagra. Pellagra is classically associated with the four "Ds": dermatitis, diarrhea, dementia, and death. However, diffuse hair loss, along with weakness, glossitis, and stomatitis, may be early manifestations.[2,3] Niacin deficiency is rare in developed countries, and isolated hair loss in the absence of the other signs and symptoms of pellagra have not been reported.[16] The most common cause of pellagra in developed countries is alcoholism. Other causes include malabsorption disorders and drug-induced deficiency (e.g., isoniazid).[15] Pellagra can be treated with dietary modification or oral supplementation.

Given their role in cellular energy processes, bioactive forms of niacin are important in rapidly dividing cells, such as those found in the hair follicle. Signaling through niacin receptors in the skin stimulates the release of leptin, which has downstream effects on hair follicle cycling.[17]

Topical niacin derivatives have been explored as a treatment option for patients with female pattern hair loss (FPHL). Notably, niacin is not suitable for topical application because it causes intense vasodilation and has short residence time in the skin. Derivatives such as myristyl (tetradecyl) nicotinate have a longer residence time in the skin, allowing for conversion into NAD. Octyl nicotinate stimulates blood flow to areas of application, enhances delivery of nutrients, and removes metabolic waste products. A RCT compared topical niacin derivatives (0.5% octyl nicotinate and 5.0% tetradecyl nicotinate) versus placebo in 60 patients with Ludwig types I–III FPHL.[18] Treatment efficacy was assessed by comparing standardized 35-mm photographs before and after 6 months of treatment. The group receiving niacin derivatives was noted to have increased hair fullness based on photographic assessment by a blinded investigator. However, it is unclear whether the niacin derivatives increased hair fullness by increasing density of hair follicles or by increasing the quality of existing hair. The treatment was well tolerated; mild adverse events included scalp stinging, burning, and itching. However, these adverse events were reported in both treatment and placebo groups and might therefore be attributable to the vehicle.

Biotin (vitamin B7)

Biotin is a cofactor for carboxylase enzymes found in the mitochondria and is required for fatty acid synthesis.[19] Biotin is found in foods rich in vitamin B, including cereal, legumes, nuts, meats, and dairy. Because intestinal bacteria can synthesize adequate levels of biotin, deficiency is rare. Alterations in gut flora, excess consumption of raw egg whites, ingestion of some antiepileptic drugs, and hereditary biotinidase deficiency are rare causes of biotin deficiency.[20,21] Biotin deficiency presents with several mucocutaneous manifestations including alopecia, scaly erythematous dermatitis, glossitis, and candidiasis.[20] The exact role of biotin in hair biology is unknown, but in vitro studies have suggested that biotin does not affect proliferation and differentiation of normal follicular keratinocytes.[22]

Biotin is one of the most commonly listed components of hair supplements, despite the fact that there are currently no clinical trials investigating the effect of biotin supplementation on hair growth. However, daily oral supplementation with 2.5 mg biotin was shown to increase nail thickness and improve nail texture in brittle nails and onychoschizia.[23] This finding may have stimulated the cross-marketing claim that biotin supplements promote both nail and hair health. One study of 541 healthy women suggested that 38% of those presenting with hair loss have biotin deficiency (<100 ng/L), but this was confounded by other factors, including gastrointestinal disease and medication use.[24] Although there are over a dozen cases of improvement in hair and nail growth after biotin supplementation (10–30 mg daily) in individuals with known biotin deficiency, the role of biotin supplementation in normal, healthy individuals is unknown.[25]

Vitamin D

Vitamin D is a fat-soluble compound that promotes calcium absorption in the gut and is important in calcium and phosphorus homeostasis. In addition to maintaining bone mineralization, vitamin D is involved in modulating cell growth as well as neuromuscular and immune function. Sources of vitamin D include dietary intake and sun exposure. There are limited dietary sources of vitamin D. The highest sources are fatty fish (e.g., salmon, tuna) and fish liver oil. Beef liver, cheese, and egg yolks contain small amounts. In the United States, fortified foods such as milk provide the most vitamin D in the diet. Sun exposure is an additional source of vitamin D. Ultraviolet (UV) light converts 7-dehydrocholesterol in the skin to previtamin D3, which is ultimately converted to vitamin D3. Although UV light promotes vitamin D synthesis, it is important to limit sun exposure to decrease the risk of skin cancer. Severe vitamin D deficiency causes rickets in children and osteomalacia in adults, and long-term insufficiency can contribute to osteoporosis. Risk factors for vitamin D deficiency include lack of UV exposure, exclusively breastfed infants, darker skin pigmentation, and fat malabsorption syndromes.[26] Excess vitamin D can lead to hypercalcemia, which causes weakness, nausea, and vomiting.

The vitamin D receptor is important in Wnt and Hedgehog signaling pathways that regulate hair follicle cycling and anagen initiation.[27] In fact, mice lacking vitamin D receptors have permanent hair loss with follicular disintegration.[9] Although the receptor is known to be critical in the normal hair cycle, the role of vitamin D itself is unclear.

Low serum levels of vitamin D have been associated with several types of alopecia, but it is also important to note that vitamin D deficiency is relatively common in the general population. There is some evidence that patients with AA have lower serum 25-hydroxy vitamin D levels than healthy matched controls, and serum vitamin D levels correlate inversely with disease severity.[28,29] In addition, the prevalence of vitamin D deficiency may be higher in patients with AA than in the general population.[29] However, an analysis based on the Nurses' Health Study cohort of over 50,000 women in the US found that there was no significant association between vitamin D intake and incidence of AA.[30] Finally, studies have suggested that patients with FPHL have lower levels of serum vitamin D3 than healthy controls,[31] and that patients with telogen effluvium (TE) may have a high prevalence of vitamin D deficiency.[32]

Topical vitamin D derivatives have been investigated as treatment options for AA. In a retrospective study of 48 patients with mild-to-moderate AA, 69.2% of patients responded (improved Severity of Alopecia Tool [SALT] score) after treatment with calcipotriol cream twice daily for 12 weeks.[33] A single-arm prospective study of 22 patients with patchy AA (<40% involvement) evaluated the effects of calcipotriol lotion 0.005% applied twice daily. After 12 weeks, 59.1% of patients had improvement in SALT score, and the mean onset to regrowth was 4.2 weeks. Notably, patients who had a lower baseline serum vitamin D level showed a better treatment response.[34] Studies investigating the role of oral vitamin D supplementation in patients with alopecia are lacking.

Vitamin E
Vitamin E is a group of fat-soluble compounds, including tocotrienols and tocopherols. These compounds have antioxidant properties and decrease the production of reactive oxygen species during fatty acid oxidation. Dietary sources of vitamin E include nuts, seeds, and vegetable oils.[35] Deficiency of vitamin E is rare, but is characterized by peripheral neuropathy, ataxia, myopathy, retinopathy, and impaired immunity. Because vitamin E is fat-soluble, individuals with fat malabsorption are at higher risk for deficiency. The exact role of vitamin E in hair biology is not known.

A RCT investigated the effects of twice daily oral supplementation with mixed tocotrienol (50 mg capsule containing 30.8% α-tocotrienol, 56.4% γ-tocotrienol, 12.8% δ-tocotrienol, and 23 IU of α-tocopherol) versus placebo in healthy volunteers without alopecia.[36] After 8 months, the treatment arm had a 34.5% increase in the number of hairs in a predetermined scalp area, compared with a 0.1% decrease in the placebo arm. The role of vitamin E supplementation in patients with alopecia is uncertain. However, excess supplementation with vitamin E has well-documented toxicities, including increased risk of bleeding and hypothyroidism, the latter of which can itself present with hair loss.

Minerals
Humans require essential trace elements in amounts ranging from 50 μg to 18 mg a day.[37] Zinc and iron are the trace elements that have been most studied in patients with hair loss, and supplementation has been explored as treatment options in smaller studies.

Zinc
Zinc is a cofactor for over one hundred metalloenzymes involved in DNA synthesis, protein synthesis, cell division, immune function, and wound healing.[38] Red meat and poultry, beans, nuts, whole grains, and dairy products are dietary sources of zinc. Manifestations of severe zinc deficiency include growth retardation, appetite loss, and decreased immune function.[39,40] Etiologies of deficiency can be nutritional (e.g., parenteral nutrition), hereditary (autosomal recessive acrodermatitis enteropathica), or iatrogenic (e.g., antihypertensive or antiepileptic medications). Other groups at risk include pregnant women, exclusively breastfed infants, and vegetarians. The exact role of zinc in hair follicle cycling is unclear, although low zinc levels have been associated with hair loss.

There is some evidence that zinc levels may be lower in patients with TE and AA than in healthy controls. In a study of 312 alopecia patients (AA, male pattern hair loss, FPHL, and TE), AA and TE patients had lower zinc levels than controls.[41] Furthermore, a recent meta-analysis of over 750 patients with AA showed that serum zinc levels in AA patients are significantly lower than those of healthy controls.[42]

Oral zinc supplementation has been studied as a treatment option in TE and AA. In a small cohort of five patients with zinc deficiency–related TE, daily oral supplementation with zinc, 150 mg for 6–12 months, improved or cured hair loss, with corresponding normalization of serum zinc levels.[43] For AA, a RCT compared the effects of twice daily zinc sulfate supplement (220 mg) with placebo in 42 patients for 3 months. The treatment group had increased serum zinc levels but no clinical improvement.[44] Thus, there is currently a lack of evidence to support oral zinc supplementation in the absence of deficiency. Importantly, oversupplementation of zinc has associated toxicities. Acute toxicity can present with gastrointestinal symptoms (e.g., vomiting, diarrhea) and chronic zinc excess can interfere with iron absorption.

Topical zinc in the form of zinc pyrithione, a common ingredient found in antidandruff shampoos, has also been studied for treatment of hair loss. Zinc pyrithione releases zinc ions, which has anti-inflammatory and antioxidant properties. Zinc ions also inhibit 5α-reductase in the skin.[45] A RCT compared 5% minoxidil (twice daily), 1% zinc pyrithione (once daily), a combination of both, and placebo in 200 patients with AGA. In the group treated with zinc pyrithione alone, there was a significant increase in total visible hair count by fiber optic microscopy and computer-assisted hair counts after 9 weeks. However, there was no clinically meaningful global improvement noted by either the investigator or the patients. Minoxidil alone or in combination with zinc was more efficacious than zinc shampoo alone.[45]

Iron

Iron is a key component of hemoglobin and myoglobin, and is also a cofactor for the rate-limiting step in DNA synthesis. Lean meats, seafood, nuts, beans, vegetables, and grains are dietary sources of iron. Iron is the most common nutritional deficiency in the world and may present with or without anemia. Patients with iron deficiency anemia have impaired immune function, cognition, and exercise or work tolerance. Groups at risk for iron deficiency include infants, pregnant women, women with heavy menstrual periods, cancer patients, and individuals with gastrointestinal disease or malabsorption. Iron supplementation can be delivered orally, intravenously, or parenterally.[46] Because iron is involved in DNA synthesis, it is critical in rapidly dividing cells, such as those in the hair follicle. However, iron's precise role in hair biology is unknown.[47]

Studies exploring the association between iron deficiency and hair loss have reported conflicting conclusions. Although some studies suggest that iron deficiency may be more prevalent in patients with AA, AGA, TE, and diffuse hair loss, others do not support this association.[48] In addition, most studies are limited to female patients with nonscarring alopecia. Given the inconsistencies and limitations of current studies, a consensus does not exist regarding iron deficiency screening for patients with hair loss. One center reported that they screen all patients with alopecia (both scarring and nonscarring types, in men and women) for iron deficiency.[48] Laboratory workup for iron deficiency should include a complete blood count as well as iron studies. Serum ferritin is the favored test, because it has high sensitivity and specificity for detecting low iron stores.[49] In cases of documented iron deficiency, the etiology of iron deficiency should be investigated; the most common causes of blood loss are from gastrointestinal or genitourinary tracts, but malabsorption or dietary deficiency should also be considered. Patients with iron deficiency and anemia should be treated either with iron supplementation or with dietary modification. However, a consensus does not exist regarding management of patients who are iron deficient without anemia. Some centers report that based on their experience, iron-deficient patients (with or without anemia) who receive iron supplementation have a better response to alopecia treatment.[48,49] Oral supplementation can be with either ferrous sulfate or ferrous gluconate, 60 mg two to three times daily, and iron studies are expected to improve within 1 month of initiation. Some recommend that ferritin levels be greater than 50 µg/L,[49] whereas others suggest keeping levels higher than 70 µg/L.[48] Patients should be monitored, as there are toxicities associated with excess supplementation and iron overload. Acute toxicity from iron intake of more than 20 mg/kg can cause gastrointestinal symptoms, including constipation, nausea, abdominal pain, and vomiting. Severe overdose (e.g., iron intake over 60 mg/kg) can lead to multisystem organ failure, coma, convulsions, and death.[46]

Currently, the studies evaluating the efficacy of iron supplementation in iron-deficient patients with alopecia are limited in number and size. An early study of 18 women with diffuse hair loss and iron deficiency without anemia found that all patients experienced hair regrowth with oral iron therapy. Hair loss recurred once iron supplementation was discontinued.[50] Another RCT of 12 women with iron deficiency and chronic TE (over 6 months duration) compared treatment with a combination of oral iron (72 mg/day) and L-lysine (1.5 g/day) versus placebo. The combination treatment decreased the percentage of hairs in the telogen phase by over 30% and it is believed that L-lysine increases iron absorption.[51]

MACRONUTRIENTS
Amino Acids and Proteins

In extreme protein malnutrition states such as kwashiorkor, hair has been described as being short, dull, thin, and soft. The anagen bulbs are atrophied and hairs are easily plucked.[1,2,52]

The role of amino acid or protein supplementation for treatment of alopecia is not well studied. There is some evidence that L-lysine (1.5–2 g/day) increases absorption of oral iron and may be of use in iron-deficient alopecia patients who do not respond to oral iron therapy alone.[51] However, protein supplements may hinder treatment efficacy in AGA. For example, creatine monohydrate, the most common physical performance–enhancing supplement, contains the amino acids arginine, glycine, and methionine. Creatine monohydrate has been shown to increase dihydrotestosterone (DHT) during training periods, and arginine itself increases DHT by increasing 5α-reductase activity.[53] Thus, concurrent supplementation with creatine monohydrate may interfere with the pharmacologic effects of 5α-reductase inhibitors in patients with AGA.

Fatty Acids

The essential fatty acids (EFAs) include polyunsaturated α-linoleic acid (ω-3) and linoleic acid (ω-6). ω-3 fatty acids are important components of cell membranes and ω-6 fatty acids form eicosanoids that mediate inflammation, vasoconstriction, and platelet aggregation. EFAs are consumed in the diet in the forms of plant and fish oils.[54] Deficiency of EFAs (e.g., from malabsorption or inappropriately administered parenteral deficiency) has been associated with diffuse hair loss of the scalp and eyebrows.[55,56] There is some evidence to suggest that fatty acids may be a treatment option for hair loss. For example, an in vitro study showed that select unsaturated fatty acids inhibit 5α-reductase and may therefore play a role in regulating androgen activity.[57] In addition, arachidonic acid promoted hair growth by inducing and prolonging anagen in mice.[58] A RCT of 120 women with FPHL demonstrated that when compared with placebo, 6-month oral supplementation with a combination of ω-3 and ω-6 fatty acids (fish and blackcurrant seed oils) and antioxidants (lycopene, vitamin C, vitamin E) increased hair density and reduced percentage of hairs

in telogen, hair loss, and the proportion of miniaturized anagen hair.[59]

NONVITAMIN NONMINERAL PRODUCTS
Caffeine

Caffeine inhibits the enzyme phosphodiesterase, thereby increasing cyclic adenine monophosphate and decreasing the effects of DHT on the hair follicle. This ultimately promotes hair proliferation by stimulating cell metabolism.[60] Caffeine penetrates the hair follicle after 2 min of topical application[61] and has been used in small single-arm prospective studies to treat patients with AGA. A nonrandomized prospective study of 40 men with AGA treated with caffeine lotion daily for 4 months showed that caffeine increases hair tensile strength as measured by a decreased number of hairs pulled in a hair pull test.[62] Another nonrandomized prospective study of 30 men with AGA showed that caffeine in a shampoo formulation used once daily for 6 months similarly increases hair tensile strength.[63] Topical caffeine treatment was well tolerated in both studies. The role of oral caffeine in treating hair loss is unknown.

Melatonin

Melatonin has antiandrogenic and antioxidant effects at the hair follicle that is mediated by signaling through the melatonin receptor.[64] There are several studies exploring the efficacy of topical melatonin in treatment of alopecia. One RCT compared the effects of 0.1% melatonin-alcohol solution versus placebo solution applied once daily for 6 months in 40 women with diffuse alopecia or AGA.[65] Trichograms were used to assess changes in anagen and telogen hairs during the treatment period. When compared with the placebo group, women with AGA in the treatment arm were noted to have increased anagen hairs in the occipital scalp with no effect in the frontal scalp. An opposite pattern was observed in women with diffuse hair loss who were treated with the melatonin solution; when compared with placebo, these patients experienced increased anagen hairs in the frontal scalp with no effect on the occipital scalp. Other nonrandomized single-arm studies with topical melatonin have shown mostly positive effects in early stage AGA. The evaluation of efficacy differed across studies, including subjective questionnaires, changes in hair pull test, and trichograms.[66] The largest of these studies involved over 1800 men and women with AGA who were treated with melatonin solution daily for 90 days. After the treatment period, the proportion of patients with a two- to three-fold positive hair pull test decreased, and the proportion of patients with a negative hair pull test increased. Once-daily topical application does not significantly alter serum melatonin levels, and the treatment is well tolerated.[66] The role of oral melatonin in treating hair loss has not been investigated.

Botanical Products

Phytosterols, such as β-sitosterol and phytosterol glycosides, are plant-derived 5α-reductase inhibitors and have been used for treatment of benign prostatic hyperplasia and AGA.[67] A RCT of 26 patients with mild-to-moderate AGA compared a combination of β-sitosterol 50 mg and phytosterol glycoside (saw palmetto berry extract) 200 mg twice daily for 5 months versus placebo.[68] Efficacy was assessed subjectively by investigator and patient questionnaire. There was improvement in 60% of patients who received the active ingredients versus 11% of those who received the placebo. The sample size of this study was small and was not aimed to establish statistical significance. The treatment was generally well tolerated, although one patient experienced loss of appetite. Notably, the evidence for efficacy of botanical products in hair loss is lacking and long-term safety is unknown. Given the variable ingredient compositions of botanical extracts, it is important that future clinical studies use botanical extracts with well-defined components for reproducibility.

MARINE COMPLEXES

Originally identified from the fish and protein-rich diets of Scandinavian Inuits in the 1980s, marine extracts have been investigated as the primary active ingredient in oral supplements for the treatment of hair loss.[69] A novel proprietary oral supplement containing extracellular matrix components of shark and mollusks blended with vitamin C, zinc, horsetail extract, and flaxseed extract has demonstrated efficacy in treating both men and women with hair loss.[70-72] The mechanism through which marine extracts promote hair growth is under investigation, but there is some evidence that they enhance proliferation of dermal papilla cells and increase expression of alkaline phosphatase, a key marker of anagen.[69]

Multiple RCTs of women with self-perceived hair thinning demonstrated that compared to those in the placebo group, patients taking the oral marine supplement had increased number of terminal hairs within target areas, increased hair diameter, decreased hair

shedding, and improved quality of life after 3–6 months of treatment.[71,72] A similar RCT with the same marine protein supplement was conducted in 60 men with AGA. After 6 months, men receiving the oral supplement had increases in total hair count and total and terminal density and fewer hairs removed by hair pull test.[70] In current studies, marine protein supplements are well tolerated without adverse events.

CONCLUSIONS

Nutritional deficiencies can result from a myriad of etiologies, some of which include inadequate dietary intake, genetic diseases, or iatrogenic causes. Obtaining a detailed history during evaluation of a patient presenting with hair loss may reveal the etiology of nutrient deficiencies. Patients with a known deficiency should be treated appropriately with oral supplementation or dietary modification. However, the role of nutrient supplementation in the absence of deficiency is unclear at this time.

There are many hair supplements available on the market that do not require a prescription. Patients should be encouraged to communicate with their healthcare providers if they are taking hair supplements. Likewise, physicians should be prepared to counsel patients about the general lack of available evidence supporting positive effects of oral nutrient supplementation on hair health. In addition, patients should be advised that excess supplementation could cause serious toxicities. Nonetheless, some existing studies suggest that topical or oral formulations of dietary ingredients and their derivatives may be useful adjuncts for treating patients with alopecia. Treatment with hair supplements should be directed by a healthcare provider to ensure safety. Further, appropriately controlled and powered studies are necessary to determine the utility of hair supplements in treating patients with alopecia (Table 28.1).

REFERENCES

1. Sims RT. Hair growth in kwashiorkor. *Arch Dis Child.* 1967;42(224):397–400.
2. Finner AM. Nutrition and hair: deficiencies and supplements. *Dermatol Clin.* 2013;31(1):167–172.
3. Spivak JL, Jackson DL. Pellagra: an analysis of 18 patients and a review of the literature. *Johns Hopkins Med J.* 1977;140(6):295–309.
4. Galimberti F, Mesinkovska NA. Skin findings associated with nutritional deficiencies. *Cleve Clin J Med.* 2016;83(10):731–739.

5. FDA Basics. https://www.fda.gov/AboutFDA/Transparency/Basics/default.htm.
6. Vitamin A – Health Professional Fact Sheet. https://ods.od.nih.gov/factsheets/VitaminA-HealthProfessional/ -en2.
7. Schiltz JR, Lanigan J, Nabial W, Petty B, Birnbaum JE. Retinoic acid induces cyclic changes in epidermal thickness and dermal collagen and glycosaminoglycan biosynthesis rates. *J Invest Dermatol.* 1986;87(5):663–667.
8. Soler-Bechara J, Soscia JL. Chronic hypervitaminosis A. Report of a case in an adult. *Arch Intern Med.* 1963;112:462–466.
9. Holler PD, Cotsarelis G. Retinoids putting the "a" in alopecia. *J Invest Dermatol.* 2013;133(2):285–286.
10. Duncan FJ, Silva KA, Johnson CJ, et al. Endogenous retinoids in the pathogenesis of alopecia areata. *J Invest Dermatol.* 2013;133(2):334–343.
11. Everts HB, Silva KA, Montgomery S, et al. Retinoid metabolism is altered in human and mouse cicatricial alopecia. *J Invest Dermatol.* 2013;133(2):325–333.
12. Bazzano GS, Terezakis N, Galen W. Topical tretinoin for hair growth promotion. *J Am Acad Dermatol.* 1986;15(4 Pt 2): 880–883, 890–893.
13. Ferry JJ, Forbes KK, VanderLugt JT, Szpunar GJ. Influence of tretinoin on the percutaneous absorption of minoxidil from an aqueous topical solution. *Clin Pharmacol Ther.* 1990;47(4):439–446.
14. Shin HS, Won CH, Lee SH, Kwon OS, Kim KH, Eun HC. Efficacy of 5% minoxidil versus combined 5% minoxidil and 0.01% tretinoin for male pattern hair loss: a randomized, double-blind, comparative clinical trial. *Am J Clin Dermatol.* 2007;8(5):285–290.
15. Wan P, Moat S, Anstey A. Pellagra: a review with emphasis on photosensitivity. *Br J Dermatol.* 2011;164(6):1188–1200.
16. Hegyi J, Schwartz RA, Hegyi V. Pellagra: dermatitis, dementia, and diarrhea. *Int J Dermatol.* 2004;43(1):1–5.
17. Sano S, Itami S, Takeda K, et al. Keratinocyte-specific ablation of Stat3 exhibits impaired skin remodeling, but does not affect skin morphogenesis. *EMBO J.* 1999;18(17):4657–4668.
18. Draelos ZD, Jacobson EL, Kim H, Kim M, Jacobson MK. A pilot study evaluating the efficacy of topically applied niacin derivatives for treatment of female pattern alopecia. *J Cosmet Dermatol.* 2005;4(4):258–261.
19. Zempleni J, Hassan YI, Wijeratne SS. Biotin and biotinidase deficiency. *Expert Rev Endocrinol Metab.* 2008;3(6):715–724.
20. Wolf B. Biotinidase deficiency. In: Pagon RA, Adam MP, Ardinger HH, et al., eds. *GeneReviews*®. Seattle, WA; 1993.
21. Castro-Gago M, Perez-Gay L, Gomez-Lado C, Castineiras-Ramos DE, Otero-Martinez S, Rodriguez-Segade S. The influence of valproic acid and carbamazepine treatment on serum biotin and zinc levels and on biotinidase activity. *J Child Neurol.* 2011;26(12):1522–1524.
22. Schulpis KH, Georgala S, Papakonstantinou ED, Michas T, Karikas GA. The effect of isotretinoin on biotinidase activity. *Skin Pharmacol Appl Skin Physiol.* 1999;12(1–2):28–33.
23. Colombo VE, Gerber F, Bronhofer M, Floersheim GL. Treatment of brittle fingernails and onychoschizia with biotin: scanning electron microscopy. *J Am Acad Dermatol.* 1990;23(6 Pt 1):1127–1132.
24. Trueb RM. Serum biotin levels in women complaining of hair loss. *Int J Trichology.* 2016;8(2):73–77.
25. Patel DP, Swink SM, Castelo-Soccio L. A review of the use of biotin for hair loss. *Skin Appendage Disord.* 2017;3(3):166–169.
26. Vitamin D – Health Professional Fact Sheet. 2016.
27. Amor KT, Rashid RM, Mirmirani P. Does D matter? The role of vitamin D in hair disorders and hair follicle cycling. *Dermatol Online J.* 2010;16(2):3.
28. Bakry OA, El Farargy SM, El Shafiee MK, Soliman A. Serum vitamin D in patients with alopecia areata. *Indian Dermatol Online J.* 2016;7(5):371–377.
29. Cerman A, Sarikaya Solak S, Kivanc Altunay I. Vitamin D deficiency in alopecia areata. *Br J Dermatol.* 2014;170(6):1299–1304.
30. Thompson JM, Li T, Park MK, Qureshi AA, Cho E. Estimated serum vitamin D status, vitamin D intake, and risk of incident alopecia areata among US women. *Arch Dermatol Res.* 2016;308(9):671–676.
31. Banihashemi M, Nahidi Y, Meibodi NT, Jarahi L, Dolatkhah M. Serum vitamin D3 level in patients with female pattern hair loss. *Int J Trichology.* 2016;8(3):116–120.
32. Cheung EJ, Sink JR, English Iii JC. Vitamin and mineral deficiencies in patients with telogen effluvium: a retrospective cross-sectional study. *J Drugs Dermatol.* 2016;15(10):1235–1237.
33. Cerman AA, Solak SS, Altunay I, Kucukunal NA. Topical calcipotriol therapy for mild-to-moderate alopecia areata: a retrospective study. *J Drugs Dermatol.* 2015; 14(6):616–620.
34. Narang T, Daroach M, Kumaran MS. Efficacy and safety of topical calcipotriol in management of alopecia areata: a pilot study. *Dermatol Ther.* 2017;30(3).
35. Vitamin E – Health Professional Fact Sheet. https://ods.od.nih.gov/factsheets/VitaminE-HealthProfessional/.
36. Beoy LA, Woei WJ, Hay YK. Effects of tocotrienol supplementation on hair growth in human volunteers. *Trop Life Sci Res.* 2010;21(2):91–99.
37. Mertz W. The essential trace elements. *Science.* 1981;213 (4514):1332–1338.
38. Zinc – Health Professional Fact Sheet. https://ods.od.nih.gov/factsheets/Zinc-HealthProfessional/ -h5.
39. MacDonald RS. The role of zinc in growth and cell proliferation. *J Nutr.* 2000;130(5S suppl):1500S–1508S.
40. Prasad AS. Zinc: an overview. *Nutrition.* 1995;11(1 suppl):93–99.
41. Kil MS, Kim CW, Kim SS. Analysis of serum zinc and copper concentrations in hair loss. *Ann Dermatol.* 2013;25(4):405–409.
42. Jin W, Zheng H, Shan B, Wu Y. Changes of serum trace elements level in patients with alopecia areata: a meta-analysis. *J Dermatol.* 2017;44(5):588–591.

43. Karashima T, Tsuruta D, Hamada T, et al. Oral zinc therapy for zinc deficiency-related telogen effluvium. *Dermatol Ther.* 2012;25(2):210–213.

44. Ead RD. Oral zinc sulphate in alopecia areata-a double blind trial. *Br J Dermatol.* 1981;104(4):483–484.

45. Berger RS, Fu JL, Smiles KA, et al. The effects of minoxidil, 1% pyrithione zinc and a combination of both on hair density: a randomized controlled trial. *Br J Dermatol.* 2003;149(2):354–362.

46. Dietary Supplement Fact Sheet: Iron. https://ods.od.nih.gov/factsheets/Iron-HealthProfessional/.

47. Kantor J, Kessler LJ, Brooks DG, Cotsarelis G. Decreased serum ferritin is associated with alopecia in women. *J Invest Dermatol.* 2003;121(5):985–988.

48. Trost LB, Bergfeld WF, Calogeras E. The diagnosis and treatment of iron deficiency and its potential relationship to hair loss. *J Am Acad Dermatol.* 2006;54(5):824–844.

49. St Pierre SA, Vercellotti GM, Donovan JC, Hordinsky MK. Iron deficiency and diffuse nonscarring scalp alopecia in women: more pieces to the puzzle. *J Am Acad Dermatol.* 2010;63(6):1070–1076.

50. Hard S. Non-anemic iron deficiency as an etiologic factor in diffuse loss of hair of the scalp in women. *Acta Derm Venereol.* 1963;43:562–569.

51. Rushton DH. Nutritional factors and hair loss. *Clin Exp Dermatol.* 2002;27(5):396–404.

52. McLaren DS. Skin in protein energy malnutrition. *Arch Dermatol.* 1987;123(12): 1674–1676a.

53. Rinaldi S, Bussa M, Mascaro A. Update on the treatment of androgenetic alopecia. *Eur Rev Med Pharmacol Sci.* 2016;20(1):54–58.

54. Omega-3 Fatty Acids – Health Professional Fact Sheet. https://ods.od.nih.gov/factsheets/Omega3FattyAcids-HealthProfessional/.

55. Delahoussaye AR, Jorizzo JL. Cutaneous manifestations of nutritional disorders. *Dermatol Clin.* 1989;7(3):559–570.

56. Goldberg LJ, Lenzy Y. Nutrition and hair. *Clin Dermatol.* 2010;28(4):412–419.

57. Liang T, Liao S. Inhibition of steroid 5 alpha-reductase by specific aliphatic unsaturated fatty acids. *Biochem J.* 1992;285(Pt 2):557–562.

58. Munkhbayar S, Jang S, Cho AR, et al. Role of arachidonic acid in promoting hair growth. *Ann Dermatol.* 2016;28(1):55–64.

59. Le Floc'h C, Cheniti A, Connetable S, Piccardi N, Vincenzi C, Tosti A. Effect of a nutritional supplement on hair loss in women. *J Cosmet Dermatol.* 2015;14(1):76–82.

60. Fischer TW, Hipler UC, Elsner P. Effect of caffeine and testosterone on the proliferation of human hair follicles in vitro. *Int J Dermatol.* 2007;46(1):27–35.

61. Otberg N, Teichmann A, Rasuljev U, Sinkgraven R, Sterry W, Lademann J. Follicular penetration of topically applied caffeine via a shampoo formulation. *Skin Pharmacol Physiol.* 2007;20(4):195–198.

62. Bussoletti C, Mastropietro F, Tolaini MV, Celleno L. Use of a cosmetic caffeine lotion in the treatment of male androgenetic alopecia. *J Appl Cosmetol.* 2011;29(4):167–179.

63. Bussoletti C, Mastropietro F, Tolaini MV, Celleno L. Use of a Caffeine shampoo for the treatment of male androgenetic alopecia. *J Appl Cosmetol.* 2010;28:153–162.

64. Fischer TW, Slominski A, Tobin DJ, Paus R. Melatonin and the hair follicle. *J Pineal Res.* 2008;44(1):1–15.

65. Fischer TW, Burmeister G, Schmidt HW, Elsner P. Melatonin increases anagen hair rate in women with androgenetic alopecia or diffuse alopecia: results of a pilot randomized controlled trial. *Br J Dermatol.* 2004;150(2):341–345.

66. Fischer TW, Trueb RM, Hanggi G, Innocenti M, Elsner P. Topical melatonin for treatment of androgenetic alopecia. *Int J Trichology.* 2012;4(4):236–245.

67. Reuter J, Merfort I, Schempp CM. Botanicals in dermatology: an evidence-based review. *Am J Clin Dermatol.* 2010;11(4):247–267.

68. Prager N, Bickett K, French N, Marcovici G. A randomized, double-blind, placebo-controlled trial to determine the effectiveness of botanically derived inhibitors of 5-alpha-reductase in the treatment of androgenetic alopecia. *J Altern Complement Med.* 2002;8(2):143–152.

69. Hornfeldt CS, Holland M, Bucay VW, Roberts WE, Waldorf HA, Dayan SH. The safety and efficacy of a sustainable marine extract for the treatment of thinning hair: a summary of new clinical research and results from a panel discussion on the problem of thinning hair and current treatments. *J Drugs Dermatol.* 2015;14(9):s15–s22.

70. Ablon G. A 6-month, randomized, double-blind, placebo-controlled study evaluating the ability of a marine complex supplement to promote hair growth in men with thinning hair. *J Cosmet Dermatol.* 2016;15(4):358–366.

71. Ablon G. A 3-month, randomized, double-blind, placebo-controlled study evaluating the ability of an extra-strength marine protein supplement to promote hair growth and decrease shedding in women with self-perceived thinning hair. *Dermatol Res Pract.* 2015;2015:841570.

72. Ablon G, Dayan S. A randomized, double-blind, placebo-controlled, multi-center, extension trial evaluating the efficacy of a new oral supplement in women with self-perceived thinning hair. *J Clin Aesthet Dermatol.* 2015;8(12):15–21.

CHAPTER 29

What Should the Hair Clinician Know About Hair Transplants?

ROBIN UNGER, MD • RUEL ADAJAR, MD

OVERVIEW OF HAIR TRANSPLANTATION FOR DERMATOLOGISTS

As dermatologists have learned, hair loss is most commonly caused by exposure of the hair follicle to dihydrotestosterone (DHT), a metabolite of testosterone that is produced when the hormone reacts with 5α-reductase. The affected follicles start miniaturizing, producing hairs that become finer and shorter with each growth cycle, eventually leading to follicular loss causing alopecia. This is most commonly seen in androgenetic alopecia. A classification of the different patterns of male pattern baldness (MPB) was developed by Norwood[1] and is now used as a reference for physicians to categorize the patient's current and future MPB. Genetics plays an important role in how severe the patient's hair loss will be over time. Although androgens and genetics play a central role in androgenetic alopecia, their effects are not as pronounced and defined in female pattern hair loss (FPHL).[2] Hair transplantation is an effective treatment for MPB and FPHL, because hair in the occipital rim (and in males, also the parietotemporal regions) is much less affected by DHT. This was confirmed when the first hair transplant surgery was successfully done by Dr. Orentreich in the 50s when he proved that donor hair taken from these regions continued to grow when they were moved to the balding areas on top of the head and remained insensitive to the effects of DHT. He referred to this property as "donor dominance." Further studies on the donor area were carried out, and in 1995 Dr. Walter Unger was able to map out the boundaries of the donor area,[3] which he termed as the "safe donor area" (SDA) (Fig. 29.1). Hairs taken within these boundaries are minimally affected by the DHT and retained this characteristic even when moved to the recipient areas. The follicular unit extraction (FUE) method allows a slight expansion of the original donor limits but should not be exceeded by too large a margin.[3]

Dermatologists frequently face patients complaining of hair loss. Often this is the first time the patient has mentioned his/her concerns. The initial assessment is beyond the topic of this chapter but may include blood tests, hormonal analyses, dermoscopy, and sometimes a scalp biopsy. If the cause is determined to be androgenetic, commonly the best first-line treatment is medical therapy. Medical treatment most commonly includes 5α reductase inhibitors (finasteride or dutasteride), antiandrogens in women, and minoxidil 5% for both men and women.[4] New experience with oral minoxidil suggests this may be a good alternative for patients who cannot tolerate the topical formulas.

Patients seeking a significant improvement will often benefit from hair transplant surgery, provided their donor regions have sufficient hair to meet their goals and expectations. In the United States, thousands of hair transplantations are being done annually. Although the majority of patients having hair transplants are still male, there is an increasing number of women who undergo the procedure for their hair loss. As the technique evolves, hair transplant surgeons are able to provide their patients results that more or less mimic the "natural look." Despite these great improvements in technique, hair transplant surgeons continue to search for new approaches to provide their patient with the best possible result.

THE PROCEDURE: EVOLUTION

In the early days of hair transplanting, Dr. Orentreich popularized the "**standard punch grafting**" technique, which used 4 mm biopsy punches to harvest grafts from the donor area. These grafts ("plugs") contained as many as 20–30 hairs each and were placed into recipient sites that were also made using biopsy punches, but only a limited number (50–100) of grafts could be safely placed at a time. These "plugs" produced the unnatural "dolls head" appearance associated with the technique and also thinned the donor area leaving an unsightly checkerboard pattern of scars (Fig. 29.2).

These factors led hair transplant physicians to abandon the technique and improve the procedure. By the late 1980s to early 1990s, the "**combination mini-micro grafting technique**" became the most

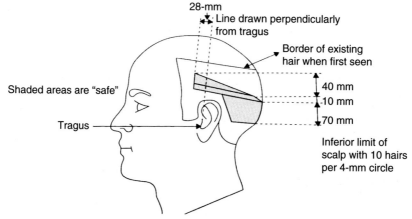

FIG. 29.1 Unger's safe donor area.

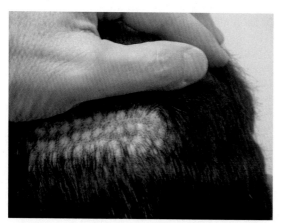

FIG. 29.2 The checkerboard pattern appearance of scars in the standard punch grafting method of donor harvest.

commonly performed hair surgery. This technique involved donor harvesting using a single strip of donor tissue (strip harvest) from which grafts containing 4–12 hairs were obtained. The grafts were placed into recipient sites made by using small slit incisions (which decreased the vascular trauma initially associated with the round grafts), and the procedure allowed for an increased number of grafts (400–800) that could be placed per session.[5] The technique also significantly improved the aesthetics of the donor area, leaving only a single linear scar at the back of the head and no perceptible decrease in density.

Hair transplant surgeons continued to look for improvement. Given that hair grows in follicular units, which are naturally occurring groups of 1–4 hairs bound by adventitial tissue, the next major advancement tried to mimic nature. The technique was called follicular unit transplantation (FUT). The grafts are obtained using the strip method of harvesting. The strip is then divided into single follicular thick slices ("slivers"), which are then divided into their naturally occurring groupings (follicular units) with the aid of microscope or loupes. The recipient sites for these grafts are so small that they enabled the hair transplant surgeons to put the grafts closer together to achieve a more natural result. The tiny recipient sites also cause less vascular trauma to the recipient area so it became possible to transplant 1000–3000 grafts in one session without fear of graft loss because of compromised blood supply. Some surgeons even pushed for "mega sessions" of 4000–5000 grafts in one session, although the survival rate of grafts in these very large surgeries remains somewhat unclear. FUT became, and remains, the preferred technique used today to produce natural results and cover larger areas of alopecia.

FOLLICULAR UNIT TRANSPLANTATION

FUT is the main method used by hair restoration surgeons worldwide. At present, there are two primary methods for harvesting grafts for FUT surgery (Fig. 29.3):

1. The traditional "strip method" in which donor hair is removed from the fringe area in a single strip. The area is then closed with sutures or staples and the individual grafts are produced by careful dissection of the strip.
2. The FUE method, which utilizes a very small punch to harvest one follicular unit at a time. The recipient area is transplanted in much the same way, regardless of the harvest method.

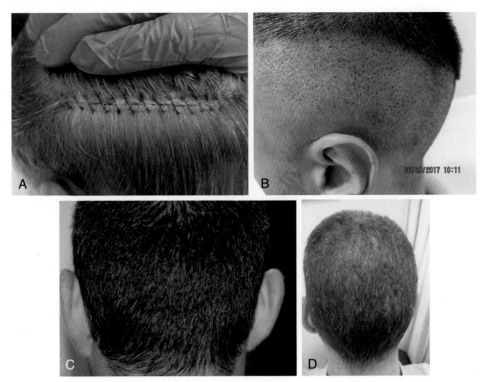

FIG. 29.3 Comparison between the two types of harvest for FUT, both FUE and FUT: **(A)** The strip method immediate post-op after closure. **(B)** The FUE method performed with a 0.9 mm punch at appropriate density, immediately post-op. **(C)** The appearance of the donor area in a patient 10 months after a strip harvest. **(D)** The appearance of the donor area in a patient at 6 months after FUE harvest. *FUE,* follicular unit extraction; *FUT,* follicular unit transplantation.

Strip Method Harvest

The goal of the strip method of harvesting grafts is to maximize the number of relatively permanent hairs that can be obtained from the fringe (the SDA), while minimizing the amount of scar tissue (Fig. 29.3A and C). The donor is excised using a single scalpel, taking care to avoid transecting the follicles, and the two lateral ends are tapered. The defect is then closed using either staples or sutures. In most patients, this results in a relatively narrow linear scar (Fig. 29.4A). However, there are situations that can lead to a widened scar; there may be patient-specific healing characteristics or surgical technique errors that can lead to this undesirable outcome (Fig. 29.4C), and this was the motivation for developing the alternative FUE harvest method.

The elliptical section that is removed is then divided into thin slices (much as a loaf of bread is sliced). The individual slivers are then further divided into follicular units containing between 1 and 4 hairs and follicular groupings that may have up to six hairs.

Follicular Unit Extraction Method Harvest

FUE is performed by harvesting each graft using a small punch (Figs. 29.3B,C and 29.4B,D). Current techniques generally use 0.8–1.0 mm punches to make a small circular incision around the follicular unit. There are many different designs of these punches, and these do have an impact on the size of the graft obtained, the amount of traction necessary for removal, the amount of protective tissue left intact, and of course the size of the punctuate scar left behind.[6] There is both an internal and an exterior diameter, which impact the quality of FUE. It is important to note that this is not a scarless procedure. Each defect produced by the graft removal creates a small scar, thus there is actually a significant amount of scar produced. However, it is not a linear scar, and therefore, if performed properly and responsibly, FUE-harvested regions can be worn in very short styles without visibility of the scars (Fig. 29.4C).

The grafts extracted are sorted and graded and occasionally trimmed. They are generally more fragile than grafts produced from a strip in which protective tissue remains surrounding the bulge region; therefore, the

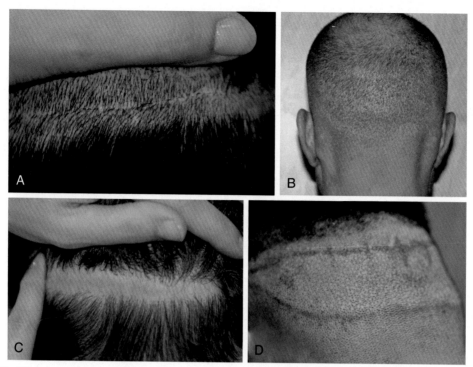

FIG. 29.4 A comparison of the scars from both harvest methods. **(A)** Single thin linear scar from strip method harvest performed skillfully in a patient with high scalp and hair color contrast. **(B)** Almost invisible scars from FUE performed with a small punch, in the appropriate donor area, and with appropriate density of extraction. **(C)** Widened scar from strip harvest method—the reason for so much fear! This may have been caused by poor technique, poor patient healing characteristics, and incomplete postoperative follow-up. **(D)** Very visible punctate scars produced by FUE method. *FUE*, follicular unit extraction.

handling of the grafts is very important. The use of implanters to reduce trauma during graft insertion will likely improve the results.

Table 29.1 clarifies some of the differences between the two harvest techniques. The most important points to highlight is that both techniques can produce better or worse scars (Fig. 29.4A–D), neither one is fool proof, and that the surgeon needs to be very skilled and up to date with the latest advances.

The most important advantages for FUE are that the technique, when properly performed, allows patients to wear very short hair styles without visibility of the scars and allows *some* expansion of the donor area to include areas where a linear scar would be visible or does not lend itself to a strip excision. Its most important drawback is that it lowers the density in the donor area and does not allow for maximum harvest from the most permanent region in the fringe.[7] There is also limited data on the survival of these grafts, and the limited studies performed thus far indicate that graft survival is lower after FUE as compared to strip harvest.[7]

The most significant benefit to the strip harvest technique is the large number of relatively permanent hairs that can be transplanted in one surgery while making no visible impact on the density in the donor area and its long-lasting results in the recipient area. Its most significant drawback is that patients are limited as to how short they can wear their hair.

Recipient Site Creation and Graft Placement

Despite all the attention garnered by harvest technique, this step remains the most important. Recipient sites may be created using small blades customized to the size of the grafts or various sizes of needles. The sites should be made in a pattern that imitates nature, following the direction and angle of the preexisting hair and producing irregularities as opposed to straight lines. There also should be a natural gradient of hair density: with a feathered looking hairline and increasing density as the eye moves to the central area of the caudal scalp (Fig. 29.5A–C). Any preexisting native hair should be protected

TABLE 29.1

Comparison of the Advantages and Disadvantages Between the Two Types of Harvests Being Used in Follicular Unit Transplantation (FUT)

Type of Harvest	Advantages	Disadvantages
Strip harvest	• Higher FU yield • Narrow donor area • Higher follicle survival • More protective tissue surrounding hair follicles • Harvest stays within the confines of the SDA • Ability to choose the size of the grafts • No perceptible change in donor hair density • One linear scar regardless of number of grafts/procedures	• Long linear scar that may be visible when the hair is cut short • More painful post-op period • Longer post-op healing period • Potential for loss of dormant follicles greater in unrecognized cases of telogen effluvium
FUE	• Shorter post-op healing • Less painful post-op period • Minute round scars that are less visible even with the hair worn short, especially with less contrast between hair and scalp color • A good complement technique when scalp laxity is limited or for repairs • Can somewhat expand scalp donor harvest in the temporal and occipital regions • Less tissue discarded with potential dormant follicles • Can use other potential sources of grafts (beard, chest, etc.) also called BHT[a]	• Lesser FU yield, more so with the "long hair" FUE technique • Immediate post-op, more noticeable donor area when using the shaven technique • Wider donor area harvested (some HRS extending past the SDA to achieve higher graft yield) • Less tissue around hair follicles (skinny grafts) contributing to lower follicle survival • Inappropriately referred to as "minimal incision surgery"[b] • Growth issues with BHT • Appreciable change in density in donor rim after harvest, especially with multiple procedures—a scar left for every follicle excised

[a]BHT should ideally be used when the donor reserve hair in the scalp has been exhausted and in areas where previously transplanted scalp hair already exists.
[b]FUE has recently been inappropriately referred to as "minimal incision surgery". If the total dimensions of each approach were taken into consideration, to produce 2000 FU, FUE would require 2000 1-mm diameter punch incision ($2 \times 3.14 \times 0.5$) that totals to 628 cm, whereas a 24-cm long strip that could frequently be expected to produce 2000 FU would only require 48 cm of incision length (24 cm × 2 sides).
BHT, body hair transplant; *FUE*, follicular unit extraction.

and undamaged by the hair transplant. The authors believe that it is also important to treat future areas of alopecia that will develop as the patient ages to avoid an unnatural hair distribution in the future. Other surgeons treat current areas of loss and will treat future areas as they evolve.

Grafts must be stored carefully from the time of extraction, until the placement time. Various holding solutions are used with the most common being normal saline, lactated ringers, and HypoThermosol with/without adenosine triphosphate.[8] The authors use the latter holding solution and also use platelet-rich plasma (PRP) to bathe the grafts prior to placement and to inject into the recipient area. Although clinical objective data regarding the intraoperative benefits of PRP is limited, anecdotal experience strongly indicates that this addition speeds recovery and improves the rate of growth.

Graft placement is also a very important step. If not performed carefully and precisely, the procedure will not produce great results. Small jewelers' forceps are used to grasp the graft at the base and then slide it gently into the site. The right size graft needs to be placed in the right location, the fit has to be snug but not tight, and the graft should sit flush with the epidermis.

Implanters are being used more frequently in hair transplant surgery. They may be used in one of two ways: sharp implanters that create the site and simultaneously insert the graft and dull implanters that allow the surgeon to premake the sites and still delegate placement with implanters.

Postoperative Course

In general, the procedure is very safe with very few postoperative problems. Forehead edema occurs in

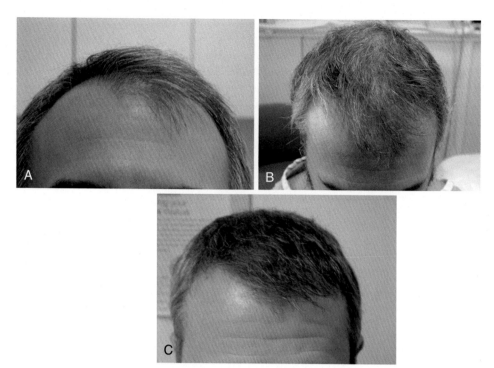

FIG. 29.5 A male patient aged 42 years with a retained frontal forelock. **(A)** The patient before surgery. **(B)** The same patient 5 months after surgery. **(C)** One year after surgery with full growth.

about 20% of patients and usually lasts about 3 days. Some patients develop postoperative folliculitis. Rarely, patients may develop minor bleeding, infection, or discomfort in the donor area. All these complications are usually mild and easily treatable.

In about 20% of patients, a complication called "shock loss" or telogen effluvium occurs. This describes when a percentage of the preexisting native hair in the recipient area before native hair in the recipient area goes into a telogen effluvium following surgery. Usually this is a temporary loss and the shocked hair will regrow. However, sometimes a percentage of the shocked hair (if very miniaturized already) will not regrow. There is more risk of shock loss in patients who have only early thinning and a significant amount of preexisting native hair. Shock loss is also more common in women. Patients with preexisting hair need to be warned about this potential complication. There is belief among some surgeons that the use of PRP during surgery can minimize the incidence of telogen effluvium.

The time frame for results is gradual. The transplanted hair usually sheds by about 2–3 weeks, at which time the patient looks like she/he did before surgery. The grafts begin to grow back at about 3 months, and between 3 and 6 months a notable change occurs. It is estimated that most patients have achieved about 60% of the effect

by this time. Improvement continues for up to 1 year but by the end of a year improvements usually taper off.

SCALP REDUCTIONS, FLAPS, TISSUE EXPANDERS

Scalp reductions, flaps, and tissue expanders are other procedures used to treat areas of alopecia on the scalp. These procedures are currently used most frequently in reconstructive cases: to treat patients with burns, posttrauma, or congenital abnormalities. They are also sometimes used as a first step in hairline lowering procedures, followed by follicular unit grafting to soften the anterior hairline.

ACHIEVING PATIENT SATISFACTION

The most important step in hair transplant surgery is actually nonsurgical: it is the consultation in which the patient is given a thorough explanation of the procedure, the various approaches that may be used, and the thinking involved in surgical planning for the long term. Many patients presenting to a surgeon want immediate gratification and are not particularly concerned about the future impact of today's choices. It is the hair transplant surgeon's obligation to educate the patient and present realistic objectives. A hairline placed low, dense, and straight in a young man with early onset MPB will undoubtedly look unnatural as he ages. A woman using her limited donor hair in the vertex whorl will regret that choice as she ages and her frontal frame becomes thinner and more receded.

The size area to be treated and the density with which it can be treated are largely determined by the amount of donor hair the patient has over the long term. Surgical plans should incorporate this information, regardless of the age of presentation. The average number of follicular units available for transplantation varies from 4000 to 10,000. A surgeon should be able to approximate the number of hairs available over the patient's lifetime, and use this information to decide what size region can be transplanted. As mentioned previously, some men also have available donor hair in the beard region that can be used to thicken areas when mixed with scalp hair and used in the central caudal scalp.

Current techniques in hair transplant surgery can produce incredibly natural results. The small grafts can be used to create natural, feathered hairlines and light coverage over larger areas of alopecia or concentrated areas of strategic density.

PRACTICAL APPLICATIONS OF HAIR TRANSPLANTATION

Originally, when large grafts were all that were available, hair transplantation was used almost exclusively to treat MPB. However, with the introduction of follicular unit grafting and tiny 1–3 hair grafts, the indications have broadened. Hair transplantation can now be used to treat delicate areas of hair loss on the face, such as eyebrows, eyelashes, beards, and mustaches. Other indications include secondary scarring on the scalp from accidents, burns, and surgery. Although controversial, transplantation can even be used to treat some forms of primary cicatricial and inflammatory alopecias. In this section, we will discuss both the common and less commonly thought of applications for hair transplantation.

Male Pattern Baldness

MPB, also known as androgenic alopecia, is the most common cause of hair loss in men and where FUT is most commonly used (Fig. 29.6A–D). Most men can achieve excellent results with modern techniques as long as they have realistic expectation and a sufficient donor area. Extremely natural results are achieved with careful surgical planning and execution.[9]

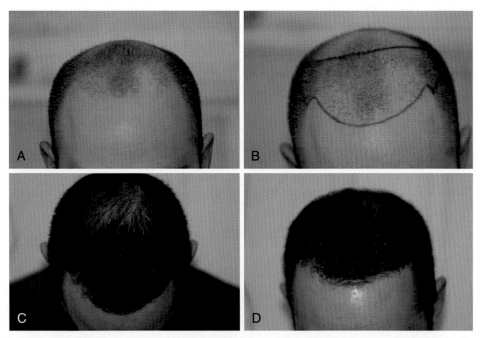

FIG. 29.6 **(A** and **B)** Surgical plan for a hair transplant procedure to the frontal area in a 32-year-old male. Note that the borders extend into the lateral rims of existing hair that are destined to be lost in the future. The central forelock with persisting hair was treated as though it was already alopecic, as any existing hair will be lost as the patient ages. **(C** and **D)** Same patient 10 months after hair transplantation to the frontal area with a fairly dense result.

Female Pattern Baldness

The incidence of female pattern baldness (FPB, FPHL) is greater than most people realize (Fig. 29.7A–D). Norwood reported that female pattern alopecia is as high as 30% in females over 30 years of age.[10,11] One reason why this is not generally appreciated is that females are very good at hiding thinning with various hairstyles, products, and hairpieces. In our society, it is socially acceptable for a man to lose his hair and is considered a variation of *"normal."* Hair loss in females is not as socially acceptable as in men. With FPB, women feel *"abnormal"* and find themselves in a position that makes them extraordinarily uncomfortable. The number of females seeking hair restoration surgery is on the rise.

The pattern of hair loss in FPHL is usually different than MPB, although some women do develop frontotemporal recessions. The majority of women have more diffuse thinning behind a relatively intact hairline. Ludwig created a scale in which she divides FPHL into Ludwig Type 1, Type 2, and Type 3, with severity getting progressively worse as we move from types 1 to 3. Olsen described a "Christmas tree" pattern of loss, which begins as a "widened part" but evolves into a zone of hair loss

that is widest anteriorly at the hairline and gradually narrows more posteriorly.[12]

It is important to note that females are more susceptible to the postoperative complication of "shock loss" than men. Postoperative shock loss occurs when preexisting native hair is triggered to go into a telogen (resting) phase by the local stressors of hair transplant surgery. In men this can occur from 10% to 20% of the time, whereas in females it occurs more frequently, almost 30%–50% of the time. In general, this shock loss is temporary, occurring about 2–3 months after surgery and resolving in 4–6 months.

A good surgical candidate will have reasonable expectations and sufficient donor hair. A minority of women are not candidates for surgery, because their hair loss is universally diffuse, affecting all scalp regions. More frequently, there is a limited zone of hair largely unaffected by hair loss that can be strategically placed in the recipient area to give the patient more satisfactory coverage. The best female candidate is one with moderate hair loss that is easily noticeable when she exposes the area.

One special scenario in females involves the high hairline. There are women with congenital high

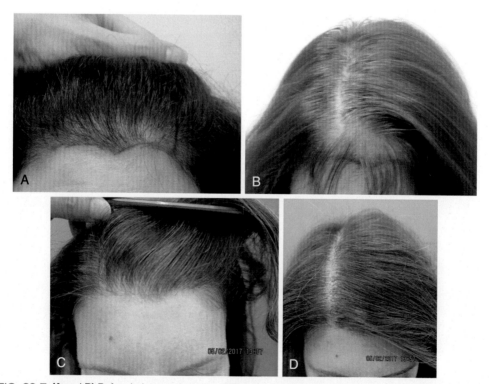

FIG. 29.7 **(A** and **B)** Before hair transplantation (HT) to frontal area and part line for FPHL. The area of greatest cosmetic significance was identified and the HT focused density in those regions. **(C** and **D)** Same patient 4 years after HT for FPHL. *FPHL,* female pattern hair loss.

hairlines who want to have them lowered. This can be accomplished with hair transplantation, but may use all or most of their donor hair supply and may be a decision they come to regret if they develop FPHL. There is also the option of a hairline advancement procedure, which can be softened frontally with some transplanted grafts.

Eyebrows and Eyelashes

Eyebrows play an essential role in facial aesthetics. Many women and some men seek treatment options for thinning or absent eyebrows. With the refinement in FUT, normal appearing eyebrows can often be restored.[13] Loss of eyebrow hair may be due to trauma, such as burns and avulsions; medical conditions such as hypothyroidism; genetics; or frontal fibrosing alopecia (FFA). It may also be self-inflicted because of long-term eyebrow plucking or trichotillomania, which is an obsessive-compulsive hair pulling disorder. It is important to treat and stabilize any underlying condition before transplantation, and monitoring and treatment will need to be continued after transplantation. Patients have to be told that the hair will grow long like normal scalp hair and that they will need to trim the hair to the desired length on a regular basis. If after surgery the shape of the eyebrow is not exactly what the patient wanted, it can be sculpted afterwards with electrolysis. Most patients obtain excellent results and are extremely satisfied.

Eyelash transplantation has also been promoted for cosmetic enhancement of thinning eyelashes not due to trauma or disease. There is still some controversy over the appropriateness of doing this procedure because of the potential complications that may occur, such as eyelid infection, distortion of the lid, injury to the tarsal plate, and misdirected hair damaging the cornea. However, innovations have been made in eyelash transplantation that allow better control of hair direction as well as more gentle insertion into the lid margins.

Beards and Mustaches

Many men have localized areas of alopecia or weak patches of hair in their beard or mustache. FUT is ideal for filling in these areas. Normal facial hair usually consists of very thick and coarse one-hair units. It is hard to find this degree of coarseness in the occipital donor area. Therefore, two-hair grafts are usually used instead of one-hair grafts in an attempt to match the thinness of the coarse beard hair. A common use for this procedure is to cover the defect resulting on the lip from a cleft palate repair or scars from trauma.

Scar Tissue Caused by Physical Trauma

Hair transplantation can be used to treat areas of scarring caused by different types of trauma, including burns, explosions, or accidents (Figs. 29.8 and 29.9). Sometimes the scarring is iatrogenic and produced by

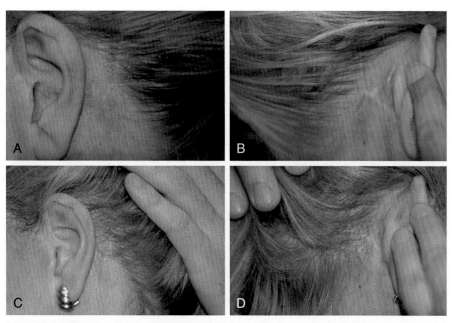

FIG. 29.8 **(A** and **B)** Before hair transplantation (HT) to repair scars and areas of alopecia in the postauricular area after a face-lift. **(C** and **D)** Nine months after the hair transplant surgery, showing excellent camouflage of the scars and filling of the alopecia. The patient is now able to wear her hair in an upswept style.

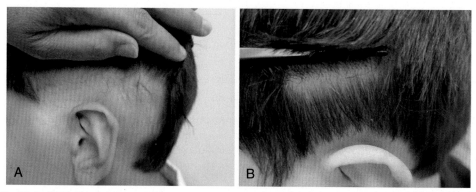

FIG. 29.9 **(A)** Before hair transplantation (HT) to a patient who had hair loss following irradiation for a tumor. **(B)** Same patient just 6 months after HT.

surgical procedures, such as face-lifts, brow lifts, radiation treatment, or the removal of a scalp tumor. Special considerations are needed when transplanting into areas of scarring.[14]

The issue of adequacy of the blood supply to the scar tissue often arises. In addition to leading to poor graft survival, this limited blood supply can potentially leave the recipient area more vulnerable to infection, further ischemia and necrosis. Although these are legitimate concerns, experience has shown that the blood supply in scar tissue is often sufficient to accommodate the appropriate placement of FU grafts. However, certain precautions and modifications should be taken. Primarily, the surgeon needs to assess the blood supply by evaluating the blood flow as sites are made and adjusting the depth and density of sites accordingly.

In general, one should always perform the first transplant with a smaller number of grafts placed further apart so as not to stress the blood supply. With scar tissue it is better to plan on doing multiple, smaller sessions that succeed, rather than one large session that fails. It is also prudent to wait longer in between sessions. We have noticed that after the first conservative transplant into an area of atrophic scarring, the tissue characteristics improve and become more favorable for a second transplant procedure. The tissue becomes thicker, softer, and more vascular. It may be that the FU grafts act like multiple tiny skin grafts and may stimulate angiogenesis.

One should always consider surgical excision as an alternative or adjunct to transplantation for areas of alopecia in the scalp. If the area of scarring is relatively small and the surgeon is confident that the scar can be removed by an excision alone, then it should be considered. If an area of scarring is very large, it is sometimes better to first excise a portion of the scarred area, leaving a smaller area to be later transplanted.

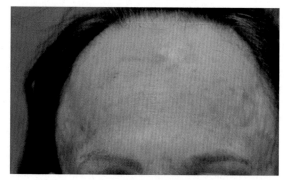

FIG. 29.10 A patient suffering from frontal fibrosing alopecia that also involved the eyebrows.

Primary Cicatricial Alopecia

The term *cicatricial alopecia* refers to scarring alopecias caused by inflammatory processes, such as central centrifugal cicatricial alopecia, pseudopelade, lichen planopilaris (LPP), FFA, discoid lupus erythematosus, etc. (Fig. 29.10). Transplanting into inflammatory cicatricial alopecia is controversial.[15]

The current philosophy amongst hair transplant physicians is to be certain the disease process has "burned out" before undertaking the procedure. A general rule of thumb is to wait until there are no signs of active disease for at least 1 or 2 years. A biopsy from the area to be transplanted to document an absence of inflammation may be helpful. There are physicians who recommend concurrent maintenance therapy for patients with cicatricial alopecia undergoing hair transplants.

The risk of surgery is that the disease process could reactivate and destroy the transplanted hairs or worse, reactivate, and continue to spread. There are not enough examples of hair transplants in these types of patients to get statistically significant numbers. Anecdotal reports exist of both success and failures. Sometimes the results may last for 2–3 years and then thin again. Others have reported results lasting up to 10 years.[16]

Over the past 10 years, the incidence of LPP and FFA has been observed more frequently amongst hair transplant surgeons. An unanswered question is whether the incidence is truly rising or if we are just more aware. Not uncommonly, it is diagnosed after an initial successful hair transplant begins to thin, for no apparent reason, a few years later and a biopsy shows LPP. This has occurred enough to raise the following question: Do hair transplants trigger the onset of new LPP or did we just miss the initial diagnosis?

Platelet-rich plasma

PRP is an autologous plasma that can contain anywhere from one to eight times the physiologic platelet concentration. The process of obtaining PRP involves a centrifugation protocol of the patient's whole blood with a separation of red and white blood cell from the plasma. This plasma is the component of blood rich in growth factors, cytokines and chemokines, which are essential for tissue repair and angiogenesis. PRP has been proved to aid in healing in other areas of medicine (dental, orthopedic, etc.). Its use in hair loss and hair transplantation has been more recent and the benefits controversial with very limited studies.[17] Currently hair transplant physicians use PRP in one of two ways: (1) intraoperatively and (2) as a nonsurgical, stand-alone treatment.

Intraoperatively, the PRP is injected into the grafted recipient area with the hope of stimulating faster healing and more robust hair growth. It has been used similarly in the donor area.

Nonsurgically, PRP has been used to treat miniaturized hair by using the mesotherapy technique of multiple superficial injections into the areas of thinning scalp. The benefits of this therapy are still controversial with limited studies available; however, anecdotal evidence is quite encouraging.

ACell Matristem

Acell is an extracellular matrix derived from porcine urinary bladder. It can be bought commercially. It contains a network of collagens and proteins and has been used in other areas of medicine to assist with wound healing.[18] It contains growth factors and is known to recruit progenitor cells possibly helping in tissue regeneration and helping follicles regenerate.[19] It has been used intraoperatively both in the recipient area and donor area with the hope of promoting healing and stimulating more hair growth.

Many hair transplant physicians have reported more impressive results when combining Acell and PRP together for both intraoperative and as a stand-alone treatment for hair loss. Further studies are needed in this area before it can be recommended as standard therapy.

REFERENCES

1. Nordstrom R. Classification of androgenetic alopecia. In: Unger W, Unger R, Shapiro R, Unger M, eds. *Hair Transplantation*. 5th ed. New York, NY: Informa; 2011:37–39.
2. Mubki T, Rudnicka L, Olszeska M, Shapiro J. Evaluation and diagnosis of the hair loss patient. *J Am Acad Dermatol*. 2014;71:415–428.
3. Devroye J. The safe donor area. In: Unger W, Unger R, Shapiro R, Unger M, eds. *Hair Transplantation*. 5th ed. New York, NY: Informa; 2011:225–262.
4. Varothai S, Bergfeld W. Androgenetic alopecia: an evidence-based treatment update. *Am J Clin Dermatol*. 2014;12:217–230.
5. Shapiro R, Callender VD. Hair transplantation for dermatologist. In: McMichael A, Hordinsky M, eds. *Hair and Scalp Diseases: Medical, Surgical and Cosmetic Treatments*. 2nd ed. Taylor and Francis; 2008.
6. Josephitis D, Shapiro R. A side by side study of 20 consecutive FUE patients comparing the use of a 0.9 mm sharp vs. 0.9 mm. *Blunt Punch*. 2016;26(5):256–259.
7. Beehner M. MFU grafts and strip harvesting. *Hair Transpl Forum Int*. 2014;24(4):125–126.
8. Cooley J. Bio-enhanced hair restoration. *Hair Transpl Forum Int*. 2014;24(4):121–130.
9. Unger WP. Planning and organization. In: Unger WP, Shapiro R, Unger RH, Unger M, eds. *Hair Transplantation*. 5th ed. New York: Marcel Dekker; 2011:106–152.
10. Ludwig E. Classification of the types of androgenetic alopecia (common baldness) occurring in the female sex. *Br J Dermatol*. 1977;97:247–254.
11. Unger R. Female hair restoration. In: Konior R, Gabel S, eds. *Facial Plastic Surgery Clinics of America*. vol. 21. 2013:407–417.
12. Olsen EA. Androgenetic alopecia. In: Olsen EA, ed. *Disorders of Hair Growth: Diagnosis and Treatment*. New York: McGraw-Hill; 1994:257–283.
13. Epstein Jeffrey. FAC eyebrow transplantation. *Hair Transpl Forum*. 2006;16(4):121–123.
14. Unger W, Unger R, Wesley C. The surgical treatment of cicatricial alopecia. *Dermatol Ther*. 2008;21:295–311.
15. Bolduc C, Sperling L, Shapiro J. Primary cicatricial alopecia. *J Am Acad Dermatol*. 2016;75(6):1101–1117.

16. Dahdah M, Iorizzo M. The role of hair restoration surgery in primary cicatricial alopecia. *Skin Appendage Disord.* 2016;2:57–60.

17. Alves R, Grimalt R. Randomized placebo-controlled, double-blind, half-head study to assess the efficacy of platelet-rich plasma on the treatment of androgenetic alopecia. *Derm Surg.* 2016;42:491–497.

18. Brown B, Lindberg K, Reing J, et al. The basement membrane component of biologic scaffolds derived from extracellular matrix. *Tissue Eng.* 2006;12(3):519–526.

19. Gentile P, Garcovich S, Bielli A, Scioli MG, Orlandi A, Cervellia V. The effect of platelet-rich plasma in hair regrowth: a randomized placebo-controlled trial. *Stem Cells Transl Med.* 2015;4(11):1317–1323.

Index

A

a6b4 integrin, 185
AA. *See* Alopecia areata (AA)
AA totalis (AAT), 59
AA universalis (AAU), 59, 188
AAI. *See* Alopecia areata incognito/
   incognita (AAI)
AANS. *See* Alopecic and aseptic nodules
   of scalp (AANS)
AAT. *See* AA totalis (AAT)
AAU. *See* AA universalis (AAU)
ACC. *See* Aplasia cutis congenita
   (ACC)
Acell matristem, 315
Acetazolamide, 254t
N-Acetylcysteine (NAC), 101
Acitretin, 181
Acne keloidalis nuchae (AKN), 36, 36f,
   163, 173, 174f
  alopecia patch, 174f
  clinical findings, 173–174
  differential diagnosis, 174–175
  epidemiology, 173
  pathogenesis, 173
  pathology, 174
  prognosis, 176
  treatment, 175, 175t–176t
  trichoscopy, 174
Acne necrotica varioliformis, 163
Acquired systemic amyloidosis
   (AL amyloidosis), 183–185
ACTH. *See* Adrenocorticotrophin
   (ACTH)
Acute cutaneous LE, 187
Acute stage, 24–26
  of alopecia areata, 27f, 214
Acute TE, 83, 89
Acute telogen effluvium, 85
Adalimumab, 170
Adipose-derived stem cells therapy
   (ADSCs therapy), 263–264
  adverse effect, 264
  mechanism of action, 263
  studies, 263–264
Adrenal hormones, 16
Adrenocorticotrophin (ACTH),
   11, 16
ADSCs therapy. *See* Adipose-derived
   stem cells therapy (ADSCs therapy)
African patients, hair morphology and
   practices with, 127
Afro-textured hair (AT hair), 135
AGA. *See* Androgenetic alopecia (AGA)

Aging, 15, 224
  population, 219
AKN. *See* Acne keloidalis nuchae
   (AKN)
AL amyloidosis. *See* Acquired systemic
   amyloidosis (AL amyloidosis)
Alkaline straighteners, 238
Alkyl iminopropionates, 286
Allergic contact dermatitis, 223
Allergy, shampoos and, 288
Allopurinol, 246t
Alopecia, 10, 13, 104, 135–136, 151,
   183, 231, 247, 263
  burden of disease in, 267
  level of evidence of therapies in
    nonscarring and scarring alopecia,
    268t
  types, 229
Alopecia areata (AA), 24–28, 43, 59,
   71–72, 96, 153, 185, 193–194, 295
  age, 193
  associated diseases, 63
  association with comorbidities, 193
  clinical features, 59–61
  clinical presentation, 193–194
  diagnosis, 61–62
  differential diagnosis, 62–63
  etiopathogenesis, 59
  management, 194
  negative prognostic factors linked
    up with, 60t
  pathology, 194
  pediatric patient with, 194f
  treatment, 63–65, 194t
  trichoscopy, 194
Alopecia areata incognito/incognita
   (AAI), 28–29, 60–61, 61f
Alopecia areata totalis, 193
Alopecia areata universalis, 193
Alopecia neoplastica (AN), 188–189
Alopecia universalis (AU), 185, 251
Alopecic and aseptic nodules of scalp
   (AANS), 169
American Hair Loss Association,
   267
Amicrobial pustulosis of folds, 180
(Amido) betaines, 286
Amino acids, 299
Amiodarone, 246t
Ammonium thioglycolate, 239
Amphoteric surfactants, 285–286
Amyloidosis, 183–185, 184f
AN. *See* Alopecia neoplastica (AN)

Anagen, 3, 83–84
  Anagen I, 9
  Anagen II, 9
  Anagen III, 9
  Anagen IV, 9
  Anagen V, 9
  Anagen VI, 9
  effluvium, 200, 245, 254
  follicles, 23, 214
  growth, 59
  stage, 9–10
    hair follicle stem cells, 9–10
    phases, 9
    regulatory pathways/molecules, 9
Analgesics/anti-inflammatories, 246t
ANAs. *See* Antinuclear antibodies
   (ANAs)
Androgen receptor (AR), 69–70
  type 2, 268–271
Androgen(s), 246t, 305
  androgen-mediated alopecia, 67
  metabolism, 115
Androgenetic alopecia (AGA), 24, 29,
   44, 67, 71t–72t, 88f, 115, 174, 179,
   259, 276–282. *See also* Nonscarring
   alopecia; Scarring alopecia
  clinical and histologic presentation,
    67–69
  clinical trial in alopecia, 277t–278t
  epidemiology, 69
  etiology and pathogenesis, 69–70
  management
    diagnosis and differential, 70–72
    prevention, treatment,
      mechanisms of action, and
      prognosis, 72–74
  pathogenesis, mechanisms of
    disease, and proposed areas of
    treatment
    animal models of human andro-
      genetic alopecia, 77
    cell therapy, 76
    genetic/genomic targets, 74–75
    signaling targets, 75–76
  phase 2 and phase 3 clinical trial for,
    279t–281t
  trichotillomania, 29
Angiotensin-converting enzyme
   inhibitors, 246t, 250
Animal models of human
   androgenetic alopecia, 77
Anionic surfactants, 285
Anisotrichosis, 115

Note: Page numbers followed by "f" indicate figures, "t" indicate tables.

Anthralin, 64
Anti-TNF blocker–induced
  psoriasiform skin lesions, 231–233
Antiandrogens, 132
Antibiotic sensitivity test, 163
Anticoagulants, 250
  clinical presentation, 250
  trichoscopy, 250
Anticoagulants, 246t
Antidandruff
  shampoos, 146–147
  substances, 289
Antiepileptics, 246t
Antifungal agents, 219
Antihistamines, 219
Antihypertensive agents, 250–251
  clinical presentation, 250
  trichoscopy, 251
Antiinflammatory
  effects, 260–261
  shampoos, 146–147
Antimalarials, 132, 147, 156
Antineoplastic agents
  antitarget drugs, 247–249
  classic-traditional antimitotic drugs,
    245–247
Antinuclear antibodies (ANAs), 152
Antioxidant(s), 299
  genes, 75
  properties, 297
Antipsychotics, 246t
Antiresidue shampoos, 292
Antiretrovirals, 252
Antiseptic solutions, 175
Antistaphylococcal topical antibiotics,
  164
Antitarget drugs, 246t, 247–249
  clinical presentation, 248–249
    diffuse alopecia involving total
      hair body, 248f
    telogen effluvium leading to
      diffuse hair thinning, 248f
    trichoscopy of total hair regrowth
      after drug withdrawal, 249f
  trichoscopy, 249
Antithyroid drugs, 246t
Aplasia cutis congenita (ACC), 193,
  196
  association with comorbidities, 196
  clinical presentation, 196
  management, 196
  pathology, 196
  trichoscopy, 196
APM. See Arrector pili muscle (APM)
Apoptosis, 151–152
  focal, 3
  of follicular epithelial cells, 117
  keratinocytes in bulb, 83
AR. See Androgen receptor (AR)
5AR inhibitors. See 5α-Reductase
  inhibitors (5AR inhibitors)
Argan oil, 287
Argan tree (Argania spinosa [L.]), 287

Argentic, 48, 49f
Arrector pili muscle (APM), 5–6
Asebia mouse, 143–144
Asian hair, 290–291
Asian perm hair, 291
AT hair. See Afro-textured hair (AT hair)
Atherosclerosis, 287
Atopic dermatitis, 146–147, 222
Atrichia with papular lesions, 63
Atrophic/atrophy, 37, 105–106, 156
  cutaneous, 105–106
  dermatosis, 186–187
  epidermal, 154
  hemifacial, 186
  peripilar cupular, 115
  scarring, 314
  scars, 152–153
  sebaceous glands, 183–185, 231
  skin, 47, 109–110, 179
  steroid, 146
AU. See Alopecia universalis (AU)
Auber's critical level, 3
Autoimmune
  bullous disorders, 185
  comorbidities, 193
  disorders, 179
  etiology, 103
Autologous bone marrow–derived
  mononuclear cells, 264
Axel Munthe's syndrome, 118
Azathioprine, 253
  clinical presentation, 253
  dermoscopic aspect, 253
Azoles, 289
Azythromycin, 170

B

B-lymphocyte stimulator (BLyS), 152
Bacterial cultures, 163
Bacterial folliculitis, 163
Bamboo hair. See Trichorrhexis
  invaginata (TI)
Baricitinib, 65
Basal cell carcinoma (BCC), 223
Basement membrane zone, 185
  BP180, 185
  BP230, 185
BCC. See Basal cell carcinoma (BCC)
Bcl-2, 10–11
Beards, 313
Benzimidazoles, 246t
Bevacizumab, 248
Bimatoprost, 254t, 273
Biologic agents, 157
Biopsy, 145–146
  findings in TA, 139–140
  from late-stage lesions, 169f
  report on horizontal sections, 26t
  skin, 163
Biotin, 296–297, 301t–302t
Björnstad syndrome, 202
BKT. See Brazilian keratin treatment
  (BKT)

"Black button" sign, 99
Black dots, 47, 47f, 61, 62f
Black piedra, 211
Black to brown eumelanin, 13
Blaschko's lines, 186
Blastoconidia, 213
Bleached hair, 289
  with Brazilian keratin treatment, 290
Bleaching, 239, 289
β-Blockers, 71t, 246t, 250
Blonde, 235
Blow-dryers, 237
Blow-drying, 240
Blue-gray dots, 50f
BLyS. See B-lymphocyte stimulator
  (BLyS)
Bone morphogenetic protein (BMP), 3
Botanical products, 300
Botanically derived phytosterols,
  301t–302t
Brachytherapy, 170
Braided hairstyles, 237
Braids, hair care with, 291
Brazilian keratin treatment (BKT), 239
  bleached hair with, 290
"Bridge" treatment, 146–147
Broken hairs, 52–53, 53f, 62, 195
Bromocriptine, 246t
Brownish-grey plaques, 180
Bubble hair, 202, 242
Bulge, 5
  activation hypothesis, 10
  stem cells, 11
Bullous disease, 185. See also Connective
  tissue disease
  EB, 185
  pemphigoid, 185
  pemphigus, 185
Bullous pemphigoid, 185
"Burnt matchstick" sign, 99
Buspirone, 246t

C

CA. See Cicatricial alopecia (CA)
Cadaverized hairs, 59
Caffeine, 299, 301t–302t
Caffeine, niacin amide, panthenol,
  dimethicone, and an acrylate
  polymer (CNPDA), 91
Calcineurin inhibitors, 156
Calcipotriene, 221
Calcipotriol, 221
Calcium hydroxide, 238
"Carpet tack" sign, 152–153
Catagen, 3, 83
  phases, 10
  regulatory pathways/molecules,
    10–11
  stage, 10–11
Catagen follicles, 23–24, 214
β-Catenin, 14, 84
Cathepsin L, 12
Cationic bridging agents, 287

Cationic surfactants, 285–286
CCCA. *See* Central centrifugal cicatricial alopecia (CCCA)
Ccl20, 3
CCLE. *See* Chronic cutaneous lupus erythematosus (CCLE)
Ccr6, 3
Cell
  of ORS, 5
  therapy, 76
  viability, 13
Central centrifugal cicatricial alopecia (CCCA), 33, 34f, 49, 97, 118, 127, 163, 174, 198–199, 222–223, 267. *See also* Androgenetic alopecia (AGA)
  clinical presentation, 128–129
    CCCA grade 1, 128f
    CCCA grade 2, 128f
    CCCA grade 3, 129f
    CCCA grade 4, 129f
    CCCA grade 5, 130f
  dermoscopy, 129–130, 130f
  differential diagnosis, 131
  epidemiology, 128
  etiopathogenesis, 128
  general measurement, 131
  hair morphology and practices with African patients, 127
  histology, 130–131
  history and terminology, 127–128
  management, 131
  medical treatment, 131–132
  surgical treatment, 132
Central nervous system (CNS), 7
Cervical spine disease, 224
Cetuximab, 254t
Chemical damage, 237–240
  hair dye, 237–238
  hair straightening, 238–240
Chemically treated hair, 289
Chemokines, 152
  differential hair cycle–dependent release, 5–6
  receptors, 152
Chemotherapy
  chemotherapy-induced hair loss, 245–246
  permanent alopecia after, 39, 39f
Chemotherapy-induced alopecia (CIA), 245, 247
Chilblain lupus erythematosus, 151
Children, 95
  hair loss in, 193
    diffuse alopecia in childhood, 199–201
    hair shaft disorders, 201–203
    patchy alopecia in childhood, 193–197
    scarring alopecias, 197–199
  with seborrheic dermatitis, 292
  shampoos for
    children with curly or textured hair, 291–292

Children *(Continued)*
    children with seborrheic dermatitis, 292
    hair care in children, 291
    hair care with braids or dreadlocks, 291
    straight caucasian hair and Asian hair, 291
Chloramphenicol, 246t
Chloroquine, 147, 156, 254–255
  clinical presentation and trichoscopy, 255
Cholestyramine, 246t
"Christmas tree" pattern of loss, 312
Chronic AA, 59, 60f
Chronic actinic damage, 179
Chronic cutaneous lupus erythematosus (CCLE), 151, 187
Chronic folliculitis, 249
Chronic granulomas, 169
Chronic pruritus, 224
Chronic scalp pruritus, 219
Chronic stage, 28
Chronic starvation, 88
Chronic TA, 139, 141
Chronic TE, 83
Chronic telogen effluvium, 29, 29f, 85–86
CIA. *See* Chemotherapy-induced alopecia (CIA)
Cicatricial alopecia (CA), 110, 127, 143, 153–154, 295, 314
Cicatricial lymphocytic alopecias, 131
Cicatricial pattern hair loss, 115–120
  CCCA/fibrosing alopecia in pattern distribution, 120f, 124f
  chronic graft-versus-host disease, 117f
  fibrosing alopecia in pattern distribution, 116f
    in man, 123f
    in women, 121f–122f
Cicatricial pemphigoid (CP), 185
Cidofovir, 246t
Cimetidine, 246t
Ciprofloxacin, 170
Circadian clock system, 7–9
CLASI tool. *See* Cutaneous lupus area and severity index tool (CLASI tool)
Classic pseudopelada of Brocq, 163
Classic-traditional antimitotic drugs, 245–247, 246t
  clinical presentation, 245–247
    dystrophic hair shafts, 247f
    total alopecia due to chemotherapy, 246f
  trichoscopy, 247
CLE. *See* Cutaneous lupus erythematosus (CLE)
Clindamycin, 164, 170
Clotrimazole, 246t
CM. *See* Cutaneous mastocytosis (CM)

CNPDA. *See* Caffeine, niacin amide, panthenol, dimethicone, and an acrylate polymer (CNPDA)
CNS. *See* Central nervous system (CNS)
Coagulase-negative staphylococci, 167
Coal tar, 289
Coconut oil, 287
Coiled hairs, 62–63, 98, 195
Collagen type IV stain, 185
"Combination mini-micro grafting technique", 305
Comma hairs, 54, 62–63, 196
Conditioning agents, 285, 289
Conditioning shampoo, 286–287
Congenital syndromes, hair shafts in, 54–56
Congenital triangular alopecia, 63, 138–139
Connective tissue disease, 186–187. *See also* Bullous disease
  DM, 186–187
  LE, 187
  scleroderma, 186
Corkscrew hairs, 54, 62–63, 196
Corticosteroids, 115, 131, 254t, 271, 289
Corticotropin-releasing hormone (CRH), 11
Cosmetic factors, 240
Cosmetic shampoos
  antiresidue shampoos, 292
  for children, 291–292
  considerations on hair washing and grooming procedures, 292
  different types, 288–292
  hair care guidelines for different hair types, 288–289
  seborrheic dermatitis in different hair types, 289–290
  for special scenarios, 290–291
Cosmetic treatments, 90
Coudability hairs, 53, 62
CP. *See* Cicatricial pemphigoid (CP)
"Crawling snake" appearance, 203
CRH. *See* Corticotropin-releasing hormone (CRH)
Cri-saborole ointment, 146–147
Cryosurgery, 175
Cryotherapy, 175
CsA. *See* Cyclosporin A (CsA)
CTCL. *See* Cutaneous T-cell lymphoma (CTCL)
Cumulative nephrotoxic side effects, 148
Curly hair
  children with, 291–292
  hair care in children, 291
Cutaneous LE, 187
Cutaneous lichen planus, 147
Cutaneous lupus area and severity index tool (CLASI tool), 157
Cutaneous lupus erythematosus (CLE), 118, 151

Cutaneous lupus lesions, treatment of, 156
Cutaneous mastocytosis (CM), 189
Cutaneous T-cell lymphoma (CTCL), 188, 223
   CTCL-related alopecia universalis, 188
Cuticle, 235
Cutis verticis gyrata, 169
Cyclosporin A (CsA), 148, 254
Cyclosporine, 132, 222–223, 254t
Cyproterone acetate, 115
Cystic fibrosis, 295
Cytokines, 5, 259
   T-cell secretion of proinflammatory, 148
   Th1, 251

D

Dabrafenib, 247
DAM. *See* N,N-Diallylmelamine (DAM)
DAM N-oxidase (DAMN-O), 276
Danazol, 246t
Dandruff, 14, 210, 216
Danger signals, 5
Dapsone, 181
5% Dapsone gel, 181
Dark hair, 235–236
Dasatinib, 248
DC. *See* Dissecting cellulitis of scalp (DC)
Deep infectious folliculitis, 175
Defolliculation, 143–144
DEGs. *See* Differentially expressed genes (DEGs)
Delayed anagen release, 84
Demodex brevis (D. brevis), 215
Demodex folliculitis, 215
   clinical presentation, 215
   dermoscopy, 215
   etiology, 215
   pathology, 215
   treatment, 215
Demodex folliculorum (D. folliculorum), 215
Demodex spp., 173, 215, 215f
Dermal papilla (DP), 2, 75
Dermatitis, diarrhea, dementia, and death (Four Ds), 296
Dermatitis herpetiformis, 185
Dermatologic pruritus, 219
Dermatomyositis (DM), 183, 186–187, 187f, 222
Dermoscopy, 43, 89, 89f, 129–130, 130f, 187–189
   of acute patch of alopecia areata, 62f
   aspect, 253
   Demodex folliculitis, 215
   features of FAPD, 117
   of LPP, 145, 145f
   moth-eaten alopecic patch, 214f
   PC, 210
   Piedra spp., 213

Dermoscopy *(Continued)*
   Seborrheic dermatitis, 216
   syphilis, 214
   TC, 207–208
Desmoglein 1, 185
Detangling process, 291–292
DHT. *See* Dihydrotestosterone (DHT)
Diabetes, 224
Diabetes mellitus, 224
   type 2, 120
Diagnostic and Statistical Manual of Mental Disorders, Fifth Edition (DSM-5), 95
N,N-Diallylmelamine (DAM), 276
Diazoxide, 246t
Dickkopf-1–related protein, 84
Dietary
   ingredients, 295
   supplements, 273–274
DIF. *See* Direct immunofluorescence (DIF)
Differentially expressed genes (DEGs), 151
Diffuse alopecia, 44, 214. *See also* Patchy alopecia
   in childhood, 199–201
      Anagen effluvium, 200
      diagnosis, 202t
      LAS, 200–201
      short anagen syndrome, 201
      telogen effluvium, 199
Diffuse follicular hyperkeratosis, 248
Diffuse hypertrichosis, 253
Diffuse LPP, 144
"Diffuse pattern", 104, 255
Digital dermoscopes, 43–44
Dihydrotestosterone (DHT), 11, 16, 70, 299, 305
Dimethicone, 286–287
Diode laser, 175
Diphenylcyclopropenone (DPCP), 64
Direct immunofluorescence (DIF), 155, 187
Discoid lupus erythematosus (DLE), 30–31, 32f, 46, 50f, 131, 151–153, 162–163, 186, 198
   clinical findings, 152–153
   dermatoscopic findings, 153–154
   early lesion of DLE on scalp, 152f
   epidemiology, 151
   etiology and pathogenesis, 151–152
   histopathologic findings, 154–155, 154f–155f
   patient management, 155–157
      first-line therapy, 156
      second-line therapy, 156–157
Dissecting cellulitis of scalp (DC), 35–36, 35f, 164, 167
   associating conditions, 169
   comorbidities in dissecting cellulitis, 169t
   clinical features, 167
   differential diagnosis, 169

Dissecting cellulitis of scalp (DC) *(Continued)*
   epidemiology, 167
   etiology, 167
   pathology, 168–169
   prognosis, 170
   treatment, 169–170
      corticosteroids, 170
      oral antibiotics, 170
      oral retinoids, 170
      other treatments, 170
   trichoscopy, 167–168
Dithranol. *See* Anthralin
Diuretics/antiandrogen therapies, 273
Dixyrazine, 246t
Dizygotic (DZ), 95
Dkk-1, 3
DLE. *See* Discoid lupus erythematosus (DLE)
DM. *See* Dermatomyositis (DM)
DM2. *See* Type 2 diabetes mellitus (DM2)
"Donor dominance", 305
Double-blind studies, 276
Doxycycline, 109, 115
DP. *See* Dermal papilla (DP)
DPCP. *See* Diphenylcyclopropenone (DPCP)
DQB1*03 alleles, 143
Dreadlocks, hair care with, 291
Dry hair, 289
   oily scalp and, 289
   with patchy alopecia, 202
Dry virgin hair, 288
DSM-5. *See* Diagnostic and Statistical Manual of Mental Disorders, Fifth Edition (DSM-5)
Dutasteride, 73, 115, 268–271, 271t–272t
Dystrophic EB, 185
DZ. *See* Dizygotic (DZ)

E

Early AGA, 69
Early catagen, 10
EB. *See* Epidermolysis bullosa (EB)
ECDS. *See* En coup de sabre (ECDS)
Ectothrix anthropophilic infections, 207
Ectothrix infection (*Microsporum canis*), 38
EDA2R gene, 69–70
EFAs. *See* Essential fatty acids (EFAs)
Elbow hairs, 62
Elderly, pruritus in, 224
Electrosurgery, 175
Embryology, 1–3
   molecular and genetic basis of hair follicle embryogenesis, 3
   stages of hair follicle formation, 1–2
En coup de sabre (ECDS), 186, 186f
Encapsulated arthroconidia, 213
Encephalopsin, 7
Endogenous factors, 83

Endothrix infection (*Trichophyton tonsurans*), 38, 207
Environmental factors, 104
EPDS. *See* Erosive pustular dermatosis of scalp (EPDS)
Epidermal growth factor, 259
  inhibitors, 248
Epidermis, 161
Epidermoid keratinization, 5
Epidermolysis bullosa (EB), 185
Epiluminescence microscopy, 43
Epithelial stem cells, 5, 76
Erlotinib, 249, 254t
Erosive pustular dermatosis of scalp (EPDS), 36, 163–164, 179, 186
  clinical findings, 179–180
  differential diagnosis, 180
  epidemiology, 179
  pathogenesis, 179
  pathology, 180
  precipitating factors in relation with, 180t
  prognosis, 181
  treatment, 180–181
  trichoscopy, 180
Erythrodermic psoriasis, 231
Essential fatty acids (EFAs), 299
Essential SA, 213–214
17-β Estradiol, 11
Estrogen, 103
Ethambutol, 246t
Ethionamide, 246t
Etiopathogenesis, 59
Excessive inflammation, 271
Excessive wetting, 236–237
Excimer laser, 110, 273
Exclamation mark hairs, 53, 59, 61, 99
Exogen, 11–12
Exogenous factors, 83
Eyebrow(s), 312–313
  loss, 108
Eyelashes transplantation, 312–313
"Eyes and goggles" signs, 29–30

F

F-MF. *See* Folliculotropic MF (F-MF)
Facial area, 161
Facial vellus hairs, 106–107
False-negative hair pull test, 89
FAPD. *See* Fibrosing alopecia in pattern distribution (FAPD)
Fatty acids, 299, 301t–302t
ω-3 Fatty acids, 299
ω-6 Fatty acids, 299
Favic infections, 207
Favus, 207
FD. *See* Folliculitis decalvans (FD)
FDA. *See* United States Food and Drug Administration (FDA)
Female pattern alopecia, 311
Female pattern baldness (FPB), 311–312

Female pattern hair loss (FPHL), 15, 67, 128, 131, 296, 305
Fetal skin development, 1
FFA. *See* Frontal fibrosing alopecia (FFA)
FFASI. *See* Frontal Fibrosing Alopecia Severity Index (FFASI)
Fibroblast growth factor (FGF), 3, 84, 259, 263
Fibronectin, 263
Fibrosing alopecia. *See also* Central centrifugal cicatricial alopecia (CCCA)
  cicatricial pattern hair loss, 115–120
  patterned hair loss, 115
Fibrosing alopecia in pattern distribution (FAPD), 115
Fibrosis, 154
Fibrous streamers. *See* Follicular streamers
Finasteride, 73, 115, 170, 268–271, 271t–272t
First-line therapy, 156
  antimalarials, 156
  topical/intralesional steroids and calcineurin inhibitors, 156
"Flag sign" of Kwashiorkor, 88
Flame hairs, 62, 97, 98f, 195
Flaps, 310
Fluconazole, 209
Fluid retention, 147
Fluoxetine, 246t
Follicle. *See* Hair follicle
Follicular
  activity, 83
  counts, 24
  degeneration syndrome, 118–119, 127–128
  density, 33
  hyperkeratosis, 144–145, 152–153
  inflammation and fibrosis, 115
  length, levels along, 24
  melanogenesis, 10
  pustules, 163
  streamers, 24
  triad, 31–33
  trochanter, 6
Follicular lichen planus. *See* Lichen planopilaris (LPP)
Follicular red dots (FRDs), 43
Follicular signs, 46–48
  dots
    black, 47, 47f
    red, 47, 47f
    white, 47, 47f
    yellow, 46, 46f
  keratotic plugs, 46, 46f
  loss of follicular openings, 48
Follicular unit extraction method (FUE method), 305–306
  harvest, 307–308
    advantages and disadvantages, 309t
    scars from both harvest methods, 308f

Follicular unit transplantation (FUT), 306–311
  harvest
    FUE method, 307–308
    strip method, 306, 307f
  postoperative course, 309–310
  recipient site creation and graft placement, 308–309
"Folliculate épilante" disease, 161
Folliculitis, 146
Folliculitis decalvans (FD), 33–35, 35f, 161, 165, 169, 174
  clinical presentation, 161–162
  diagnosis, 162–163
    bacterial cultures, 163
    clinical history, 162
    dermatologic examination, 162–163
    differential, 163–164
    photography, 163
    skin biopsy, 163
  disease, 161
  epidemiology, 161
  etiopathogenesis, 161
  histopathology, 162, 163f
  history and definition, 161
  prognosis, 165
  treatments, 164
    local, 164
    oral, 164, 164t
  trichoscopy, 162, 162f
Folliculitis keloidalis nuchae. *See* Acne keloidalis nuchae (AKN)
Folliculotropic MF (F-MF), 188
Four Ds. *See* Dermatitis, diarrhea, dementia, and death (Four Ds)
FPB. *See* Female pattern baldness (FPB)
FPHL. *See* Female pattern hair loss (FPHL)
FRDs. *See* Follicular red dots (FRDs)
"Friar Tuck" sign, 96–97
"Fringe sign", 135–136
Frontal fibrosing alopecia (FFA), 31–33, 33f, 103, 106f–107f, 117–118, 138–139, 143, 198, 312–313
  clinical features, 104–108
    glabellar red dots, 107f
    loss of vellus hairs in hairline, 108f
    skin between old and new hairlines, 106f
    trichoscopy shows perifollicular scaling, 107f
  diagnosis, 108
  epidemiology, 103
  follow-up, 110–111
  pathogenesis, 103–104
    autoimmune etiology, 103
    environmental factors, 104
    genetics, 104
    hormonal etiology, 103
    lipid metabolism dysfunction, 104
    neurogenic inflammation, 104

Frontal fibrosing alopecia (FFA)
(*Continued*)
treatment, 108–110
patient with, 110f
Frontal Fibrosing Alopecia Severity
Index (FFASI), 110–111
Frontal hairlines, 135–136
FUE method. *See* Follicular unit
extraction method (FUE method)
Fungal infection, 162–163
Fusidic acid, 164
FUT. *See* Follicular unit transplantation
(FUT)

G
GARD. *See* National Institute of
Health's Genetic and Rare Diseases
Information Center (GARD)
Gasdermin 3, 143–144
Gastrointestinal upset, 147
Gefitinib, 249, 254t
and erlotinib, 255
therapy, 179
Genetic(s), 104, 305
basis of hair follicle embryogenesis,
3
genetic/genomic targets, 74–75
Genodermatoses, 199
Genome Wide Association Studies
(GWAS), 59, 69–70
Genuine
alopecia areata, 233
telogen effluvium, 229
Glatiramer acetate, 246t
Glibenclamide, 246t
Global photography, 163
Glutamate, 224
Glutamine, 11
Glyoxylic acid, 239
hair fiber treated with, 239–240
treatment, 240
Goggles, 145–146
signs, 29–30
Graft placement, 308–309
Graft-versus-host disease (GvHD), 117,
190
Graham-Little-Piccardi-Lasseur syn-
drome, 143, 145
Granulomatous dermatitis, 187–188
leprosy, 188
sarcoidosis, 187–188, 188f
Gray hair, 236
Great imitator. *See* Syphilis
Growth factors, 260
Guanidine carbonate, 238
GvHD. *See* Graft-versus-host disease
(GvHD)
GWAS. *See* Genome Wide Association
Studies (GWAS)

H
Habit reversal training (HRT), 224
Habit-tic disorder, 224

Hair, 267
accessory, 138
anatomy, 235
dry trichoscopy, 236f
tricorrhexis nodosa, 236f
bulb, 4, 9, 24
casts, 107–108, 139
changes to drugs
hair and drugs, 245–255
pathophysiology, 245
counts, 23–24
cycle, 83
hair cycle–dependent changes, 11
length, 12
density, 14
dermoscopy, 129
diameter, 14
variability, 44
dye, 237–238
extensions, 237, 238f
germ, 2
graying, 14
matrix, 3, 9
morphology and practices with
African patients, 127
placode, 2
problems, 245
research, 1
shampoo pH and hair frizz, 287–288
shedding, 12
straightening, 127, 238–240
shaft with loss of cuticle and
cortex exposure, 240f
Hair and drugs
anticoagulants, 250
antihypertensive agents, 250–251
antineoplastic agents, 245–249
antiretrovirals, 252
azathioprine, 253
chloroquine, 254–255
CsA, 254
drugs acting on nervous system,
252–253
interferons, 251
minoxidil, 253
oral contraceptives, 252
permanent alopecia to chemotherapy,
255
prostaglandin analogs, 254
radiation therapy, 249–250
retinol and retinoids, 251–252
strontium ranelate, 253–254
thallium, 254
Hair and scalp
dermatoscopy
patient evaluation, 44–45
trichoscopic signs and patterns,
46–56
trichoscopy devices and
particularities, 43–44, 44f
trichoscopy helping clinician, 43
infections, 207
demodex folliculitis, 215

Hair and scalp (*Continued*)
PC, 209–211
Piedra spp., 211–213
seborrheic dermatitis, 215–217
TC, 207–209
Hair care
with braids or dreadlocks, 291
in children, 291
guidelines for different hair types
bleached hair, 289
dry virgin hair, 288
normal hair, 288
oily hair and scalp, 288
oily scalp and dry hair, 289
"Hair collar sign", 196
Hair cosmeceuticals
different types of cosmetic shampoos, 288–292
mineral and vegetable oils, 287
shampoos, 285–287
and allergy, 288
pH and hair frizz, 287–288
Hair follicle (HF), 1, 3, 23–24, 83, 103
cycling, 7–13, 8f
anagen stage, 9–10
catagen stage, 10–11
differences of HF cycling in anatomic locations, 12–13
exogen, 12
kenogen, 12
metabolism during cycling, 13
role of oxidative damage, 13
telogen stage, 11
dermal papilla, 4
formation, 1
stages, 1–2
immunologic components, 5–6
inferior, 4
melanogenesis, 13
molecular and genetic basis of HF
embryogenesis, 3
morphology, 4f
neuroendocrinology, 15–16
telogen, 12
types, 7
vellus, 7
Hair follicle stem cells (HFSCs), 1,
9–10, 14
Hair loss, 103, 136, 145, 185, 187,
189, 229, 245, 246t, 267
in children, 193
diffuse alopecia in childhood,
199–201
hair shaft disorders, 201–203
patchy alopecia in childhood,
193–197
scarring alopecias, 197–199
novel treatment modalities for
ADSCs therapy, 263–264
LLLT, 260–262
mesotherapy, 262
microneedling, 262–263
PRP, 259–260

Hair loss disorders, clinical trials for
  androgenetic alopecia, 276–282
  burden of disease in alopecia, 267
  clinical study design, 276
  clinical testing, 275
  devices, 273
  dietary supplements and nutraceuti-
    cals, 273–274
  drugs, 267–273
    development and FDA approval
      process, 274, 274f
    diuretics/antiandrogen therapies,
      273
    immunomodulators, 271–273
    prostaglandin agonists, 273
    5α-reductase inhibitors, 268–271
    vasodilator, 268
  IDE, 275–276
  IND, 275
  NDA, 276
  phase 1 clinical studies, 275
  phase 2 clinical studies, 275
  phase 3 clinical studies, 275
  phase 4 clinical studies, 275
  preclinical testing, 274–275
Hair pathology
  alopecia
    nonscarring, 24–29
    scarring, 29–36
  follicular counts, 24
  hair follicles and hair counts, 23–24
  horizontal sections, 23
  levels along follicular length, 24
  miscellaneous
    lichen simplex chronicus, 37–38,
      37f
    permanent alopecia after
      chemotherapy, 39, 39f
    scalp psoriasis, 37, 37f
    seborrheic dermatitis, 36, 36f
    syphilitic alopecia, 38–39
    tinea capitis, 38, 38f
  scalp biopsy, 23
"Hair powder" sign, 97, 195
Hair pull test, 71–72, 89, 201, 300
Hair shaft disorders, 45, 201–203
  with increased fragility, 201–203
    bubble hair, 202
    monilethrix, 201
    Pili torti, 202
    TI, 201–202
    TN, 203
    TTD, 202–203
  without increased fragility, 203
    Pili annulati, 203
    Pili trianguli et canaliculi, 203
    Woolly hair, 203
Hair shaft(s), 51–56, 235
  abnormalities, 193
  broken hairs, 52–53, 53f
  comma hairs and corkscrew hairs, 54
  in congenital syndromes, 54–56
  damage, 240

Hair shaft(s) *(Continued)*
  diameter, 115
  diameter variability, 51
  exclamation mark hairs and coud-
    ability hairs, 53
  SRHs, 51–52, 52f
  types of, 7
Hair supplements
  macronutrients, 299
  marine complexes, 300
  micronutrients, 295–299
  nonvitamin nonmineral products,
    299–300
Hair transplantation, 110, 305
  achieving patient satisfaction,
    310–311
  for dermatologists, 305
    SDA, 306f
  evolution, 305–306
  FUT, 306–310
  practical applications, 311–315
    Acell Matristem, 315
    beards and mustaches, 313
    eyebrows and eyelashes, 312–313
    FPB, 311–312
    MPB, 311
    primary cicatricial alopecia,
      314–315
    scar tissue caused by physical
      trauma, 313–314
Hair weathering, 235
  causes of weathering, 235–240
  clinical examination, 240–242
    findings, 240–242
    trichorrhexis nodosa, 240–241
  diagnosis, 240
  hair anatomy, 235
  treatment, 242
HairMax LaserBand, 273
HairMax LaserComb, 261, 273
Hairstyle diversification, 140
Haloperidol, 246t
Hamburger sign, 29, 99
Handheld dermoscopes, 43–44
Hashimoto thyroiditis, 179
HCQ. *See* Hydroxychloroquine (HCQ)
Hedgehog pathways, 84
Hedgehog signaling pathways, 297
Helicobacter pylori (H. pylori), 143
Hematologic
  changes, 147
  malignancies, 223–224
Hemifacial atrophy, 186
Hepatic growth factor (HGF), 84
Hepatitis C virus, 143
Hepatocyte growth factor, 263
Heredity, 67
Herlitz junctional EB, 185
Herpes simplex virus 2, 143
HF. *See* Hair follicle (HF)
HF density (HFD), 7
HFSCs. *See* Hair follicle stem cells
  (HFSCs)

HGF. *See* Hepatic growth factor (HGF)
Hidradenitis suppurativa (HS), 167,
  175
Hispanic hair, hair care in children,
  291
Histologic and fluorescence-activated
  cell sorting analysis, 76
Histology, TA, 139–140
Histopathologic
  features of traction alopecia, 139t
  findings, 154–155, 154f–155f, 162
HIV. *See* Human immunodeficiency
  virus (HIV)
HLA DRB1*11 alleles, 143
Honeycomb pattern, 48–49, 49f
Horizontal section(s), 23, 69
  of biopsy, 29, 37–38
Hormonal
  etiology, 103
  influence, 167
Hormones, 67
"Hot comb alopecia", 118–119, 127
HoVert technique, 145–146
HRT. *See* Habit reversal training (HRT)
HS. *See* Hidradenitis suppurativa (HS)
"Hugging pattern", 130–131
Human
  differences between humans and
    mouse hair follicles morphology,
    15
  papillomavirus, 143
  scalp
    in different ages, 14–15
    HFs, 7
Human androgenetic alopecia, animal
  models of, 77
Human HF, 1
  anatomy and cytology of pilosebaceous
    unit, 3–7
    immunologic components of HF,
      5–6
    other constituents of pilosebac-
      ceous unit, 6–7
  cycling, 7–13
    differences between humans and
      mouse HF morphology and, 15
  embryology, 1–3
    molecular and genetic basis of HF
      embryogenesis, 3
    stages of HF formation, 1–2
  human scalp in different ages, 14–15
  melanogenesis, 13
  neuroendocrinology, 15–16
  normal human scalp characteristics
    in different races, 13–14
  types, 7
Human immunodeficiency virus
  (HIV), 143, 207
Humidity, 289
Hydroxides, 239
Hydroxychloroquine (HCQ), 109, 147,
  156, 222–223
Hydroxypyridones, 289

Hyperpigmenation, 48–49, 138–139
Hypertrichosis, 276
Hypogranulosis, 231–233
Hypothalamic–pituitary–adrenal axis supression, 146

I

IDE. *See* Investigational device exemption (IDE)
IFN. *See* Interferon (IFN)
IGF. *See* Insulin-like growth factor (IGF)
IGF-1. *See* Insulin growth factor-1 (IGF-1)
IgG. *See* Immunoglobulin G (IgG)
IL. *See* Interleukin (IL)
Imatinib, 248
Immediate anagen release, 84
Immune system, 143
Immunoglobulin G (IgG), 152
Immunoglobulins, 246t
Immunomodulators, 271–273
Immunosenescence, 224
Immunosuppressants, 132
Inciting factor removal, 90
IND. *See* Investigational new drug (IND)
Indinavir, 246t
Infectious
    pediculosis capitis, 223
    tinea capitis, 223
Inflammatory/inflammation, 145–146
    allergic contact dermatitis, 223
    atopic dermatitis, 222
    attack, 143
    dermatomyositis, 222
    lesions, 163
    processes, 314
    scalp psoriasis, 220–221
    scarring alopecia, 115, 222–223
    seborrheic dermatitis, 219
    TC, 169, 207, 208f
Infliximab, 170
Infundibular keratinization, 5
Infundibulum, 5–6, 24, 108
Inner root sheath (IRS), 2, 185
Institutional Review Board (IRB), 275–276
Insulin, 11
Insulin growth factor-1 (IGF-1), 11, 84
Insulin-like growth factor (IGF), 259, 263
Interferon (IFN), 2, 246t, 251, 251f
    clinical presentation, 251
    gene expression, 152
    interferon-α2b, 254t
    interferon-γ, 148
    system, 152
    trichoscopy, 251
Interfollicular, 48
    epidermis, 185, 231
    interface dermatitis, 154–155
    patterns

Interfollicular *(Continued)*
    hyperpigmenation, 48–49
    perifollicular erythema, 48, 48f
    peripilar sign, 48
    scaling, 48
    white-gray halo, 49
Interleukin (IL), 2
    IL-1, 251, 259
    IL-2, 251
Intermediate hairs, 7
Internal root sheath (IRS), 127
Intraepithelial components, 185
Intralesional
    corticosteroids, 110, 164
    steroids, 63, 156
    therapies, 146–147
    triamcinolone, 175
Intraoperatively PRP, 315
Intravenous IG (IVIG), 157
Investigational device exemption (IDE), 275–276
Investigational new drug (IND), 275
IRB. *See* Institutional Review Board (IRB)
Iron, 297–299, 301t–302t
    deficiency, 91
IRS. *See* Inner root sheath (IRS); Internal root sheath (IRS)
Isotretinoin, 170
Isthmus, 24, 108, 109f
Itchy scalp. *See also* Scalp psoriasis
    dermatologic pruritus, 219
    primary cutaneous diseases, 219–224
    pruritus without associated skin findings, 224–225
IVIG. *See* Intravenous IG (IVIG)

J

Janus Kinase (JAK), 64–65
Junctional EB with pyloric atresia, 185

K

K81 hair keratins, 201
K86 hair keratins, 201
Kenogen, 12
Keratin, 287
    hydrolysates, 287
    keratin 6, 5
    keratin 16, 5
Keratinocyte growth factor, 263
Keratolytics, 219
Keratotic plugs, 46, 46f
Kerion, 196
Kerion celsi, 169, 207, 208f
Ketoconazole, 219, 289
Klippel-Feil syndrome, 179
Kwashiorkor, 88, 295, 299

L

Laminin 332, 185
Laminin 5, 185

Laminins 311, 185
Langerhans cells, 2
Lanugo hairs, 7
LAS. *See* Loose anagen syndrome (LAS)
Laser therapy, 64, 164
Latanoprost, 254t, 273
Late catagen, 10
LE. *See* Lupus erythematosus (LE)
Leflunomide, 246t
LEP. *See* Lupus erythematosus profundus/panniculitis (LEP)
Leprosy, 188
"Less-aggressive sulfate-free" surfactants, 291
Levodopa, 246t, 253
Lichen planopilaris (LPP), 29, 31–33, 32f, 48, 103, 115, 131, 143, 151, 162–163, 186, 198, 199f, 222, 267, 314
    clinical features, 144–145
    dermoscopy, 145, 145f
    epidemiology, 143
    etiology, 143
    histopathology, 145–146, 146f
    management, 146–148
        systemic therapies, 147–148
        topical/intralesional therapies, 146–147
    pathogenesis, 143–144
    treatment options for, 146t
Lichen Planopilaris Activity Index (LPPAI), 110–111
Lichen planus pigmentosus (LPPigm), 107
Lichen planus spinulosus, 145
Lichen simplex chronicus, 37–38, 37f
Lichenoid interface perifolliculitis, 145–146
Light stimulation, 74
Linear IgA bullous dermatosis, 185
Linear LPP, 145
"Linear pattern", 104
Lipid
    bonding, 12
    metabolism, 144
    metabolism dysfunction, 104
Lisinopril-induced alopecia, 250
Lithium, 246t
LLLT. *See* Low-level laser/light therapy (LLLT)
Localized scleroderma, 186
"Lonely hairs", 105, 105f, 138–139
Loose anagen syndrome (LAS), 200–201, 201f
    hair pull test, 201
Loss of follicular openings, 48
Low-level laser/light therapy (LLLT), 74, 260–262, 261f, 273
    mechanism of action, 260–261
    studies, 261
    treatments for AGA, 261–262
Low-level light therapy. *See* Low-level laser/light therapy (LLLT)

LPP. *See* Lichen planopilaris (LPP)
LPPAI. *See* Lichen Planopilaris Activity Index (LPPAI)
LPPigm. *See* Lichen planus pigmentosus (LPPigm)
Lupus erythematosus (LE), 183, 187
Lupus erythematosus profundus/panniculitis (LEP), 151
Lupus panniculitis, 153
Lycopene, 299
Lymphocytic cicatricial alopecia, 143
Lymphoproliferative disorders, 188

M

M-TAS Score. *See* Marginal Traction Alopecia Severity Score (M-TAS Score)
Macrolides, 170
Macronutrients
    amino acids and proteins, 299
    fatty acids, 299
Major histocompatibility complex (MHC), 5
Malassezia spp., 1, 173, 217, 219
Male pattern baldness (MPB), 305, 311
Male pattern hair loss (MPHL), 15, 67
Malfunctioning of HF immune privilege, 5–6
Maprotiline, 246t
Marginal alopecia, 45
Marginal presentation, 136
Marginal TA, 135–136, 136f
Marginal Traction Alopecia Severity Score (M-TAS Score), 135–136, 137f
Marine complexes, 300, 301t–302t
Marrocan argan oil, 287
Mast cells, 2
Master regulator
    of genes, 13
    protein, 144
Mastocytosis, 189
Matrical cells, 5
Matrix keratinocytes, 245
Mature follicles, 76
MEA. *See* Methyl eicosanoic acid (MEA)
Melanin, 235–236
    production, 2, 9
    types, 13
Melanocytes, 5
    stem cells, 14
Melanogenesis in hair follicle, 13
Melatonin, 299–300, 301t–302t
Menkes syndrome, 202
Mesalazine, 246t
Mesenchymal cell aggregation, 2
Mesotherapy, 262, 262f
    caveats, 262
    mechanism of action, 262
    studies, 262
Methotrexate, 229, 273
Methyl eicosanoic acid (MEA), 235
Methylene glycol, 239
Methylprednisolone, 64

Methysergide, 246t
MF. *See* Mycosis fungoides (MF)
MHC. *See* Major histocompatibility complex (MHC)
Microarray technique, 144
Microinflammation, 115
Microneedling, 262–263, 263f, 273
    alopecia, 263
    mechanism of action, 262–263
    studies, 263
Micronutrients
    minerals, 297–299
    vitamins, 295–297
Microsporum canis. *See* Ectothrix infection *(Microsporum canis)*
Microsporum species, 196–197, 209
    M canis, 207
    M. gypseum, 38
Mid-catagen, 10
Mild thinning, 145
Mineral(s), 297–299
    iron, 298–299
    oils, 287
    zinc, 298
Miniaturization, 69
Minoxidil, 72–73, 84, 91, 115, 131, 246t, 253, 254t, 268, 269t–270t, 276–282
    clinical presentation and trichoscopy, 253
    development, 1
Mitochondrial membrane potential, 13
MMF. *See* Mycophenolate mofetil (MMF)
Molecular basis of hair follicle embryogenesis, 3
Molecular controls of HF induction and morphogenesis, 3
Monilethrix, 54–55, 55f, 201
Monozygotic twin (MZ twin), 95
Morphea. *See* Localized scleroderma
Morse code hairs, 196
Moth-eaten or patchy alopecia, 214
Mouse hair follicles morphology and cycling, differences with humans and, 15
MPB. *See* Male pattern baldness (MPB)
MPHL. *See* Male pattern hair loss (MPHL)
Mucinous fibrosis, 31–33
Multidrug therapy, 188
Multitargeted receptor TKIs, 248
Mupirocin, 164
Mustaches, 313
Myalgia, 147
Mycobacterium leprae (M. leprae), 188
Mycologic culture, 208–209
Mycophenolate mofetil (MMF), 132, 147–148, 222–223
Mycosis fungoides (MF), 188
Myristyl (tetradecyl) nicotinate, 296
MZ. *See* Monozygotic (MZ)

N

NAC. *See* N-Acetylcysteine (NAC)
NAD. *See* Nicotinamide adenine dinucleotide (NAD)
NADP. *See* Nicotinamide adenine dinucleotide phosphate (NADP)
National Institute of Health's Genetic and Rare Diseases Information Center (GARD), 73
Natural African hair, 289–290
Natural curly hair, 290
NDA. *See* New drug application (NDA)
Natural African hair, 289–290
Necrosis, 151
Neoplastic processes, 219, 223–224
Nerve compression, 224
Nervous system, drugs acting on, 252–253
    clinical presentation, 253
    trichoscopy, 253
Netherton syndrome, 201–202
Neuroendocrinology of hair follicle, 15–16
Neurogenic inflammation, 104
Neuropathic
    cervical spine disease, 224
    diabetes mellitus, 224
    PHN, 224
    treatment for neuropathic pruritus, 224
Neuropeptides, 104
Neurotrophins, 7
New drug application (NDA), 275–276
Niacin, 296, 301t–302t
Nicotinamide adenine dinucleotide (NAD), 296
Nicotinamide adenine dinucleotide phosphate (NADP), 296
Nioxin, 91
Nitrofurantoin, 246t
Nits, 210
Non-Herlitz junctional EB, 185
Noncicatricial alopecia, 153–154
Noninflammatory
    black dot pattern, 207, 207f
    SD type, 207
    tinea capitis, 223
Nonionic surfactants, 285–286
Nonmarginal presentation, 135
Nonmarginal traction alopecia, 136, 138f
"Nonmarginal" distribution, 136
Nonpolarized lights, 44
Nonscarring alopecia, 24–29, 83, 135, 138, 183, 187–188, 267. *See also* Androgenetic alopecia (AGA); Scarring alopecia
    alopecia areata, 24–28
        incognito, 28–29
    androgenetic alopecia, 29
        trichotillomania, 29
    chronic telogen effluvium, 29
Nonscarring alopecic patches, 193
Nonsurgically PRP, 315

Nontraditional demographic groups, 135
Nonvitamin nonmineral products
  botanical products, 300
  caffeine, 299
  melatonin, 299–300
Noonan syndrome, 200–201
Noonan-like syndrome, 200–201
Normal hair, 288
Normal human scalp characteristics in different races, 13–14
Nrf2. *See* Nuclear factor (erythroid-derived 2)-like 2 (Nrf2)
NRTI. *See* Nucleoside reverse transcriptase inhibitor (NRTI)
Nuclear factor (erythroid-derived 2)-like 2 (Nrf2), 13
Nucleoside reverse transcriptase inhibitor (NRTI), 252
Nutraceuticals, 273–274
Nutritional supplementation, 91

O

Occasional congenital alopecia, 185
Occipital region, 104, 105f
Octreotide, 246t
Octyl nicotinate, 296
Ocular abnormalities, 63
Oils, 287
Oily hair, 288–289
Oily scalp, 288
  and dry hair, 289
  wavy/curly relaxed hair with dry tips and, 291
  wavy/curly virgin hair with dry tips and, 290
Oily straight caucasian virgin hair, 290
  with dry tips, 290
Onion-shaped indentation, 4
Onycholysis, 231–233
Ophiasis, 60
Ophthalmologic damage, 147
Optimal scalp biopsy, 89
Oral
  antibiotics, 164, 170, 175
  antihistamines, 221
  clinical presentation and trichoscopy of oral contraceptives, 246t, 252
  cyclosporine, 64
  dexamethasone, 64
  hydroxychloroquine, 115
  prednisolone, 64
  retinoids, 170
    therapy, 147
  treatment, 164
Organ-cultured human HFs, 11
ORS cells. *See* Outer root sheath cells (ORS cells)
Osteomyelitis, 170
Outer root sheath cells (ORS cells), 2, 5, 185
Owl eyes, 145–146
Oxidative damage role, 13

P

P-cadherin-mediated signals, 11
p21CIP1 protein, 5
p27KIP1 protein, 5
p57KIP2 protein, 5
Panitumumab, 254t
Panniculitis-like lymphoma, 153
Panopsin, 7
Papular lesions, atrichia with, 63
PAR. *See* Protease-activated receptor (PAR)
Paroxetine, 246t
Patch of acute and active AA, 59
Patch test, 132
Patchy alopecia, 44–45. *See also* Diffuse alopecia; Scarring alopecias
  in childhood, 193–197
    ACC, 196
    alopecia areata, 193–194
    diagnosis, 200t
    tinea capitis, 196–197
    traction alopecia, 197
    TTA, 195–196
    TTM, 194–195
Patchy LPP, 144
Patterned hair loss, 115
Patterned LPP, 144
Pazopanib, 248
PC. *See* Pediculosis capitis (PC)
PCOS. *See* Polycystic ovarian syndrome (PCOS)
PDGF. *See* Platelet-derived growth factor (PDGF)
PDT. *See* Photodynamic therapy (PDT)
Pediatric AA, 59
Pediatric alopecia, 193
Pediculosis capitis (PC), 209–211, 211f, 223. *See also* Tinea capitis (TC)
  clinical presentation, 209–210
  dermoscopy, 210
  etiology, 209
  treatment, 210–211, 212t
Pediculus humanus capitis, 223
PEG–IFN-α. *See* Pegylated interferon α (PEG–IFN-α)
Pegylated interferon α (PEG–IFN-α), 251
Pellagra, 296
Pemphigoid, 185
Pemphigus, 185
Pemphigus foliaceus (PF), 185
Pemphigus vegetans, 185
Pemphigus vulgaris (PV), 185, 186f
Penicillamine, 254t
Perifollicular, 48
  dermis, 161
  erythema, 48, 48f, 138–139, 144–145
  fibrosis, 108, 115
  patterns
    hyperpigmentation, 48–49
    perifollicular erythema, 48, 48f
    peripilar sign, 48

Perifollicular *(Continued)*
    scaling, 48
    white-gray halo, 49
Peripheral blood monocytes, 152
Peripheral HPA axis, 16
Peripilar salmon-colored halos, 183–185
Peripilar sign, 48
Permanent alopecia
  after chemotherapy, 39, 39f, 200
  due to chemotherapy, 255
    clinical presentation, 255
    trichoscopy, 255
  due to radiation, 249, 250f
Permanent hair coloring damages hair cuticle, 237
Peroxisome biogenesis, 144
Peroxisome proliferator–activated receptor γ (PPAR-γ), 104, 144
PF. *See* Pemphigus foliaceus (PF)
PFS. *See* Postfinasteride syndrome (PFS)
PGD2. See Prostaglandin D2 (*PGD2*)
Phenytoin, 254t
PHN. *See* Postherpetic neuralgia (PHN)
Phosphodiesterase 4 inhibitor, 146–147, 222
Photo dermoscopy, 163
Photochemical degradation, 235
Photodynamic therapy (PDT), 164, 170
Photoprotection, 156
Photoreceptors OPN2, 7
Photoreceptors OPN3, 7
Phototherapy, 64
Physical damage, 237
  hair extensions, 237
Physical trauma, scar tissue caused by, 313–314
Phytosterol glycosides, 300
Phytosterols, 300
Piedra spp., 211–213, 213f
  clinical presentation, 211
  culture, 213
  dermoscopy, 213
  etiology, 211
  P. hortae, 211
  treatment, 213
Pigmented casts, 29
Pili annulati, 55, 55f, 203
Pili torti, 55, 202
Pili trimanguli et canaliculi, 56, 203
Pilosebaceous unit, 6, 6f, 143
  anatomy and cytology, 3–7
    immunologic components of hair follicle, 5–6
    other constituents of pilosebaceous unit, 6–7
Pioglitazone, 147
Piroxicam, 246t
Pityriasis simplex capitis. *See* Dandruff
Plasmacytoid dendritic cells, 155
Platelet lysis, 259

Platelet-derived growth factor (PDGF), 259, 263
Platelet-rich plasma (PRP), 259–260, 308, 315
  male with androgenetic alopecia, 261f
  mechanism of action, 259
  studies, 259–260
  telogen effluvium, 260
PMR. *See* Progressive muscle relaxation (PMR)
Pohl-Pinkus constrictions, 54–55, 245–246
Polarized lights, 44
Polycystic ovarian syndrome (PCOS), 70
Polypeptides, 286
Polypharmacy, 224
Polysiloxane polymers, 287
Polytrichia, 162
POMC. *See* Proopiomelanocortin (POMC)
Post-menopausal osteoporosis, 253
Posterior hairlines, 135–136
Posterior scalp, 197–198
Postfinasteride syndrome (PFS), 73
Postherpetic neuralgia (PHN), 224
Postmenopausal women, 103
Postoperative alopecia (PA). *See* Pressure-induced alopecia
Postoperative course, 309–310
  scalp reductions, flaps, tissue expanders, 310
Postoperative radiation therapy, 175
Potassium thiocyanate, 246t
PPAR-γ. *See* Peroxisome proliferator–activated receptor γ (PPAR-γ)
Premature desquamation of IRS, 131
Pressure alopecia. *See* Postoperative alopecia (PA)
Pressure-induced alopecia, 99–101, 189, 190f, 197–198
Primary alopecia, 183
Primary cicatricial alopecia, 161, 314–315
  PRP, 315
Primary cutaneous diseases
  infectious, 223
  inflammatory, 219–223
  neoplastic, 223–224
Primary lymphocytic cicatricial alopecia, 103
Progressive muscle relaxation (PMR), 225
Proinflammatory cytokines, 148
"Proinflammatory toxic" lipids, 144
Prominent facial papules, 106–107, 106f
Proopiomelanocortin (POMC), 15
Propionibacterium acnes (P. acnes), 167
Prostaglandin
  agonists, 273
  analogs, 254
  PGF2A analog bimatoprost, 75

Prostaglandin D2 (*PGD2*), 75
Protease-activated receptor (PAR), 222–223
  PAR-2, 222–223
Protein(s), 235, 299
  malnutrition, 295
  precursors, 263
Proximal trichorrhexis nodosa, 240–241
PRP. *See* Platelet-rich plasma (PRP)
PRP combined with dalteparin (PRP-DP), 259
Pruritus, 223
  without associated skin findings
    in elderly, 224
    neuropathic, 224
    psychiatric conditions, 224–225
    underlying systemic disease, 224
Pseudo 'fringe sign' pattern, 104, 105f
Pseudo-monilethrix hairs, 62
Psoralen and ultraviolet A radiation (PUVA), 64
Psoralens, 254t
Psoriasiform
  alopecia, 229
  epidermal hyperplasia, 231–233
  rash on scalp, 222
Psoriasis, 183, 285, 287
  of scalp and psoriasiform alopecia, 229
Psychiatric conditions
  stress and scalp itch, 225
  trichotillomania, 224
Psychologic support, 90–91
Punch biopsy, 23, 193
PUVA. *See* Psoralen and ultraviolet A radiation (PUVA)
PV. *See* Pemphigus vulgaris (PV)
Pyridostigmine, 246t

Q

Quality of life (QOL), 131
Quinacrine, 147
Quinolones, 170

R

Radiation, 246t
  radiation-induced alopecia, 249
  therapy, 249–250
    clinical presentation, 249
    trichoscopy, 250
Radiotherapy, 164, 245–246, 249
Randomized controlled trials (RCTs), 271, 296
Ranibizumab, 248
Raynaud's phenomenon, 151
RBV. *See* Ribavirin (RBV)
RCTs. *See* Randomized controlled trials (RCTs)
Reactive oxygen species (ROS), 13
Recipient site creation, 308–309
Red dots, 47, 47f
Red hair, 235

5α-Reductase inhibitors (5AR inhibitors), 103, 115, 132, 268–271, 299, 305
Refractory AKN case, 175
Refractory phase, 11
Regulating pathways/molecules
  of anagen stage, 9
  of catagen stage, 10–11
  of telogen stage, 11
Regulatory T cells (Treg cells), 3
Relaxed African hair, 290
  seborrheic dermatitis, 290
Renbök phenomenon, 231
Restoration surgery, 164
Retinoids, 229, 246t, 251–252
  clinical presentation, 252
  trichoscopy, 252
Retinol, 246t, 251–252
Reversible alopecia, 135
Reversible hair discoloration, 254–255
Rheumatoid arthritis, 179, 221
Rhodopsin, 7
Ribavirin (RBV), 251
Ribociclib, 248
Rifampicin, 164, 170
Ringed hair. *See* Pili annulati
Risperidone, 246t
Rodents, 15
ROS. *See* Reactive oxygen species (ROS)
Rosiglitazone, 147
Ruxolitinib, 65, 273

S

SA. *See* Syphilitic alopecia (SA)
SADBE. *See* Squaric acid dibutylester (SADBE)
Safe donor area (SDA), 305, 306f
Salicylates, 246t
Salicylic acid, 189, 289
SALT score. *See* Severity of Alopecia Tool score (SALT score)
Sarcoidosis, 187–188, 188f
Scaling, 48
Scalp, 96–97, 194, 219, 229, 245
  biopsy, 23, 33, 89
  itch, 225
  pruritus, 219, 220t
  reductions, 310
  resection, 170
  trichoscopy of active DLE, 153, 154f
Scalp psoriasis, 37, 37f, 220–221.
  See also Itchy scalp
  clinical patterns, 229
  course and prognosis, 229–231
  degree of sebaceous hypoplasia, 230–231
  histopathology, 231
  psoriasis of scalp and psoriasiform alopecia, 229
  treatment, 231–233

Scanning electron microscopy (SEM), 235, 240
Scar tissue caused by physical trauma, 313–314
Scarring, 145–146, 154
  alopecic patches, 163
  process, 145–146
Scarring alopecia, 29–36, 104, 128, 131, 138–139, 143, 152–153, 183, 197–199, 214, 222–223, 231–233. *See also* Androgenetic alopecia (AGA); Nonscarring alopecia; Traction alopecia (TA)
  acne keloidalis nuchae, 36, 36f
  in African Americans, 127
  CCCA, 198–199
  central centrifugal cicatricial alopecia, 33, 34f
  discoid lupus erythematosus, 30–31, 32f
  dissecting cellulitis of scalp, 35–36, 35f
  DLE, 198
  EPDS, 36
  folliculitis decalvans, 33–35, 35f
  frontal fibrosing alopecia, 31–33, 33f, 198
  genodermatoses, 199
  lichen planopilaris, 31–33, 32f, 198
  pressure-induced alopecia, 197–198
  traction alopecia, 33, 34f
SCC. *See* Squamous cell carcinoma (SCC)
Scleroderma, 186
Sclerotic state, 138–139
Scutula, 207
SD. *See* Seborrheic dermatitis (SD)
SDA. *See* Safe donor area (SDA)
Sebaceous gland(s), 108, 143–144, 174, 229–230
  dysfunction, 144
  number and size, 14
Sebaceous hypoplasia degree, 230–231
Seborrheic dermatitis (SD), 36, 36f, 207, 215–217, 216f, 231, 285
  children with, 292
  clinical presentation, 216
  dermoscopy, 216
  in different hair types, 289–290
    Asian hair, 290
    chemically treated hair, 289
    dry hair, 289
    natural African hair, 289–290
    natural curly hair, 290
    oily hair, 289
    relaxed african hair, 290
  etiology, 215–216
  pathology, 216
  treatment, 217, 217t
Sebum, 285
Second-line therapy, 156–157
  biologic agents, 157

Secondary alopecia, 183
  amyloidosis, 183–185, 184f
  bullous disease, 185
  common conditions associating with, 183t
  connective tissue disease, 186–187
  granulomatous dermatitis, 187–188
  malignancy, 188–189
    AN, 188–189
    cutaneous T-cell lymphoma, 189f
    lymphoproliferative disorders, 188
  miscellaneous, 189–190
    GVHD, 190
    mastocytosis, 189
    PA, 189, 190f
Secondary germ, 10
Secondary hair germ cells, 11
Secondary peripheral edema, 147
Secondary surfactants, 285
Secretory granules, 13
Selenium disulfide, 289
Self-induced hair loss, 135
SEM. *See* Scanning electron microscopy (SEM)
Semilunar tissue expander, 175
Semitranslucent epidermis, 196
Senescent alopecia, 15
Serial clinical photography, 89
Serotonin reuptake inhibitors, 246t
Serum ferritin, 298–299
Severity of Alopecia Tool score (SALT score), 297
Sexual maturity, 7
Sezary syndrome (SS), 188
Shampooing, 240
Shampoos, 285–287
  and allergy, 288
  amphoteric surfactants, 286
  anionic surfactants, 285
  cationic surfactants, 286
  for children, 291–292
  conditioning shampoo, 286–287
  nonionic surfactants, 286
  pH and hair frizz, 287–288
  for special scenarios
    Asian perm hair, 291
    bleached hair with Brazilian keratin treatment, 290
    oily straight Caucasian virgin hair, 290
    relaxed African hair, 290
    wavy/curly relaxed hair with oily scalp and dry tips, 291
    wavy/curly virgin hair with dry tips and oily scalp, 290
  surfactants, 285, 286t
"Shock loss", 309
Short anagen syndrome, 84, 201. *See also* Loose anagen syndrome (LAS)
Short regrowing hairs (SRHs), 51–52, 52f, 62
Signaling targets, 75–76
Silica, 286

Silicon dioxide. *See* Silica
Silicones, 286, 292
Single nucleotide polymorphisms (SNPs), 74
Sisaipho, 60
β-Sitosterol, 300
Skin, 117
  biopsy, 163
  hyperpigmentation, 147
  skin-softening effect, 221
SLE. *See* Systemic lupus erythematosus (SLE)
Small telogen follicles, 28–29
SNPs. *See* Single nucleotide polymorphisms (SNPs)
Soap, 285
Sonic hedgehog, 3
Spironolactone, 73–74, 115, 246t, 273
Splaying of hair shaft or split ends. *See* Trichoptilosis
Spun glass hair, 203
Squamous cell carcinoma (SCC), 223
Squaric acid dibutylester (SADBE), 64
SRHs. *See* Short regrowing hairs (SRHs)
SS. *See* Sezary syndrome (SS)
"Standard punch grafting" technique, 305
Staphylococcus aureus (*S. aureus*), 161, 167, 173
Staphylococcus epidermidis (*S. epidermidis*), 167
Stearyl-coenzyme A desaturase gene, 143–144
Stemoxydine, 91
Steroid acne, 146
Steroid atrophy, 146
Straight caucasian hair, 291
Streptomycin, 254t
Stress and scalp itch, 225
Strip method
  harvest, 306, 307f, 309t
  of harvesting, 306
Strontium ranelate, 253–254
  clinical presentation and trichoscopy, 254
Subacute cutaneous LE, 187
Subacute stage, 28
Subdermis, 30–31
Subungual hyperkeratosis, 231–233
Sudden whitening of hair, 60
Sulfate-free shampoo, 285
Sulphasalazine, 246t
Sun exposure, 297
Sunflower oil, 287
Sunitinib, 248
Sunlight, 235–236
  blonde and red hair, 235
  dark hair, 235–236
  gray hair, 236
Supercontraction, 238
Superficial mycoses, 211

Superoxide dismutase, 263
Suprabulbar portion, 4
Surfactants, 285, 286t
Surgical excision, 203
"Swarm of bees", 24–26, 27f, 36, 39f, 194
Symptomatic SA, 213–214, 213f
Syphilis, 143, 213–215
  clinical presentation, 213–214
  dermoscopy, 214
  pathology, 214
  treatment, 214–215
Syphilitic alopecia (SA), 38–39, 213
Systemic anti-inflammatory agents, 115
Systemic lupus erythematosus (SLE), 151, 187
Systemic steroids, 64
Systemic therapies, 147–148, 156

T

T cells, 2, 151–152
TA. *See* Traction alopecia (TA)
Tacrolimus, 254t
Takayasu arteritis, 179
Tamoxifen, 246t
TC. *See* Tinea capitis (TC); Trichotillomania (TC)
TCIs. *See* Topical calcineurin inhibitors (TCIs)
TCs. *See* Topical corticosteroids (TCs)
TE. *See* Telogen effluvium (TE)
Telangiectasia, 156, 186–188
Telogen, 3, 83
  follicles, 24, 214
  stage, 11
    regulating pathways/molecules, 11
Telogen effluvium (TE), 83, 199, 245, 250, 252–253, 260, 297, 309
  causes, 85t
  clinical features, 85–86
    acute telogen effluvium, 85
    chronic telogen effluvium, 85–86
  diagnosis, 88–89
    cosmetic treatments, 90
    dermoscopy, 89, 89f
    differential diagnoses, 89, 90t
    emerging treatments, 91
    hair pull test, 89
    history, 88, 88t
    investigations, 89
    management, 89–91
    nutritional supplementation, 91
    physical examination, 88–89
    psychologic support, 90–91
    removal of inciting factor, 90
    topical minoxidil, 91
    Wood's light examination, 89
  epidemiology, 83
  histopathology, 86–88
  pathogenesis
    inciting factors, 84–85

Telogen effluvium (TE) *(Continued)*
    pathophysiology of telogen effluvium, 84
    physiology of hair shedding, 83–84
  prognosis, 91
Telogen germinal unit (TGU), 24
Temporal triangular alopecia (TTA), 138–139, 193, 195–196
  age, 195
  association with comorbidities, 195
  clinical presentation, 195
  management, 196
  pathology, 195
  trichoscopy, 195
Temporary hair coloring techniques, 237
Terbinafine, 210, 196, 209, 246t
Terfenadine, 246t
Terminal hairs, 7
Test hair shaft, 3
Testosterone, 16
Tetracyclines, 132, 164, 170
Textured hair
  children with, 291–292
  hair care in children, 291
TGF. *See* Transforming growth factor (TGF)
TGU. *See* Telogen germinal unit (TGU)
Thalidomide, 132, 156–157, 222–223
Thallium, 254
  clinical presentation, 254
  trichoscopy, 254
THD. *See* Total hair density (THD)
Thiamphenicol, 246t
Thioglycolate, 239
Thyroid hormones, 11, 16, 99–101
Thyrotropin-releasing hormone (TRH), 11
TI. *See* Trichorrhexis invaginata (TI)
"Tiger-tail" banding, 202–203
Tinea capitis (TC), 38, 38f, 63, 99–101, 128, 163, 193, 196–197, 197f, 207–209, 209f, 223, 231. *See also* Pediculosis capitis (PC)
  age, 196
  clinical presentation, 196, 207
  culture, 208–209
  dermoscopy, 207–208
  etiology, 207
  management, 196–197, 209
  oral antifungals used in treatment, 210t
  pathology, 208
  trichoscopy, 196
Tiny vellus follicles, 7
Tissue expanders, 310
TKI. *See* Tyrosine kinase inhibitor (TKI)
TN. *See* Trichorrhexis nodosa (TN)
TNF. *See* Tumor necrosis factor (TNF)
Tofacitinib, 65, 221, 273
Tonsure pattern, 96–97, 96f
Topical antibiotics, 175
Topical calcineurin inhibitors (TCIs), 131, 146–147

Topical corticosteroids (TCs), 146, 156, 164
Topical immunotherapy, 64
Topical minoxidil, 91
Topical potent corticosteroids, 181
Topical steroids, 63, 156
Topical tacrolimus 0.1% ointment, 181
Topical therapies, 146–147
Topiramate, 254t
Total hair density (THD), 14
Traction alopecia (TA), 33, 34f, 99–101, 131, 135, 141, 197
  clinical presentation, 135–138, 197
  demographic factors, 135
  diagnostic workup, 139–140
    histology, 139–140
    trichoscopy, 139, 139f
  differential diagnosis, 138–139, 138t
  histopathologic features of traction alopecia, 139t
  management, 197
  risk factors, 138t
    for traction alopecia, 138t
  treatment, education, and prognosis, 140–141
  trichoscopy, 139, 197
Traction-based hairstyle, 138
Traditional "strip method", 306
Trametinib, 247
Transcription factor, 143–144
Transforming growth factor (TGF), 3, 230, 259
  TGF-β, 84
    TGFβ-1, 11, 263
    TGFβ-2, 11
Transient amplifying cells, 9
Transmission electron microscopy, 240
Transverse sections. *See* Horizontal sections
Traumas, 179
Traumatic hair care practices, 128
Treg cells. *See* Regulatory T cells (Treg cells)
Treponema pallidum (T. pallidum), 213
TRH. *See* Thyrotropin-releasing hormone (TRH)
Triamcinolone acetonide, 63, 146–147
Triazoles, 246t
Trichobezoar, 96
Trichoclasis, 241
Trichodaganomania, 96
Trichograms, 299–300
Trichomalacia, 29, 99, 100f
Trichophagia, 96
Trichophyton species, 196–197, 209
  T. schoenleinii, 207
  T. tonsurans, 207
Trichophyton tonsurans. See Endothrix infection *(Trichophyton tonsurans)*

Trichoptilosis, 202, 241, 241f–242f
Trichorrhexis invaginata (TI), 55,
    201–202
Trichorrhexis nodosa (TN), 202–203,
    240–241, 241f
    bubble hair, 242
    hair shaft with brushlike ends,
        241f
    trichoclasis, 241
    trichoptilosis, 241, 241f
    trichoschisis, 241
Trichoscopy, 43, 54, 89, 110–111, 129,
    193, 201, 240, 245
    ACC, 196
    acute telogen effluvium, 250–251
    AKN, 174
    alopecia areata, 194, 251
    anticoagulants, 250
    antihypertensive agents, 251
    chemotherapy-induced hair loss,
        247
    chloroquine, 255
    devices and particularities, 43–44,
        44f
    dissecting cellulitis of scalp,
        167–168, 168f
    drugs acting on nervous system, 253
    EPDS, 180
    examination of eyebrows, 45
    from female child presenting with
        severe alopecia, 55f
    folliculitis decalvans, 162, 162f
    helping clinician, 43
    interferons, 251
    minoxidil, 253
    oral contraceptives, 252
    permanent alopecia, 250
        due to chemotherapy, 255
    radiation therapy, 250
    retinol (vitamin A) and retinoids,
        252
    signs and patterns, 46–56
        follicular signs, 46–48
        hair shafts, 51–56
        peri-and interfollicular patterns,
            48–49
        vascular patterns, 49
    strontium ranelate, 254
    structures, 46
    telogen effluvium, 249
    thallium, 254
    tinea capitis, 196
    traction alopecia, 139, 139f, 197
    trichotillomania, 97–99, 97t
    TTA, 195
    TTM, 195
Trichosporon asahii (T. asahii), 211
Trichosporon inkin (T. inkin), 211
Trichosporon mucoides (T. mucoides),
    211
Trichosporon ovoides (T. ovoides), 211
Trichoteiromania, 96

Trichothiodystrophy (TTD),
    202–203
Trichotillomania (TC), 95, 100t
    children and adults, 95
    clinical presentation, 96–97
    differential diagnosis, 99–101
        patchy alopecia in children, 101t
    etiology, 95–96
        trichodaganomania, 96
        trichophagia and trichobezoar, 96
        trichoteiromania, 96
        trichotemnomania, 96
    management, 101
    pathology, 99
    trichoscopy, 97–99
Trichotillomania (TTM), 29, 62–63,
    138, 169, 193–195, 224, 312–313
    age, 194
    association with comorbidities, 194
    clinical presentation, 194–195
    management, 195
    pathology, 195
    trichoscopy, 195
Tricyclic antidepressants, 246t,
    252–253
TSH receptor (TSH-R), 16
TSH-R. *See* TSH receptor (TSH-R)
TTA. *See* Temporal triangular alopecia
    (TTA)
TTD. *See* Trichothiodystrophy (TTD)
TTM. *See* Trichotillomania (TTM)
Tufted folliculitis, 161, 185
Tufted hairs, 161–162, 162f, 174f
Tulip hairs, 97t, 98, 195
Tumor necrosis factor (TNF), 2
    TNF-α blocker–induced psoriasiform
        alopecia, 231–233
    TNF-α inhibitors, 143, 152, 170, 229
    TNF-α production, 152
Type 2 diabetes mellitus (DM2), 224
Tyrosine kinase inhibitor (TKI), 247

U

Ultraviolet (UV), 13–14, 297
    irradiation, 151, 235
    light, 151, 273
UMC. *See* Uppsala Monitoring Centre
    (UMC)
Uncombable hair syndrome. *See* Pili
    trianguli et canaliculi
Underlying systemic disease, 224
United States dollars (USD), 267
United States Food and Drug Adminis-
    tration (FDA), 72–73, 101, 146–147,
    267–268, 295
Unsaturated fatty acids, 299
Uppsala Monitoring Centre (UMC),
    250
USD. *See* United States dollars (USD)
Ustekinumab, 157, 231–233
Utero, 1
UV. *See* Ultraviolet (UV)

V

"V-sign", 97t, 98, 195
van der Waals force, 287
Vascular endothelial growth factor
    (VEGF), 259, 262–263
Vascular patterns, 49
Vasodilator, 268
Vasopressin, 246t
Vegetable oils, 287
VEGF. *See* Vascular endothelial growth
    factor (VEGF)
Vellus hair shaft, 7
Vemurafenib, 247–248, 248f
Vertex of scalp, 13–14, 44, 255
Videodermatoscopes (VM), 43–44
Visceral malignancy, 188–189
Vitamin A, 251–252, 273–274,
    295–296, 301t–302t
Vitamin A. *See* Retinol
Vitamin B3. *See* Niacin
Vitamin B7. *See* Biotin
Vitamin C, 299
Vitamin D, 297, 301t–302t
    receptor, 297
Vitamin E, 297, 299, 301t–302t
Vitamins, 295–297
    biotin, 296–297
    micronutrients, 295–296
    niacin, 296
    vitamin A, 295–296
    vitamin D, 297
    vitamin E, 297
VM. *See* Videodermatoscopes (VM)
Vogt-Koyanagi-Harada disease, 185

W

Water content, 235
Water retention index (WRI), 240
Wavy hair, hair care in children,
    291
Wavy/curly relaxed hair with oily scalp
    and dry tips, 291
Wavy/curly virgin hair with dry tips
    and oily scalp, 290
Weathering, causes of
    age, 240
    chemical damage, 237–240
    excessive wetting, 236–237
    physical damage, 237
    sunlight, 235–236
Weaves, 127–128, 237, 291
Wet combing, 210
White dots, 47, 47f
White piedra, 211, 213f
White-gray halo, 49, 50f
WHO. *See* World Health Organization
    (WHO)
WIHN. *See* Wound-induced hair
    neogenesis (WIHN)
Wnt pathway, 84, 297
Wnt signaling, 3, 75
WNT10B genes, 69–70, 262–263

Wood's light examination, 89
Woolly hair, 203
World Health Organization (WHO), 250
Wound-induced hair neogenesis (WIHN), 77
WRI. *See* Water retention index (WRI)

Y

Yellow dots, 46, 46f, 61, 62f, 194, 250f
Yellow to reddish-brown pheomelanin, 13

Z

Zidovudine, 254t

Zigzag hairs, 196, 207–208
Zinc, 297–298, 301t–302t
    deficiency, 85, 298
Zinc pyrithione, 289, 292, 298, 301t–302t

Printed in the United States
By Bookmasters